KIDNEY TRANSPLANTATION

KIDNEY TRANSPLANTATION

Luis H. Toledo-Pereyra

Chief, Transplantation
Director, Research
Mount Carmel Mercy Hospital
Detroit, Michigan

F.A. DAVIS COMPANY • Philadelphia

Printed in the United States of America

NOTE: As new scientific information becomes available through basic and clinical research, recommended treatments and drug therapies undergo changes. The author(s) and publisher have done everything possible to make this book accurate, up-to-date, and in accord with accepted standards at the time of publication. However, the reader is advised always to check product information (package inserts) for changes and new information regarding dose and contraindications before administering any drug. Caution is especially urged when using new or infrequently ordered drugs.

Library of Congress Cataloging-in-Publication Data

Kidney transplantation.

    Includes bibliographies and index.
    1. Kidneys—Transplantation.   I. Toledo-Pereyra,
Luis H. [DNLM: 1. Kidney—transplantation.
WJ 368 K457]
RD575.K52 1988   617'.4610592   88-3727
ISBN 0-8036-8504-1

Foreword

It was only 33 years ago, in 1954, that doctors at the Peter Bent Brigham Hospital performed the first successful kidney transplant. This was a living related kidney transplant between identical twins where there were no immunologic barriers. But it was not until several years later that the first successful kidney transplant between nonidentical twins was performed. Non-HLA-identical sibling and cadaver transplants were truly remarkable achievements when one considers not only the strong immunologic barriers against which these transplants were carried out but also the then minimal understanding of how to circumvent these barriers.

The subsequent achievements accomplished in the field of kidney transplantation are essentially unsurpassed in medicine, so that the development of kidney transplantation can be characterized as one of the truly outstanding medical developments of this century. Against what were initially perceived as insurmountable immunologic barriers, kidney transplantation has today in good part achieved its primary goal—it has been able not only to alleviate suffering but also to provide meaningful life and quality rehabilitation for many patients who have now returned to normal, productive lives with their families and society. The magnitude of this accomplishment can best be appreciated by the fact that just two decades ago, almost all patients with end-stage kidney failure succumbed to their illness.

The improving utility and success of kidney transplantation is most clearly and elegantly presented in this book edited by Dr. Luis Toledo-Pereyra. This is a most comprehensive and broad-based exposition of the current status of the field. It begins with the basic considerations of histocompatibility, kidney retrieval, and evaluation of potential transplant recipients. Subsequent chapters, in logical sequence, discuss the important aspects of anesthesia and surgical techniques. But today's successes in kidney transplantation are also due to a better understanding of risk factors and management of the transplant recipient, including the important immunologic considerations that relate to graft rejection and its control. The immunobiology of transplantation is carefully considered in this text, and it is this area that today portends the future of kidney transplantation.

This book, therefore, presents a very thoughtful, in-depth consideration of the many factors involved in successful kidney transplantation. It is scientific in its approach, yet extremely practical, so that it can provide an easy reference to students, residents in training, fellows, and even current practitioners in the field. The book's ultimate objective is a focus on the patient. It provides the pertinent information for achieving the best possible results in kidney transplantation, whether the donated kidney is from a living or cadaveric source.

Finally, the achievements and accomplishments of kidney transplantation chronicled in this book, and which were realized during a very short period of time following the first successful transplant, serve to underscore tremendous optimism for additional future successes. More specifically, we expect a further unraveling of the mysteries of the human immune response, eventually allowing more selective control of the body's response to the allografted kidney, whereby kidney transplantation can then be performed with nearly 100 percent success and negligible morbidity.

We are deeply indebted to Dr. Toledo-Pereyra for a very lucid and accurate portrayal of the current status of kidney transplantation in modern medicine and its unfolding potential for the successful treatment of essentially all patients with end-stage renal failure.

OSCAR SALVATIERRA, JR., M.D.
Professor of Surgery and Urology
Chief, Transplant Service
University of California, San Francisco

Preface

Kidney transplantation has reached maturity in the last few years. Refinements in the use of current immunosuppressive drugs, including antilymphocyte globulin preparations, cyclosporine, and, recently, the use of monoclonal antibodies, have provided the transplantation specialist with a wide variety of resources. The results have considerably improved since the introduction of cyclosporine, and it is not unusual to obtain greater than 70 percent graft survival of first cadaver allografts. Schemes have been developed to overcome the potential toxic effects of cyclosporine. However, nephrotoxicity is still with us. In our hands, use of continuous intravenous low doses of cyclosporine has greatly resolved part of the problem.

In spite of better means of preserving kidneys, we continue to see a moderately high level of acute posttransplant renal failure nowadays, that is, 25 to 40 percent. An important factor is the prolongation of preservation time and acceptance of some questionable organs. However, the number of nonviable kidneys has decreased. Because long-term results continue to improve, various groups are dealing with more consistent ways to improve immediate function.

Our perspectives constantly change as to the contribution of various parameters to the outcome of transplantation. Although once considered to be important, random pretransplant blood transfusions appear to be of less value for increasing cadaver allograft survival in the cyclosporine era. However, donor-specific blood transfusions are still being used for living related transplants. Similarly, the importance of donor-recipient histocompatibility in cadaver transplants is being questioned. However, it is still a significant parameter in the success of living related renal transplants. Procedures for more accurately determining kidney graft status, such as cyclosporine monitoring, percutaneous needle biopsy, and fine-needle aspiration biopsy, are being assessed at the present time. New combinations of immunosuppressive therapy are being tested that will, we hope, enable us to tailor these drugs to each patient's immunologic needs.

In kidney transplantation, in general, we are at the point of assessing long-term survival (5 to 10 years) expectations of cadaver and living related recipients. Nevertheless, the future is bright, and today kidney transplantation is a firm therapeutic modality.

Finally, why do we need another book on kidney transplantation, especially when several books are on the market? We believe that to further scientific knowledge, we must stimulate new ideas and express various points of view. Because each group of specialists has a potentially different perspective on a broad topic like transplantation, our book represents a fresh approach to the subject. Furthermore, we have attempted here to present the American side of kidney transplantation; all coauthors are established in the United States.

In closing, I would like to thank all my associates and our hard-working transplant group, who have provided support in the endeavor. This book would not have been possible without the daily input of our transplant nephrologists, nurses, dialysis personnel, and patients with end-stage kidney disease. The contributions of Debra A. Gordon in the development of this work are appreciated. Thank you all.

LUIS H. TOLEDO-PEREYRA, M.D.
Ph.D. (SURGERY)
Ph.D. (HISTORY OF MEDICINE)

Contributors

J. Michael Cecka, Ph.D.
Department of Surgery
University of California at Los Angeles
  School of Medicine
Los Angeles, California

Mark I. Evans, M.D.
Assistant Professor
Department of Obstetrics and Gynecology
Department of Molecular Biology and
  Genetics
Director
Division of Reproductive Genetics
Wayne State University School of
  Medicine/Hutzel Hospital
Detroit, Michigan

Ronald M. Ferguson, M.D., Ph.D.
Associate Professor
Director, Division of Transplantation
Department of Surgery
Ohio State University Hospitals
Columbus, Ohio

Duane T. Freier, M.D.
Chairman
Department of Surgery
Danbury Hospital
Danbury, Connecticut

Mitchell L. Henry, M.D.
Assistant Professor
Division of Transplantation
Department of Surgery
Ohio State University Hospitals
Columbus, Ohio

Thomas H. Hostetter, M.D.
Associate Professor of Medicine
Director, Renal Division
University of Minnesota School of
  Medicine
Minneapolis, Minnesota

Eleanor Lederer, M.D.
Assistant Professor of Medicine
Baylor College of Medicine
Houston, Texas

Clara J. Linke, M.D.
Formerly Associate Professor of
  Anesthesiology
University of Rochester School of
  Medicine
Rochester, New York

Vijay K. Mittal, M.D.
Transplant Surgeon
Mount Carmel Mercy Hospital
Detroit, Michigan

David A. Ogden, M.D.
Chief, Renal Section
University of Arizona College of Medicine
Tucson, Arizona

Israel Penn, M.D.
Professor of Surgery
University of Cincinnati Medical Center
Chief of Surgery
Cincinnati Veterans Administration
  Medical Center
Cincinnati, Ohio

Theodore A. Reyman, M.D.
Director of Laboratories
Mount Carmel Mercy Hospital
Detroit, Michigan

Mark E. Rosenberg, M.D.
Instructor
Division of Renal Disease
Department of Medicine
University of Minnesota School of
  Medicine
Minneapolis, Minnesota

J. Thomas Rosenthal, M.D.
Head, Renal Transplantation
Division of Urology
University of California at Los Angeles
  Medical Center
Los Angeles, California

Oscar Salvatierra, Jr., M.D.
Professor of Surgery and Urology
Chief, Transplant Service
University of California, San Francisco
San Francisco, California

Robert J. Sokol, M.D.
Professor, Chairman, and Chief
Department of Obstetrics and Gynecology
Wayne State University/Hutzel Hospital
Detroit, Michigan

Donald R. Steinmuller, M.D.
Head, Section of Medical Transplantation
Department of Hypertension and
  Nephrology
Cleveland Clinic
Cleveland, Ohio

Wadi N. Suki, M.D.
Professor of Medicine, of Physiology, and
  of Molecular Biophysics
Baylor College of Medicine
Chief, Renal Section
The Methodist Hospital
Houston, Texas

Paul I. Terasaki, Ph.D.
Professor of Surgery
University of California at Los Angeles
  School of Medicine
Los Angeles, California

**Luis H. Toledo-Pereyra, M.D., Ph.D.,
  Ph.D.**
Chief, Transplantation
Director, Research
Department of Surgery
Mount Carmel Mercy Hospital
Detroit, Michigan

Ruben L. Velez, M.D.
Director of Acute Hemodialysis
Methodist Medical Center
Staff Physician
Dallas Transplant Institute
Dallas, Texas

Pedro Vergne-Marini, M.D.
Clinical Professor of Medicine
University of Texas Southwestern Medical
  School
Medical Director of Transplantation
Methodist Medical Center and Dallas
  Transplant Institute
Chief of Nephrology
Methodist Medical Center
Dallas, Texas

Robert A. Welch, M.D.
Assistant Professor
Department of Obstetrics and Gynecology
Division of Maternal-Fetal Medicine
Wayne State University School of
  Medicine/Hutzel Hospital
Detroit, Michigan

James I. Whitten, M.D.
Chief, Vascular Surgery
Department of Surgery
Mount Carmel Mercy Hospital
Detroit, Michigan

Contents

SECTION IV. LIVING RELATED TRANSPLANTATION

SECTION I

PREPARATIONS FOR TRANSPLANTATION

Chapter 1

Tissue Typing and Histocompatibility

J. MICHAEL CECKA
PAUL I. TERASAKI

The Structure of HLA: Genes and Antigens
Inheritance of the HLA Antigens
Tissue-Typing Techniques
  Cytotoxicity Testing
  Cellular Typing—Mixed Lymphocyte Culture (MLC)
  Cellular Typing—Primed Lymphocyte Typing (PLT)
  New Technologies for Tissue Typing
Applications of Tissue Typing to Kidney Transplantation
  The Crossmatch Test and Panel-Reactive Antibodies
The Role of HLA Matching in Renal Transplantation
The Role of HLA Matching in the Cyclosporine Era

The major barrier to transplantation of any tissue or organ from one individual to another of the same species is a group of cell-surface antigens collectively referred to as "major histocompatibility antigens." Our understanding of this system of antigens has developed dramatically over the past 20 years, but its foundations date back considerably farther. The difficulties associated with grafting skin from one person to another, for example, were appreciated by surgeons well before the turn of the century. In the early 1900s Carrel[51] carried out extensive organ grafting experiments in dogs and cats and established that autografts (organs transplanted to another site in the same animal) were far more successful than allografts (organs exchanged between individuals). During this same pe-riod, Jensen[52] and Loeb[53] observed that tumors arising in one inbred strain of mice could not be transplanted into mice of another inbred strain. Tyzzer[54] and Little,[55,56] also working on the mouse system, made similar observations and showed that the rejection of allogeneic tumors was under the control of dominant genes. The first description of the antigen system that would later become known as the major histocompatibility system did not appear until the late 1930s. Peter Gorer[57,58,59] showed that tumors transplanted between mouse strains elicited an antibody response and that these antibodies could be used serologically to identify the tissue antigens responsible for the rejection of the incompatible tumor. In the mid-1940s, Medawar, Billingham, Brent, and others[60,61] extended these findings to the rejection of normal skin grafts in rabbits and mice and showed that graft rejection was an immune response mounted in the recipient to the histocompatibility gene products of the donor. The term "major histocompatibility gene" was introduced in 1956 by George Snell[62] to distinguish between genes associated with acute rejection of allogeneic tumors or tissue grafts in mice from "minor histocompatibility genes" associated with chronic rejection of mouse skin grafts. The pioneering work of Little, Gorer, Snell, Medawar, and others in developing inbred strains of mice, serological techniques, and the basic laws of transplantation established the groundwork for the study of histocompatibility systems in many species.

Our understanding of the major histocompatibility system in humans has evolved in parallel with studies in the mouse and in other mammalian species, with considerable sharing of techniques and ideas. In fact, the remarkable similarities between the major histocompatibility systems of the various mammalian species studied[1] has played a significant role in the rapid development of the field over the past 30 years. The major histocompatibility complex (MHC) remains a target of study among researchers in a variety of fields who are intrigued by the extensive polymorphisms of the antigens encoded and controlled by genes within the complex. It has often been pointed out that the MHC probably evolved with some other purpose than that of frustrating transplantation surgeons, and although some might suggest that we are very close to appreciating the "true" function of these genes and molecules, the fact remains that one major application of our knowledge of the MHC harks back to the roots of its discovery—transplantation.

The first human MHC antigen, MAC, was described in 1958 by Dausset[2] based on the reaction pattern of leukoagglutinating antibodies from the sera of parous women. MAC later became HLA-A2. The first allelic pair of human antigens was described by van Rood[3] in 1962. These were called 4a and 4b.

In 1964 an international group of investigators met in Durham, North Carolina, with the idea of establishing a framework to assemble, analyze, and discuss data related to the human MHC. This idea has grown and developed through nine international workshops as summarized in Table 1–1.

By 1970 the HLA (human leukocyte antigen) system had been established as a dominant autosomal gene complex consisting of at least two separate loci called HLA-A and HLA-B. A third locus was also described at the 1970 workshop,[4] but no antigenic specificities were assigned to the HLA-C locus until the 1975 workshop. One of the major advances associated with the 1970 workshop was the adoption of a standard microcytotoxicity assay system that allowed laboratories from all over the world to test and compare antisera. This standardized test allowed the development of the HLA serology and nomenclature that persists today. Antigens that mapped into the HLA-D region were described in 1973 using cellular techniques.[5,6] The assignment of serologic specificities to the D-related region (DR) did not come until the 1977 workshop in Oxford. The D-DR region remains something of a puzzle, as it contains specificities defined by both serologic and cellular techniques, and the degree of overlap is not yet completely determined. We know from the molecular genetics that the D region contains genes coding for some 13 polypeptide chains, and from molecular biology that some of these polypeptides may associate with one another in complicated assortments, but the correspondence among serologic specificities, cellular-determined specificities, and molecular structures throughout the D region is only recently beginning to be established.[7]

At the time of the last workshop in 1984, nearly 100 serologic specificities associated with five distinct HLA gene loci had been accepted. These are listed in Table 1–2 together with the frequency with which each antigen occurs in three major racial groups. Although the serology has undergone several refinements over the years, it now appears that almost all the major antigens at the HLA-A and HLA-B loci have been identified. The frequency of blanks (an antigen not identified) at each of these loci is now less than 1 percent in whites. The HLA-C and HLA-D loci, on the other hand, are expected to yield more, as yet undefined, specificities.

Table 1–1 Summary of the Development of HLA Serology Through Nine International Workshops

Workshop	Location	Organizer	WHO-Recognized Antigens			
			A Locus	*B Locus*	*C Locus*	*D Loci*
I 1964	Durham	DB Amos				
II 1965	Leiden	JJ van Rood				
III 1967	Torino	R Ceppellini				
IV 1970	Los Angeles	PI Terasaki	1–3, 9–11, 19, 28	5, 7, 8, 12–15, 17, 18, 22, 27		
V 1972	Paris	J Dausset	23–26 29–32	16, 21, 35 (W5)		
VI 1975	Aarhus	F Kissmeyer-Nielsen	33, 34 36, 43	37–42	1–5	
VII 1977	Oxford	WF Bodmer		44–54	6	1–7
VIII 1980	Los Angeles	PI Terasaki		55–63	7, 8	8–10
IX 1984	Munich	ED Albert	66, 68, 69	64, 65, 67		11–14, 52, 53
		WR Mayr		70–73		DQw1–3, DPw1–6

THE STRUCTURE OF HLA: GENES AND ANTIGENS

Because of the fascination that HLA (and the other mammalian MHC systems) holds for investigators across a variety of disciplines, these gene complexes are among the best-studied mammalian genetic systems. A detailed review of the molecular biology and molecular genetics is beyond the scope of this chapter; however, a number of up-to-date reviews are available.[8,9] Figure 1–1 summarizes current knowledge of the organization at both the genetic and molecular level of the human MHC. The genes encoding the MHC antigens are located on the short arm of chromosome 6 in humans. Two distinct classes of cell-surface histocompatibility antigens are encoded in this gene complex. The class I molecules are the major transplantation antigens (HLA-A, B, C), which consist of a heavy chain of 45,000 daltons molecular weight noncovalently associated with β-2 microglobulin. The class I antigens are expressed on all nucleated cells in the body, with the highest concentration found on lymphocytes and platelets. In the kidney, the class I antigens are found on all cells,[10] and in high concentration on the vascular endothelium, dendritic cells, tubules, and mesangium.[11]

The class II antigens (HLA-DP, DQ, DR) are heterodimers comprised of a "heavy" (α) chain of 35,000 daltons molecular weight noncovalently associated with a "light" (β) chain of 31,000 daltons molecular weight. The class II antigens have a more restricted tissue distribution than do the class I antigens. They are expressed on B lymphocytes, monocytes, dendritic cells, and some activated T lymphocytes. In the kidney the class II antigens are found on the glomerular endothelium, intertubular capillaries, and some tubular cells.[12]

Class I and class II antigens are distinct from one another at the molecular level, but they share certain characteristics in their genetic and domain structures which include both in the immunoglobulin "superfamily."[13] Studies at the levels of DNA and protein sequence suggest that the variability that gives rise to the extensive polymorphism of these antigens is restricted to the two external domains (shaded in Fig. 1–

Table 1-2 HLA Serologic Phenotypes and Population Frequencies c1984

HLA-A Locus

HLA-A Locus	% Population Frequency*		
	W†	A	B
A1	26	2	16
A2	49	48	32
A3	25	3	13
A11	12	22	4
A23 ⎤ A9‡	3	1	15
A24 ⎦	20	53	9
A25 ⎤ A10	5	0	0
A26 ⎦	6	14	9
A28	9	4	19
A29 ⎤	6	1	10
A30	7	4	21
A31 ⎦ A19	6	10	3
A32	8	1	4
Aw33	3	12	8
Aw34	1	1	10
Aw36	1	1	6
Aw43	0	0	2
Aw66	1	1	1
AX§	1	3	10

HLA-B Locus

HLA-B Locus	% Population Frequency		
	W	A	B
B7	22	9	23
B8	18	1	11
B13	6	7	3
B18	11	1	8
B27	7	3	4
B35	20	19	14
B37	3	1	2
B38 ⎤ B16	5	1	3
B39 ⎦	4	1	0
B41	2	1	4
B42	1	1	11
B44 ⎦ B12	23	12	15
B45 ⎤	1	1	5
Bw46	1	7	0
Bw47	1	1	0
Bw48	0	3	0
B49 ⎤ B21	4	1	5
B50 ⎦	2	1	1
B51 ⎤ B5	12	15	4
B52 ⎦	4	14	1
Bw53	1	1	13
Bw54	1	13	0
Bw55 ⎤ B22	3	4	0
Bw56 ⎦	2	3	1
Bw57 ⎤ B17	6	1	6
Bw58 ⎦	0	2	0

HLA-C Locus

HLA-C Locus	% Population Frequency		
	W	A	B
Cw1	6	30	2
Cw2	8	2	22
Cw3	24	47	16
Cw4	22	10	26
Cw5	13	1	6
Cw6	16	7	24
Cw7	43	23	42
Cw8	7	1	7
CX	44	56	38

HLA-B Locus (cont.)

HLA-B Locus (cont.)	% Population Frequency		
	W	A	B
Bw59	0	4	1
Bw60 ⎤ B40	8	13	4
Bw61 ⎦	4	22	3
Bw62 ⎤ B15	12	18	5
Bw63 ⎦	1	0	4
Bw64 ⎤ B14	2	0	3
Bw65 ⎦	5	1	3
Bw67	0	1	0
Bw71	1	1	2
Bw72	1	1	14
Bw73	1	1	0
BX	1	3	3

HLA-D Locus

HLA-D Locus	% Population Frequency		
	W	A	B
DR1	18	10	10
DR2	29	28	28
DR3	23	4	28
DR4	24	39	15
DR7	23	6	25
DRw8	6	14	2
DRw9	2	22	3
DRw10	2	1	4
DRw11 ⎤ DR5	23	8	30
DRw12 ⎦	4	14	7
DRw13 ⎤ DRw6	10	6	7
DRw14 ⎦	8	13	20
DR52	54	49	76
DR53	49	69	36
DRX	15	25	10
DQw1	54	51	64
DQw2	33	10	41
DQw3	41	55	43
DQX	46	54	23

*Calculated from gene frequencies listed in Bauer, MP, et al: Population analysis on the basis of deduced haplotypes from random families. In Albert, ED, et al (eds): Histocompatibility Testing 1984. Springer-Verlag, Berlin, 1984, p 333.
†W = White, A = Asian, B = Black.
‡Brackets indicate "splits" of an antigen.
§X denotes the frequency of an unidentified antigen at the locus.

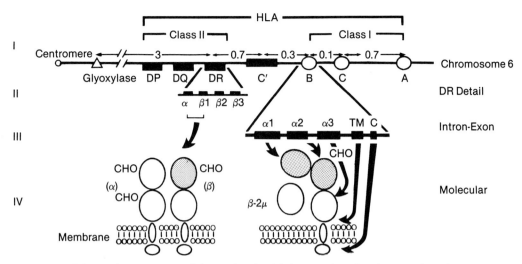

Figure 1-1. Schematic summary of the molecular biology and molecular genetics of HLA. Level I shows the overall organization of gene loci on chromosome 6, including the order of class I and class II loci and the recombination frequencies. Level II shows the genes that make up the DR locus. One alpha gene product associates with one of three beta gene products to produce the DR heterodimer. Level III shows the genetic fine structure for an HLA-B locus gene. The intron (thin line)-exon (thick line) structure corresponds to the domain structure of the HLA molecule, including the three external domains ($\alpha1$, $\alpha2$, $\alpha3$), the transmembrane (TM), and the cytoplasmic (C) domains. Level IV shows the molecular structure of these transmembrane antigens and the location of carbohydrate (CHO) groups. Probable antigenic regions are shaded. (See references 13 through 17.)

1) of the class I heavy chain, and to the external domain of the class II light chain.[14–17]

Recognition of the class I and class II HLA antigens, serologically using antibodies, by lymphocytes in cellular typing, or in a developing immune response to an allograft, is complex. On the one hand, class I antigens are structurally similar to one another, so that some determinants may be shared by many different antigens, while single amino acid changes may define determinants that can discriminate between two individual antigens that are otherwise identical. In addition, the production of an antibody, or any other immune response, will be dictated by the immunogenic difference between the antigen that stimulates the response and the antigen that the responder's immune system tolerates as "self."

INHERITANCE OF THE HLA ANTIGENS

The recombination frequency over the entire HLA region is 1.8 percent (1 percent between HLA-A and HLA-B and 0.8 per-

cent between HLA-B and HLA-DR). Each individual carries two HLA haplotypes, one set of loci on each chromosome. Because the frequency of recombination is low, offspring usually inherit one intact haplotype from each parent. Thus, a child will be identical to each parent for at least one A locus antigen, one B locus, one C locus, and one of each of the D locus antigens. Siblings generally show a typical Mendelian inheritance of the HLA complex as a single unit. Thus, if the mother carries the haplotypes H and J, and the father carries K and L, the offspring will express one of the four possible combinations: HK, HL, JK, or JL, and the probability that two siblings will be identical at both haplotypes is 25 percent.

TISSUE-TYPING TECHNIQUES

Cytotoxicity Testing

The backbone of the HLA system is serologic testing. Sera from multiparous women are the major sources of HLA antibodies used to identify the specificities listed in Table 1–2. These antibodies are produced by the mother in response to paternal antigens of the fetus. As a rule these sera contain relatively low titers of HLA antibodies, and the spectrum of specific antibodies may range from narrow to rather broad. Other types of human sera from skin-grafted immunized volunteers[18] or from recipients of multiple blood transfusions[19] have also been shown to contain anti-HLA antibodies, but sera from multiparous women continue to be the primary sources of HLA typing antibodies.

The first microcytotoxicity test was described in 1964 by Terasaki and McClelland.[20] This test took advantage of the fact that many of the HLA antibodies produced by parous females were able to kill lymphocytes (cytotoxic) in the presence of rabbit complement. This test also required very small amounts of antiserum, which was a distinct advantage, since the reagents were generally of low titer and were available in limited quantities. The test was modified[21] to its current standard form as schematically outlined in Figure 1–2. This test is sometimes called the NIH test because a group of investigators met at the NIH to agree on the standard set of conditions for testing.

Testing for the HLA-A, -B, and -C specificities is typically performed on peripheral blood lymphocytes or T lymphocytes purified from buffy coat cells by any of a variety of techniques. Typing for the HLA-DR specificities must be performed using purified B lymphocytes, as the DR antigens are not expressed on the bulk of peripheral blood lymphocytes. The reaction of each typing antiserum with the target lymphocytes is scored according to the percentage of cells that are killed. A reaction of 1 indicates no cells or less than 10 percent of cells were dead on completion of the test and a reaction of 8 indicates that all cells or nearly all cells have been killed. Each typing tray contains control sera that will either kill no cells or that will kill all cells to provide reference wells and to control for problems of complement toxicity, which may arise under some conditions. Partial reactions may occur and may reflect heterogeneity in the cells (antigen density, susceptibility to lysis) or extra reactivities in the typing sera. Some sera directed

against an A or B specificity, for example, may also contain antibodies to DR. In most cases the contaminating anti-DR antibodies do not interfere because relatively few B cells are present. However, if a cell sample has 40 percent B cells, the contaminating antibodies will cause a partial killing.

In the normal situation, HLA typing is relatively straightforward, although there may be some variation when typing is performed at two different laboratories. This is especially true in the case of particularly rare or difficult specificities. Tissue-typing a kidney donor and sometimes a potential recipient may present special difficulties. Patients receiving steroids or on dialysis may be leukocytopenic and/or have "fragile" lymphocytes, making typing difficult. Patients receiving frequent blood transfusions may present a confusing picture if blood is drawn too soon after a transfusion. Kidney donors can be typed from spleen or lymph node cells; however, this requires that typing wait until the time of organ harvest, which may delay the identification of a suitable recipient. With skill it is possible to type essentially all donors and recipients with 20 ml of fresh blood for the HLA-A, -B, and -DR antigens.

Cellular Typing—Mixed Lymphocyte Culture (MLC)

When lymphocytes from two unrelated individuals are mixed in tissue culture, both sets of cells are stimulated to proliferate. The HLA-D specificities (listed as DW1-19 as of 1984) were defined on the basis of stimulation of lymphocytes by a series of homozygous typing cells (HTC). The latter are homozygous at a single D determinant. Lymphocytes that share the D determinant with a particular HTC will not be stimulated in culture.

Cellular Typing—Primed Lymphocyte Typing (PLT)

The PLT test is a secondary MLC reaction. The test measures the ability of lymphocytes primed in vitro to be restimulated, either by the priming cell or by a second test cell.

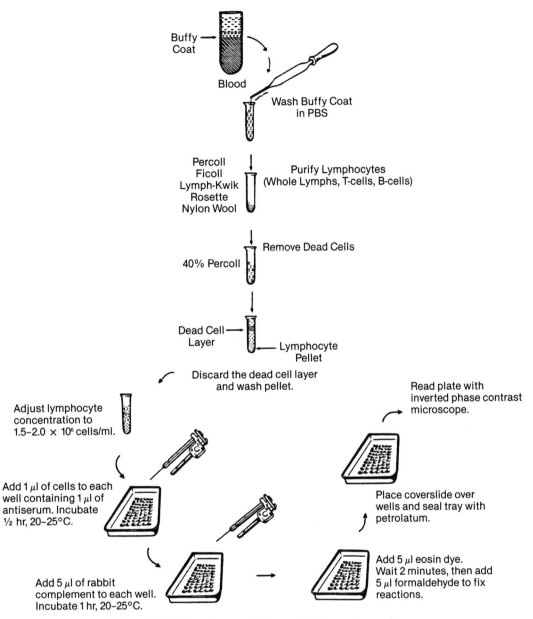

Figure 1–2. The microdroplet cytotoxicity test procedure.

Both of these cellular typing techniques identify determinants present on molecules encoded in the HLA-D region. The correspondence between the DW specificities defined by MLC reactivity and the serologically defined DR specificities is quite good but not complete. HTC typing suggests that the serologically defined DR4 specificity is heterogeneous and will eventually be subdivided as better serologic reagents are found. Primed lymphocyte typing has defined the DP antigens.

New Technologies for Tissue Typing

In the 1984 workshop several new approaches were introduced for typing.[7,22,23] The molecular genetic technology allows one to examine genes directly in the DNA without having to extrapolate from a phenotype. This technology has provided the excellent resolution of the HLA-D region. The development of monoclonal antibody reagents has contributed considerably to the sorting out of the D-region serology in combination with molecular biological approaches (two-dimensional gel analysis) as well as refining some of the HLA-A locus specificities. Of these new technologies monoclonal reagents may make even more substantial contributions in the future.

APPLICATIONS OF TISSUE TYPING TO KIDNEY TRANSPLANTATION

The Crossmatch Test and Panel-Reactive Antibodies

One of the hard and fast rules of kidney transplantation is that no kidney should be transplanted into a recipient who has circulating antibodies directed against the HLA antigens of the donor. Early experience showed that such transplants were almost invariably rejected in a hyperacute fashion.[24–26] Thus, the crossmatch test prior to transplantation has become a standard screening test. It is performed using the microdroplet cytotoxicity test outlined in Figure 1–2, except that serum from the potential kidney recipients is tested against lymphocytes (particularly against T lymphocytes) from the donor. A positive crossmatch is a contraindication for the transplant. Similarly, sera from potential transplant recipients are often tested against panels of lymphocytes from random individuals in order to ascertain the immune status of patients awaiting transplants and to identify patients for whom a suitable transplant may be difficult to obtain.

The origin of anti-HLA antibodies in potential kidney recipients is not always evident, although some factors have been identified. As with typing antibodies, it is clear that pregnancy and birth are potent immunogenic stimuli, particularly when coupled with blood transfusions.[27–29] The combination of pregnancies and transfusions accounts for the majority of potential recipients of first cadaver kidney trans-

plants who have broadly reactive cytotoxic antibodies measured on random panels of lymphocytes.[27] Other factors that may lead to the production of panel-reactive antibody (PRA) include previous transplants[30] and blood transfusions.[27–30] To some extent the PRA is an indicator of the probability of a positive crossmatch. Patients who have no PRA are likely to be crossmatch-negative for the majority of donors, and finding a suitable kidney for these patients will be less difficult than for a patient who has antibodies reactive with a high percentage of random panel cells. Although it is generally accepted that antibodies reactive to T lymphocytes lead to hyperacute rejection, it appears that not all antibodies in the serum of a potential recipient reactive with donor lymphocytes are deleterious (reviewed in reference 31). Antibodies in the serum may also vary with time so that when several separate bleedings are compared, a patient may show a developing antibody response as a result of transfusion, for example, or a broad response that becomes narrow or disappears with time. The significance of these variations has been the subject of several studies.[32–35] However, more studies will be required before definitive conclusions can be drawn.

THE ROLE OF HLA MATCHING IN RENAL TRANSPLANTATION

There is no doubt that the HLA system is the major histocompatibility complex in man and that the MHC antigens play a significant role in kidney graft survival. This role is most clearly illustrated in the clinical context by considering transplants from living related donors as reported by this laboratory in 1969[36] and as shown in Figure 1–3. There is a striking correlation between the number of haplotypes shared between donor and recipient and kidney graft survival over the entire 5-year period shown. Since 1978 there have been very few transplants between monozygotic twins, but these grafts have excellent survival prognosis, and none of the grafts between twins have been lost during the period of this study. Transplants between HLA-identical siblings had a 5-year survival rate of nearly 80 percent. Within this group no antigens

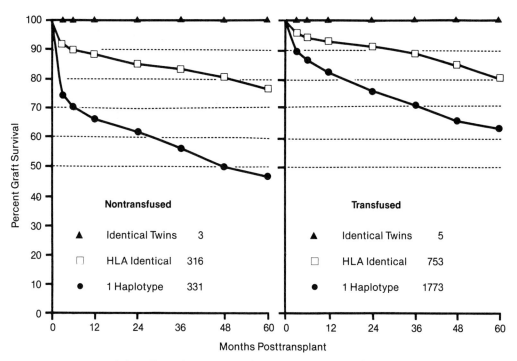

Figure 1–3. The beneficial effect of HLA matching on the survival of first kidney grafts from living related donors. Actuarial graft survival over a 5-year period was significantly higher in recipients of kidney grafts from donors who were identical to the recipient for all HLA antigens than in recipients of grafts from donors identical for only one HLA haplotype, whether the recipient was given pretransplant transfusions or not. All transplants were performed between 1978 and 1985. One-haplotype-mismatched grafts among transfused recipients included 715 sibling donors, 879 parent donors, and 180 offspring donors. The survival curves for the three categories of one-haplotype-mismatched donors were contiguous in each case.

in the MHC are mismatched between donor and recipient, and yet some grafts are lost. It is difficult to know precisely what factors contribute to the loss of these grafts. Some may be lost because of rejection reactions directed against antigens that are not associated with HLA. Probably not all are lost for immunologic reasons, however. The analysis also considers the death of a patient as a graft loss, even if the graft was functioning at the time of death. Transplants between donors and recipients who share only one HLA haplotype (one-haplotype-identical siblings, parent to offspring and offspring to parent) had a five-year graft survival rate of less than 50 percent as shown on the left of Figure 1–3. Thus, recipients whose grafts were completely matched for their HLA antigens had about 30 percent higher graft survival over 5 years than did recipients given grafts that were not completely matched. On the right-

hand side of Figure 1–3 the effect of a second factor, pretransplant blood transfusions, was also considered. These transfusions increased the graft survival rate for one-haplotype-matched recipients to 62 percent at 5 years. They also increased graft survival among recipients of HLA-identical grafts within the 5-year period, although the difference in survival at the end of 5 years is not significant. The effect of HLA matching was reduced because of the increase in graft survival attributable to transfusions, but completely matched grafts still had a much better (15 to 20 percent) survival rate than mismatched grafts.

The value of HLA matching in cadaver donor transplants, on the other hand, remains somewhat controversial. The controversy stems from two major categories of considerations. First, it is difficult to know with certainty what to match. In the case of living transplants between HLA-identical siblings, it is clear that the HLA molecules are identical because they are products of the same inherited genes. In the case of cadaver transplants, matching must rely on serologically defined specificities that may be broad (including several slightly different HLA molecules) or that may be very narrow (identifying a single molecular species). The finer the specificity one demands, the less often a perfect match will be found. Some authors have recently reported that matching for broader specificities may be as effective in terms of graft survival as matching for more narrow specificities.[37] It may also be that not all mismatches have equal value in all patients and that the particular constellation of antigens present in the recipient plays a role in determining what constitutes a significant mismatch.[38] Compounding these problems is the quality of tissue typing; that is, whether all antigens can be typed with confidence and whether two different tissue typing laboratories will have concordant results.

Second, the kidney transplant is an extremely complex clinical situation. In addition to matching and blood transfusions, a few factors are immunosuppressive therapy, sensitization, original disease leading to end-stage renal disease, age, sex, and race of the recipient. The relative contributions of these factors to graft survival varies between the transplant centers and within a single center between recipients. In Figure 1–3, for example, the effect of pretransplant blood transfusions is larger in the one-haplotype-matched recipients than in the HLA-identical recipients. In cadaver donor transplants, the effect of HLA-A and -B matching has been reported to be larger in sensitized recipients[39] and in male recipients who are blood groups A, B, or AB and not blood group O.[40,41] Thus, patient demographics may play a role in the evaluation of any single factor.

There exists extensive literature on the various aspects of HLA matching and its effect on survival of cadaver kidney grafts (reviewed in reference 42), but there is little agreement overall regarding the effectiveness of matching. Multicenter studies that involve large numbers of transplants[43,44] generally find a significant improvement in graft survival associated with well-matched transplants. Small studies and single-center studies vary considerably in their assessment of the effectiveness of HLA matching, and this may be due to the statistical variations inherent in small sample sizes as argued by Mickey.[38] Data from the UCLA Transplant Registry have consistently shown a beneficial effect of HLA matching for cadaver kidney transplants.[38,45,46] These data are updated in Figure 1–4, which shows the results of matching for the various combinations of HLA antigens in first cadaver kidney transplants performed since 1978. The curves show the actuarial graft survival over 5 years, without consideration for other factors that might influence graft survival except that all recipients were given pretransplant blood transfusions. In each of the matching categories, patients who received grafts with no antigens mismatched had the highest survival rates. The optimum graft survival was obtained in patients who had no antigens mismatched at any of the HLA-A, -B, or -DR loci. If antigens at the A locus were ignored, patients who had no mismatches at the -B or -DR loci also had very high graft survival rates, followed in order by patients with no mismatches at -A or -DR (ignoring the -B locus) and then patients with no mismatches at -DR and finally those with no mismatches at -A or -B. At the same time, recipients of grafts that were completely mismatched in each of the matching groups had the poorest outcome, with 5-year graft survival about 40 percent in each case. The rather remarkable 30 percent increase in graft survival at 5 years in recipients of grafts with no antigens mismatched at the HLA-A, -B, and -DR loci convincingly demonstrates that HLA matching plays a significant role in the survival of cadaver kidney grafts. However, such well-matched donor-recipient combinations are rare (123 of 6000, or about 2 percent) and once a single mismatch is introduced, the effect of matching becomes less dramatic. There still remains a tendency within each matching group shown in Figure 1–4 toward a graded effect of matching. That is, one mismatch results in higher graft survival than four mismatches. This suggests that as tissue typing techniques and reagents improve, the effect of HLA matching on graft survival will increase.

This has been the case historically. In 1970, only 28 HLA-A, B specificities were

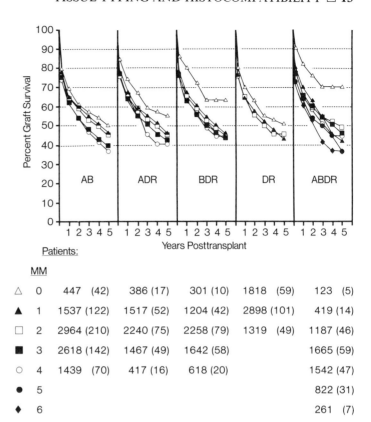

Figure 1–4. The beneficial effect of HLA matching on the survival of first cadaver donor kidney grafts. Actuarial survival of first cadaver kidney grafts over a 5-year period suggests that kidney allografts that had no antigens mismatched from the recipient in each of the HLA mismatch groups shown had higher survival rates than those that had one or more antigens mismatched. All transplants were performed between 1978 and 1985. All recipients were given preoperative blood transfusions. The number of patients in each group is shown below the section. Numbers in parentheses are the number of patients with surviving grafts who were followed for the entire 5-year period.

	MM	AB	ADR	BDR	DR	ABDR
△	0	447 (42)	386 (17)	301 (10)	1818 (59)	123 (5)
▲	1	1537 (122)	1517 (52)	1204 (42)	2898 (101)	419 (14)
□	2	2964 (210)	2240 (75)	2258 (79)	1319 (49)	1187 (46)
■	3	2618 (142)	1467 (49)	1642 (58)		1665 (59)
○	4	1439 (70)	417 (16)	618 (20)		1542 (47)
●	5					822 (31)
♦	6					261 (7)

known. At that time, no convincing correlation was found between HLA matching and transplant outcome.[47] In 1980, even with many more HLA specificities identified, the correlation between matching and transplant survival was difficult to demonstrate. By 1984 nearly 100 HLA-A, B, C, DR specificities had been identified, and in the 1984 workshop study,[48] a significant correlation was found between HLA matching and cadaver kidney graft survival.

THE ROLE OF HLA MATCHING IN THE CYCLOSPORINE ERA

Cyclosporine, an immunosuppressive agent, has had an impressive impact on kidney transplantation over the past three years in the United States and somewhat longer in Europe. The increased graft survival in recipients given this potent drug has raised the question as to which of the factors contributing to increased graft survival are still important in patients receiving cyclosporine. Many centers appear to have adopted the position that the greater degree of immunosuppression associated with cyclosporine overrides the effect of matching for HLA antigens. This position allows a center to transplant cadaver kidneys with very short ischemia times and to curtail expensive organ-sharing programs required to increase the recipient pool size so that well-matched transplants are possible. This position also reduces the ability of centers that do not harvest their own kidneys to perform transplants.

Two large multicenter studies, one from the collaborative transplant study in Europe[49] and one from the UCLA Transplant Registry[50] have recently reported that matching for the HLA-B and -DR antigens significantly improves survival of cadaver kidney grafts in recipients treated with cyclosporine. Both of these studies (each with approximately 2000 cyclosporine-treated recipients) found a 15 to 20 percent increase in 1-year graft survival among recipients with no mismatches at HLA-B or -DR. In each of these studies the effect of cyclosporine alone was a 10 percent increase in graft survival at 1 year. In the short term at least, it would appear that the effect of matching for HLA antigens is additive to the potent immunosuppressive action of cyclosporine. The relative contributions of HLA matching and cyclosporine treatment to the long-term survival of kidney grafts remain to be seen. Late nephrotoxic side effects of cyclosporine may lead to increased difficulties over longer periods of follow-up for kidney transplant recipients. If this proves to be the case, the effect of matching may take on even greater importance, since it may be that better matched transplants will require lower doses of drug to maintain a sufficient level of immunosuppression.

SUMMARY

The major histocompatibility complex is a genetic region that encodes a series of cell-surface glycoproteins that are intimately involved in the control and signaling of the immune system in all mammalian species. The molecules controlled by genes of the MHC also represent the major barrier to the transplantation of any tissue or organ from one individual to another of the same species because these molecules vary antigenically between individuals. Over the past 20 years, our understanding of the structure, function, and genetics of the human MHC (HLA) has increased dramatically. The ability to identify the HLA antigens serologically has continuously improved, and new technologies promise further to refine our definitions of these important antigens. The role of the HLA antigens as they relate to kidney transplantation is twofold: first as the targets of a crossmatch test that measures pre-existing antibodies in the recipient directed against HLA antigens of the potential donor, and second as the targets of the immune response that may develop in the recipient after transplantation. This latter aspect of the role of HLA is the object of some controversy. Matching the HLA antigens of the donor to those of the recipient limits the potential targets of a rejection reaction, and this effect is clearly evident in transplants from living related donors where matching can be complete. Immunosuppressive drugs given at the time of the transplant

can prevent or reduce the development of a rejection response, and this effect may or may not override the effect of HLA matching. In fact, these factors appear to complement one another, and optimum survival of kidney transplants is obtained through minimizing antigenic differences between graft and recipient and effectively suppressing the immune response to those that do exist.

REFERENCES

1. Goetze, D (ed): The Major Histocompatibility System in Man and Animals. Springer-Verlag, New York, 1977.
2. Dausset, J: Iso-leuko-anticorps. Acta Haematol (Basel) 1958, 20:156.
3. van Rood, JJ: Leukocyte Grouping: A Method and Its Application (thesis). Leyden, 1962.
4. Sandberg, L, et al: Evidence for a third sublocus within the HLA chromosomal region. In Terasaki, PI (ed): Histocompatibility Testing 1970. UCLA Tissue Typing Laboratory, Los Angeles, 1970, p 165.
5. van den Tweel, JG, et al: Typing for MLC (LD): I. Lymphocytes from cousin marriage offspring as typing cells. Transplant Proc 5:1535, 1973.
6. Dupont, B, et al: Typing for MLC determinants by means of LD-homozygous and LD-heterozygous typing cells. Transplant Proc 5:1543, 1973.
7. Bodmer, WF: The HLA system: 1984. In Albert, ED, et al (eds): Histocompatibility Testing 1984. Springer-Verlag, Berlin, 1984, p 11.
8. Möller, G (ed): Molecular genetics of class I and II MHC antigens: 1. Immunological Reviews 84, Munksgaard, Copenhagen, 1985.
9. Möller, G (ed): Molecular genetics of class I and II MHC antigens: 2. Immunological Reviews 85, Munksgaard, Copenhagen, 1985.
10. Daar, AS, et al: The detailed distribution of HLA-A, B, C antigens in normal human organs. Transplantation 38:287, 1984.
11. Fuggle, SV, et al: Localization of major histocompatibility complex (HLA-ABC and DR) antigens in 46 kidneys: Differences in HLA-DR staining of tubules among kidneys. Transplantation 35:385, 1983.
12. Daar, AS, et al: The detailed distribution of MHC class II antigens in normal human organs. Transplantation 38:293, 1984.
13. Larhammar, D, et al: Alpha chain HLA-DR transplantation antigens is a member of the

same protein super-family as the immunoglobulins. Cell 30:153, 1982.

14. Kaufman, JF, et al: The class II molecules of the human and murine major histocompatibility complex. Cell 36:1, 1984.

15. Kaufman, JF and Strominger, JL: HLA-DR light chain has a polymorphic N-terminal determinant region and a conserved Ig-like C-terminal region. Nature 297:694, 1982.

16. Kaufman, JF and Strominger, JL: The extracellular region of the light chains from human and murine MHC class II antigens consists of two domains. J Immunol 130:808, 1983.

17. Jordan, DR, et al: Transformation of murine LMTK- cells with purified HLA class I genes: III. Human HLA class I antigens coded by hybrid genes constructed in vitro indicate association of serologic reactivities with the first two domains of the molecule. Immunogenetics 18:165, 1983.

18. Thorsby, E: IIL-A antigens on human granulocytes studied with cytotoxic isoantisera obtained by skin grafting. Scand J Haematol 6:119, 1969.

19. Ferrara, GB: Production of isoantisera for HL-A typing by planned immunization: A four year experiment. Symp Serol Immunobiol Stand, 18:20, 1973.

20. Terasaki, PI and McClelland, JD: Microdroplet assay of human serum cytotoxins. Nature 204:998, 1964.

21. Terasaki, PI: Microdroplet testing for HLA-A, -B, -C, and -D antigens. Am J Clin Pathol 69:103, 1978.

22. Dausset, J and Cohen, D: HLA at the gene level. In Albert, ED, et al (eds): Histocompatibility Testing 1984. Springer-Verlag, Berlin, 1984, 22.

23. Crumpton, MJ: Biochemistry of class II antigens: Workshop report. In Albert, ED, et al (eds): Histocompatibility Testing 1984. Springer-Verlag, Berlin, 1984, 29.

24. Kissmeyer-Nielsen, F, Olsen, S, and Petersen, VP: Hyperacute rejection of kidney allografts associated with pre-existing humoral antibodies against donor cells. Lancet 2:662, 1966.

25. Williams, GM, et al: "Hyperacute" renal homograft rejection in man. N Engl J Med 279:611, 1968.

26. Patel, R and Terasaki, PI: Significance of the positive crossmatch test in kidney transplantation. N Engl J Med 280:735, 1969.

27. Opelz, G, et al: Lymphocytotoxic antibody responses to transfusions in potential kidney transplant recipients. Transplantation 32:177, 1981.

28. Scornik, JC, et al: Assessment of the risk for broad sensitization by blood transfusions. Transplantation 37:249, 1984.

29. Fehrman, I, Ringden, O, and Möller, E:

Blood transfusions as pretreatment for kidney transplantation: Immunization rate and effect on cellular immune response in vitro. Transplantation 35:339, 1983.

30. Thick, M, et al: Sensitization following kidney graft failure and blood transfusion. Transplantation 37:525, 1984.

31. Ting, A: The lymphocytotoxic test in clinical renal transplantation. Transplantation 35:403, 1983.

32. Sanfilippo, F, et al: Cadaver renal transplantation ignoring peak reactive sera in patients with markedly decreasing pretransplant sensitization. Transplantation 38:119, 1984.

33. Sanfilippo, F, et al: Influence of changes in pretransplant sensitization on patient and graft survival in cadaver renal transplantation. Transplantation 38:124, 1984.

34. Cardella, CJ and Falk, JA: Graft outcome in patients with antibodies reactive with donor T and B cells. Transplant Proc, 15:1142, 1983.

35. Fuller, TC, Forbes, JB, and Delmonico, FL: Renal transplantation with a positive historical donor crossmatch. Transplant Proc, 17:113, 1985.

36. Singal, DP, Mickey, MR, and Terasaki, PI: Serotyping for homotransplantation. XXIII. Analysis of kidney transplants from parental versus sibling donors. Transplantation 7:246, 1969.

37. Delmonico, FL, et al: New approaches to donor crossmatching and successful transplantation of highly sensitized patients. Transplantation 36:629, 1983.

38. Mickey, MR: HLA matching in transplants from cadaver donors. In Terasaki, PI (ed): Clinical Kidney Transplants. UCLA Tissue Typing Laboratory, Los Angeles, 1985, p 45.

39. Busson, M, et al: Influence of HLA-A, B, and DR matching on the outcome of kidney transplant survival in preimmunized patients. Transplantation 38:227, 1984.

40. Opelz, G and Terasaki, PI: Influence of sex on histocompatibility matching in renal transplantation. Lancet 2:419, 1977.

41. D'Amaro, J, et al: Influence of sex and ABO blood group on HLA-A, B, and DR matching in renal transplantation. Transplant Proc 17:758, 1985.

42. Tiwari, JL. Review: Kidney transplantation and HLA. In Terasaki, PI (ed): Clinical Kidney Transplants. UCLA Tissue Typing Laboratory, Los Angeles, 1985, p 233.

43. Rosansky, SJ and Sugimoto, T: An analysis of the United States renal transplant population and organ survival characteristics: 1977–1980. Kidney Intl 22:685, 1982.

44. Sanfilippo, F, et al: Benefits of HLA-A and HLA-B matching on graft and patient out-

come after cadaveric-donor renal transplantation. N Engl J Med 311:358, 1984.

45. Opelz, G, Terasaki, PI, and Graver, B: Correlation between the number of pretransplant blood transfusions and kidney graft survival. Transplant Proc 11:145, 1979.

46. Ayoub, G and Terasaki, PI. HLA-DR matching in multicenter, single typing-laboratory data. Transplantation 33:515, 1982.

47. Mickey, MR, et al: Analysis of the HL-A incompatibility in human renal transplants. Tissue Antigens 2:57, 1971.

48. Opelz, G. Ninth international histocompatibility workshop renal transplant study. In Albert, ED, Baur, MP, and Mayr, WR (eds): Histocompatibility Testing 1984. Springer-Verlag, New York, 1984, p 342.

49. Opelz, G. Correlation of HLA matching with kidney graft survival in patients with or without cyclosporine treatment. Transplantation 40:240, 1985.

50. Cicciarelli, J, Teresaki, PI, and Mickey, MR: The effect of zero HLA class I and II mismatching in cyclosporine-treated kidney transplant patients. Transplantation 43:636, 1987.

51. For biography see Surgery and Life, The Extraordinary Career of Alexis Carrel by Theodore I Malinin. Harcourt Brace Jovanovich, New York, 1979.

52. Jensen, CO: Experimentelle Untersuchung über Krebs bei Maüsen. Centralblatt Bakteriol Parasitenk Infectionskrankh 34:28, 1903.

53. Loeb, L: Über Entstehung eines Sarcoms nach Transplantation eines Adenosarcoms einer japanischen Maus. Zeitschr f Krebsforschung 7:80, 1908.

54. Tyzzer, EE: A study of inheritance in mice with reference to their susceptibility to transplantable tumors. J Med Res 21:519, 1909.

55. Little, CC: A possible Mendelian explanation for a type of inheritance apparently non-Mendelian in nature. Science 40:904, 1914.

56. Little, CC and Tyzzer, EE: Further experimental studies on the inheritance of susceptibility to a transplantable tumor, carcinoma (JWA) of the Japanese waltzing mouse. J Med Res 33:393, 1916.

57. Gorer, PA: The genetic and antigenic basis of tumor transplantation. J Pathol Bacteriol 44:691, 1937.

58. Gorer, PA: Further studies on the antigenic differences in mouse erythrocytes. Brit J Exp Pathol 18:31, 1937.

59. Gorer, PA: The antigenic basis of tumor transplantation. J Pathol Bacteriol 47:231, 1938.

60. Medawar, PB: The behavior and fate of skin autografts and skin homografts in rabbits. J Anat Lond 78:176, 1944.

61. Billingham, RE, Brent, L, Medawar, PB, and Sparrow, EM: Quantitative studies on tissue transplantation immunity: I. The survival times of skin homografts exchanged between members of different inbred strains of mice. Proc Roy Soc (London) B 143:43, 1954.

62. Counce, S, Smith, P, Barth, R, and Snell, GD: Strong and weak histocompatibility gene differences in mice and their role in the rejection of homografts of tumors and skin. Ann Surg 144:198, 1956.

Chapter 2

Cadaver Kidney Donation

DUANE T. FREIER

Need for Cadaver Donors
Most Available Donor
Legislation: Greatest Boon in Public Acceptance
  Public Law 98-507, National Organ Transplant Act
  Required-Request Law
  Brain-Death Legislation
  Uniform Anatomical Gift Act
  Public Law 92-603, End-Stage Renal Disease Medicare
    Coverage
  Public Law 95-292, Coverage of Organ Retrieval
Brain Death: Medical and Ethical Facts
Transplantation Coordination: Liaison That Makes Transplan-
    tation Possible
Ethics and the Shortage: Changing Opinion
Medical Barriers: Dislodged by Discussion and Education
Public Barriers
Transportation Barriers

Recent passage of landmark organ donation legislation affirms that public acceptance of organ donation has caught up with medical transplantation advances. But the conservative attitudes of physicians and health care personnel, coupled with the mistrust of family members at the time of donation, are leaving a vast resource—cadaveric kidneys—untapped as an unlimited donor source.

Today, 30 years after the first renal transplant, one of the largest challenges facing kidney transplantation has still not been hurdled. The unmet need for renal transplantation as a result of the shortage of donor organs is overwhelming. Awareness of issues affecting kidney transplantation may help reduce organ shortages. What are

the physician's and the public's roles in new legislation? What are the legal, medical, and ethical facts in determining brain death? What support structures exist within hospitals to facilitate cadaver donations?

Increasing the number of actual cadaver donors from the pool of potential ones requires the full backing of all physicians and families of brain-dead patients. To win their support, hospitals need to dedicate an organ procurement staff to help facilitate the many related duties and procedures of donation and retrieval. Also, broad sweeping public and professional education is needed to dispel misunderstandings of the ethical and moral issues. It is in the medical realm that reform of attitude can create the most significant effect on the growing number of patients suffering from end-stage kidney disease.

NEED FOR CADAVER DONORS

Today the growing population of dialysis patients in the United States exceeds 85,000, but only 7 percent of dialysis patients receive cadaveric kidneys (Tables 2–1 and 2–2). At least half of dialysis patients could benefit from renal transplantation, yet only 7000 patients receive a transplant. Since 50 percent of all dialysis patients are expected to die within 5 years after beginning treatment, aggressive procurement of cadaveric kidneys could benefit tens of thousands of dialysis patients.

Recent reports by the U.S. Department of Health and Human Services show a 62 percent increase in the number of patients receiving dialysis over the past 6 years (1980–1985) and a similar 70 percent in-

Table 2–1			
	Number of Patients* Receiving Living Related Kidneys	Number of Patients* Receiving Cadaveric Kidneys	Rate of Cadaveric Kidneys Based on Total Patients Transplanted
1980	1275	3422	73%
1981	1456	3427	70%
1982	1667	3681	69%
1983	1784	4328	71%
1984	1704	5264	76%
1985	1875	5819	76%
(Percent of 6-Yr Increase)	(47)	(70)	(3)

*Personal communication, Bureau of Management and Strategy, Health Care Financing Administration, Department of Health, Education and Welfare
(From End State Renal Disease Systems Branch, Annual ESRD Facility Survey, Baltimore, MD 1980–1985.)

Table 2–2			
	Number of Patients* on Hemodialysis	Number of Patients* Receiving Cadaveric Kidneys	Rate of Cadaveric Kidneys Based on Number of Patients on Hemodialysis (%)
1980	52,364	3422	6.5
1981	58,924	3427	6
1982	65,765	3681	5.5
1983	71,987	4328	6
1984	78,483	5264	7
1985	84,797	5819	7
(Percent of 6-Yr Increase)	(62)	(70)	(0.5)

*Personal communication, Bureau of Management and Strategy, Health Care Financing Administration, Department of Health, Education and Welfare
(From End Stage Renal Disease Systems Branch, Annual ESRD Facility Survey, Baltimore, MD 1980–1985.)

crease in the number of organ transplants from a cadaveric source during that same period. Staying even is not making progress.

MOST AVAILABLE DONOR

Living related organ donors, sparse in opportunity and numbers, create medical and psychologic risk to the donor, who must live with only one kidney. For the recipient, however, a living-related donor is the ideal.[1]

A recipient of a well-matched living related kidney donor can expect the new body part to function for as long as 20 years, compared with the much shorter expected life-span of the cadaver organ. But the greatest check on the use of living donor organs is their limited supply. Thousands of patients die each year waiting for a donor.

Because of the certainty of death, cadaver organs are not so limited. Most cadaveric donors double the gift by providing two kidneys for a possible transplantation match. A cadaveric donor creates less emotional stress in the recipient. And in many cases the organ gift of a deceased loved one has been comforting to survivors. Cost of transplantation compared with that of sustained dialysis is also a continuing incentive. Recent innovations in drug therapies have further reduced costs for organ transplantation, compared with escalating costs of dialysis. General acceptance of cadaver organ donation has been heightened by new legislation, by government funding for procurement agencies, and by positive publicity on transplant candidates and recipients.

LEGISLATION: GREATEST BOON IN PUBLIC ACCEPTANCE

During the past 5 years, public awareness and acceptance of organ transplantation has been extrinsically reflected by the passage of welcome legislation. Important new laws affecting organ donation are "required request" statutes and a national law addressing organ donation and distribution. While both are now widely accepted, the new rulings, however progressive in intent, are at best educational. They are empowered by only sporadic means of enforcement. Actual enactment of the laws is determined by individual physician practice and hospital directives. However, a clear understanding of the legal facts regarding organ donation may spur a voluntary commitment from physicians and health care teams to encourage organ donation in their institution.

Public Law 98-507, National Organ Transplant Act

Enacted in 1984, the National Organ Transplant Act established a national task force to address the medical, legal, ethical, economic, and social issues of organ procurement and transplantation. The law prohibits the sale of any organ because it is considered unethical by the national medical community.

The 25-member task force concerns itself with matters about kidney, liver, heart, lung, pancreas and bone marrow transplants. Grants have been established for the legislation of start-up operational costs and expansion of organ procurement services throughout the country. In addition, a national network to coordinate a recipient registry and organ exchange was created.

Required-Request Law

More than 15 states in the United States have enacted required-request or routine-inquiry statutes, which require hospitals to adopt policies that facilitate identification of all potential organ or tissue cadaver donors at the time of death.

New York State has a strict regulatory approach for its required-request law. The New York State Public Health Law mandates hospitals to file a certificate that documents the efforts of the hospital staff in requesting and investigating possible organ donations for each death. Under this provision any designated hospital staff member, not just physicians, may request donations from families of dying patients. Proper execution of the mandate requires extensive in-service training, hospital guidelines about donor criteria for various organs, and established medical protocols on the suitability of donors. Local organ procurement agencies have sponsored programs to assist hospitals with the challenging educational aspects of the new law.

The effectiveness of required-request laws has not been documented, but organ procurement agencies report that tissue donation (bone, skin, corneas, etc.) has increased substantially over the few years since the law's inception. However, organ donation that requires a brain-dead donor has not increased.

Brain-Death Legislation

One great legal and ethical debate stirred by organ transplantation is the determination of brain death. Thirty-six states have defined brain death and legislatively accepted it.[2] The other 14 states have opted for judiciary rather than legislative determination of brain death based on case-by-case precedent.

Laws regarding the determination of brain death first emerged 17 years ago, when the Kansas state legislature passed the first brain-death statute in 1970. Other states soon afterward adopted similar statutes. The historic Kansas law states that a physician may declare brain death if the pronouncement of death is made before artificial respiratory and circulatory functions are terminated and before any vital organ is removed for transplantation.

Unfortunately, some brain-death laws were amended to the Uniform Anatomical Gift Act, a 1968 law calling for the donor's or his family's predetermined or "explicit consent" to donation of organs. This created the impression that brain-death laws applied only to cases of potential organ donation. Consequently, appropriate discontinuation of respiratory support for cases not involving organ donation were not addressed.

Advances in artificial respiration and transplantation techniques spurred medical associations to look more stringently at explicit-consent laws. The American Medical Association has held that physicians could declare death according to accepted medical standards. This ethical premise was usually upheld in court, but as society grew

more litigious, many physicians were unwilling to risk pronouncing a patient brain dead without strong legal support. AMA members lobbied for the security of an "explicit-death law."

An effort to combine the ethical acceptance of brain-death criteria with state brain-death laws occurred in 1980. The President's Commission for the Study of Ethical Problems in Medicine and Biomedical and Behavioral Research met with physician and lay sponsors of existing laws to draft the Uniform Determination of Death Act. Their hope was to create a uniform statement that would be accepted by all 50 states. It reads:

> An individual who has sustained either (1) irreversible cessation of circulation and respiratory functions, or (2) irreversible cessation of all functions of the entire brain, including the brain stem, is dead. A determination of death must be made in accordance with accepted medical standards.[5]

The two-sentence statement, adopted by many states, was a much anticipated legal-medical milestone. It tersely captured a widespread and ethically acceptable medical practice that had been used widely in every state for years. Through the Uniform Determination of Death Act, brain death is legally defined, but it awaits to be legislatively adopted in all states.

Uniform Anatomical Gift Act

The oldest and a pivotal organ donation law, the Uniform Anatomical Gift Act was approved by the National Conference of Commissioners on Uniform State Laws in 1968. Less than 6 years later all 50 states in the country had passed a version of the law. The speed of its acceptance alone was revolutionary, marking the "fastest enactment of a uniform statute in history.... "[6]

The law requires "explicit consent," rather than implied consent from the donor or his survivors. This may be granted through a premortem mechanism such as a driver's license, where individuals indicate their desire to donate their organs and designate the recipient (individual, physician, hospital, medical school, or tissue bank).

The law also allows individual donors to revoke their organ donation decision.

Guidelines set for the medical community, according to the Uniform Anatomical Gift Act, require any attending physician other than the doctor or surgeon removing or transplanting the organ to certify the time of death.

A definition of brain death was omitted from the law because of the anticipated controversies. Stipulations that the law must not interfere with the duties of the medical examiner have led to many confrontations between medical examiners and transplantation physicians. The medical examiner fears destruction of evidence by the donation process if foul play is suspected in the case. Communication, trust, and cooperation between the parties have eliminated the problem in most communities through the efforts of transplantation physicians and organ procurement agency personnel.

Public Law 92-603: End-Stage Renal Disease Medicare Coverage

End-stage renal disease (ESRD) received significant social and political relevance with the passage of this law in 1972. It extended Medicare benefits to all ESRD patients regardless of age. It made no economic provisions for the cost of organ donation, but the law did provide financial support for transplantation activity through a system of ESRD networks.

Public Law 95-292: Coverage of Organ Retrieval

The implementation of this law in 1979 called for expanded coverage through Medicare of all medical services related to donor retrieval.[7] In addition, the law expanded federal payment of donor expenses through the Health Care Financing Administration (HCFA) and its chosen intermediary, Aetna Life Insurance Company. By 1986 more than 50 independent organ procurement agencies nationwide had received certification under Medicare for organ retrieval services.

BRAIN DEATH: MEDICAL AND ETHICAL FACTS

State laws have endowed medical practice with the responsibility for establishing the criteria for declaring brain death. The advent of the mechanical respirator, which prolongs maintenance of brain-dead, heart-beating patients, forced the issue of death declaration based on evidence other than cessation of circulation.

In 1968 the Ad Hoc Committee of the Harvard Medical School to Examine the Definition of Brain Death was the first group to publish standards defining irreversible coma.[8] The committee stated that irreversible coma must be determined by a physical examination and readily available tests.

The report described the "permanently nonfunctioning brain" as totally unreceptive and unresponsive to all external and internal stimuli. All central reflexes were considered to be totally absent, and "as a rule" the stretch of tendon reflexes could not be elicited. A misinterpretation of the language "as a rule" created uncertainty. Clinicians confused central reflexes such as ocular movement and blinking in response to head turning and irrigation of the ears with ice water with such peripheral reflexes as tendon stretching. Central reflexes must be absent before brain death can be proclaimed, but peripheral reflexes can be present. Dilated and fixed pupils were established criteria for brain death. Body movements such as swallowing, yawning, vocalization or decerebrate posturing were evidence contrary to the diagnosis. Lack of spontaneous respiration was considered another essential criterion for brain-dead status.

The Harvard criteria instruct that physicians allow the patient to breathe without the assistance of a respirator for at least 3 min, providing that the carbon dioxide tension was within normal range at the start of the trial period and also that the patient had been breathing room air for at least 10 min. A flat electroencephalogram (EEG) was recommended by the Harvard standards but not considered essential. They stated that if an EEG was not available, purely clinical signs were sufficient to judge the condition. Also, an acceptable practice was noting the absence of cerebral circulation by judging the standstill of blood in retinal vessels. Today nuclear imaging or angiographic methods determine this graphically.

The Harvard standards required the series of tests to be repeated in 24 hours to rule out hypothermia and nervous system depressants and to provide evidence that the patient's condition remained unchanged. The 24-hour criterion is unrealistic because it is often impossible to sustain circulation that long.

The Harvard standards, upheld for 14 years, were updated by the President's Commission for the Study of Ethical Problems in Medicine in 1982. The commission report and a separate publication of the commission's medical consultants addressed many objections of the earlier recommendations.[5,9] Most important, the new standards defined cessation of cerebral and brainstem functions and irreversibility.[5]

Recent studies by Rohling concluded that testing for apnea is often done incorrectly; an adequate apnea test was performed on only 1 of 28 donors examined through the study.[10] To address that point, the earlier President's commission specifically recommended:

Adequate testing for apnea is very important. An accepted method is ventilation with pure oxygen or an oxygen and carbon dioxide mixture for 10 minutes before withdrawal of the ventilator, followed by passive flow of oxygen. (This procedure allows $PaCO_2$ to rise without hazardous hypoxia.) Hypercarbia adequately stimulates respiratory effort within 30 seconds when $PaCO_2$ is greater than 60 mm Hg. A 10 minute period of apnea is usually sufficient to attain this level of hypercarbia. Testing of arterial blood gases can be used to confirm this level. Spontaneous breathing efforts indicate that part of the brainstem is functioning.[9]

The cause of the coma must be established and be sufficient to account for the clinical state. Reversible conditions such as sedation, hypothermia, neuromuscular blockage, and shock must be ruled out. If no sufficient cause is identified, prolonged observation and extensive testing should be performed.

Special tests for confirmation of brain death have always been sought despite the

acceptance that brain death can be established reliably by clinical criteria alone.[11] The electroencephalogram, with all its previously noted problems, is the earliest test used. Cerebral pan angiography is acceptable but also has similar problems of availability, reliability, and convenience.

Radionuclide scanning is considered satisfactory by many centers but has been questioned by Link et al because the brainstem cannot be adequately evaluated[12,13]. These authors recommend adding brainstem auditory evoked potential (BAEP) testing to supplement cerebral perfusion scintigraphy (CPS). Evoked potential studies can be supplemental in cases of intoxications but will not rule out the other misleading conditions of hypothermia and young age.[14]

Awareness of the special tolerance of infants and children under 5 years of age to cerebral ischemia was emphasized in the President's commission report. The complicating conditions of drug and metabolic intoxication, hypothermia, and shock also received appropriate detailed discussion.

Any medical facility can confidently document brain death. The rules are flexible as long as they are satisfactory to local physicians and clearly stated in a written document specific for that facility. The best guidelines are simple, practical ones that can be adapted to special needs. The unethical practice of "breathing a cadaver" make brain death standards necessary for all hospitals with respirator and intensive care capability regardless of organ donation intentions.

A summary of the basic criteria for brain death:

1. Absence of spontaneous respiration, thoroughly determined and documented
2. Absence of response to all stimuli
3. Absence of any spontaneous movement
4. Absence of central reflexes
5. Presence of fixed and dilated pupils
6. Presence of a plausible etiology with elimination of hypothermia, drugs, or metabolic causes that could be reversible
7. Consideration that the time of observation is compatible with the reversibility of etiology, with special consideration of the regeneration of brain function in children
8. Prudent but not mandatory use of rea-

sonable and practical methods of documentation such as the EEG, nuclear imaging, arteriography, and evoked potentials

TRANSPLANTATION COORDINATION: LIAISON THAT MAKES TRANSPLANTATION POSSIBLE

Donation of cadaver organs requires cooperation among hospital administrators, physicians, transplant coordinators, laboratory technicians, and operating room teams from multiple hospitals, often thousands of miles apart. Coordination of these systems grew more sophisticated with the 1978 passage of Public Law 95-292, which provided Medicare funding to cover organ retrieval and expanded federal payment of donor expenses through HCFA and Aetna Life Insurance Company.

Before this legislation many organ donation expenses were underwritten as research costs, and physicians waived their professional fees. Transportation was donated by local and state police forces, and coordination of reimbursement was haphazard. A few local and regional associations were developed, including models such as the Southeastern Organ Procurement Foundation in 1969 and the Transplantation Society of Michigan in 1972.

Under the leadership of these pioneering associations, independent organ procurement agencies (IOPAs) began to emerge. Supported in part through federal money, they assumed the coordination efforts and cost of organ donation, and in 1986, 57 IOPAs nationwide had received certification by Medicare.

Functioning independently of patient care providers, IOPAs are governed by boards composed of physicians, health care administrators, nurses, clergy, and transplant recipients themselves. Most of the work is done by small, dedicated full-time IOPA staff, including an administrator, coordinators, educators, and secretaries. Serving as a liaison between multiple transplantation centers and donating hospitals, the IOPAs' specific functions often include:

1. Operating a 24-hour call service for information

2. Coordinating all activities of procurement

3. Identifying suitable donors

4. Educating professionals and the lay public

5. Scheduling procurement teams

6. Preserving and transporting organs

7. Assuring proper histocompatibility testing

8. Keeping records and accounts

9. Affiliating with other state and national programs

10. Promulgating standards and guidelines

11. Monitoring and evaluating outcomes through peer review and audits

12. Compiling and computing recipient listings

13. Reimbursing all related costs through third-party carriers

14. Administrating day-to-day affairs

15. Obtaining letters of agreement from all participating hospitals.[15]

Hospitals with no access to a freestanding agency like an IOPA often assign donation and retrieval duties to existing staff members. Since patient care responsibilities take priority over organ donation, this alternative is less effective than an IOPA.

Not only have IOPAs improved organ donation and transplantation, but also they have implemented the complex responsibilities in a cost-effective way. Reports from Aetna Life and Casualty Insurance Company show that IOPAs have kept kidney donation costs surprisingly stable over the past 3 years. From 1982 to 1985 the average cost of donation and retrieval per kidney has risen only 3 percent, from $7764 to $7997. Another indication of the effectiveness of IOPAs is their success in transplanting available organs. The number of kidneys wasted, or donated and not transplanted, has dropped from 15 percent in 1982 to 10 percent in 1985.

The 1984 National Organ Transplant Act made available significant grant money to support the establishment of IOPAs throughout the country. The law defines them as nonprofit, with a decentralized organizational structure and self-reliant operations. Each contains its own administrative, accounting, and reimbursement expertise and operates within a defined service area. Policy development and major decision-making draw on the experience of an advisory board made up of health care personnel and physicians, community leaders, and lay people.

The National Organ Procurement and Transplantation Network, also established by the legislation, maintains a national waiting list of organs and coordinates organ matching throughout the country.

ETHICS AND THE SHORTAGE: CHANGING OPINION

Twice as many individuals are on cadaver waiting lists as receive a cadaver kidney each year. Referring to organ shortage as a "shortage in the face of plenty," Bart and associates[3] estimated that the usage of potential donors is about 20 percent.[3] Ironically, as more donors are available, more recipients appear on the waiting list. Some of them are patients requiring a retransplantation; this group becomes difficult to match because of increased sensitivity to antigens. Most of the group creating this phenomenon are dialysis patients who notice the increased activity and decreased waiting time and request transplantation.

Today approximately 7 percent of patients with end-stage renal disease receive a cadaver kidney (Table 2–2). Doubling that number would make a significant contribution to the large number of patients in the dialysis pool.

In 1980, 3422 cadaver transplants were done; in 1985, 5819 were done. This is a 70 percent increase of transplants from a cadaveric source in 6 years. But the recipient pool is growing just as fast and little gain has been made. Living related donors have been a relatively stable pool since 1980. Two options are available to provide more kidneys, and both should be pursued: (1) retrieve cadaver donor kidneys at a higher rate than now, and (2) move on to the living nonrelated potential pool. This is not a consideration this chapter purports to discuss, but I wish to suggest it.[10,16,17]

To gain on the number of kidney disease patients waiting for a transplant, physical and psychological barriers must be overcome. The barriers most affecting kidney donations involve medical ethics, public opinion, transportation, and distribution, according to the Minister's Task Force on Kidney Donation of Ontario, Canada.[18]

Required-request laws are beginning to solve some of the hospital barriers. To be truly effective, these new laws must be adapted to mandate all hospitals, not just transplant and dialysis centers, to assert the issue of donation with the family members of all dying patients. The enforcement of strong hospital policy mandating active surveillance of patients and medical records will do the most to further this effort, recommend Bart and associates.[4]

MEDICAL BARRIERS: DISLODGED BY DISCUSSION AND EDUCATION

Today a serious impediment to kidney donation is physician practice and attitude. Investigation of two New York City hospitals confirmed that half of the kidneys potentially available were never evaluated.[16] Why? Lack of physician referral, concluded the study.

Another evaluation by the Canadian Task Force surveyed 118 Ontario hospitals and interviewed the ICU personnel, including nurses, chaplains, residents, neurosurgeons, and neurologists.[18] Some 75 percent reported that lack of coordination assistance, firm guidelines on donation criteria, and the time demand were significant deterrents to promoting donation. Only 65 percent of the respondents said they knew the telephone number to call for organ donation and procurement assistance. Some 44 percent of the neurosurgeons polled said that they would initiate or become involved in a donation. Qualitative analysis showed that physician reluctance stemmed from fear of legal liability and lack of incentive to dedicate the time required to organize the organ gift.

To overcome these medical barriers, transplant physicians must convince their colleagues of the social and health benefits of transplantation. This can be achieved through casual discussion, educational opportunities, grand rounds, staff meetings, and staff-directed awareness programs.

The social benefits of transplantation versus continued dialysis treatment:

1. Sustaining a life
2. Improved quality of life
3. Reduced government-subsidized health care costs to society
4. The psychological rewards of donation

Physician committees have rejected such financial incentive programs as awarding a finder's fee, stating that it is unethical. Increased awareness of the social and psychological benefits to the patient and health care team must suffice as incentive-building tools. Awareness campaigns that project the urgent need for donor kidneys and relay success stories are needed on all professional levels and within the community.

PUBLIC BARRIERS

The Gallup Poll on Organ Donation, sponsored by the National Kidney Foundation, showed that public awareness of organ transplantation is high.[19] Some 93 percent of respondents said they have heard of organ transplant cases and are aware of the individual's and family's rights regarding permission for donation. Although 72 percent are willing to give permission to donate the kidneys of a loved one, more specific questions revealed that only 50 percent would grant permission to donate the kidneys of their own child; only 24 percent said they would donate their own kidneys.

Racial differences in the willingness to donate organs was significant, according to the poll. Only 10 percent of the blacks polled said they would donate their own kidneys, compared with 27 percent in the white population. The discrepancy is a serious one. The incidence of end-stage renal disease in the urban black population is greater than the national average. One urban institution reports that 41 of 47 cadaver kidneys transplanted into black recipients were donated by nonblacks.[20] Similarly, donation patterns in Chicago show that the retrieval rate was 34 percent for the total population but only 17 percent in the black population.[21] A striking 91 percent of the cases showed lack of family consent as the predominant reason for the low organ retrieval rate among the black sector. The elicited contributing factors included

1. Lack of knowledge
2. Opposing religious beliefs
3. Fear of complications
4. Lack of adequate communications between laypersons and the health provider

Public attitudes cannot be legislated, but public education can be effective. Grants through the National Organ Transplantation Act are available for public education and media awareness campaigns.

TRANSPORTATION BARRIERS

Advances in medical techniques have reduced many of the transportation complications that affected organ donation and transplantation only 5 years ago. The acceptable use of inexpensive portable ice storage for transporting organs replaced cumbersome perfusion machines and eliminated the need for a technician to travel with the organ. Also, the establishment of a national clearing agency through the National Transplant Act increased the accessibility of organs and resolved many transportation problems.

CONCLUSION

Medical technology has provided a means through sophisticated transplantation techniques not only to sustain the lives of chronic kidney disease sufferers, but also to greatly improve their ability to lead fulfilling lives. Government programs and laws have made renal transplantation available to all end-stage renal disease patients, yet many patients die each day waiting for a donor kidney. Others wait a long time for the procedure that will free them of dependence on dialysis.

The next step in improving the management of renal disease is providing kidneys to all who could benefit from renal transplantation. It is a step that science, technology, and government cannot coerce. Physicians and consenting family members hold the most important contribution: a reform of attitude and greater willingness to participate in this life-giving gift. Only then will significantly more cadaver donations be available for transplantation. Massive educational programs for the professional and public sectors are needed to reach the modest goal of doubling the number of cadaver donations within the next 5 years.

REFERENCES

1. Rapaport, FT and Cortesini, R: The past, present and future of organ transplantation with special reference to current needs in kidney procurement and donation. Transplant Proc (Suppl 2)17:3, 1985.
2. Youngstein, KP (ed): Statutory Regulation of Organ Donation in the United States, ed 2. Southeastern Organ Procurement Foundation, Richmond, VA, 1986.
3. Bart, KJ, et al: Cadaveric kidneys for transplantation. Transplantation 31:379, 1981.
4. Bart, KJ, et al: Increasing the supply of cadaveric kidneys for transplantation. Transplantation 31:383, 1981.
5. President's Commission for the Study of Ethical Problems in Medicine: Defining Death: A Report on the Medical, Legal, and Ethical Issues in the Determination of Death (1982-371-059/8192). United States Government Printing Office, Washington, DC, 1982.
6. Youngstein, KP (ed): Statutory Regulation of Organ Donation in the United States, ed. 1. Southeastern Organ Procurement Foundation, Richmond, VA, 1979.
7. Health Care Financing Administration: Second Annual Report to Congress (1980-311-168-149). US Government Printing Office, Washington, DC, 1980.
8. Report of the Ad Hoc Committee of the Harvard Medical School to Examine the Definition of Brain Death: A definition of irreversible coma. JAMA 205:337, 1968.
9. Report of the Medical Consultants on the Diagnosis of Death Problems in Medicine and Biomedical and Behavioral Research: Guidelines for the determination of death. JAMA 246:2184, 1981.
10. Rohling, R, et al: Apnea test: Pitfalls and correct handling. Transplant Proc (Suppl 3)18:388, 1986.
11. Canadian Neurosurgery Society Guidelines for the Determination of Brain Death (Version of 18 Feb. 1985). Transplant Proc 17:64, 1985.
12. Goodman, JM, Heck, LL, and Moore, BD: Confirmation of brain death with portable isotope angiography: A review of 204 consecutive cases. Neurosurgery 16:492, 1985.
13. Link, J, et al: Diagnosis of brain death by BAEP and CPS? Transplant Proc 18:385, 1986.
14. Cuerit, JM and Marieu, P: Are evoked potentials a valuable tool for the diagnosis of brain death? Transplant Proc 18:386, 1986.
15. Freier, DT: Kidney donation. In Toledo-Pereyra, LH (ed): Basic Concepts of Organ Procurement, Perfusion, and Preservation for Transplantation. Academic Press, New York, 1982, p 48.
16. Sales, CM and Burrous, L: Cadaveric organ procurement: An investigation of a source of kidney shortage. Transplant Proc (Suppl 3)18:416, 1986.
17. Burley, JA and Stiller, CR: Emotionally related donors and renal transplantation. Transplant Proc (Suppl 3)17:123, 1985.
18. Robinette, MA and Stiller, CR: Summary of task force findings. Transplant Proc (Suppl 3)17:62, 1985.
19. Robinette, MA, et al: Gallup poll on behalf of the National Kidney Foundation. Transplant Proc (Suppl 3)17:62, 1981.
20. Callender, CO, et al: Attitudes among blacks toward donating kidneys for transplantation: A pilot project. J Nat Med Assoc 74:807, 1982.
21. Pollak, R, et al: Donor referral and organ procurement patterns in a large metropolitan area: A single center prospective study. Transplant Proc 18:399, 1986.

Chapter 3

Kidney Harvesting and Preservation

LUIS H. TOLEDO-PEREYRA

Adequate methods for renal harvesting and preservation are essential for satisfactory graft function after transplantation. Several recent practices, such as increased organ sharing between transplant centers and longer distances between donor and recipient hospitals, necessitate the development of methods for safely extending preservation times without compromising kidney viability. Also, multiple organ harvesting from a single donor may present challenges to organ procurement teams experienced only with kidney retrieval. This chapter will review the development of renal preservation and offer current and future perspectives in organ procurement and preservation.

HISTORICAL PERSPECTIVES

The first documented attempts at maintaining the viability of various tissues and organs outside the body were published in the 1800s. Physiologists such as Legallois,[1] von Cyon,[2] Ringer,[3] and Langendorff[4] studied the effects of ex vivo normothermia on various organs.[5,6] They determined that certain blood components were necessary for maintenance of the organs at room temperature. At the beginning of this century, Carrel and Lindbergh[7] were able to unify many of the concepts begun in the 1800s. Using a pump and perfusion apparatus, they perfused some organs for 20 to 40 days with normothermic serum. When blood was added to the perfusate, the maximum time for preservation of kidneys was about 2 days. Viability was assessed by measuring oxygen and glucose consumption. Preservation of architecture was analyzed by histologic studies. Carrel and Lindbergh's work was disrupted, however, by the beginning of World War II.

Lefebvre and Nizet[8] introduced the idea of low-temperature perfusion in 1952. In 1960 the first canine kidney autograft was transplanted, after 24 hours of hypothermic preservation.[9] The organ was first perfused for 1 hour with cooled whole blood, kept in the cold (2 to 4°C) for 24 hours, and then reperfused with warm blood for 1 hour prior to reimplantation.

A few years later, Humphries and colleagues[10] successfully used an alternative method of continuous perfusion of kidneys to preserve canine kidneys for 24 hours.

Cooled diluted blood (10°C) was pumped at a pressure of 40 mmHg to supply oxygen and nutrients to the tissue.

Belzer and his associates obtained consistent function after 72 hours of canine kidney preservation by means of continuous pulsatile perfusion at 10°C with a canine cryoprecipitated plasma (CPP) preparation.[11] To prepare CPP, plasma was frozen, thawed and filtered to remove some of the labile lipoproteins.

The use of intracellular crystalloid solutions for renal hypothermic storage was introduced, in 1969, by Collins and Terasaki.[12] Using these solutions, excellent results were obtained after hypothermic storage of canine kidneys for up to 30 hours. Their results encouraged the use of hypothermic storage as an alternative to hypothermic pulsatile perfusion for renal preservation. Variations of these intracellular crystalloid solutions are still used clinically.

In 1972 Johnson and colleagues[13] reported successful preservation of both canine and human kidneys using a new perfusate, human plasma protein fraction (PPF). Subsequent work by this group produced successful 7- and 8-day preservation in two of five and two of seven kidneys, respectively. PPF was prepared to be free of fibrinogen, lipoproteins, gamma globulins, isoagglutinins, cytotoxic antibodies, complement, and hepatitis agents. This preparation is still used routinely for perfusion preservation.

In 1973 we[14] introduced a new process for removing labile lipoproteins, cholesterol, and fibrinogen from plasma used for perfusion. Silica gel was added to the plasma before freezing, thawing, and filtering it. The resulting fraction was called silica gel fraction, or SGF. Excellent results have been obtained using SGF both experimentally and clinically for perfusion of kidneys.[15–17] One drawback to the routine widespread use of SGF has been the high cost and limited commercial availability of this preparation. Most clinicians prefer commercially available plasmanate or albumin solutions for perfusion.

Since the development of the original SGF preparation, we have developed other hyperosmolar colloid (SGF-base) solutions (TP-series) that have proven valuable for preservation of kidneys. They are especially useful after ischemic damage[18] and are adaptable for preservation by either hypothermic storage or pulsatile perfusion. Some of these preparations have also been used for preservation of heart, pancreas, and liver allografts.[18] The composition of the TP-series solutions is discussed in the section New Preservation Solutions.

In the past decade experimental efforts have continued to extend renal preservation times. Van der Wijk and colleagues,[19] for example, were able to obtain 6-day hypothermic machine perfusion of canine kidneys by the use of intermittent normothermic ex vivo perfusion between the kidney and the donor animal. Work by Rijkmans and associates[20] has investigated the use of intermittent normothermic blood perfusion to extend preservation times of perfused kidneys. After hypothermic perfusion for 2 days kidneys were placed on normothermic (37°C) blood perfusion for 3 hours, followed by hypothermic perfusion for a total of 6 days of preservation. Life-sustaining function was observed in 9 of 11 animals transplanted with these kidneys.

DONOR MAINTENANCE, ORGAN PROCUREMENT, AND PRESERVATION CONSIDERATIONS

Donor Maintenance

Protection of the kidneys from ischemic damage begins during donor maintenance procedures prior to organ harvesting and continues during the organ procurement procedure (Fig. 3–1; Table 3–1). It is important to maintain optimal circulation up to the time of organ removal, when a potential organ donor is identified. The donor blood pressure should be stabilized by appropriate fluid replacement. Colloid and crystalloid solutions may be used alone or together to correct hypovolemic hypotension due to dehydration and other associated factors. If a vasopressor is necessary to maintain blood pressure >100 mmHg, despite volume expansion, dopamine is the drug of choice. Urinary output should be replaced milliliter by milliliter on an hourly basis, when blood pressure is stabilized. Furosemide or mannitol may be administered if diuretics are necessary to maintain adequate diuresis. Good hydration of the donor is ultimately related to good organ perfusion.

The potential donor is declared brain dead when the absence of brainstem or cortical activity has been demonstrated.[21] The Harvard criteria have been widely applied since 1968 for this determination; however, other modifications have been made at some centers.[21] More detail regarding brain death and kidney donation may be found in Chapter 2.

Organ Procurement

After declaration of brain death, family permission should be obtained and the donor should be taken to the operating suite as soon as possible. Kidneys should be quickly dissected and removed. It is important to minimize the length of warm ischemia between cross-clamping the circulation and organ removal. Prolonged warm ischemia is related to an increased incidence of delayed posttransplant function and irreversible tissue damage. Some transplant teams choose to flush the donor in situ with cold flush solution via an aortic catheter to avoid this problem.[22] This allows for organ cooling before removal. In situ flushing is especially useful when extrarenal organs are also harvested. At our cen-

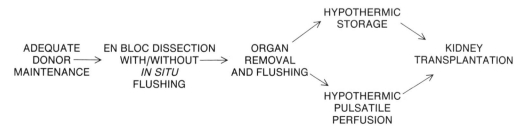

Figure 3–1. To achieve optimal results after cadaver kidney transplantation, it is necessary to protect the renal allograft from ischemic damage during each step of organ procurement and preservation.

Table 3–1 Protection of Kidneys from Ischemic Damage

Kidneys obtained from heart-beating cadaver donors with good hydration, diuresis, and cardiovascular stability
Cautious use of vasoactive drugs
Use of colloids, heparinization, and metabolic and cell protectants
Avoidance of toxic drugs
Meticulous organ procurement techniques and atraumatic organ removal
Minimum of warm ischemia
Use of appropriate preservation method

---

ter we do not rely on this technique for minimizing warm ischemia. Although the kidneys may be removed singly, most transplant centers prefer to remove them en bloc with a segment of aorta and vena cava. This provides for maximum arterial length and prevents intimal damage to the renal artery. This technique is especially useful, since it permits the use of a Carrel patch, which includes a patch of aorta and the origins of multiple renal arteries. The choice of preservation technique depends on the conditions of donor maintenance and organ harvesting as well as on the particular preference of the transplant team.

Metabolic Considerations

Early efforts in organ procurement and preservation were made without a clear understanding of the many changes occurring as a result of organ ischemia. Investigators have attempted to improve organ viability during ischemia by either inhibiting or maintaining cellular metabolism (Table 3–2). Current research continues to probe the details of the physiology of ischemia to achieve better viability after preservation.

Metabolic Inhibition

Hypothermia has been widely applied in renal preservation to reduce renal metabolic needs. Studies by Levy[23] in 1959 demonstrated that hypothermia significantly decreases the kidney's oxygen demand. Oxygen use is reduced 84 percent at 20°C and 95 percent at 10°C as compared with body temperatures. The use of surface cooling or hypothermic storage and cooling by perfusion have evolved from this concept. Cry-

opreservation or organ freezing has also been tested as a means of accomplishing long-term preservation.

Other methods of metabolic inhibition include the use of pharmacologic agents.[24] Vasoactive drugs such as phenoxybenzamine,[25] propanolol,[26] furosemide,[24] glucagon,[27] and prostaglandins[28,29] have been tested to prevent vasoconstriction and promote vasodilation. Glycerol[30] and mannitol[31] have been used to prevent edema. Corticosteroids[32,33] have also been applied as membrane stabilizers. Another recent approach has been the use of oxygen-free radical scavengers, discussed later in this chapter. Some of these drugs, such as methylprednisolone, phenoxybenzamine, and furosemide, have been incorporated into routine clinical use at many centers. Others have been used only sporadically in clinical applications or have remained entirely experimental.

Table 3–2 Strategies for Improving Kidney Viability During Ischemia

Metabolic Inhibition
Hypothermia
Pharmacologic agents
  Vasodilators
  Propanolol
  Furosemide
  Prostaglandins
  Prostaglandin inhibitors—indomethacin
  Corticosteroids
  Oxygen-free radical scavengers
  Calcium channel blockers

Metabolic Maintenance
Energy substrates and precursors
  Adenosine triphosphate (ATP)
  Adenine nucleotides

Metabolic Maintenance

An alternative approach has been to provide for the organ's metabolic needs rather than attempting to reduce organ metabolism during preservation. Several studies have attempted to do this by supplying energy substrates and precursors such as adenosine triphosphate (ATP) and adenine nucleotides during preservation.[34,35] Success with these methods, however, has been inconsistent.

HYPOTHERMIC STORAGE

Practical Considerations

Hypothermic storage is an attractive preservation method because it is simpler and less expensive than hypothermic pulsatile perfusion. Its outcome and reliability, however, are dependent on the length of preservation and the type of solution used. Hypothermia is initiated by a cold intra-arterial flush combined with surface cooling. If kidneys are obtained from heart-beating cadaver donors with minimal ischemia, preservation by hypothermic storage after flushing is usually reliable for 24 hours. If preservation is extended beyond 24 hours,

storage is much less effective than perfusion. One center, however, has reported successful hypothermic storage for up to 95 hours.[36]

The degree of warm ischemia involved during organ procurement may have an important effect on the outcome of renal preservation. Delayed immediate function or ATN is seen in about half of the cases where kidneys are stored for 24 hours even with minimal or no warm ischemia. These results, however, are not substantially different from those obtained after pulsatile perfusion.

One disadvantage in using hypothermic storage is that it is not possible to evaluate kidney viability during storage. When perfusion methods are employed, flows and perfusion pressures may be monitored as needed.

Storage Solutions

Solutions developed for clinical hypothermic storage include both iso-osmolar and hyperosmolar and crystalloid and colloid preparations. Various combinations of electrolytes have been used, including K^+, Mg^+, Na^+, Cl^-, and mannitol. The effectiveness of each solution for hypothermic

Table 3–3 Composition of Preservation Solutions for Hypothermic Storage			
Collins (C-2)		**Sacks II**	
KH_2PO_4	2.05 g/L	KH_2PO_4	2.05 g/L
$K_2HPO_4\ 3H_2O$	9.7 g/L	K_2HPO_4	9.7 g/L
KCl	1.12 g/L	KCl	1.12 g/L
$NaHCO_3$	0.84 g/L	$NaHCO_3$	0.84 g/L
Glucose	25 g/L	Mannitol	37.5 g/L
$MgSO_4\ 7H_2O$	7.38 g/L	$MgCl_2$	16 mEq/L
Osmolarity	~320 mOsm/L	Osmolarity	~430 mOsm/L
Euro-Collins*		**Euro-Collins†**	
KH_2PO_4	2.05 g/L	KH_2PO_4	2.05 g/L
K_2HPO_4	7.40 g/L	K_2HPO_4	7.40 g/L
KCl	1.12 g/L	KCl	1.12 g/L
$NaHCO_3$	0.84 g/L	$NaHCO_3$	0.84 g/L
Glucose	35 g/L	Glucose	70.7 g/L
Osmolarity	~357 mOsm/L	Osmolarity	~529 mOsm/L

*Original formulation for Euro-Collins solution.
†Recently additional glucose has been added to increase the osmolarity.

storage is generally related to its composition as well as the length of warm ischemia and preservation time. Numerous experimental and clinical studies have shown the value of hyperosmolar, hyperkalemic, and hypermagnesemic flush solutions for the storage of rabbit, pig, dog, and human kidneys, with good preservation of structure and function for 72 hours or more. The longest reported period of hypothermic storage for human kidneys was 95 hours,[36] although practical range is between 1 and 2 days maximum. Several solutions are routinely used for clinical hypothermic storage preservation (Table 3–3). These include Collins' solutions (C-2), Sacks, and Euro-Collins solution. We[18] use colloid hyperosmolar solutions for kidneys procured by our team and transplanted at our center.

HYPOTHERMIC PULSATILE PERFUSION

Practical Considerations

The longest experimental and clinical renal preservation times have been accomplished using hypothermic pulsatile perfusion. This method reduces the metabolic function, oxygen demand, and nutritional requirements of the kidney. Oxygenated plasma solution is pumped through the kidney to supply the residual metabolic needs. Under ideal conditions of harvesting and preservation, ATP, ADP, and AMP are stabilized at near-normal levels. However, cellular metabolism is slightly abnormal.[37] Hypothermic pulsatile perfusion appears to be useful even for ischemically damaged kidneys. Clinical perfusion, however, is more costly and complex. It is sometimes inconvenient to transport of kidneys between centers, and specially trained personnel are needed. The majority of clinical perfusion uses pulsatile methods, although a few centers apply nonpulsatile methods. Hypothermic conditions are used for all perfusion methods in clinical transplantation.

Development of Perfusion Machines

By 1967 Belzer[11] developed a pulsatile pump for kidney preservation (Fig. 3–2).

The first kidney perfusion machine was marketed in 1968 by Life-Med Corporation. By June 1970, more than 30 kidneys had been preserved using this system for periods averaging 24 hours. Further efforts in perfusion technology were centered on simplifying the methodology and reducing the costs to procure, preserve, and transport human kidneys. Although the Belzer machine was an innovation in preservation, it was bulky and expensive. Cost and size were later reduced through the use of the Mini-Belzer, which is no longer used.

During the 1970s several other types of perfusion apparatus were developed and marketed. Travenol offered the Viacell, which included diastolic and pulse pressure control mechanisms. Travenol stopped production in 1972 and concentrated on the development of solutions for preservation. The Gambro machine, a nonpulsatile set-up manufactured in Sweden, is still used at some European centers. The most popular and widely used pulsatile perfusion machine in the United States at present is made by Waters Instruments (Fig. 3–3). The disposable organ cassettes are interchangeable between portable machines, which greatly facilitates the logistics of organ sharing between centers.

In our laboratories work on prototype perfusion machines has included the development of two unique nonpulsatile units.[38] The T.P.-1 is designed to simplify previous perfusion models. It uses a nonpulsatile pump and is a compact, self-contained, portable unit (Fig. 3–4). The recently developed AED-KPU-100 unit features a nonpulsatile system with convenient digital displays for temperature, pressure, flow, and voltage (Fig. 3–5).

During hypothermic pulsatile perfusion, plasma or a plasma-derived solution is circulated through the organ at 4 to 7°C by a pulsatile pump. The most commonly used clinical perfusates are cryoprecipitated plasma (CPP), albumin, plasma protein fraction or plasmanate (PPF), silica gel fraction (SGF), and the Belzer perfusate (Table 3–4). Although all these have shown acceptable long-term results, the final decision as to the choice of perfusate is based on several factors such as simplicity, storage capability, and cost. Many centers use a particular perfusate based more on subjective observation than on objective testing.

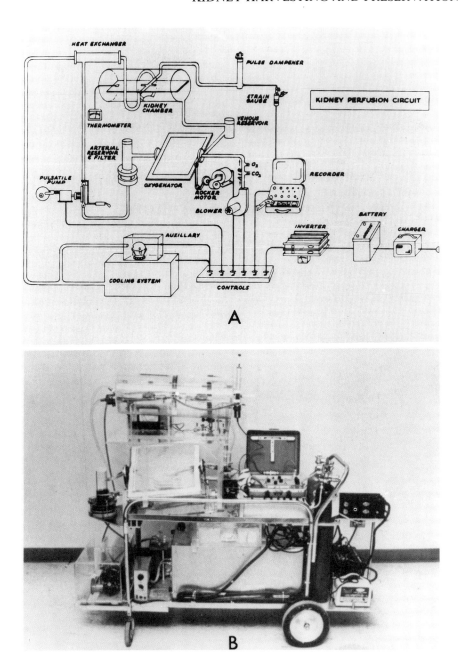

Figure 3–2. Belzer pulsatile perfusion machine: (*A*) Schematic view. (*B*) complete exterior view. From Belzer, FO, et al: Isolated perfusion of organs. In Norman, JC (ed): *Organ Perfusion and Preservation.* Appleton Century Crofts, New York, 1968, p 9.

Perfusion Parameters

Few studies have analyzed the effects of specific parameters on kidney perfusion (Table 3–5). In our laboratories we[39] have determined that kidneys perfused at a neutral pH of 7.4 did better than renal allografts perfused at acidic or alkaline pH. This has also been confirmed in our clinical experience. No prospective or randomized studies have indicated the best level of osmolarity for perfusion. However, we have observed that hyperosmolarity appears to offer some protection. No clear attempts have been made to define the role of electrolytes during perfusion. Empirically, an extracellular concentration of electrolytes has been used. Of the various drugs that

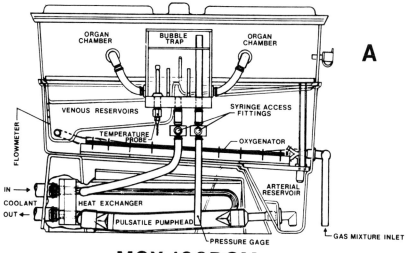

MOX-100DCM

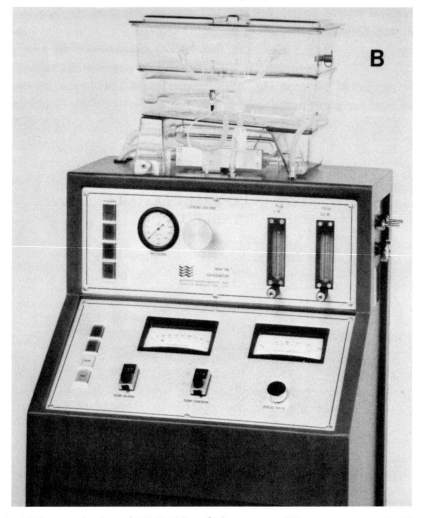

Figure 3–3. (*A*) Schematic view of MOX-100 perfusion cassette (Waters Instruments). (*B*) MOX-100 perfusion machine with organ cassette in place.

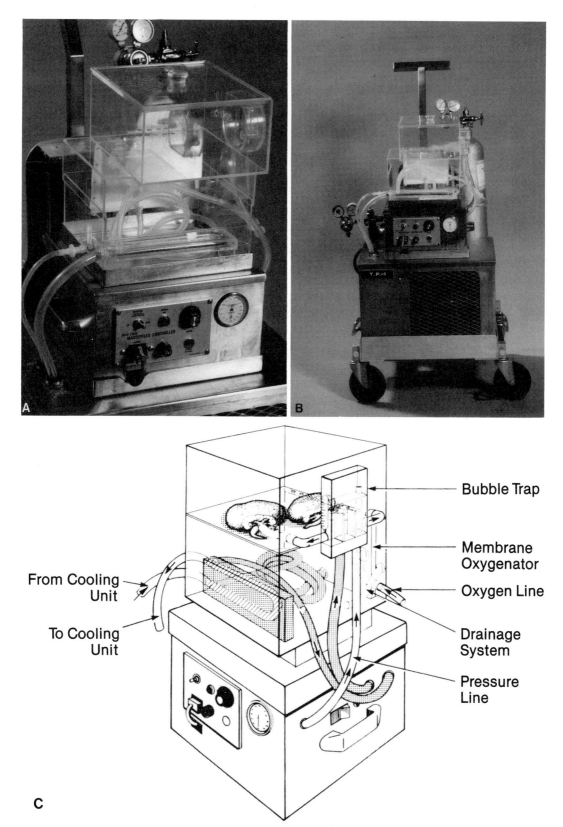

Figure 3–4. Prototype of T.P.-1, a nonpulsatile perfusion unit. (*A*) Close-up view of organ cassette. (*B*) Schematic view of T.P.-1 unit. (*C*) Schematic view of T.P.-1 organ cassette and cooling unit.

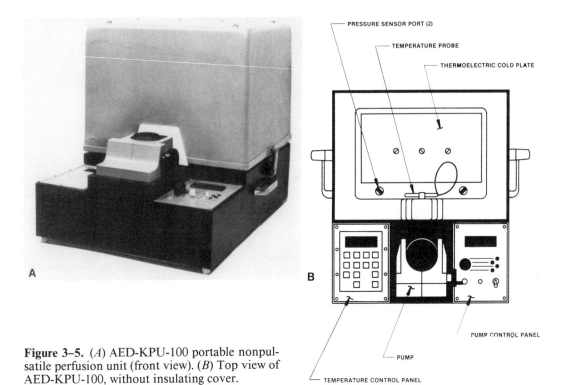

Figure 3–5. (*A*) AED-KPU-100 portable nonpulsatile perfusion unit (front view). (*B*) Top view of AED-KPU-100, without insulating cover.

Table 3–4 Composition of Clinical Perfusates				
Cryoprecipitated Plasma (1 L)			**Albumin (250 ml)**	
Cryoprecipitated plasma	1 L		25% Albumin	250 ml
K^+	4.0 mEq		$MgSO_4$	8 mEq
Na^+	137 mEq		Regular insulin	100 U
Cl^-	103 mEq		Penicillin G	5000 U
$MgSO_4$	8 mEq		PSP dye	4 ml
Mannitol	5 gm		Dextrose 5%	7 g
Regular insulin	80 U		NaCl (0.9%)	115 mEq
Penicillin G	250,000 U		KCL	5.4 mEq
PSP dye	2 ml		$NaHCO_3$	13.8 mEq
Solu-medrol	1 gm		Sterile water	56.2 ml
			Solu-medrol	250 g
Plasma Protein Fraction (PPF) (500 ml)			**Silica Gel Fraction (SGF) (900 ml)**	
Plasma protein fraction	500 ml		Silica gel fraction	900 ml
$MgSO_4$	4 mEq		K^+	4 mEq/L
Regular insulin	40 U		Na^+	145 mEq/L
Penicillin G	250,000 U		Protein	65 g/L
PSP dye	2 ml			
Solu-medrol	250 mg			
NaCl	25 mEq			
KCL	4 mEq			
$NaHCO_3$ (pH to 7.4)	8 ml			

Table 3–5 Guidelines for Optimizing Renal Perfusion

pH	Neutral pH (7.4) better than acidic or alkaline pH
Osmolarity	No prospective or randomized studies; hyperosmolar may be beneficial depending on conditions of donor maintenance and harvesting
Electrolytes	Empirically extracellular concentrations used with acceptable results
Temperature	4–7°C standard for clinical preservation; cyropreservation to as low as −196°C has been used experimentally
Length of warm ischemia	No specific guidelines established. In clinical experience up to 20 minutes may be tolerated depending on other conditions. Higher incidence of ATN with >20 min warm ischemia

have been added to perfusates, methylprednisolone appears to play an important role. Other drugs, such as oxygen-free radical scavengers (allopurinol, superoxide dismutase, and catalase), have been recently investigated in experimental applications and will be discussed later.

Although no specific guidelines have been established as to the length of warm ischemia tolerated by renal grafts, clinical experience has shown that up to 20 min may be acceptable if other conditions are ideal. This is dependent on other factors such as harvesting technique. When warm ischemia exceeds 20 min, a higher incidence of acute posttransplant renal failure or acute tubular necrosis (ATN) is observed. Periods of warm ischemia >40 min increase the risk of irreversible renal failure.

In general, the major advantage to hypothermic perfusion is that kidneys are preserved under aerobic conditions, so mitochondria are better maintained. During perfusion the clinician or perfusionist is better able to assess function and viability of the kidney in vitro. In clinical practice, hypothermic pulsatile perfusion is reliable up to 72 hours.

PRESERVATION DAMAGE

Organ damage during preservation may result from several factors (Table 3–6). Several studies have shown that oxygen tensions during continuous perfusion may lead to mitochondrial damage and to peroxidation of lipids.[40] Electrolyte transport may also be impaired with elevated oxygen tension,[50] toxicity from oxygen may become a limiting factor in long-term preservation and may be diagnosed by chemi-

Table 3–6 Causes of Impaired Renal Viability During Preservation

Oxygen toxicity
Denaturation of albumin
Bacterial or pyrogen contamination
Perfusion damage
Rapid cooling
Inappropriate pH
Release of lysosomal enzymes
Impaired mitochondrial function
Damage to polysomes
Decreased RNA synthesis
Edema, cellular swelling
Accidental injury; human error (trauma to organ during handling, perfusion of air, etc.)
Warm ischemia
Formation of oxygen-free radicals

luminescence or malondialdehyde determinations. Southard and associates[41] have observed that kidneys may be damaged during long-term preservation by denaturation of albumin in the perfusate. This could be diagnosed by polyacrylamide disk gel electrophoresis of the perfusate during preservation. Coriell[42] has noted that bacterial or pyrogen contamination may be associated with damage to the vascular endothelium in addition to contributing to postoperative morbidity and mortality. Although perfusate culture results are not always available prior to transplantation, bacteria may be detected by other assays such as Lymulus lysate and radioimmunoassay tests.

High perfusion pressures may cause damage to the vascular endothelium during preservation by pulsatile perfusion. Factors contributing to this type of injury may include temperature, osmolarity, perfusion pressure, length of perfusion, and the presence of antibodies in the perfusate.[43] Improper cannulation techniques may also cause renal artery damage. Endothelial damage ranges from minute breaks to complete denudation to expose collagen. The clotting sequence is thereby activated, resulting in platelet and fibrin deposition.

The nature of damage attributed to warm ischemia has been extensively researched. Ischemia has been shown to produce a release of lysosomal enzymes[44] and impairment of mitochondrial function.[45] Polysomes are also affected by warm ischemia and disassociation into ribosomes upon reperfusion.[46] Thus protein synthesis is stopped. The nucleus of the cell is also affected both morphologically and biochemically.[47] A reduction in ribonucleic acid synthesis[48] is observed. Warm ischemia has also been associated with endothelial damage and cellular swelling, leading to redistribution of blood flow in the organ.[49]

It is important to remember that many potential viability problems can be reversed during preservation. The pH and pressure, for example, can be corrected, and the perfusate can be changed. Various agents that have been tested to prevent warm ischemic injury include aprotinin (Trasylol), steroids, inosine, furosemide

and coenzyme Q10.[43] All have been used with some success. Other substances that have been tested are prostaglandins,[28,29] mannitol,[31] calcium channel blockers,[43] propranolol,[26] oxygen-free radical scavengers,[50,51] and chlorpromazine.[52,53] A combination of Mg and ATP has been found to improve the function of canine kidneys after prolonged ischemia.[35] Although there is variation between the histologic and physiologic changes occurring in each individual kidney stored for a given period of time, some generalizations can be made regarding this pathology. These are discussed in the section entitled Risks of Long-Term Preservation.

ASSESSMENT OF VIABILITY

The development of reliable methods for assessing the viability of kidneys prior to transplantation is important to minimize organ wastage, while maximizing kidney function after surgery. Unfortunately, no one method can determine with perfect accuracy whether a given organ will support the life of a patient after transplantation. Many tests, however, appear to be good indicators of subsequent function, and possibly a combination of several could be used to determine a viability index with predictive value.

Several approaches to assessment of kidney graft viability prior to transplantation have been taken (Table 3–7). Noninvasive methods include analysis of perfusion and perfusate characteristics during hypothermic preservation and evaluation of physiological performance during normothermic perfusion. Invasive methods include obtaining biopsy specimens for microscopic examination, tests of cellular integrity, and energy metabolism. The results of these tests may give an indication of an individual organ's future performance. In general, however, alone they are not reliable enough to be used to decide whether a kidney should be transplanted after preservation, since some changes may be reversible upon reperfusion. Possible approaches for determining renal viability prior to transplantation include nuclear magnetic resonance,[43] positron emission tomography,[54] redox imaging,[55] and vascular imaging.[56]

Table 3–7 Renal Viability Assessment

Noninvasive Methods
Perfusion Characteristics
   Vascular resistance
   Blood flow distribution
   Urine output
Perfusate Characteristics
   Metabolite, enzyme, electrolyte profiles
   pH
   Redox potential
Physiologic Performance
   Normothermic in vitro perfusion

Invasive Methods
Cellular Tests (Biopsy)
   Microscopic examination
   Tests of cellular integrity, energy metabolism
      Energy metabolism (assessment of ATP, ADP, and adenine nucleotide levels)
      Membrane permeability (K^+/Na^+ ratios)
      Enzyme activity (ATPase, etc.)
      Membrane transport

New Approaches
Nuclear magnetic resonance
Positron emission tomography
Redox imaging
Vascular imaging

NEW CONCEPTS IN RENAL PRESERVATION

Investigation continues in an effort to extend safe preservation beyond its present limits, especially when warm ischemia is involved. This work has led to an increased understanding of the biochemical and physiologic changes occurring during renal preservation. This has resulted in new methods and techniques for improving viability and achieving longer preservation periods, especially after warm ischemia. Areas of study have included the use of oxygen-free radical scavengers, combining hypothermic storage and perfusion, normothermic perfusion, non-pulsatile perfusion, and cryopreservation.

New Preservation Solutions

Recently several preservation solutions have been developed as alternatives to the standard formulations. Belzer and colleagues[35] have introduced a preservation solution containing gluconate, albumin, and adenosine. In experimental trials they were able to perfuse canine kidneys for 48 hours and subsequently store them for an additional 24 hours with satisfactory function after transplantation. Later reports[57] indicated that the Belzer solution also yielded acceptable results in clinical application (Fig. 3–6). An 80 percent immediate function rate and a 97 percent 1-month graft survival rate were obtained in 87 transplants.

Two additional formulations for preservation solutions have also been recently tested by the same group: Belzer-II solution, which has been tested for perfusion; and UW solution, which has been tested in cold-storage settings. Both of these solutions utilize hydroxyethyl starch as an additional component (Table 3–8). The UW solution also incorporates K^+-lactobionate, raffinose, and allopurinol into formula.[71]

Our institution has recently developed and used hyperosmolar colloid flush preparations (TP series, SGF based)[18] (Table 3–9), as an alternative to the crystalloid solu-

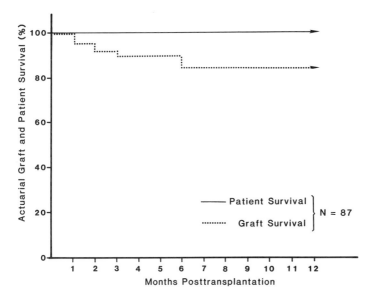

Figure 3–6. Actuarial graft and patient survival of 87 consecutive cadaver transplants perfused with Belzer solution for a mean of 35 hours (range 22–60 hours). Data from Belzer et al: Beneficial effects of adenosine and phosphate in kidney preservation. Transplantation 36:633, 1983.

tions for hypothermic storage, with excellent experimental and clinical results, especially after prolonged warm ischemia. In recent trials[58] the efficacy of TP-II storage has been compared with conventional perfusion methods (Fig. 3–7). Kidney pairs from the same cadaver donor were split; one kidney was flushed with TP-II and stored, while the other kidney was placed on perfusion with plasmanate solution. Only 2 of 10 patients receiving kidneys preserved with TP-II for a mean ($\pm$SD) of 22 hours 44 min ($\pm$ 10 hours) required dialysis within the first week after transplantation. In the group receiving kidneys preserved for a mean ($\pm$SD) of 19 hours 29 min ($\pm$ 2 hours 53 min), 5 of 10 patients were dialyzed in the first week after transplantation. The long-term outcomes of grafts and patients in the TP-II group were also slightly better than those in the perfused group. TP-IV and TP-V have also been used for clinical renal preservation at our center with satisfactory results. The solutions designated TP-VI-X are currently being tested to protect organs from ischemic damage and reperfusion injury.

Oxygen-Free Radical Scavengers and Xanthine Oxidase Inhibition

Recent work has indicated that oxygen-free radicals, generated during ischemia via the xanthine–uric acid pathway, are responsible for damage to various organs during ischemia. Our own work[50] and that of others[51] has indicated that allopurinol, which inhibits xanthine oxidase, and oxygen-free radical scavengers such as superoxide dismutase, and catalase can sometimes protect organ grafts from this type of damage (Fig. 3–8).

Oxygen Persufflation

Gaseous oxygen perfusion or persufflation has been successfully used by several groups to protect stored kidneys, even after ischemic damage.[59] Satisfactory function was obtained after 30 min of warm ischemia and 48 hours of hypothermic storage using oxygen perfused via either the renal artery or the vein.

Cryopreservation

Successful freezing or cryopreservation would provide an attractive means of achieving long-term storage or long-term organ banking prior to transplantation. Although techniques for freezing single cells and tissues have been developed, it has been difficult to obtain consistent results with whole organs such as the kidney.[60,61] Perhaps improvement in freezing techniques will someday provide long-term preservation.

Table 3–8 Belzer Solutions for Preservation

Belzer-1		Belzer-II		UW Solution	
H₂O	850 ml	HES	5 g/dl	K⁺-lactobionate	100 mmol
Sodium gluconate	17.5 g/L	Sodium or potassium gluconate	80 mM	KH₂PO₄	25 mmol
KH₂PO₄	3.4 g/L			MgSO₄	5 mmol
Glucose	1.5 g/L	Potassium phosphate	25 mM	Raffinose	30 mmol
Glutathione	0.9 g/L	Glucose	10 mM	Adenosine	5 mmol
Adenosine	1.3 g/L	Glutathione	3 mM	Glutathione	3 mmol
HEPES	4.7 g/L	Magnesium gluconate	5 mM	Insulin	100 U
NaOH (5M)	10 ml	HEPES	10 mM	Bactrim	0.5 ml
Penicillin	200,000 U	Penicillin	2 × 10⁵U	Dexamethasone	8 mg
Dexamethasone	8 mg	Dexamethasone	12 mg	Allopurinol	1 mM
Phenosulphathelein	12 mg	Phenol red	12 mg	Hydroxyethyl starch	50 g
Insulin	40 U	Insulin	100 U		
Human Serum Albumin	150 ml	Calcium chloride	1.5 mM		
MgSO₄	1 g/2 ml				

Table 3–9 Composition of TP-Preservation Solutions

TP-I

Silica gel fraction base

K^+	80–100 mEq/L
Na^+	140 mEq/L
Cl^-	125 mEq/L
Albumin	4.1 g/dl
Total protein	6.2 g/dl
Glucose	800–1000 mg/L
Osmolarity	~450 mOsm/L

TP-II

Silica gel fraction base

KH_2PO_4	4.05 g/L
K_2HPO_4	3.7 g/L
Dextrose	40 g/L
Osmolarity	~520 mOsm/L

TP-III

Plasma protein fraction base

KH_2PO_4	4.05 g/L
K_2HPO_4	3.7 g/L
Sucrose	40 g/L
Osmolarity	~500 mOsm/L

TP-IV

Silica gel fraction base

KH_2PO_4	4.05 g/L
K_2HPO_4	3.7 g/L
Sucrose	40 g/L
Osmolarity	~430 mOsm/L

TP-V

Silica gel fraction base

Dextrose	20 g/L
Sucrose	50 g/L
ATP	393.4 mg/L
$MgCl_2$	145 mg/L
Osmolarity	~500 mOsm/L

TP-VI

Silica gel fraction base

Sodium gluconate	17.5 g/L
KH_2PO_4	3.4 g/L
Glucose	1.5 g/L
HEPES buffer	4.7 g/L
Dexamethasone	8.0 g/L
Magnesium sulfate	1.0 g/L
Adenosine	1.3 g/L
Glutathione	0.9 g/L

TP-VII

Same as TP-V, plus

Allopurinol	500 mg/L
Catalase	5000 mg/L

TP-VIII

Same as TP-V, plus

Trifluoperazine	8.0 mg/L

TP-IX

Same as TP-V, plus

Allopurinol	500 mg/L
Catalase	5000 mg/L
Trifluoperazine	8 mg/L

TP-X

Same as TP-IX, plus

Diphosphoglycerate

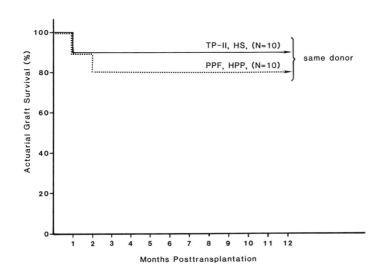

Figure 3–7. Comparative actuarial graft survival for cadaver renal allografts procured from the same donor and preserved with either TP-II (hypothermic storage) or plasmanate (PPF) (hypothermic pulsatile perfusion), respectively. Mean preservation time was 22 hours 44 min ±10 hours (range 13–46 hours) for the TP-II stored kidneys and 19 hours 29 min ±2 hours 53 min (range 16–24 hours) for the PPF perfused kidneys.

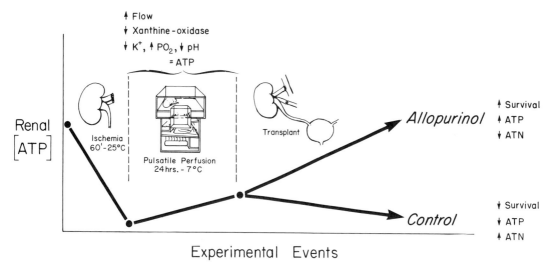

Figure 3–8. In kidneys exposed to 60 min of warm ischemia at 25°C, prior to 24 hours' hypothermic pulsatile perfusion, the addition of allopurinol to the perfusate increased survival and renal adenosine triphosphate (ATP) levels while reducing delayed renal function (ATN) after transplantation.

LONG-TERM PRESERVATION

Considerations for Success

The success of long-term preservation of kidney allografts (hypothermic storage >24 hours and pulsatile perfusion >36 hours) is dependent on many factors. Adequate donor maintenance and proper harvesting techniques may contribute to ultimate renal function. Administration of prostaglandins and oxygen-free radical scavengers may also be beneficial for safely extending preservation times, especially when long-term preservation is coupled with significant periods of warm ischemia.

Mechanisms of Injury

Several mechanisms can affect long-term preservation. Nonviability after prolonged preservation may be due to impairment of energy metabolism during storage or perfusion. This may be caused by a lack of substrates and accumulation of waste products. Studies by Southard and colleagues[62–64] analyzed the effects of 3-day and 5-day perfusion on the in vitro metabolism of canine kidneys (Table 3–10). It was found that tissue goes through several identifiable changes during this period. There is a loss of adenosine nucleotides, a reduction in respiration and ATP synthesis, and an uncoupling of oxidation and

Table 3–10 Comparison of 3-Day (Viable) and 5-Day (Nonviable) Hypothermic Pulsatile Perfusion*	
Effects on Metabolism and Cell Function	
No Differences	*Significant Differences*
Average respiration rate	Cell volume regulation
Mitochondrial function	Na^+/K^+ pump function
Cell saccharide permeability	Lysosomal enzyme release
Phospholipid loss	
*Kidney tissue slices in vitro evaluation. From Southard et al.[63]	

Table 3–11 Reversible Pathologic Changes During Long-Term Preservation*

Hypothermic Storage (>24 hr preservation)
Edema caused by entrance of water into the basement membrane
Widening of endothelial fenestrations along foot processes
No mechanical endothelial damage

Hypothermic Pulsatile Perfusion (>36 hr preservation)
Mechanical endothelial cell damage
Endothelial cells degenerated
Subendothelial glomerular basement membrane damage

*<5 min warm ischemia.

---

phosphorylation in mitochondria. After 5 days' perfusion, significant differences were observed in cell volume regulation, sodium/potassium pump function, and lysosomal enzyme release. Buhl and colleagues[65] have studied the changes in perfused rabbit kidneys. They observed a progressive fall of adenosine nucleotide content in anaerobically perfused kidneys and a complete regeneration of these nucleotides during 1 hour of perfusion with oxygen. Methods to ameliorate respiratory injury during long-term preservation have included the addition of adenosine,[35] ATP,[18] and oxygen perfusion.[59]

Pathological Changes During Long-Term Preservation

Table 3–11 shows the reversible pathologic changes that occur during long-term preservation of kidneys exposed to <5 minutes of warm ischemia. As the length of preservation increases, clinical and physiologic manifestations of injury may be identified (Table 3–12). Early degenerative changes during the first 12 hours involve the renal tubules. This is followed by changes in the glomerular epithelial cells and swelling and blunting of the foot processes between 12 and 24 hours. The physiologic evidence of these changes is seen as minor graft dysfunction or as unrecognized reversible perfusion abnormalities. As the preservation time increases to 24 to 48 hours, disruption of the organelles in the epithelial cells occurs. This may be associated with an ATN or near-ATN condition. When preservation time exceeds 48 hours, cell damage results in cellular necrosis and ATN.

The spectrum of mechanical endothelial injury occurring in perfused kidneys was detailed earlier under Hypothermic Pulsatile Perfusion. There is a close association

---

Table 3–12 Pathologic Changes During Preservation and Their Clinical and Physiologic Manifestations

Preservation Time	Clinical or Physiologic Manifestations	Pathologic Outcome
<12 hr	No clinical representation, unknown changes	Early degenerative changes or tubules. Progression of tubular damage
12–24 hr	Minor graft dysfunction, Na^+ tubular reabsorption ↓, free water clearance ↓, GFR ↓, unrecognized reversible renal perfusion abnormalities	Glomerular epithelial cells with degenerative changes and swelling, blunting of foot processes. Elevation or detachment of endothelial cells from glomerular basement membrane.
24–48 hr	ATN or nearly ATN	Disruption of epithelial and endothelial cell organelles.
>48 hr	ATN	Cell necrosis.

Table 3–13 Risks of Long-Term Preservation

Physiologic	↑ pressure, ↓ flow, ↑ renal vascular resistance
Biochemical	Functional parameters; ↓ creatinine clearance
	Enzymes: LDH, etc. ↓
	Glomerular filtration rate ↓
Pathologic	Vascular endothelium damage, thrombosis of small vessels, tubular injury (necrosis)
Immunologic	Rejection, hyperacute or acute
Clinical	Renal dysfunction (ATN); cyclosporine modulation
Overall	Comprehensive assessment of all of above parameters with final determination regarding function (nephrectomy)

between the length of preservation and perfusion-related injuries. Scanning microscopic studies of perfused kidneys have identified capillary and arterial endothelial damage in perfused human kidneys.[66] In addition to tubular necrosis and fused glomerular visceral epithelial foot processes, changes in the glomerular and endothelial surfaces were noted.

Risks of Long-Term Preservation

The most obvious risk of long-term preservation is the possibility of compromising the function of an otherwise viable, transplantable organ. Sometimes logistics require use of long-term preservation. However, when the surgeon is able to choose the time of the transplant, loss of viability should be avoided if possible, especially when the recipient is highly sensitized (high cytotoxic antibody levels) and has been awaiting transplant for a long time or when the patient is considered to be at high risk or top medical priority and should be urgently transplanted.

There are multiple risks of long-term preservation (Table 3–13) as evidenced by physiologic, biochemical, pathologic, immunologic, and clinical changes. Identifiable physiologic and biochemical changes include an increase in renal pressure, a decrease in flow and an increase in renal vascular resistance. There are also significant elevations in serum creatinine and a reduction in creatinine clearance as well as the glomerular filtration rate. The pathologic risks during long-term preservation include changes in the vascular endothelium, thrombosis of small vessels, and tubular injury leading to tubular necrosis. Whether cellular damage during long-term preservation may increase the immunologic risk of rejection is controversial, since some studies have reported prolongation of graft survival after perfusion.[67]

Many factors determine whether extension of preservation alone increases the incidence of acute tubular necrosis (ATN). There is generally more ATN in stored kidneys than in kidneys perfused for the same period of time (Table 3–14). In studies by Spees and associates[68] there was significantly more ATN in stored kidneys preserved a mean of 19.7 hours than in kidneys perfused for a mean of 26.5 hours. However, there was no significant differ-

Table 3–14 Relationship Between Incidence of ATN and Preservation Time (Mount Carmel Experience)

Preservation Time	Incidence of ATN/ATN Recovery	
	Perfused Kidneys (n = 178)	*Stored Kidneys (n = 47)*
0–12 hr	40%/100%	0%/—
12–24 hr	29%/78%	16%/100%
24–36 hr	36%/76%	78%/80%
36–48 hr	53%/70%	37%/92%
>48 hr	55%/60%	—/—

		Table 3–15 Incidence of ATN in Precyclosporine and Cyclosporine Eras		
Group	**N**	**Mean Preservation Time (hr)**	**Incidence of ATN (%)**	
All HS	236	24.0	52.2	
All HPP	275	25.7	43.6	
Pre-CyA era—HS	100	25.5	62.0	
Pre-CyA era—HPP	106	25.2	56.5	
CyA era—HS	136	22.3	44.9	
CyA era—HPP	169	26.1	35.5	

HS = hypothermic storage.
HPP = hypothermic pulsatile perfusion.

ence in 1-year graft survival between the two groups. At our center and in other studies when kidneys were preserved for more protracted periods, the incidence of ATN was shown to increase in kidneys stored for >24 hours and in those perfused >36 hours (Table 3–11). However, the recovery from ATN was not significantly different between short- and long-term storage.

It is often difficult, in retrospective clinical studies, to separate the effects of long-term preservation from the other factors that may ultimately contribute to graft function. Some long-preserved kidneys are obviously eliminated from eligibility based on the subjective criteria of the transplant center; thus, their function is never evaluated in vivo. Although it was once felt that long-term preservation increased the incidence of ATN, in recent years clinical data from many centers indicate that the rate of ATN does not necessarily increase as the period of preservation is lengthened. A more accurate comparison is to assess the function at 30 days and thereafter to determine the rate of recovery from ATN.

The recent use of cyclosporine for immunosuppression has added caution to the use of long-term renal preservation procedures. Since this drug may be nephrotoxic,[69] the clinician may have difficulty in determining the contribution of cyclosporine nephrotoxicity to impaired renal function when ATN is also present. This is avoided by reduction or elimination of the cyclosporine dosage in the immediate transplant period. When we compared the incidence of ATN in the precyclosporine and cyclo-

sporine eras,[40] we found no significant difference in the incidence of ATN or the ATN recovery rate when a conservative approach to cyclosporine administration is used (Table 3–15).

SUMMARY

Continuing work in renal preservation has been successful in extending the limits of preservation by both storage and perfusion. Although some new concepts are not readily applied to clinical practice, better methods for safely extending preservation times are being developed. This is a result of gaining a better understanding of the physiologic and biochemical changes that occur during preservation. Therefore prospects for reducing the incidence of ATN and improving renal function in the immediate posttransplant period are good, even in kidneys preserved for long periods.

REFERENCES

1. Legallois, CJ: Experiences sur le Principle de la Vie, Notament sur Celui Mouvements du coeur et sur le Siege de se Principe: Suivies du Rapport Fait à la Premier Classe de L'Institut sur Celles Relatives aux mouvements du Coeur. D'Hautel, Paris, 1812.
2. von Cyon, E: Die physiologischem Hertzgifte. IV Thiel. Alte and Neue Methoden zum Studium der isolirten intraund extracardialen Nervencentra. Pfleugers Arch Ges Physiol 77:215, 1899.

3. Ringer, S: Concerning the influence exerted by each of the constituents of blood on the contraction of the ventricle. J Physiol (Lond) 3:380, 1881.
4. Langendorff, O: Untersuchungen am uberlebendun Saugthierherzen. Pfleugers Arch Ges Physiol 61:291, 1895.
5. Toledo-Pereyra, LH: A study of the historical origins of cardioplegia. Thesis, University of Minnesota, April 1984.
6. Humphries, AH and Dennis, AJ: Historical developments in preservation. In Toledo-Pereyra, LH (ed): Basic Concepts of Organ Procurement, Perfusion, and Preservation for Transplantation. Academic Press, New York, 1982, p 1.
7. Carrel, A and Lindbergh, CA: The culture of whole organs. Science 81:621, 1935.
8. Lefebvre, L and Nizet, E: Shunt vasculaire dans les reins de chien perfuses et conserves à basse temperature. Arch Int Pharmacodyn 92:119, 1952.
9. Lapchinsky, AG: Recent results of experimental transplantation of preserved limbs and kidneys, and possible use of this technique in clinical practice. Ann NY Acad Sci 87:539, 1960.
10. Humphries, AL, et al: Successful reimplantation of canine kidneys after 24 hour storage. Surgery 54:136, 1963.
11. Belzer, FO, et al: Twenty-four and 72-hour preservation of canine kidneys. Lancet 2:536, 1967.
12. Collins, GM, Bravo-Shugarman, M, and Terasaki, PE: Kidney preservation for transplantation. Lancet 2:1219, 1969.
13. Johnson, RWG, et al: Evaluation of a new perfusion solution for kidney preservation. Transplantation 13:270, 1972.
14. Toledo-Pereyra, LH and Condie, RM: Comparison of Sack's and a new colloid hyperosmolar solution for hypothermic renal storage. Transplantation 26:166, 1978.
15. Toledo-Pereyra, LH, et al: Long-term kidney preservation with a new plasma perfusate. Proceedings of the Clinical Dialysis and Transplant Forum 3:88, 1973.
16. Toledo-Pereyra, LH, et al: A fibrinogen-free plasma perfusate for preservation of kidneys for 120 hours. Surg Gynecol Obstet 138:901, 1974.
17. Toledo-Pereyra, LH, et al: Improvement of silica gel fraction for hypothermic pulsatile perfusion: New trends in cadaver kidney preservation. Minn Med 60:243, 1977.
18. Toledo-Pereyra, LH: A new generation of colloid solutions for preservation. Dialysis and Transplantation 14:143, 1985.
19. Van der Wijk, J, et al: Successful 96- and 144-hour experimental kidney preservation: A combination of standard machine preservation and newly developed normothermic ex vivo perfusion. Cryobiology 17:473, 1980.
20. Rijkmans, BG, Burrman, WS, and Kootstra, G: Six-day canine kidney preservation: Hypothermic perfusion combined with isolated blood perfusion. Surg Res 18:99, 1975.
21. Stuart, FP: Brain death: Diagnostic criteria and legal status. In Toledo-Pereyra, LH (ed): Basic Concepts of Organ Procurement, Perfusion and Preservation for Transplantation. Academic Press, New York, 1982, 34.
22. Rosenthal, JT, et al: Principles of multiple organ procurement from cadaver donors. Ann Surg 198:617, 1983.
23. Levy, MN: Oxygen consumption and blood flow in the hypothermic perfused kidney. Am J Physiol 197:1111, 1959.
24. Santiago-Delpin, EA: Pharmacological principles during harvesting. In Toledo-Pereyra, LH (ed): Basic Concepts of Organ Procurement, Perfusion, and Preservation for Transplantation. Academic Press, New York, 1982, 73.
25. Chatterjee, SN: Pharmacologic agents of potential value in protecting kidneys from ischemic damage. Transplant Proc 9:1579, 1977.
26. Stowe, N, et al: Protective effect of propanolol in the treatment of ischemically damaged canine kidneys prior to transplantation. Surgery 84:265, 1978.
27. Kazmers, A, et al: Glucagon and canine mesenteric hemodynamics:. Effects on superior mesenteric arteriovenous and nutrient capillary blood flow. J Surg Res 30:372, 1981.
28. Maixner, W, et al: The peripheral hemodynamics of exogenously administered prostaglandin E_1, during major venous occlusion in the dog. J Surg Res 30:563, 1981.
29. Seelig, RF, Kerr, JC, and Hobson, RW: Effects of prostaglandin E_1 injections and infusions on canine femoral hemodynamics. J Surg Res 30:293, 1981.
30. Jacobsen, IQ: Cooling of rabbit kidneys permeated with glycerol to subzero temperatures. Cryobiology 16:24, 1979.
31. Diethelm, AG, et al: Large volume diuresis as a mechanism for immediate maximum renal function after transplantation. Surg Gynecol Obstet 138:869, 1974.
32. McCabe, R, et al: Reduction of acute tubular necrosis (ATN) by furosemide and steroids in cadaveric kidney recovery. Am J Surg 129:246, 1975.
33. Miller, HC and Alexander, JW: Protective effect of methylprednisolone against ischemic injury to the kidney. Transplantation 16:57, 1973.

34. Lytton, B, et al: Improved renal function using adenosine triphosphate-magnesium chloride in preservation of canine kidneys subjected to warm ischemia. Transplantation 31:187, 1981.
35. Belzer, FO, et al: A new perfusate for kidney preservation. Transplantation 33:322, 1982.
36. Haberal, M, et al: Cadaver kidney transplantation with cold ischemia time from 48 to 95 hours. Transplant Proc 16:1330, 1984.
37. Cunarro, JA, et al: Metabolic consequences of low temperature preservation. J Lab Clin Med 88:873, 1976.
38. Toledo-Pereyra, LH: A new machine for organ preservation. Henry Ford Hospital Medical Journal 26:53, 1978.
39. Toledo-Pereyra, LH, MacKenzie, GH, and Frier, DT: The role of pH monitoring during kidney preservation: Experimental and clinical observations. Proceedings of the Clinical Dialysis and Transplant Forum 10:211, 1980.
40. Southard, JH, et al: Toxicity of oxygen to mitochondrial respiratory activity in hypothermically perfused canine kidneys. Transplantation 29:459, 1980.
41. Southard, JH, et al: Denaturation of albumin: A critical factor in long-term kidney preservation. J Surg Res 30:80, 1981.
42. Coriell, LL; Contamination Control, In Karow, AM and Pegg, DE (eds): Organ Preservation for Transplantation, ed 2. Marcel Dekker, New York, 1981, 85.
43. Fahy, GM: Viability concepts in organ preservation for transplantation. In Toledo-Pereyra, LH (ed): Basic Concepts of Organ Procurement, Perfusion, and Preservation for Transplantation. Academic Press, New York, 1982, 121.
44. Horpacsy, G, et al: Lysosomal and ATP changes after renal-stalk clamping in rats. Circ Shock 4:55, 1977.
45. Daniel, AM and Beudoin, JG: Evaluation of mitochondrial function in the ischemic rat liver. J Surg Res 17:19, 1974.
46. Morimoto, K and Yanagihara, T: Cerebral ischemia in gerbils: Polyribosomal function during progression and recovery. Stroke 12:105, 1981.
47. Trump, BF, Strum, JM, and Bulger, RE: Studies on the pathogenesis of ischemic cell injury. I. Relations between ion and water shifts and cell ultrastructure in rat kidney slices during swelling at 0–4 degrees. Virchows Arch Abt B Cell Path 16:1, 1974.
48. Lazarus, HM: Isolation of cell nuclei from ischemic renal tissue: Biochemical characteristics of these nuclei. J Surg Res 12:394, 1972.
49. Balint, P and Szocs, E: Intrarenal hemodynamics following temporary occlusion of the renal artery in the dog. Kidney Int (Suppl)6:A128, 1976.
50. Toledo-Pereyra, LH, et al: Clinical effect of allopurinol on preserved kidneys: A randomized double-blind study. Ann Surg 185:128, 1977.
51. Koyama, I, et al: The role of oxygen free radicals in mediating the reperfusion injury of cold-preserved ischemic kidneys. Transplantation 40:590, 1985.
52. Eyal, Z, et al: Successful in vitro preservation of the integrity of the small bowel, including maintenance of mucosal integrity with chlorpromazine, hypothermic, and hyperbaric oxygenation. Surgery 57:259, 1965.
53. Toledo-Pereyra, LH, Simmons, RL, and Najarian, JS: Comparative effects of chlorpromazine, methylprednisolone and allopurinol during small bowel preservation. Am J Surg 126:631, 1973.
54. Sokoloff, L, et al: The (14C) deoxyglucose method for the measurement of local cerebral glucose utilization: Theory, procedure, and normal values in the conscious and anesthetized albino rat. J Neurochem 28:897, 1977.
55. Franke, H, Barlow, CH, and Chance, B: Oxygen delivery in perfused rat kidney: HADH fluoresence and renal functional state. Am J Physiol 231:1087, 1976.
56. Fordham, EW: The complementary role of computerized axial transmission tomography and radionuclide imaging of the brain. Semin Nucl Med 7:137, 1977.
57. Belzer, FO, et al: Combination perfusion-cold storage for optimum cadaver kidney function and utlization. Transplantation 39:118, 1985.
58. Toledo-Pereyra, LH, MacKenzie, GH, and Baughman, RD: Comparative results of prolonged hypothermic storage of canine kidneys preserved with hyperosmolar colloid (TP-II) or crystalloid (Euro-Collins) solution. J Urol 129:166, 1983.
59. Ross, H, and Escott, ML: Renal preservation with gaseous perfusion. Transplantation 33:206, 1982.
60. Guttman, FM, et al: Survival of canine kidneys after treatment with dimethyl-sulfoxide, freezing at −80°C and thawing by microwave illumination. Cryobiology 14:559, 1977.
61. Toledo-Pereyra, LH: Factors involved in successful freezing of kidneys for transplantation. J Surg Res 28:563, 1980.
62. Southard, JH, et al: Effects of hypothermic perfusion of kidneys on tissue and mitochondrial phospholipids. Cryobiology 21:20, 1984.
63. Southard, JH, et al: Comparison of the effect of 3- and 5-day hypothermic perfusion

on metabolism of tissue slices. Cryobiology 21:285, 1984.

64. Pavlock, GS, et al: Lysosomal enzyme release in hypothermically perfused dog kidneys. Cryobiology 21:521, 1984.

65. Buhl, MR, and Jensen, MH: Metabolic inhibition. In Karow, AM and Pegg, DE (eds): Organ Preservation for Transplantation. Marcel Dekker, New York, 1981, 497.

66. Evan, AP, et al: Glomerular endothelial injury related to renal perfusion. Transplantation 35:436, 1983.

67. Payne, WD, et al: Effects of pulsatile perfusion on the immunogenicity of renal allografts. J Surg Res 22:380, 1977.

68. Spees, EF, et al: Preservation methods do not affect cadaver renal allograft outcome. The SEOPF prospective study 1977–1982. Transplant Proc 16:177, 1984.

69. Flechner, SM, et al: The nephrotoxicity of cyclosporine in renal transplant recipients. Transplant Proc (Suppl 1)15:2689, 1983.

70. Mittal, VK, et al: Role of preservation and cyclosporine: An updated study. Transplant Proc 18:572, 1986.

71. Wahlberg, JA, et al: 72-Hour preservation of the canine pancreas. Transplantation 43:5, 1987.

Chapter 4

Pretransplantation Evaluation

RUBEN L. VELEZ
PEDRO VERGNE-MARINI

The pretransplant evaluation of a kidney recipient has evolved with the recent advances in immunosuppressive therapy and the changing dialysis population. In view of this, most transplant programs are changing their criteria for recipient evaluation and acceptance. It is our purpose in this chapter to review the new recipient population and to recommend some guidelines for work-up.

CHANGING DIALYSIS POPULATION

The dialysis patient population has changed over the past 10 years as progress in treatment modalities evolved. Hull and associates[1] have reviewed the trends of the dialysis population in the Dallas area over a 10-year period. As Table 4–1 shows, the percentage of patients over 55 years of age

Table 4–1 Changes in End-Stage Renal Disease (ESRD) Patient Profiles Between 1970 and 1980 in 3-Year Increments, Compared With Those Entering in 1981

	1970–74	1974–77	1977–80	1981
Average age at initiation of dialysis (yr)	40	46.5	47	51.8
Number of patients over 55 yr of age at initiation of dialysis	61 (18%)	143 (35%)	260 (45%)	(54%)
Diabetic (insulin) patients enrolled	20 (5.8%)	74 (18%)	125 (20%)	(25.3%)
Average age of potential transplants (yr)	33	33.5	32.5	38.6
Number of potential transplants	217 (63%)	186 (45%)	181 (35%)	

at initiation of dialysis has had a significant change from 18 percent early in the 1970s to approximately 55 percent in the early 1980s. At the same time the average age of potential transplant recipients has increased from 33 to 39 by the early 1980s. In comparison, during 1985, 48 percent of the patients initiating dialysis in the Dallas area were above 55 years of age, and 31 percent of those initiating dialysis were diabetics. This essentially means that approximately 79 percent of the potential transplant pool was in high-risk categories.

The latter was reflected in the transplant population. Thirty-one patients (19 percent) were above the age of 50, and 25 patients (16 percent) of those transplanted were diabetics. These trends are consistent with the changes noted by the Registry of the European Dialysis and Transplantation Association,[2] which also reflected the increase in age and the number of transplanted diabetic patients. Because of the higher risk and mortality, the work-up in these patients has to be more comprehensive. This will be discussed in later sections.

GENERAL ASSESSMENT

Selection and a thorough evaluation of the recipient are of utmost importance in obtaining a successful outcome and decreasing the complications. A transplant candidate should be suffering from irreversible renal failure; be free of any active infection, malignancy, or active renal disease; and be able to withstand the surgical procedure.

The routine pretransplant evaluation recommended is shown in Table 4–2. Although recently age per se has not been a contraindication for transplantation, the best results have been obtained among patients from 5 to 50 years of age.[3,4] Nevertheless, age as a criterion for acceptance has been relaxed, and specific situations will be discussed later.

In the initial evaluation the patient and family should be fully informed about renal transplantation, the possible medical and surgical complications, the medications, their cost, and the expected follow-up. A complete history and physical exam are the basis of the evaluation, since this is where the majority of the problems and potential complications will be diagnosed and corrected. A special emphasis on blood trans-

Table 4–2 Patient Evaluation

History and physical exam
Past history and family history
Laboratory work
  CBC
  PT, PTT
  Blood type and antibody screening
  Liver functions
  HBsAg
  VDRL
  HTLV$_3$
  HLA
TB skin test
EKG
Recent chest x-ray
Recent pelvic exam with PAP smear
Recent progress notes
VCUG

fusion history is placed on the initial interview in view of the beneficial effects reported by many groups.[5-8] A comprehensive psychosocial evaluation should be completed if warranted in view of the possible stress, and the side effects of the steroids and cyclosporine. This initial laboratory work-up recommended in Table 4–1 should include HLA typing, serum reactivity (PRA) and preformed antibody determination. Urinalysis and urine culture are specifically indicated if there is recent or previous history of urinary tract infections or calculi or if the potential recipient has urine output.

We are becoming more aware of the lethal combination of anti-HTLV III positivity and immunosuppression in transplantation. Donor kidneys from a host with positive anti-HTLV III corroborated by Western Blot or clinical AIDS cause 100 percent mortality within 6 to 12 months. Recipients with serologic findings have similar morbidity and mortality. Consequently, the following should be required:

1. All living related donors must have a negative anti-HTLV III or other satisfactory testing.

2. All cadaver donors have to be HTLV III negative.

3. Both living related and cadaveric recipients must be screened before placement on the active waiting list or completion of living related work-up.

The initial radiologic evaluation should include chest x-rays and a voiding cystourethrogram (VCUG).[27] Use of other radiologic procedures depends on the specific problems or physical findings obtained during the evaluation and will be discussed later. The work-up on women should include recent pelvic exam and Pap smear. For a nonsymptomatic, nondiabetic patient with no previous history of cardiac disease, a full cardiac evaluation is not warranted, and an electrocardiogram in conjunction with the chest x-ray should suffice. Patients with a previous cardiac history may require a complete cardiac evaluation—consultation, stress test, 2D echocardiography—up to and including cardiac catheterization and angiography if needed. Diabetic patients will be discussed separately.

SPECIAL PROBLEMS

Patients Over 50 Years of Age

Age as a criterion for transplantation has changed in response to the changing dialysis population. It is not our purpose in this chapter to discuss the pediatric population, since this information can be found in other publications.[9] On the other hand, more and more older patients are being referred for transplantation and may one day become the majority of our transplant pool. In 1971 Simmons and associates[10] reported on a small group of recipients over the age of 45 who did poorly and had a high mortality. In 1981 Sommer and colleagues[11] reported on a larger group of recipients over the age of 50. The most common cause of graft loss was death, most often secondary to sepsis (69 percent) followed by cardiovascular disease (23 percent). Rejection of the allograft accounted for only 16 percent of grafts lost. The authors made an interesting point, that only 44 percent of the cadaver allograft recipients who died of septic complication had a rejection episode. This suggests that the initial immunosuppression dose may have been too high. Baquero and associates[12] corroborated this point when he found that sepsis accounted for 50 percent of mortality and cardiovascular events for 32 percent. They again noted that 54 percent of the patients who had died as a result of septic complications never had a rejection episode.

It is well established that patients over 50 years old are in the high-risk population. Lee and Terasaki,[13] in their review of the UCLA International Transplant Registry, show a steady decline in patient survival in the older population (>50), with standard immunosuppression (azathioprine and prednisone). The use of cyclosporine A (CsA) when used with prednisone (CsA & P) or in triple therapy (CsA, AZA, & P) has shown a highly significant increase in both patient and graft survival in this group.

With the new immunosuppression combinations transplantation can be performed in this group with relative safety. In order to decrease morbidity and mortality, evaluation of these patients should be comprehensive and individualized. Barium enema

Table 4–3 Evaluation of Patients Over 50 Years of Age

Cardiac evaluation
  Cardiac stress test
  Echocardiogram
  Coronary angiography if abnormal results
Abdominal sonogram to include liver, gall-
  bladder, pancreas
Barium enema

should be included (Table 4–3) in view of the high incidence of diverticulosis and diverticulitis in this group. If significant diverticular disease is encountered, surgical correction prior to transplantation may be indicated.

Gallbladder evaluation is included because of the higher incidence of cholelithiasis. In the general population cholecystectomy for asymptomatic gallstones is a debatable issue, but we strongly recommend cholecystectomy in the high-risk group because of the added mortality of the immunosuppression regimen.

A full cardiovascular evaluation is mandatory. The evaluation should include EKG, a cardiac stress test, a 2D echocardiogram, and cardiac catheterization for symptomatic or asymptomatic patients with positive stress test or previous history. If correctable left main or coronary artery disease (CAD) is diagnosed, surgical intervention is indicated. If diffuse disease is found but the recipient is an adequate surgical risk in view of ventricular function, transplantation can be entertained if the increased risks are clearly explained to the recipient. These patients are more closely monitored by placement of Swan-Ganz catheters and observed postoperatively in ICU for the initial 72 hours. Evaluation of peripheral pulses by physical exam should be included with Doppler studies and arteriography for symptomatic patients.

Diabetic Patients

Diabetic patients are extremely difficult to manage. They represent close to 30 percent of patients entering the ESRD pro-

gram. Earlier studies[14–18] of diabetic patients on chronic hemodialysis showed a high incidence of complications, with rapid progression of cardiovascular disease (cardiac, cerebrovascular, and peripheral-vascular), retinopathy with blindness, and neuropathy. The results of transplantation as compared with those of chronic hemodialysis in this population has made the former the treatment of choice in this high-risk group.[19–21] Furthermore, the multiorgan involvement makes a comprehensive evaluation mandatory. Cardiovascular mortality as a result of CAD has been reported to be as high as 54.5 percent,[22,23] which may be lower than that of diabetic patients on hemodialysis.[17,24] Patient survival rates after transplantation are lower when compared with those of nondiabetics. Cardiovascular mortality is an important cause of graft loss.[25] The previous results in addition to the concern that noninvasive evaluation may not be sensitive enough in diabetics to diagnose asymptomatic CAD[24,26] has led some programs to rely on coronary angiography as the most important standard in determining the risk of diabetics.[22] In fact, Khauli and associates[28] found that selection of patients for transplantation on the basis of coronary angiography had a significant positive effect on patient survival.

In view of the above and as seen in Table 4–4, the cardiac evaluation includes routine history and electrocardiograms, 2D echocardiography for evaluation of heart chambers, valve and left ventricular dysfunction, and cardiac stress test or thallium stress testing.[29,30] Cardiac catheterization is highly recommended for patients over the age of 30 if there is a previous history of cardiac problems, if there is evidence of

Table 4–4 Protocol for Cardiac Evaluation for Diabetic Patients

EKG
Echocardiogram
Noninvasive evaluation
  Cardiac stress test
  Radionuclide ventriculography/stress test
Coronary angiography

coronary disease, or if left ventricular dysfunction is detected by noninvasive techniques. Some groups strongly feel it should be performed on all diabetic candidates over the age of 30.[22]

Diabetic patients have a higher incidence of peripheral vascular disease. Even after a successful transplant, diabetics have a higher incidence of amputation of digits or extremities owing to ischemic changes.[17,20,21] Whether this is due to a combination of diabetic small-vessel disease or major atherosclerotic disease[31,32] is controversial and is not the aim of this chapter. Nevertheless, evaluation of peripheral pulses with noninvasive techniques (Doppler studies) is highly recommended, and if potentially correctable lesions are noted, angiography is recommended.

Predialysis Recipient

An ever-increasing number of patients are referred to transplant programs prior to initiation of dialysis. The results of transplantation are no different than in comparable populations who have had dialysis. This group, however, presents several practical problems in evaluation both from the medical viewpoint and also from insurance entitlement by Medicare, for completion of the work-up and transplantation must occur within the time allotted by Medicare. At our institution a patient is considered a candidate when glomerular filtration rate clearance is less than 15 ml per min, without a reversible component to the renal failure. Otherwise, the patient follows the pretransplant evaluation described in this chapter. Placement of a vascular access before transplantation is strongly recommended although not mandatory. It should also be understood that the pretransplant work-up may have to be repeated if too much time elapses before the onset of clinical uremia and transplantation occurs. Medicare coverage for a predialysis patient may begin the month the individual receives a kidney transplant. The Medicare benefits may also include the pretransplant evaluation as long as it has been done no more than 3 months before the day of the transplant.[33]

Malignancy

Recently diagnosed or metastatic cancer is an absolute contraindication to transplantation.[34] More candidates with history of a previous cancer and a significant "disease-free interval" are being referred for evaluation. Penn[35] reviewed this problem and made the following observations:

1. The longer the disease-free interval, the less the chance of recurrence.

2. Patients with unsuspected asymptomatic renal malignancy show little tendency to recur.

3. The unpredictable nature of malignant melanomas and carcinomas of the breast, which may recur many years after removal of the primary, should always be considered.

In summary, patients with prior malignancy should be considered for transplantation on an individual basis, with full consideration given to the type of malignancy. In general, a disease-free interval of at least 2 years has been set by our institution and others[4] with good results.

Infections

Hemodialysis patients have a higher risk of infection in view of their chronic debilitating disease and the frequent exposure to venipunctures of arterialized blood. It is universally agreed that active infection is a contraindication for transplantation.

Specific criteria for documented infection in pre-transplant recipients are difficult to find. Some general guidelines are offered in Table 4–5. Patients with documented sepsis should be culture-negative and afebrile a minimum of 6 weeks off antibiotics after appropriate therapy has been given. The possible source of the sepsis should be completely evaluated.

Patients with active urinary tract infection (UTI) should be culture-negative and afebrile approximately 4 weeks off antibiotics after appropriate therapy. Patients with frequent UTI should have a full urologic evaluation, some leading to nephrectomies for recurrent or chronic infections, discussed later.

Superficial wound or skin infections usu-

Table 4–5 Infections in Pretransplant Patients

Patients with sepsis should be culture-negative and afebrile off antibiotics for over 6 weeks.

UTI should be culture-negative and afebrile for over 1 month off antibiotics.

Superficial wound/skin infection: afebrile off antibiotics for over 2 weeks.

Pneumonia: after radiologic clearing and afebrile over 4 weeks.

---

ally do not create a significant problem as long as they are treated with appropriate antibiotics. We recommend the clearing of the infection and off antibiotics for 2 weeks. Chronic skin or wound infections with less typical organisms (fungi, for example) require aggressive treatment and individual evaluation.

Patients with previous history of tuberculosis (pulmonary or extrapulmonary) create a special problem and need to be fully evaluated for active disease before transplant. Prophylactic therapy with antituberculosis medication should be continued posttransplant. A special word of caution should be said about potential problems of these drugs, specifically with cyclosporine A.

Patients diagnosed with recent pneumonia should have demonstrable radiologic clearing of the process and be afebrile off antibiotics for 2 to 4 weeks. Special attention should be given to patients with recurrent pneumonias, chronic smokers, and patients with chronic obstructive pulmonary disease, as they will require a more complete evaluation of their respiratory system. Patients with simple upper respiratory infections (URI) usually have minimal complications but should be afebrile for 2 to 4 weeks.

Primary Renal Disease

Renal transplantation has been carried out in many different primary renal diseases with varied success rates.[34,36,37] It is our purpose to concentrate on diseases that

may cause special problems and affect the outcome of the transplant.

Systemic Lupus Erythematosus (SLE)

It is generally accepted that in most cases the manifestation of SLE usually burns out with the development of ESRD.[38] Therefore transplantation has been attempted, even though recurrent lupus nephritis has been reported.[37,39] Renal transplantation is contraindicated in patients with active SLE (nephritis, pericarditis, cerebritis, vasculitis). These patients may also be at higher risk for both venous and arterial thrombosis, in part because of lupus anticoagulants.[40–42] A simple recommended screening test is partial thromboplastin time (PTT). If this test is prolonged, or if there is history of thrombosis such as the access thrombosis, then evaluation to include lupus anticoagulant, anticardiolipin antibody, and perhaps antithrombin III and/or protein C determination should be performed depending on the individual case. This becomes even more important when one considers the association of CsA with thrombosis.[43–45]

Antiglomerular Basement Membrane Disease (ANTI-GBM)

Patients with anti-GMB glomerulonephritis present a special problem. It is generally felt that one should wait for anti-GBM titers to become undetectable before proceeding with transplantation. In order to clear these antibodies, bilateral native nephrectomies and pretransplant and posttransplant plasmapheresis have been recommended, but recurrent disease and graft loss can occur in spite of any of these therapeutic interventions.[46–50] Specific recommendations are therefore difficult, but we wait for at least 6 months until the anti-GMB titer remains negative.

Primary Oxalosis and Fabry's Disease

Primary oxalosis and Fabry's disease have been considered as contraindications for transplantation.[38,51] Recurrence of oxalate deposits with resultant graft loss has been described by many groups.[37,52,53,54] Some programs report successful renal transplantation in these patients if aggressive therapy to minimize the oxalate deposits is strictly adhered to,[55,56] but our experience has not been similar. The same poor results have been obtained in Fabry's disease with progression of the multiorgan involvement.[36,56-58] Furthermore, the available data fail to show that renal allograft can supply the missing enzyme and prevent progression of the disease.

Amyloidosis

Renal failure owing to primary or secondary amyloidosis has been a relative contraindication in the past, but this view has changed in recent years.[51,59] Recent data showing improved results seem to justify transplantation in selected cases, especially with the addition of colchicine to decrease amyloid deposition.[55,59,60]

Polycystic Kidney Disease (PKD)

The need for pretransplant nephrectomy for PKD has decreased; it is no longer absolutely required unless there is massive enlargement causing anatomic problems or evidence of significant bleeding or chronic infection.

Other Metabolic and Inherited Diseases

Other metabolic and inherited diseases associated with renal failure, such as cystinosis, gout, Alport's syndrome, and sickle cell disease, are not contraindications for renal transplantation and have been attempted successfully.[37] In the case of sickle cell disease or trait, there appears to be a higher incidence of painful crises post-transplantation responding well to exchange transfusions with good allograft function.[61-63]

Patients with congenital abnormalities of the lower urinary tract have been successfully transplanted using other surgical strategies such as ileal conduit and are not an absolute contraindication for transplantation. A complete urologic evaluation is required, with possible native nephrectomy if significant reflux or infections are found.[34]

The latter is also true in patients with bilateral reflux alone or with evidence of ectatic or poorly draining ureters with infection. The need of nephrectomy for calculi has been debated. This procedure should be recommended if there is evidence of chronic infection or obstruction. The determination of a neurogenic bladder is not an absolute contraindication for transplantation although it makes the postoperative and long-term care more difficult. Either ileal conduits or self-catheterization are used in the latter cases.[64] Table 4-6 is a summary of urologic recommendations.

Uncontrolled hypertension is rarely seen with present-day medical therapy. The need for nephrectomy has been greatly reduced because of this. Severe hypertension in association with high plasma renin not responsive to treatment has been recommended as a criterion for nephrectomy but not corroborated by other groups.[65] If nephrectomy can be avoided, the risk of severe anemia is reduced, and blood transfusions are not necessary. This reduces the possibility of random sensitization, hepatitis, and possible exposure to AIDS.

Other Glomerulopathies

It is accepted that other forms of glomerulonephritis causing chronic renal failure may recur in the transplanted kidney; these include focal glomerulosclerosis, membranous, membranoproliferative (Types I and II), crescentic, mesangial IgA, hemolytic uremic syndrome, anti-GBM, and Henoch-Schoenlein purpura.[38,66,67] Nevertheless, these do not constitute an absolute contraindication for renal transplantation

---

Table 4-6 Urological Problems

Renal stones: nephrectomy if indicated
Severe reflux with history or evidence of infection: nephrectomy
Mild reflux, no infection: observation
Refractory UTI: full evaluation plus nephrectomy/chronic antibiotic
Evidence of obstruction: evaluation and surgery
"Neurogenic" bladder: full evaluation

unless there is evidence of active disease at the time of surgery. For this reason, an obligatory period of dialysis may be wise in some of these patients.

OTHER SPECIAL PROBLEMS

The criteria for transplantation have been relaxed, and as a consequence more patients are being referred with an increased number of other medical and surgical problems. Our purpose is to mention only the most frequent problems and to provide some guidelines for their evaluation and possible management.

Liver Disease

Liver disease is a common problem, and therefore more patients with abnormal liver function tests or hepatitis B-positive antigens (HBsAg) are being referred for transplantation. The significance of chronic hepatitis in transplantation remains controversial. Available data indicate that immunosuppression (steroids) in chronic viral hepatitis does not improve the course of the disease, but in fact may be harmful.[68,69] Degos and colleagues[70] and Weir and associates[71] reported deterioration of the diseased liver posttransplant in patients with HBsAg-positive disease. Furthermore, accelerated deterioration of liver disease posttransplant was recently reported by Parfrey and associates,[72] prompting them to recommend against transplantation for HBsAg-positive patients. More information is necessary to understand the progression of chronic viral liver disease on the immunosuppressed host. Renal transplantation should not be performed in the face of acute liver disease or recent HBsAg-positive conversion. A liver biopsy is indicated on patients with chronically abnormal liver function tests or on HBsAg-positive patients to evaluate the exact nature of the liver disease and its activity. If the findings are compatible with active or progressive liver disease (chronic active hepatitis), transplantation should not be performed. Reevaluation of patients with persistent liver abnormalities or antigen positivity may be undertaken every 4 to 6 months

with serial biopsies and chemistries. Table 4–7 summarizes the work-up.

Gastrointestinal Problems

Active peptic ulcer disease is a relative contraindication for transplantation, and these patients need a complete evaluation. Even though the new histamine antagonists (e.g., cimetidine, ranitidine) make medical therapy effective, elective pyloroplasty and vagotomy or superselective vagotomy may be preferred in view of the higher incidence of bleeding posttransplantation and the higher mortality of the latter when associated with immunosuppression.[73–75]

Patients with a previous history of peptic ulcer disease are evaluated with appropriate x-rays and endoscopy.[34] Occasionally gastric analysis with both basal and postgastrin stimulation may be helpful in determining whether surgery is indicated.

The widespread use of phosphate binders in dialysis patients appears to make them more prone to develop diverticular disease, especially in the older population. Older individuals (>50 years of age) and those with previous clinical or radiologic evidence of diverticular disease should be evaluated. Partial colectomy pretransplant may occasionally be necessary for severe involvement or previous history of perforation.

Asymptomatic cholelithiasis is also controversial,[76–78] but even more so when dealing with immunosuppressed patients, since the available literature of when to do cholecystectomy relates mostly to nonimmunosuppressed patients. Our personal experience and that of others has been fraught with catastrophic cases when the latter was

Table 4–7 Liver Problems
Abnormal liver functions for ≥ 6 months
Positive HBsAg
Work-up
Liver spleen scan
Sonogram
Liver biopsy
Antiviral titers
Serologies

not performed. Elective cholecystectomy for patients with documented cholelithiasis or gallbladder disease may be indicated even more in the high-risk population (those >50 years of age and those with diabetes). The frequent use of cyclosporine, which may be associated with cholelithiasis, hepatotoxicity, and cholestasis,[79,80] in this specific patient pool seems to make a logical argument for the recommendations.

Seizure Disorders

One of the reported complications of cyclosporine has been seizures,[79,81-84] seen in approximately 3 percent of our recipients. Whether this is related to one or a combination of factors like direct CsA neurotoxicity, vascular damage, and possible ischemic lesions, hypomagnesemia, hypocalcemia and hypertension has not been well studied. Be that as it may, transplant recipients with previous history of grand mal seizures or dialysis-induced seizures should undergo a complete neurologic evaluation including CT scan and EEG. If an epileptiform focus is identified, the use of anticonvulsant medication is strongly recommended if the patient is not under therapy. Furthermore, care should be taken to maintain CsA levels below the toxic range, to have tight control of hypertension, and to avoid hypomagnesemia.[84]

Metabolic Bone Disease

Secondary hyperparathyroidism is seen in all hemodialysis patients to a lesser or greater extent. It should be kept in mind that a small percentage of patients (fewer than 1 percent) will require surgical intervention pretransplant, since severe hypercalcemia (>12) may occur. Although there are no infallible indications, partial parathyroidectomies should be considered in patients with persistent hypercalcemia, evidence of metastatic calcifications, or pathologic fractures.[34]

It is our hope that we have provided some useful guidelines in the pretransplant evaluation of patients with renal insufficiency. The most important thoughts we can give are that each patient should be looked at as an individual and that it is better to correct any problem *before* rather than after immunosuppression.

REFERENCES

1. Hull, AR, et al: Dialysis: A ten year review. Seminars in Nephrology, 2:90, 1982.
2. Kramer, P, et al: Combined Report on Regular Dialysis and Transplantation in Europe. Presented at the XXIst Congress of EDTA, 1984.
3. Chatterjes, SN: Selection and Preparation of Recipients for Renal Transplantation. In Chatterjes, SN: Manual of Renal Transplantation. Springer Verlag, 1979, p 35–39.
4. Strom, TB, Tilney, NL, and Merill, JP: Renal transplantation: Clinical management of the transplant recipient, Chapter 51, The Kidney. p 2618.
5. Norman, DJ, Barry, JM, and Fischer, S: The beneficial effect of pre-transplant third party blood transfusion on allograft rejection in HLA identical siblings' kidney transplants. Transplantation 41:125, 1986.
6. Terasaki, PI: The beneficial transfusion effect on kidney graft survival attributed to clonal deletion. Transplantation 37:119, 1984.
7. Fine, RN, et al: Renal transplantation update. Ann Intern Med 100:246, 1984.
8. Moorhead, JF, et al: Blood transfusion for renal transplantation: Benefits and risks. Kidney Int (Suppl) (14) S-20-3, 1983.
9. Sheldon, CA, Najarian, JS, and Maver, SM: Pediatric renal transplantation. Surg Clin North Am 65:1589, 1985.
10. Simmons, RL, Kjellstrand, CM, and Buselmejer, TJ: Renal transplantation in high-risk patients. Arch Surg 103:290, 1971.
11. Sommer, BG, et al: Renal transplantation in patients over 50 years of age. Transp Proceed 23:33, 1981.
12. Baquero, A, et al: Cadaver renal transplantation in patients over 50 years of age. Transp Proceed 27:2003, 1985.
13. Lee, PC, and Terasaki, PI: Effect of age on kidney transplantation. Clin Kid Trans Chap. 8, 123, 1985.
14. Shapiro, FL, Leonard, A, and Comty, CM: Mortality, morbidity and rehabilitation results in regularly dialyzed patients with diabetes mellitus. Kid Int (Suppl) 6:S-8-14, 1974.
15. Kassissieh, SD, et al: Hemodialysis-related problems in patients with diabetes mellitus. Kid Int (Suppl 5)6:100, 1974.
16. May, KW, Masler, DS, and Brown, DC:

Hemodialysis in diabetic patients with chronic renal failure. Ann Int Med 83:215, 1975.

17. Mitchell, JC: End stage renal failure in juvenile diabetes mellitus. Mayo Clinical Proceedings 52:281, 1977.
18. Goldstein, DA, and Massry, SG: Diabetic nephropathy: Clinical course and effect of hemodialysis. Nephron 20:286, 1978.
19. Najarian, JS, et al: Kidney transplantation for patients with diabetes mellitus. Transplant Proceedings (Suppl 1)6:121, 1974.
20. Najarian, JS, et al: Ten year experience with renal transplantation in juvenile onset diabetes. Ann Surg 190:487, 1979.
21. Bentley, FR, et al: The status of diabetic renal allograft recipients who survived for ten years after transplantation. Transplantation Proceedings 27:1573, 1985.
22. Weinauch, LA, et al: A symptomatic coronary artery disease: Angiography in diabetic patients before renal transplantation. Ann Inter Med 88:346, 1978.
23. Bennett, WM, et al: Natural history of asymptomatic coronary arteriographic lesions in diabetic patients with end stage renal disease. Am J Med 65:779, 1978.
24. Braun, WE, et al: Coronary arteriography and coronary artery disease in 99 diabetic and nondiabetic patients on chronic hemodialysis or renal transplantation programs. Transplantation Proceedings 13, 128, 1981.
25. Cats, S, and Galton, J: Effect of original disease in kidney transplant outcome. In Terasaki, PI: Clinical Kidney Transplants Nineteen Eighty-Five. UCLA Tissue Typing Laboratory, p. 111, 1985.
26. Weinrauch, L, et al: Asymptomatic coronary artery disease: Angiographic assessment of diabetics evaluated for renal transplantation. Circulation 58:1184, 1978.
27. Weinrauch, LA, et al: Asymptomatic coronary artery disease: Angiography in diabetic patients before renal transplantation. Ann Int Med 88:346, 1978.
28. Khauli, RB, et al: Improved results of cadaver renal transplantation in the diabetic patient. J Urol 130:867, 1983.
29. Morrow, CE, et al: Predictive value of thallium stress testing for coronary and cardiovascular events in uremic diabetic patients before renal transplantation. Am J Surg 146:331, 1983.
30. Mueller-Brand, J, et al: Role of radionuclide ventriculography in management of kidney transplant candidates. J Med 27:579, 1986.
31. Logerfo, FW, and Coffman, JD: Vascular and microvascular disease of the foot in diabetes: Implications for foot care. N Engl J Med 311:165, 1984.
32. Blumenthal, HT: More on microvascular

disease of the foot in diabetes. N Engl J Med 313:696, 1985.
33. Special Provisions Relating to Coverage Under Medicare Program for End Stage Renal Disease. Sec. 226A (16,302) Medicare and Medicade Guide, Commerce Clearing House, Inc. 1986.
34. Briggs, JD: The recipient of a renal transplant. In Morris, PJ: Kidney Transplantation. Chapter 4, 1984.
35. Penn, I: Renal transplantation in patients with pre-existing malignancies. Transplant Proc 25:1079, 1983.
36. Kjellstrand, CM, et al: Recipient selection, medical management, and dialysis. Transplantation Chap. 12, 418, 1972.
37. Wilson, RE: Transplantation in patients with unusual causes of renal failure. Clin Neph 5:51, 1976.
38. Strom, TB, and Tilney, NL: Renal transplantation: Clinical aspects. In Brenner and Recton (eds): The Kidney, ed 3. p 1941, 1986.
39. Amend, WJC, et al: Recurrent systemic lupus erythematosus involving renal allografts. Ann Int Med 94:444, 1981.
40. Much, JR, Herbst, KD, Rapaport, SI: Thrombosis in patients with the lupus anticoagulant. Ann Inter Med 82:156, 1980.
41. Boey, ML, et al: Thrombosis in systemic lupus erythematosus: Striking association with the presence of circulating lupus anticoagulant. Br Med J 287:1021, 1983.
42. Feinstein, DI: Lupus anticoagulant, thrombosis, and fetal loss. N Engl J Med 313:1348, 1985.
43. Vanrenterghem, V, et al: Increased incidence of thromboembolic complications in cyclosporine A treated cadaveric kidney allograft recipients (abstr). Kidney International 28:701, 1985.
44. Neild, G, et al: Glomerular thrombi in renal allografts associated with cyclosporine therapy (abstr). Kidney International 27:345, 1985.
45. Cohen, DJ, et al: Cyclosporine: A new immunosuppressive agent for organ transplantation. Ann Int Med 101:667, 1984.
46. Wilson, CB, and Dixon, FJ: Antiglomerular basement membrane antibody-induced glomerulonephritis. Kidney International 3:74, 1973.
47. McPhaul, JJ, Jr, et al: Evidence suggesting persistence of nephritogenic immunopathologic mechanisms in patients receiving renal allografts. J Clin Invest 52:1059, 1973.
48. Beleil, OM, et al: Recurrent glomerulonephritis due to antiglomerular basement membrane antibodies in two successive allografts. Clin Nephrol 1:377, 1973.
49. Couser, WG, et al: Successful renal trans-

plantation in patients with circulating antibody to glomerular basement membrane: Report of two cases. Clin Nephrol 1:381, 1973.

50. Cove-Smith, JR, et al: Transplantation immunosuppression and plasmapheresis in Goodpasture's syndrome. Clin Nephrol 9:126, 1978.

51. Crosnier, J: Indications for kidney transplantation preparation treatment and supervisions of the patient. In Hamburger, J, Crosmier, J, et al: Renal Transplantation Theory & Practice. Williams & Wilkins, Baltimore, 1981, p 146.

52. Klavwers, J, Wolf, PL, and Cohn, R: Failure of renal transplantation in primary oxalosis. JAMA 209:551, 1969.

53. Saxon, A, et al: Renal transplantation on primary hyperoxaluria. Arch Int Med 133:464, 1974.

54. Toussaint, C, Goffin, Y, Potvliege, P: Kidney transplantation primary oxalosis. Clin Nephrol 5:239, 1976.

55. Whelchel, JD, et al: Successful renal transplantation in hyperoxaluria. Transplantation 35:161, 1983.

56. Groth, CG and Ringden, O: Transplantation in relation to the treatment of inherited disease. Transplantation 38:319, 1984.

57. Spence, MW, et al: Failure to correct the metabolic defect by renal allotransplantation in Fabry's disease. Ann Intern Med 84:13, 1976.

58. Maziel, SE, et al: Ten-year experience in renal transplantation for Fabry's disease. Transplant Proc 13:57, 1981.

59. Jacob, ET, et al: Renal transplantation in the amyloidosis of familial mediterranean fever. Arch Int Med 139:1135, 1979.

60. Zemer, D, et al: Colchicine in the prevention and treatment of the amyloidosis of familial mediterranean fever. N Engl J Med 314:1001, 1986.

61. Spector, D, et al: Painful crises following renal transplantation in sickle cell anemia. Am J Med 64:835, 1978.

62. Chatterjee, SN: National study on natural history of renal allografts in sickle cell disease trait. Nephron 25:199, 1980.

63. Gonzalez-Carrillo, M, et al: Renal transplantation in sickle cell disease. Clin Nephro 18:209, 1982.

64. Flechner, SM, et al: Intermittent clean catheterization: An alternative to division in continent transplant-recipients with lower urinary tract dysfunction. J Urol 130:875, 1983.

65. Craswell, PW, Hird, PA, Baillod, RA, Varghese, Z, Moorhead, JF: British Medical Journal 4, 749, 1972.

66. Glassock, RJ, et al: Human renal isografts: A clinical and pathologic analysis. Medicine 47:411, 1968.

67. Cameron, JS: Glomerulonephritis in renal transplants. Transplantation 34:237, 1982.

68. Gregory, PB, et al: Steroid therapy in severe viral hepatitis. N Engl J Med 294:681, 1976.

69. Lam, KC, et al: Deleterious effect of prednisolone in HBsAg positive chronic active hepatitis. N Engl J Med 304:380, 1981.

70. Degos, F, et al: Is renal transplantation involved in post-transplantation liver disease? Transplantation 29:100, 1980.

71. Weir, MR, Kirkman, RL, and Strom, TB: The long term effects of hepatitis B virus on renal transplant recipients: Analysis of morbidity and mortality. Transp Proceed 27:163, 1985.

72. Parfrey, PS, et al: The impact of renal transplantation on the course of hepatitis B liver disease. Transplantation 39:610, 1985.

73. Spanas, PK, et al: Peptic ulcer disease in the transplant recipient. Arch Surg 109:193, 1974.

74. Hadjiyannakis, EJ, et al: Gastrointestinal complications after renal transplantation. Lancet 2:781, 1971.

75. Sarosdy, MF, et al: Upper gastrointestinal bleeding following renal transplantation. Urology, 26:347, 1985.

76. Gracie, WA, and Ransohoff, DF: The natural history of silent gallstones. N Engl J Med 307:798, 1982.

77. Weiss, KM, and Hanis, CL: All "silent" gallstones are not silent. N Engl J Med 310:657, 1984.

78. McSherry, CK, et al: The natural history of diagnosed gallstone disease in symptomatic and asymptomatic patients. Ann Surg 202:59, 1985.

79. Laupacis, A: Complications of cyclosporine therapy: A comparison to azathioprine. Cyclosporine 532, 1984.

80. Schade, RR, et al: Cholestasis in heart transplant recipients treated with cyclosporine. Cyclosporine 541, 1984.

81. Durrant, S, et al: Cyclosporine A, methylprednisolone and convulsions. Lancet 2:829, 1982.

82. Joss, DV, et al: Hypertension and convulsions in children receiving cyclosporine A. Lancet 1:909, 1982.

83. Powell-Jackson, PR, et al: Adult respiratory distress syndrome and convulsions associated with administration of cyclosporine in liver transplant recipients. Transplantation 38:341, 1984.

84. Thompson, CB, et al: Association between cyclosporine neurotoxicity and hypomagnesemia. Lancet 2:1116, 1984.

TRANSPLANTATION PROCEDURES AND CLINICAL MANAGEMENT

Chapter 5

Anesthesia

CLARA L. LINKE

The patient with end-stage renal disease (ESRD) presents a significant challenge to anesthesiologists. Although dialysis has greatly improved the preoperative medical status of the ESRD patient, it is not a stable state. Numerous factors contribute to the instability. Intravascular volume can fluctuate widely, as anesthesia affects peripheral vascular resistance, especially in the presence of preoperative hypertension. Persistent anemia limits the oxygen-carrying capacity. Acidosis and hyperkalemia potentiate drug effects and increase cardiotoxic effects of some anesthetics. Today's halogenated inhalational anesthetics have a propensity for nephrotoxicity or hepatotoxicity. Most neuromuscular blocking drugs depend on renal excretion, and many are difficult to reverse at the close of anesthesia. Diabetes and severe coronary artery disease are more commonly encountered today as older and higher-risk patients with multisystem disease are accepted for transplantation.

HISTORY

The anesthetic management of the patient for renal transplantation has varied frequently since the first renal transplantation in 1954. Changing surgical approaches, advances in dialysis, and the introduction of new anesthetic agents all require ongoing re-evaluations of anesthetic techniques employed.

The first renal transplantation (extraperitoneally in the iliac fossa) was performed with minimal preoperative dialysis. Anesthesia for this operation was via continuous spinal.[1] Historically, spinal anesthesia had been the technique of choice for renal failure patients. It required such a small dose of local anesthetic agent that no systemic pharmacologic effects were caused. Spinal anesthesia also controlled the hypervolemic hypertension intraoperatively by decreasing the peripheral vascular resistance through sympathetic blockade. Regional anesthesia also avoided tracheal intubation, which opened the lower respiratory tract to new organisms in these uremic patients with poor defense mechanisms.

In succeeding years, it was deemed desirable to remove the native kidneys at the time of renal transplantation. Operations of such intraperitoneal magnitude carried excessive risks for renal transplant patients. They required excellent relaxation; significant extracellular fluid shifts took place; blood loss was often excessive; and postoperative pulmonary complications were frequent. Because such procedures were difficult to manage with regional anesthesia, many anesthesiologists turned to general anesthesia.

At this time new nonexplosive halogenated inhalational anesthetics such as methoxyflurane and halothane were introduced and were soon found to be more chemically active than their predecessors. These new inhalational agents are biotransformed to varying degrees of metabolism in the kidneys and liver. Methoxyflurane undergoes substantial metabolism to break down in the acid environment of the kidney to oxalic acid and fluoride. The fluoride induces the nephrotoxicity characterized by the inability to concentrate urine, manifested by a high-output renal failure. Enflurane, a more recent agent, is also metabolized to fluoride, though much less than methoxyflurane. Its use is controversial for a patient with known renal disease.[2] Halothane, although not nephrotoxic, can be hepatotoxic for some patients after multiple exposures. Nitrous oxide, while not biotransformed, does limit the oxygen-carrying capacity, which is already impaired by the persistent anemia in ESRD.

The halogenated anesthetics readily cause hypotension, as they are devoid of sympathetic stimulation. Furthermore, they are known to be direct myocardial depressants; thus, deep anesthesia must be avoided, which sacrifices good muscular relaxation. The subsequent increased use of neuromuscular blocking agents was followed by reports of prolonged paresis in patients with renal failure.

To avoid toxicity and the inability to reverse muscle relaxants, some anesthesiologists returned to regional anesthesia. This became especially applicable when the renal transplant operation was limited to an extraperitoneal iliac fossa surgical exposure. Single-dose spinal anesthesia provided excellent relaxation, and exposure was further enhanced by the constriction of the small bowel during sympathetic blockade.

However, nephrologists were also making great strides in improving fluid removal via ultrafiltration (hemofiltration). With patients less hypervolemic preoperatively, sudden and excessive hypotension occurred with the onset of spinal anesthesia. Continuous epidural anesthesia was then undertaken at some centers. Here small intermittent doses of an anesthetic agent could be given to avoid sudden hypotension, and the anesthetic block could also be prolonged through repeated doses if necessary. However, epidural techniques required much larger drug doses.

Local anesthetic agents have a shorter duration of action in ESRD patients. The ESRD hyperdynamic circulatory state secondary to anemia causes increased cardiac output and increased blood flow through the tissues, resulting in more rapid venous removal of the drug from the site of injection. While the catheter techniques permit repeated intermittent drug administration, there are risks presented by the greater total amount of drug necessary for "continuous" epidural blocks.

Lidocaine with epinephrine for epidural block has been reported to cause pulmonary edema in an ESRD patient with significant cardiac disease. The moderate increase in heart rate was sufficient to decompensate the cardiac patient with marginal reserve.[3]

Bupivacaine does not require epinephrine, since it is not as vasoactive as lidocaine. However, a high epidural concentration of 0.75 percent is necessary to provide good muscle relaxation. This can readily cause toxic effects if inadvertent rapid intravenous absorption occurs. In recent years studies have suggested that hyperkalemia enhances the cardiotoxic effects of both lidocaine and bupivacaine, but especially bupivacaine. Myocardial depression with bradycardia and hypotension preceded the cardiac arrests reported with bupivacaine.[4]

RECIPIENT ASSESSMENT

All patients with ESRD manifest similar symptoms regardless of the cause of uremia. However, there are considerable variations in their physical status when they arrive for renal transplantation.

Fluid Balance

Today most of the clinical signs of ESRD are generally well controlled by dialysis. We rarely see gross volume overload with heart failure, pulmonary edema, or pericarditis. However, hypertension may persist. To assess fluid status, time of the most recent dialysis will indicate the likelihood of a positive or negative extracellular fluid balance. To avoid severe hypotension with the induction of anesthesia, it is advisable to keep the patient somewhat hypervolemic at the last preoperative dialysis. The patient's predialysis and postdialysis weight change will also aid in this assessment.

The type of dialysis is important. Today many patients are on peritoneal dialysis. These patients generally are children or adults who have had problems maintaining patent arteriovenous fistulae and who have few remaining vascular access sites. These patients do not have an arteriovenous fistula to monitor during anesthesia. Patients on hemodialysis require very close monitoring of the AV fistula during anesthesia, as thrombosis frequently occurs in the presence of hypovolemia, hypotension, and the hypercoagulable state stimulated by surgery. Thrombosis of an AV fistula is a major complication, as dialysis may be required if postoperative kidney function is inadequate.

Electrolytes

Electrolyte studies after dialysis are generally predictable, but are required preoperatively to observe undue changes in the interval. Serum potassium is the most important. It should be below 5.5 mEq per liter at the commencement of anesthesia, as it will surely rise during anesthesia and surgery. This rise in serum potassium results from several events: succinylcholine-induced depolarization of the myoneural junction, cellular destruction with surgery, release of high-potassium preservative solution (used for cold kidney preservation) following perfusion of the transplanted kidney, and acidosis caused by ischemia of the leg if the iliac artery is occluded for the arterial anastomosis. Whole blood transfusions, when required in large volumes, also contribute to rapid rise of serum potassium.

Acid-Base Balance

A moderate metabolic acidosis is present despite dialysis. Treatment is seldom required, although sodium overload is a risk if sodium bicarbonate is administered.

Acidosis, however, may effect the pharmacokinetics of anesthetic adjuvant agents. Protein binding is perhaps the most significant factor in determining drug disposition. Because the organic acids bind to plasma proteins as part of a buffering mechanism, less unbound protein is available to bind with drugs as relaxants, narcotics, or local anesthetics. A protein-bound drug is an inert drug. When less protein is available, as in acidosis, more free drug will distribute to active sites for a more profound effect. This phenomenon is further enhanced by the relative hypoalbuminemic state of patients with ESRD.[5]

Respiratory acidosis augments neuromuscular blockade through the above mechanism and makes reversal more difficult. An increasing metabolic acidosis will also be accompanied by a rising serum potassium level, as acidosis favors extracellular rather than intracellular distribution of potassium.[2]

Hematology

Hematologic abnormalities include anemia and platelet dysfunction. The kidney normally senses the oxygen available to the tissues. If oxygen delivery is impaired, the kidney releases the hormone erythropoietin into the plasma to stimulate the erythroid marrow.[6] This nonexcretory function of the kidney is maintained to varying degrees in ESRD patients. Patients who have had bilateral nephrectomy are persistently more anemic than ESRD patients who still have their own kidneys. The difference in the degree of anemia is sufficient to require more blood transfusions for totally nephrectomized patients.

While the most important cause of anemia in ESRD patients is decreased erythropoietin, the anemia is aggravated by shortened red cell survival. Both native and transfused red cells have a shortened survival in the ESRD patient. Dialysis will not increase red cell survival. Hemolysis is not a major factor except in a small group of patients with hypersplenism.[6] Many patients are very knowledgeable about the degree of anemia they live with and know their general hematocrit levels. Some older and higher-risk patients experience dyspnea or angina when the hematocrit is too low, a worthwhile history to obtain.

In 1987 reports on the research and first use of recombinant human erythropoietin in ESRD patients showed the most promising results. This major advance significantly improved the hematocrits of most of the small group of patients treated. It may eliminate the need for most blood transfusions in ESRD patients as well as the risks of immunologic sensitization and infections as hepatitis. The patients' well-being also improved dramatically. While no direct toxic effects have been noted thus far, the increase in red cell mass in a previously anemic patient will increase the blood viscosity and may increase vascular resistance.[7]

Platelet dysfunction is the primary cause of the bleeding problems commonly observed in ESRD. The platelet defect is qualitative, not quantitative. The etiology of platelet dysfunction has been extensively studied and is still not fully understood. Decreased platelet aggregation is a factor. Uremic toxins as urea, phenols, and guanidino-succinic acid are believed to inhibit the cellular metabolism of circulating platelets.[8] Because these toxins are readily dialyzed, dialysis can significantly improve the platelet function to minimize bleeding tendencies. However, only successful renal transplantation can permanently solve this problem.

Cardiovascular System

Dialysis alleviates most of the cardiovascular symptoms of ESRD. The hypertension, secondary to fluid retention, is generally well controlled. However, a small number of patients suffer hypertension of a more ominous nature due to high renin levels, which do not respond to antihypertensive therapy. Bilateral nephrectomy to eliminate the high renin source is occasionally necessary.

Anemia affects the cardiovascular function by causing a hyperdynamic circulatory state, including increased cardiac output and increased venous pressure. Coronary artery disease due to atherosclerosis and hypertension is common at a relatively early age. Angina with worsening anemia or with hypotension may occur during dialysis. Some patients have undergone coronary artery bypass to relieve the angina.

Endocrine System

Growth retardation is a most striking sign of ESRD. The stature of the young patient will not agree with the age. Many teenagers with ESRD have the body of a young child at the age of onset of their renal failure.

Uterine bleeding secondary to ovarian dysfunction may further aggravate the anemia of ESRD. Infertility is the rule for both sexes.

Neurology

Autonomic and peripheral neuropathy are of concern whether general or regional anesthetics are to be given. Diabetic patients are more prone to develop these deficits. Autonomic neuropathy prevents the normal sympathetic response to hypotension, whether caused by hypovolemia or anesthetics. Peripheral neuropathy is most prominent in the lower extremities. Demyelinization causes sensory paresthesias and eventual motor weakness. Regional anesthesia, whether axillary block, spinal, or epidural, has not been reported to have adverse effects on the neurologic status. Successful transplantation can reverse some of these abnormalities.

Psychology

Psychologic factors cannot be ignored in ESRD patients. Anxiety concerning the prognosis of their disease, which manifests so many deficits, is common. The physical restrictions placed upon them by dialysis and their dependence on others for continuous care add to the emotional strain.

PHARMACOKINETICS OF DRUGS IN ESRD

Many drugs depend on renal function for elimination. Those of greatest concern to the anesthesiologist are local anesthetics, neuromuscular blocking agents, narcotics, antihypertensive agents, β-adrenergic blocking agents, calcium channel blocking agents, digitalis, insulin, and antibiotics.

Local Anesthetics

Local anesthetics are of two types. The esters, which include tetracaine, procaine, and chlorprocaine, are hydrolyzed primarily in the plasma by pseudocholinesterase. Enzyme dilution by hemodialysis has not been clinically observed. The amide local anesthetics lidocaine, mepivacaine and bupivacaine are metabolized in the liver. Most toxic reactions due to local anesthetics (seizures) result from rapid vascular absorption and stimulation of the central nervous system. In the presence of hyperkalemia, cardiotoxicity (severe myocardial depression) is a more frequent reaction.[4]

Perhaps the most significant effect of ESRD on local anesthetics is the shortened duration of action. Bromage[9] estimated that the duration is actually 38 percent less than in the normal population. Apparently the increased cardiac output and increased blood flow through the tissues result in more rapid removal of the drug. This parallels the 40 percent increase in cardiac index observed in ESRD patients secondary to anemia.

Neuromuscular Blocking Drugs

Until recently, neuromuscular blocking agents had been a major problem because most of them depended on renal function for elimination: Gallamine 80 to 100 percent and metocurine, pancuronium approximately 60 percent, d-tubocurarine 40 percent (Figs. 5-1 and 5-2). The inability

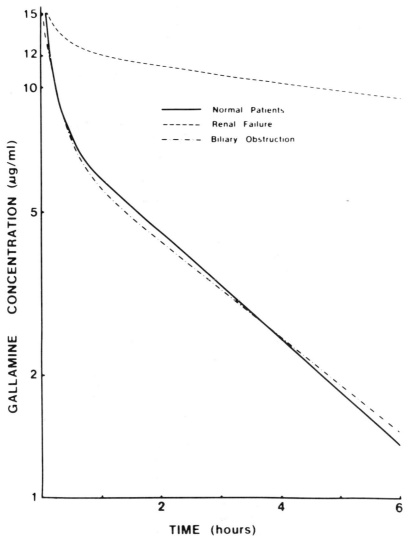

Figure 5–1. Mean plasma concentration-time profiles of gallamine in normal persons versus biliary obstruction and renal failure patients. (From Ramzan et al: Pharmacokinetics and pharmacodynamics on gallamine triethiodide in patients with biliary obstruction. Anes Analg 60:294, 1981, with permission.)

to reverse relaxants at the close of anesthesia became a common problem. Some patients required reintubation of the trachea or prolonged intubation and ventilation. There was a time when the problem was thought to be "recurarization," that the neuromuscular blocking drug would outlast the anticholinesterase reversal agent. However, studies demonstrated that the anticholinesterase neostigmine had a similar pattern of renal excretion (50 percent) as d-tubocurarine; therefore it too had a prolonged action in renal failure.[10] Difficulty

reversing the relaxants by anticholinesterases in renal failure patients lies in the decreased plasma clearance of the relaxants.[11] Excessive dosage of anticholinesterases is inadvisable. Neostigmine antagonizes only the nicotinic (skeletal muscle blocking) effects of relaxants while enhancing muscarinic effects such as bradycardia, hypotension, bronchial constriction, and increased secretions, despite the addition of the anticholinergic atropine or glycopyrrolate. Aminoglycoside antibiotics enhance neuromuscular blockade, further contributing

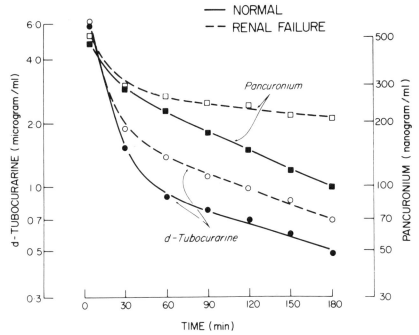

Figure 5–2. Decay of d-tubocurarine and pancuronium in patients with normal renal function and renal failure. (From Miller: Reversal of neuromuscular blockade. ASA Refresher Courses in Anesthesiology 5, 1977, with permission.)

to the problems of reversal. The newly transplanted kidney is capable of excreting relaxants and neostigmine at rates similar to normal kidneys.[12] Rejection would be expected to compromise this excretion.

After much research to discover new nondepolarizing relaxants of shorter duration that require little or no renal function for elimination, two new neuromuscular blocking agents were introduced: atracurium in 1981 and vecuronium in 1982.[13]

Atracurium was designed as an unstable molecule that undergoes rapid chemical inactivation by Hofman elimination at physiologic pH and temperature. However, another parallel enzymatic ester hydrolysis (not pseudocholinesterase-related) contributes to the molecule breakdown. Recent studies indicate that the latter may play the more dominant role in the inactivation of atracurium.[14] Atracurium causes some histamine release, which can contribute to hypotension. Its metabolic product, laudanosine (a stimulant) has in recent animal studies demonstrated arousal of the central nervous system independent of the neuromuscular blocking effect of atracurium.[15]

Impaired renal or hepatic function will not affect the elimination of atracurium. As with all relaxants, blocking effects may be enhanced by potent inhalational anesthetics. Atracurium may be administered without cumulative effects by intermittent boluses or by continuous infusion. It is readily reversed with the standard anticholinesterases[13] (Fig. 5–3; Table 5–1).

Vecuronium has a steroid nucleus similar to pancuronium and is equipotent with pancuronium, having approximately one third the duration. Its predominant route of elimination is bile, with only 10 to 25 percent excreted in the urine. Another advantage is that it does not have the vagolytic (tachycardic) effect of pancuronium. Renal failure does not prolong vecuronium's block.[13] However, prolonged effect and difficult reversal with neostigmine have been reported in a renal failure patient also receiving verapamil.[16] Calcium may influence the amount of acetylcholine released at nerve endings; therefore, calcium channel blocking drugs such as verapamil may potentiate neuromuscular blocking agents. The use of such drugs is now more frequently encountered as more patients

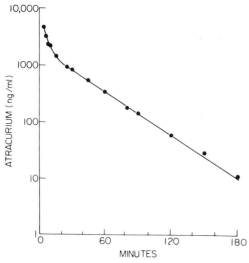

Figure 5–3. Timed atracurium levels in patients with abnormal renal function. (From Fahey et al: Pharmacokinetics and pharmacodynamics of atracurium in patients with and without renal failure. Anesthesiology 61:700, 1984, with permission.)

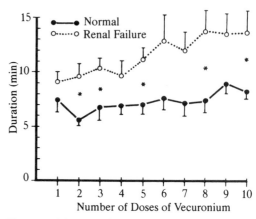

Figure 5–4. Duration of action of repeated doses of vecuronium in control versus renal failure patients. (From Bevan, et al: Vecuronium in renal failure. Can Anaesth Soc J 31:493, 1984, with permission.)

with coronary artery disease are accepted for renal transplantation (Fig. 5–4). All nondepolarizing neuromuscular blocking agents are water-soluble and readily dialyzed.

Succinylcholine still has a place in anesthesia for renal transplantation. It can safely be used after adequate dialysis when the serum potassium is within normal limits. It remains the relaxant with the shortest onset time for rapid-sequence induction and intubation when the patient is not fasting.

Narcotics

Morphine in small doses postoperatively has been observed to cause prolonged respiratory depression in uremic patients. One study found the duration of action of morphine to be more dependent on decreased plasma protein binding than on the severity of the renal failure as measured by creatinine clearance.[17] More recent studies on the pharmacokinetics of morphine in renal disease demonstrated that the elimination of morphine from the plasma correlates well with creatinine clearance immediately after successful renal transplantation. Morphine glucuronide, the primary metabolite of morphine, is normally

Table 5–1 Pharmacodynamic Data for Atracurium*				
Patient Group	N	Onset (min)	Duration (min)	Recovery Time (min)
Normal	10	1.8 ± 0.1	69.5† ± 5.2	10.5‡ ± 1.1
Renal failure	10	2.0 ± 0.4	77.4 ± 3.2	13.1 ± 3.2

*Values represent mean ± SEM.
†n = 7.
‡n = 8.
From Fahey et al: Pharmacokinetics and pharmacodynamics of atracurium in patients with and without renal failure. Anesthesiology 61:701, 1984, with permission.

excreted in the urine, although it may accumulate in ESRD patients (Fig. 5–5). The uptake and elimination of morphine by the brain are slower and more complicated than those of the plasma. Only unbound, uncharged, or nonionized lipid-soluble molecules can cross the blood-brain barrier.

Controversy has surrounded the effect of pH on brain uptake of morphine. Acidosis was believed to increase the permeability of the blood-brain barrier.[18] However, recent studies have demonstrated that respiratory alkalosis increases the percentage of uncharged morphine in the blood, thereby making it more lipid-soluble and thus more permeable to the blood-brain barrier.[19] Hyperventilation during anesthesia has been known to enhance narcotic effects. In the cerebral spinal fluid, where a lower pH prevails, ionization of the morphine takes place, making it more difficult for the morphine to exit from the brain. In animal studies the metabolite has also been observed to cross the blood-brain barrier and produce ventilatory depression.

Thus, the increased morphine effect observed in many ESRD patients may result from several factors. First, 10 percent of the morphine, which is excreted unchanged by the kidney in normal persons, is now retained in ESRD and increases the amount of drug available in the blood to cross the blood-brain barrier, perhaps including its metabolite as well.[20] A second factor is the hyperventilatory effect during anesthesia. Respiratory alkalosis increases the percentage of unchanged morphine in the plasma, making it more lipid-soluble and enhancing its permeability through the blood-brain barrier. Finally, the ionization of morphine in the brain prevents its release from the central nervous system, thereby prolonging its effect.

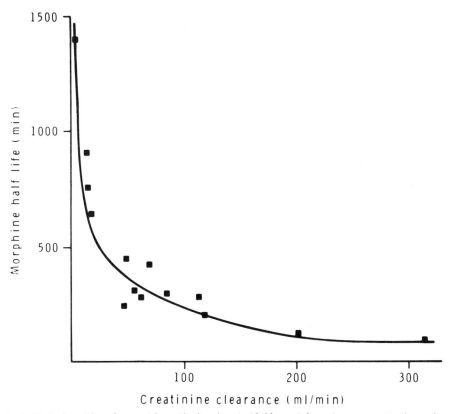

Figure 5–5. Relationship of morphine elimination half-life and first-day posttransplantation creatinine clearance. (From Sear, et al: Morphine kinetics and kidney transplantation: Morphine removal is influenced by renal ischemia. Anesth Analg 64:1069, 1985, with permission.)

Meperidine, more lipophilic than morphine, is metabolized to normeperidine in the liver. This active metabolite has a more excitatory and a less depressant effect and is excreted by the kidneys. In renal failure the metabolite can accumulate and cause convulsions. Neither morphine nor meperidine is dialyzable.[21] Overdose effects have been managed by narcotic antagonists given over an extended period.

Fentanyl, a short-acting narcotic, has a very high lipid solubility compared with morphine and meperidine. This facilitates rapid entry into and exit from the brain. Therefore, fentanyl redistributes rapidly from the brain to muscle and fat in a manner similar to thiopental. As the total fentanyl dose is raised, the narcotic effect increases until it resembles that of morphine or meperidine.[22] Prolonged respiratory depression with large doses may result from the slow release and mobilization of fentanyl from tissue stores. This is more common in patients with microvascular diseases such as diabetes.[23]

Thiopental and Etomidate

More profound effects of thiopental have been observed in renal failure patients. This appears to be related to its decreased protein binding, since thiopental normally binds strongly to plasma albumin.[24] Thus, more drug is free to act in the brain; thereafter, it will redistribute as usual, resulting in brief action.

Etomidate pharmacokinetics are similar to those of thiopental in ESRD patients.[25] Recent reports of adrenal insufficiency following etomidate administration have emerged.[26] Some ESRD patients who have had previous steroid therapy (lupus) must receive supplementation preoperatively, especially if use of etomidate is anticipated.

Antihypertensive Agents

Both propranolol and metoprolol (available parenterally) can be administered without major modification in renal failure patients.[27]

Such antihypertensive agents as clonidine, diazoxide, hydralazine, and methyldopa are eliminated more slowly by patients with renal failure; however, overdose is unlikely as long as blood pressure is carefully monitored.[27]

Cautious use of sodium nitroprusside may be required during hypertensive crises, especially immediately postoperatively in ESRD patients. The rate of metabolism of nitroprusside is the same as in normal persons. However, the metabolite thiocyanate, which is normally excreted by the kidneys, may accumulate. If prolonged (1 to 2 days) infusion of sodium nitroprusside is necessary, thiocyanate plasma levels should be monitored. Serum concentrations above 0.1 mg per ml will produce toxic symptoms such as weakness, nausea, tinnitus, muscle spasms, and disorientation.[26-28] Signs of the rarer cyanide toxicity are tachyphylaxis (decreasing effectiveness), increased oxygen tension in venous blood, and metabolic acidosis. Sodium nitroprusside is readily dialyzed.

Calcium Channel Blocking Agents

Calcium channel blocking agents such as verapamil may potentiate neuromuscular relaxants and make reversal more difficult. The amount of acetylcholine released at nerve endings is enhanced by calcium.

Cardiac Glycosides

Cardiac glycosides depend on renal excretion and therefore require dose adjustments in ESRD patients. The potency of digoxin is related to the potassium levels in the myocardium. Hyperkalemia decreases, while hypokalemia increases the sensitivity of the myocardium to digoxin.

Insulin

Insulin is normally degraded in the kidney, so less insulin may be required to regulate the diabetic ESRD patient. However, nondiabetic ESRD patients have a carbohydrate intolerance similar to maturity-onset diabetes in which the insulin, though present, is less effective in lowering blood glucose levels. Hyperglycemia is not uncommon after transplantation when steroid therapy is begun, making the management of insulin-dependent diabetic patients more difficult.

Antibiotics

The broad-spectrum high-dose antibiotics given pre- and intraoperatively have greatly reduced the incidence of wound infection. However, the potentiation of muscle relaxants by aminoglycoside antibiotics can lead to postoperative respiratory insufficiency.

PREANESTHETIC PREPARATION

Renal transplantation from a live related donor is an elective procedure, while the cadaver donor transplantation is urgent, since kidney preservation is time-limited.

The time of most recent dialysis is important to evaluate fluid status. Ideally the patient is dialyzed within 24 hours before surgery. A preoperative relative hypervolemia is desirable to prevent hypotension with the induction of anesthesia when vasodilatation occurs.

Electrolyte studies should be repeated just before anesthesia to check for an undue rise in serum potassium, which should be below 5.5 mEq per liter. Liver function studies are also desirable, as many drugs are eliminated by both the kidney and the liver. Liver disease is not uncommon in ESRD patients.

The degree of anemia should be judged in terms of the patient's usual values. A preoperative hematocrit of 25 is generally satisfactory in ESRD. Red blood cells are preferable to whole blood if a transfusion is necessary. These are most commonly infused during the last preoperative dialysis.

Preoperative coagulation studies are important. Platelet dysfunction, the most common coagulation abnormality in uremia, may be present despite a reasonable platelet count. Platelet aggregation is abnormal, so bleeding time may be prolonged.

Immunosuppression is begun preoperatively. Azathioprine can be given intravenously when there is inadequate time for oral medication before cadaver donor transplantation. Cyclosporine presents a problem in that its intravenous infusion requires several hours. The oral cyclosporine has a lipid base and is frequently given in chocolate milk or fruit juice to mask its taste. The lipid base, milk, and acid juice all present formidable problems should pulmonary aspiration occur during the induction of anesthesia.

To prevent wound infections, common in immunosuppressed patients, several broad-spectrum antibiotics are begun prophylactically before surgery. These often include an aminoglycoside, which may potentiate neuromuscular blockade.

CHOICE OF ANESTHESIA FOR RENAL TRANSPLANTATION

Most renal transplantation operations today are limited to the iliac fossa site and are extraperitoneal in adults. This exposure lends itself to either general or regional anesthetic techniques.

General Anesthesia

Choices for general anesthesia have improved remarkably as recently as 1981. New muscle relaxants that do not depend on the kidney for elimination have recently been developed. Atracurium, though short-acting and requiring many supplemental doses, does not accumulate. It can be administered by infusion if desired. Vecuronium is eliminated by the liver and should not accumulate significantly unless liver function is altered, such as during hypotension, when liver blood flow is decreased. Difficult reversal with vecuronium has recently been reported in a renal failure patient, which the authors believe was caused by verapamil. Calcium channel blocking agents have the potential to increase neuromuscular blockade. It appears that for patients receiving a calcium channel blocking drug, atracurium is more desirable because accumulation is not a factor and because potentiation can be readily monitored with a nerve stimulator.

General anesthesia using breathing circuits that are disposable, sterile, or antibacterial, including bacterial filters, may lessen the risk of pulmonary infection in the immunosuppressed patient. Isoflurane, a new inhalational anesthetic agent that has the least biodegradation of any halogenated anesthetic, is now the most commonly administered anesthetic for patients having transplantation operations. Nitrous oxide may be added to permit a lower concentration of isoflurane; however, a higher oxygen concentration is required in the face of severe anemia and hyperdynamic circulatory state.

Narcotics must be used with caution. Excessive and prolonged central nervous system depression has been reported in some renal failure patients secondary to altered protein binding and acidosis. Narcotics are not dialyzable, and prolonged use of narcotic antagonists have sometimes been required. Large doses of the short-acting narcotics can accumulate.

A rapid-sequence induction of preoxygenation, cricoid pressure, thiopental, and succinylcholine has been well tolerated by most ESRD patients. However, a smaller dose of thiopental may be advisable. There is no contraindication to the use of succinylcholine so long as the patient is not hyperkalemic.

Regional Anesthesia

Regional anesthesia is still a good choice in experienced hands. "Continuous" intermittent techniques are advisable for lengthy operations. Coagulation studies should be normal. No complications relating to coagulopathy have been reported when regional anesthesia has been administered to renal failure patients. It is important to remember the estimated 38 percent loss of duration of the local anesthetic agents secondary to the hyperdynamic circulatory state. Frequent drug supplementations may lead to drug accumulation in the plasma, which can become cardiotoxic in the presence of hyperkalemia. This is especially so when bupivacaine 0.75 percent is used to provide good muscle relaxation. Judicious sedation must accompany all regional anesthesia of lengthy duration. Supplemental oxygen is also advised, as the anemia limits the oxygen-carrying capacity of the ESRD patient. Chilling, secondary to vasoconstriction of the unanesthetized upper body, which is a common patient complaint, may be prevented by application of an automatic warming blanket over the patient's chest.

INTRAOPERATIVE MANAGEMENT

The extremity containing the arteriovenous fistula must not be disturbed by intravenous lines or restraints. However, the bruit should be constantly monitored during the operation. Additional fluids may be required to maintain adequate flow through the fistula. Loss of a fistula via thrombosis is a major complication.

An intravenous catheter of sufficient caliber to administer blood is inserted preoperatively, usually in the hand opposite the fistula, to begin antibiotic medication. The antecubital site is the first choice for a central venous pressure line. If this fails, the jugular vessels are used. Our renal failure patients have suffered a higher than usual complication rate with internal jugular insertions compared to other surgical patients. Perhaps this relates to their preoperative hypovolemic state after dialysis. It is essential to place a central venous line as a guide for intraoperative and postoperative fluid administration. The hypovolemic state is hazardous for the newly transplanted kidney as well as for the arteriovenous fistula. Acute tubular necrosis is more likely to occur if inadequate fluids are administered at the time of transplantation. Techniques such as phlebotomy, plasmapheresis, and dialysis can be instituted to remove excess extracellular fluid in the event of gross overload. A central venous pressure of 10 to 15 ml water is usually adequate.

An arterial line or pulmonary artery catheter is rarely necessary. The blood pressure is easily taken on the same arm that has the peripheral and central venous lines. Excessive blood loss is the exception rather than the rule during renal transplantation.

The electrocardiogram is the most important monitor for evaluating hyperkalemia. A recording monitor permits easier comparisons of T-wave changes, which are the earliest signs of hyperkalemia. Peaked T waves may become evident after the release of vascular clamps, although this change is usually transient. Hyperkalemia is treated by hyperventilation if the patient is under general anesthesia. Calcium (1 g) is administered to stabilize the myocardium. Sodium bicarbonate is given to counteract acidosis, which favors extracellular potassium distribution. Glucose and insulin also encourage potassium shifts into the cells. These measures cause only redistribution of potassium from the extracellular to the intracellular space; none promote its excretion. Only Kayexelate-excelate ion exchange or dialysis will actually reduce the amount of potassium in the body (Fig. 5–6).

Neuromuscular blockade is monitored via a nerve stimulator in all patients receiving general anesthesia.

Fluid Management

An adequately perfused newly transplanted kidney is an important determinant of immediate renal function and avoids postoperative acute tubular necrosis. A state of slight hypervolemia should be encouraged perioperatively. Large volumes of isotonic sodium chloride may be required after the induction of anesthesia to assure a central venous pressure of 10 to 15 ml water. Controlled fluid loading studies have produced brisk diuresis when the pulmonary capillary wedge pressure was raised to 18 torr during living and cadaver donor kidney transplants. There is risk of pulmonary edema, especially after positive pressure ventilation is discontinued at the close of anesthesia.[30,31]

Dextrose solutions are not used after the first liter, as plasma glucose rises rapidly with the stress of anesthesia, surgery, and the steroid medication given at the time of vascular clamp release. Lactated Ringer's solution is avoided because it contains potassium, although the 4 mEq per liter of potassium it contains is considered insignificant by some anesthesiologists. Insulin-dependent diabetics, necessarily fasting preoperatively, are given 10 percent dextrose in water solution at approximately 50 ml per hour. Any further fluids necessary for diabetics to maintain an adequate central venous pressure consist of isotonic sodium chloride or rarely hypotonic sodium chloride if hyperglycemia and hyperosmolarity become a problem.

In summary, the goal of the fluid administration is to maintain a central venous pressure of approximately 10 to 15 ml water, a systolic pressure above 120 mm Hg and a bounding AV fistula. Isotonic sodium chloride is primarily used. Blood transfusion policies vary with each institution. Some still prefer frozen red blood cells at transplantation to avoid cytomegalovirus infection transmission. Whole blood is given when severe bleeding occurs.

Medications administered intraoperatively include antibiotics such as penicillin and clindamycin, though other antibiotics may have preceded these preoperatively. Methylprednisolone (1 mg per kg) is given shortly before the vascular clamps are released. Mannitol (12.5 g) and furosemide (40 mg) are given before vascular clamps are released and may be repeated one hour later if there is no urine output.

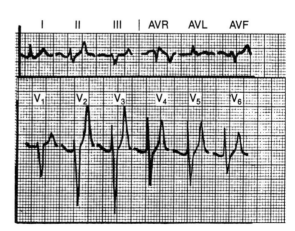

Figure 5–6. Hyperkalemia. (From Rollason: Electrocardiography for the Anaesthetist. Blackwell Scientific Publications, ed 4. Oxford, England, 1964, with permission.)

ANESTHESIA FOR DONOR NEPHRECTOMY

Living Donor

Kidney transplants from living related donors have been more successful than those from cadaver donors.[32] However, the ethical problems presented by living donors must be continually evaluated. To subject a healthy person to a major upper abdominal surgical procedure that will not improve his or her health presents a new concept in surgery. Concerns of complications from this operation loom larger. Excessive blood loss, atelectasis, pneumonitis, pulmonary embolism, infection, and even deaths have been reported.[33,34]

Anesthesiologists should have input into the selection and timing of the donor operations. While a donor may be a good tissue match for transplantation, a history of smoking and obesity in an otherwise healthy person increase the risk of postoperative complications, primarily pulmonary. We make intense efforts and have been successful in having some prospective donors stop smoking. We have requested obese donors to reduce weight to less than 20 percent over the ideal for their stature. Both of these objectives may require delays in the date of the transplantation.

The donor is hydrated for about 12 hours prior to nephrectomy with a salt-containing solution to maintain urine output. Transperitoneal nephrectomy, performed in the supine position, is less likely to result in cardiovascular instability often noted in the flexed lateral position required for the flank approach, where all four extremities are dependent. The supine position is especially beneficial should excessive bleeding occur. Intravenous fluids are given liberally until the kidney is removed. Mannitol may be administered early in the procedure to aid in maintaining urine output, to help prevent cellular swelling, and to flush the tubules of any debris that may develop during manipulations.[35] Lidocaine or papaverine is sometimes infiltrated around the renal pedicle to prevent or treat renal vasospasm resulting from surgical manipulation.

A narcotic-nitrous oxide-relaxant anesthetic technique presents minimal risk of postoperative hepatic or renal complications for the donor. Isoflurane may be added as necessary, and any relaxant may be used. Oliguria secondary to large doses of narcotics (which stimulate secretion of antidiuretic hormone) and positive pressure ventilation can be overcome by adequate hydration and intraoperative mannitol.

Cadaver Donor

The cadaver donor (brain dead) for organ transplantation needs no anesthesia but does require careful hemodynamic management. Aggressive maintenance of renal circulation during the harvesting procedure is important to ensure optimal preservation of renal tissue. Donor hydration, maintenance of normal blood pressure, and diuresis as recommended during live-donor nephrectomy are equally important during cadaver nephrectomy. However, some features are unique to the cadaver donor.

Patients with brain trauma are often dehydrated because of fluid restriction and diuretics given in an effort to control cerebral edema. Others may have abnormal fluid losses from a diabetes insipidus–like syndrome that can result from brainstem injury. Fluid replacement monitored by a central venous pressure line should begin at the time that brain death is diagnosed. The importance of adequate hydration of patients undergoing extensive abdominal surgical procedures is well established. The harvesting of two kidneys involves exposure of a large surgical field over a relatively long period (1 or 2 hours). A xyphoid-to-pubis abdominal incision is used for exposure. Both kidneys and ureters, together with a segment of the aorta and vena cava, are resected en bloc. This permits use of the full length of the renal vessels and enables identification and preservation of multiple renal arteries when present. In situ flushing of the kidneys with cold preservation solution is performed in an effort to eliminate the damaging effect of warm ischemia. The in situ flushing is done by cannulating the abdominal aorta and the vena cava just above their bifurcations. Systemic heparinization is used to prevent clotting in the cannulae. The aorta is then clamped above the renal vessels. Phentolamine or other alpha-adrenergic blocking agents such as phenoxybenzamine may be given just before aortic clamping to diminish vascular spasm, which the cold solution may otherwise stimulate. Once the kidneys have been cooled with 4°C preservation solution, the en bloc dissection can be performed without undue haste (Fig. 5–7).

The anesthesiologist's responsibility in managing such a cadaver is to maintain cardiovascular and ventilatory function and to support effective renal perfusion and oxygenation prior to aortic clamping. Fluid and blood losses, with such a large surgical dissection, require rapid replacement with several liters of lactated Ringer's solution. Blood transfusions are seldom necessary. However, an infusion of dopamine to increase renal blood flow and cardiac output may be indicated. This dose should be limited to 3 to 5 μg per kg per min. Large doses such as 10 μg per kg per min cause peripheral and renal vasoconstriction and must be avoided. Isoproterenol, another β-adrenergic agonist, may be necessary if the circulation is not satisfactorily maintained by hydration and dopamine. A dose of 1 to 2 μg per min in a 70 kg patient causes periph-

eral vasodilatation and increases the cardiac output, thus improving organ perfusion. Isoproterenol can, however, cause severe tachycardia and arrhythmias when infused too rapidly. It is perferably administered via an infusion pump. The intravascular volume must be carefully maintained because such vasodilating agents increase the vascular bed capacity. Peripheral vasoconstrictors should be avoided because of their unfavorable effects on renal hemodynamics.

Mannitol 12.5 to 25 g is given intravenously early in the operation to all donors to increase renal blood flow and to assure good urine flow until vascular occlusion. Once the oxygen supply to the kidney is interrupted, the energy-dependent ATP sodium pump begins to fail, causing sodium and water to accumulate in the cells, with resulting cellular swelling. Theoretically, mannitol increases extracellular osmolality and decreases this cellular swelling;[36] this is, however, controversial. Furosemide may be required if no urine output is evident. The urine output should be above 1.5 ml per min during harvest.

Many patients with intracranial injury will have been administered steroids in an effort to decrease brain edema. The administration of further steroids at the time of cadaver nephrectomy appears appropriate for the added stress of the procedure.

Other medications often given include heparin 15,000 units (150 mg), just prior to insertion of aortic and vena caval cannulae, and phentolamine 10 mg, an α-adrenergic antagonist to prevent renal arteriospasm when the renal arteries are perfused with iced solution.

Once the aorta is clamped above the renal vessels, ventilation is discontinued.

Multiple Organ Procurement

Multiple organ procurement at brain death is becoming more common. In addition to kidneys, heart, liver, pancreas, and eyes may be removed.

For multiple organ donation the incision is sternal splitting to pubis. This provides immediate access to the heart if there is any instability and also permits bathing the heart with warm solutions, as hypothermia can cause cardiac arrest early in the proce-

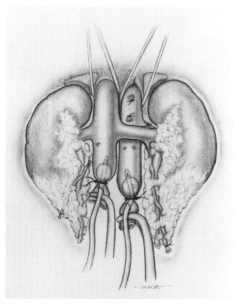

Figure 5–7. Cadaver kidney procurement, en bloc dissection. (From Linke, et al: Cadaver kidney retrieval for transplantation. Surgical Rounds 7:25, 1984, with permission.)

Table 5–2 Complications of Bilateral Nephrectomy

Pt.—Age	Etiology of End Stage Renal Disease	Indication for Bilat. Nephrectomy	Adjuvant Procedure	Complications
AL—35	Glomerulonephritis, chronic pyelonephritis	Vesicoureteral reflux, recurrent urinary tract infection	Appendectomy, bilat. ureterectomy	
RV—16	Glomerulonephritis	Malignant hypertension		Hyperkalemia
LM—43	Polycystic kidney disease	Recurrent infections, significant mass effect		Thrombosed arteriovenous fistula
TS—20	Vesicoureteral reflux, pyelonephritis	Vesicoureteral reflux, recurrent urinary tract infection	Bilat. ureterectomy	
DU—40	Obstructive uropathy	Vesicoureteral reflux, recurrent urinary tract infection	Bilat. ureterectomy	
BK-33	Glomerulonephritis, chronic pyelonephritis	Vesicoureteral reflux, recurrent urinary tract infection	Appendectomy, bilat. ureterectomy	
LP—9	Obstructive uropathy	Recurrent pyelonephritis	Appendectomy, bilat. ureterectomy	Postop. bleeding

PD—29	Posterior urethral valves, vesicoureteral reflux	Recurrent urinary tract infection	Appendectomy, bilat. ureterectomy	
BG—39	Systemic lupus erythematosus	Recurrent pyelonephritis		
TL—24	Obstructive uropathy	Recurrent pyelonephritis, hypertension	Excision ileal loop, cystoscopy	Rt. pneumothorax
MS—30	Juvenile onset diabetes mellitus	Papillary necrosis with obstruction and infection	Appendectomy	
VC—52	Polycystic kidney disease	Intractable pain, hematuria, significant mass effect	Total abdominal hysterectomy	Thrombosed arteriovenous fistula
NC—30	Glomerulonephritis	Vesicoureteral reflux, recurrent urinary tract infection	Cystoscopy, bilat. ureterectomy	
NE—18	Obstructive uropathy	Recurrent pyelonephritis		Malignant hypertension, morphine sulfate toxicity, mechanical small bowel obstruction

From Scheinfeld et al: Selective pre-transplant nephrectomy: Indications and perioperative management. J Urol 133:380, 1985, with permission.

dure. The liver and/or pancreas are mobilized first, then the kidneys. Heparinization precedes cannulation just above the bifurcation of the aorta and venae cavae as in kidney donation. The splenic vein is also cannulated for portal perfusion. Lactated Ringer's solution is first perfused via these cannulae. Close temperature monitoring at the heart level is crucial at this time. If the heart is to be removed, the pericardium is now opened and the cavae, aorta, and pulmonary arteries are mobilized. A cannula is inserted into the ascending aorta, which is then clamped, and a cardioplegic solution begun. An α-adrenergic blocking drug is given and the aorta is cross-clamped above the origin of the celiac axis. Immediately thereafter the iced flushing solutions are begun to cool the liver and kidneys. The heart is removed first, followed by the liver or pancreas with a segment of aorta and vena cava, then the kidneys en bloc, also with a portion of the aorta and vena cava.[37,38]

The anesthesiologist must realize that coordination is important if these techniques are to be successful. Surgeons from various disciplines are generally involved, sometimes from other transplantation centers. Much larger fluid volumes are necessary than for kidney donation alone. A large vascular access should be established. Blood will definitely be required (approximately 4 units per adult). Esophageal temperature monitoring is vital, and all fluids and blood should be administered via a blood warmer. Urine output must be maintained. Dopamine may again be administered to maintain kidney blood flow and blood pressure, at a rate not to exceed 10 μg per kg per min, thus avoiding renal vasoconstriction. Heparin 300 units per kg and phentolamine 10 mg per 70 kg should be at hand to administer at the proper designated time. Steroids may be added as in kidney donation.

The eyelids must be closed and protected by dressings (no ointment) during all harvesting operations, as the eyes are also included in most harvests.

BILATERAL NEPHRECTOMY

Pretransplantation bilateral nephrectomy and splenectomy have carried a high perioperative morbidity and mortality in hemodialyzed patients. In the 1960s this operation was performed, often routinely, before renal transplantation to remove the source of hypertension and infection (bilateral nephrectomy) and to decrease antibody-producing tissue (splenectomy). It reached its highest mortality, 15.4 percent, in diabetic patients.[39] With the introduction of more potent antihypertensive drugs and ultrafiltration, much of the hypertension could be medically controlled. Indeed convincing reasons for leaving the native kidneys and spleen in place were becoming evident. The anephric patient is much more anemic owing to the total lack of erythropoietin. Also, some ESRD patients secrete sufficient urine to allow more fluid intake, thereby contributing to their well-being and requiring less dialysis. Fulminant sepsis has been reported in splenectomized persons. Therefore, only specific indications should subject a patient to bilateral nephrectomy, and rarely is splenectomy indicated.

The primary indications for pretransplantation bilateral nephrectomy:

1. To remove the source of chronic infection in anticipation of immunosuppression

2. To remove the source of renin in patients with medically uncontrolled hypertension due to high renin levels

3. To remove large polycystic kidneys, creating space for the renal transplant

Preoperative and intraoperative anesthetic management is essentially the same as that used for renal transplantation prior to release of the vascular clamp and kidney perfusion. General anesthesia is given, perferably administering such agents as isoflurane with nitrous oxide, atracurium for relaxation, and sodium chloride for fluid losses. The most severe complications relating to anesthesia have been associated with thrombosis of arteriovenous fistulae when fluid replacement was inadequate; pneumothorax during internal jugular cannulation for central venous pressure monitoring; and relative narcotic overdose. A central venous pressure line is critical as a guide for fluid replacement. Dramatic fluid shifts into the retroperitoneal space occur, most frequently when large polycystic kidneys are removed. In a 5-year study the average fluid replacement until postoperative dialysis was almost 6 liters, and one patient required 11 liters to maintain a CVP at 5 ml water. Another young man suffered a hypertensive crisis (systolic 280) postoperatively. He was given morphine, hydralazine, and propranolol without significant effect. Sodium nitroprusside was then administered. At the time it was unrecognized that he came to surgery 3 kg above his estimated dry weight; he received 1400 ml fluid intraoperatively; CVP was approximately 10 ml water. Postoperative dialysis removed 4 liters of fluid, after which he was normotensive without other medications. However, in the interim he had received excessive narcotic medication, which was not dialyzable. He became stuporous and unresponsive 3 days postoperatively. The diagnosis was difficult to establish, and neurologists were consulted. Serial doses of the narcotic antagonist nalaxone reversed the morphine effects 6 days postoperatively[40] (Table 5–2).

These events emphasize the importance of fluid management. Several factors contribute:

1. Preoperative extracellular fluid volume compared to the patient's known dry weight (weight on dialysis when sufficient fluid has been removed to cause a significant blood pressure drop)

2. The size of the kidneys to be removed, exposing retroperitoneal tissues to rapid and excessive fluid losses

3. Significant vasodilation arising from renin reduction after the second renal pedicle is clamped

It is more harmful to restrict fluids in these patients than to risk overload. Loss of the AV fistula due to hypovolemia is a serious complication. Dialysis is commonly postponed until 24 hours postoperative to avoid bleeding secondary to heparinization. However, in an emergency dialysis can be instituted without heparinization. Rarely is a pulmonary artery catheter necessary unless there is poor left-ventricular function. None of the above patients demonstrated left-heart failure. Blood transfusions are given as necessary to replace losses, and whole blood will improve the oncotic pressure if necessary. Excessive blood loss has seldom been a major problem.

REFERENCES

1. Vandam, LD, et al: Anesthetic aspects of renal homotransplantation in man. Anesthesiology 23:783, 1962.
2. Stoelting, RK and Miller, RD: Basics of Anesthesia. Churchill Livingstone, New York, 1984.
3. Rooke, NT and Milne, B: Acute pulmonary edema after regional anesthesia with lidocaine and epinephrine in a patient with chronic renal failure. Anesth Analg 63:363, 1984.
4. Avery, P, et al: The influence of serum potassium on the cerebral and cardiac toxicity of bupivacaine and lidocaine. Anesthesiology 61:134, 1984.
5. Reidenberg, MM and Drayer, DE: Alteration of drug-protein binding in renal disease. Clin Pharmacokinet (Suppl 1) 9:18, 1984.
6. Eschbach, JW and Adamson, JW: Anemia in end-stage renal disease. Kidney Int 28:1, 1985.
7. Eschbach, JW, Egrie, JC, and Downing, MR: Correction of the anemia of end-stage renal disease with recombinant human erythropoietin. N Engl J Med 316:73, 1987.
8. Encke, A, Breddin, K, and Fassbinder, W: Hemostatic disorders during operative procedures in chronic renal failure. In Surgery in Chronic Renal Failure. Thieme-Stratton, New York, 1984.
9. Bromage, PR and Gertel, M: Brachial plexus anesthesia in chronic renal failure. Anesthesiology 36:488, 1972.
10. Cronnelly, R, et al: Renal function and the pharmacokinetics of neostigmine in anesthetized man. Anesthesiology 51:222, 1979.
11. Bevan, DR, et al: Reversal of pancuronium in renal failure: No recurarization. Anesthesiology 55:A212, 1981.
12. Miller, RD, et al: Influence of renal failure on the pharmacokinetics of d-tubocurarine in man. J Pharmacol Exp Ther 201:1, 1977.
13. Miller, RD, et al: Clinical pharmacology of vecuronium and atracurium. Anesthesiology 61:444, 1984.
14. Nigrovic, V, Auen, M, and Wajskol A: Enzymatic hydrolysis of atracurium in vivo. Anesthesiology 62:606, 1985.
15. Lanier, WL, Milde, JH, and Michenfelder, JD: Cerebral effects of atracurium. Anesthesiology 61:A361, 1984.
16. van Poorten, JF, Dhasmana, KM, and Kuypers, RSM: Verapamil and reversal of vecuronium neuromuscular blockade. Anesth Analg 63:155, 1984.
17. Olsen, GD, Bennett, WM, and Porter, GA: Morphine and phenytoin binding to plasma proteins in renal and hepatic failure. Clin Pharmacol Ther 17:677, 1975.
18. Fink, AD, et al: Pharmacokinetics of morphine. Anesthesiology 47:407, 1977.
19. Schulman, DS, et al: Blood pH and brain uptake of C-morphine. Anesthesiology 61:540, 1984.
20. Aitkenhead, AR, et al: Pharmacokinetics of

single-dose IV morphine in normal volunteers and patients with end stage renal failure. Br J Anaesth 56:813, 1984.
21. Brater, DC: Drug Use in Renal Disease. ADIS Health Service Press, Sydney, 1983.
22. Stanski, DR: Narcotic pharmacokinetics. Can Anaesth Soc J 30:257, 1983.
23. Gulden, D, et al: Fentanyl pharmacokinetics during renal transplantation. Anesthesiology 61:A243, 1984.
24. Goodman, LS and Gilman, AG: The Pharmacologic Basis of Therapeutics. Macmillan, New York, 1983.
25. Carlos, R, Calvo, R, and Erill, S: Plasma protein binding of etomidate in patients with renal failure or hepatic cirrhosis. Clin Pharmacokinet 4:144, 1979.
26. Wagner, RL, and White, PL: Etomidate inhibits adrenocortical function in surgical patients. Anesthesiology 61:647, 1984.
27. Rahn, KH, et al: Drug treatment in chronic renal failure. In Eigler, FW: Surgery in Chronic Renal Failure, Thieme-Stratton, Inc. New York, 1984.
28. Fabre, J, et al: Differences in kinetic properties of drugs. Clin Pharmacokinet 5:441, 1980.
29. Verbeeck, RK, Branch, RA, and Wilkinson, GR: Drug metabolites in renal failure. Clin Pharmacokinet 6:329, 1981.
30. Carlier, M, et al: Maximal hydration during anesthesia increases pulmonary artery pressures and improves early function of human renal transplants. Transplantation 34:201, 1982.
31. Grodin, W, Scantlebury, V, and Warmington N: Dopaminergic stimulation of renal blood flow and renal function after transplantation. Anesthesiology 61:A129, 1984.
32. Tilney, NL and Lazarus, JM: Surgical Care of the Patient with Renal Failure. WB Saunders, Philadelphia, 1982.
33. Friedman, EA, et al: Ethical aspects in renal transplantation. Kidney Int 23:S90, 1983.
34. Aldrete, JA, et al: Anesthesia experience with living renal transplant donors. Anesth Analg 50:169, 1971.
35. Flores, J, et al: The role of cell swelling in ischemic renal damage and the protective effect of hypertonic solute. J Clin Invest 51:118, 1972.
36. Johnson, RWG: The effect of ischemic injury on kidneys preserved for 24 hours before transplantation. Br J Surg 59:765, 1972.
37. Shaw, BW, et al: Combination donor hepatectomy and nephrectomy and early functional results. Surg Gynecol Obstet 155:321, 1982.
38. Rosenthal, JT, et al: Principles of multiple organ procurement from cadaver donors. Ann Surg 198:617, 1983.
39. Matas, AJ, et al: Lethal complications of bilateral nephrectomy and splenectomy in hemodialyzed patients. Am J Surg 129:616, 1975.
40. Sheinfeld, J, et al: Selective pre-transplant nephrectomy: Indications and perioperative management. J Urol 133:379, 1985.

Chapter 6

Surgical Techniques

JAMES I. WHITTEN
LUIS H. TOLEDO-PEREYRA

Cadaver Donor Nephrectomy
Living Related Donor Nephrectomy
Renal Transplant Technique
Pediatric Renal Transplant Technique
Transplant Nephrectomy

A variety of surgical procedures have been developed over the past two decades in relation to organ procurement, transplantation, and removal if necessary. This chapter presents an illustrated perspective of the methods that have become more or less standardized for these procedures, including cadaver and living related donor nephrectomy, adult and pediatric renal transplantation, and transplant nephrectomy. The personal preferences of the authors have also been incorporated.

CADAVER DONOR NEPHRECTOMY

The peritoneal cavity is entered through a vertical midline incision from the xyphoid to pubis. To facilitate ease of removal of organs, a horizontal incision at the level of the umbilicus may be added. The resulting four flaps can be bent backward and secured with towel clips (Fig. 6–1).

First a thorough exploration of the abdominal cavity is carried out to ensure that there is no tumor or visceral injury. The lateral peritoneal reflection of the right colon is then incised along with the hepatocolic ligament (Fig. 6–2).

The right colon is mobilized by blunt dissection and retracted both medially to the left and superiorly. The duodenum is visualized, its lateral peritoneal attachments are incised, and the duodenum is bluntly mobilized medially to the left. The vena cava, aorta, and right kidney and ureter are thus exposed in their retroperitoneal positions (Fig. 6–3).

The fibroareolar tissue overlying the aorta is incised. The inferior mesenteric artery is dissected free, isolated, divided, and tied. This will allow further retraction of the colon and the mesentery away from the aorta and iliac vessels (Fig. 6–4).

The dissection is carried superiorly along the aorta and vena cava. The aorta and vena cava are exposed to the level of the left renal vein (Fig. 6–5).

The dissection is continued above to the level of the aortic hiatus. The dissection is more difficult because of a thick nerve plexus that crosses the aorta in this region. The celiac artery and superior mesenteric

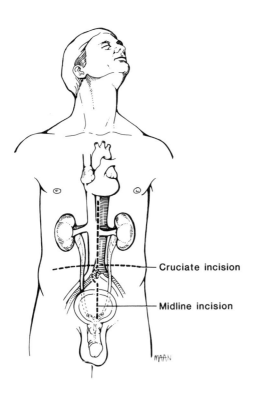

Cadaver donor

Figure 6–1

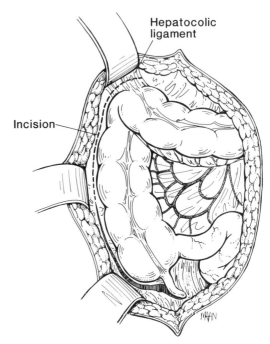

Incision along lateral peritoneal reflection
and hepatocolic ligament

Figure 6–2

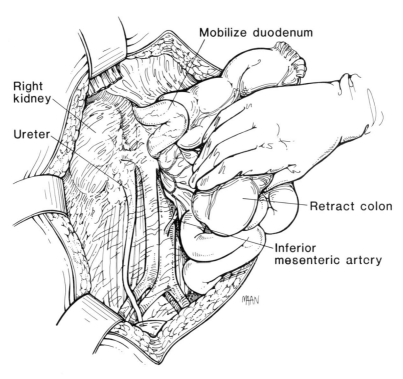

Retract viscera upward to left

Figure 6–3

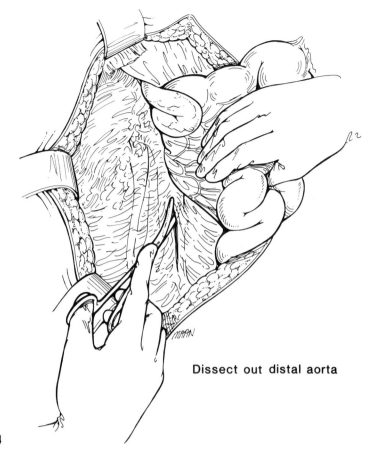

Dissect out distal aorta

Figure 6–4

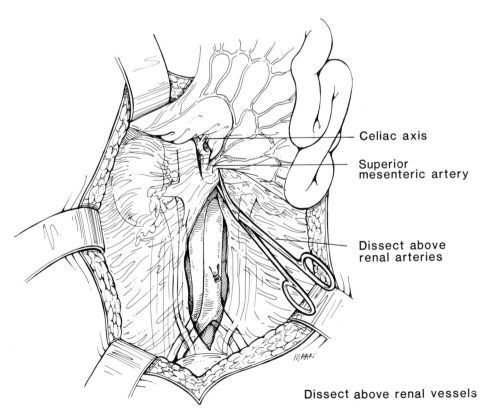

Celiac axis

Superior
mesenteric artery

Dissect above
renal arteries

Dissect above renal vessels

Figure 6–5

artery are identified, dissected free, isolated, divided, and tied (Fig. 6–6).

The dissection is carried laterally along the left renal vein until the adrenal vein and gonadal vein are identified. These are isolated, divided, and tied (Fig. 6–7).

The kidneys can then be mobilized. Gerota's fascia is incised, and by sharp and blunt dissection the kidneys are freed from the surrounding tissues. The ureters are transected below the brim of the pelvis, and notation of urine flow is made for future reference. The proximal cut end of the ureter is retracted anteriorly and superiorly. Meanwhile, the fibroareolar network of tissues surrounding the ureter is incised back to the pelvis of the kidney (Fig. 6–8).

The aorta is cannulated inferiorly either through one of the common iliac arteries or directly through the aorta. The cannula is usually secured with a ligature. The distal aorta or iliacs are clamped and divided. The proximal cut end of the aorta is lifted anteriorly and superiorly. The exposed paired lumbar vessels are seen and are subject to blunt dissection. The lumbar vessels

are ligated with hemoclips and divided. This dissection is carried beneath the aorta up to the level of the left renal vein (Fig. 6–9).

Both the aorta and the vena cava are encircled above the renal vessels. A 20,000-unit bolus of heparin is given intravenously. The aorta and vena cava can then be clamped above the level of the renal vessels. Immediately the in situ cold flush is begun. A Robinson catheter is inserted into the vena cava distally. The catheter is connected to a drainage bag, which is placed on the operating room floor. The flush is continued until the effluent is clear and the kidneys are pale and cool. Sterile iced saline slush may be added to the operating field the more rapidly to cool the kidneys (Fig. 6–10).

The proximal aorta and vena cava are divided. With the assistant elevating the mobilized kidneys and ureters anteriorly, the remaining attachments of the aorta and vena cava to the retroperitoneum are incised (Fig. 6–11).

The en bloc kidneys together with a seg-

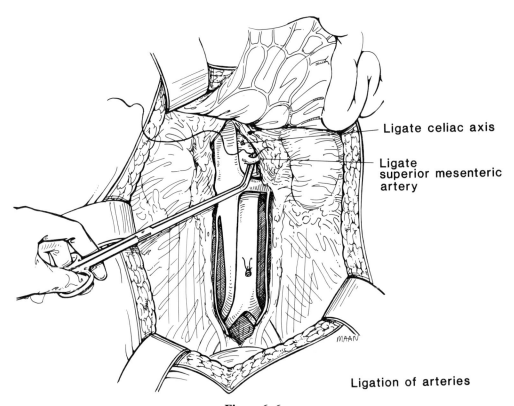

Ligate celiac axis

Ligate
superior mesenteric
artery

Ligation of arteries

Figure 6–6

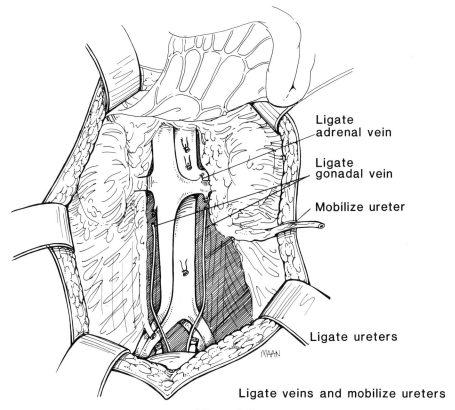

Ligate
adrenal vein

Ligate
gonadal vein

Mobilize ureter

Ligate ureters

Ligate veins and mobilize ureters

Figure 6–7

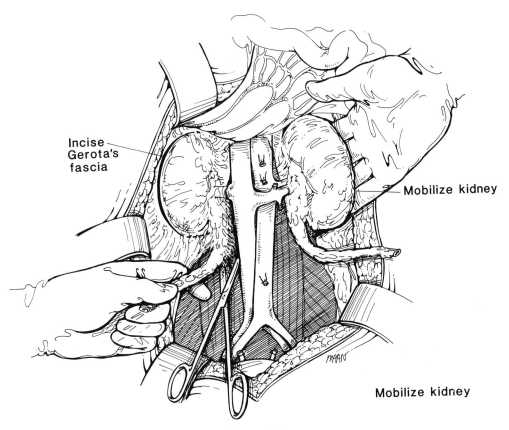

Incise
Gerota's
fascia

Mobilize kidney

Mobilize kidney

Figure 6–8

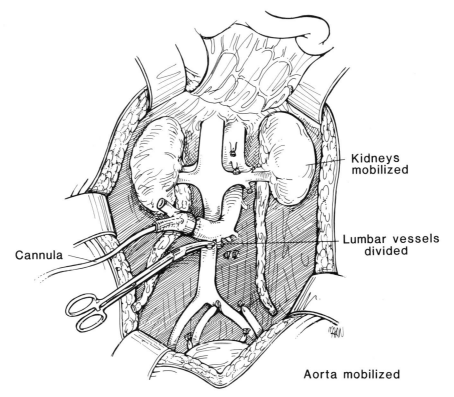

Kidneys
mobilized

Lumbar vessels
divided

Cannula

Aorta mobilized

Figure 6–9

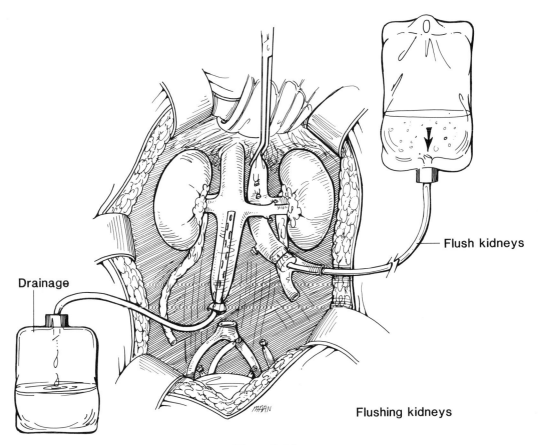

Flush kidneys

Drainage

Flushing kidneys

Figure 6–10

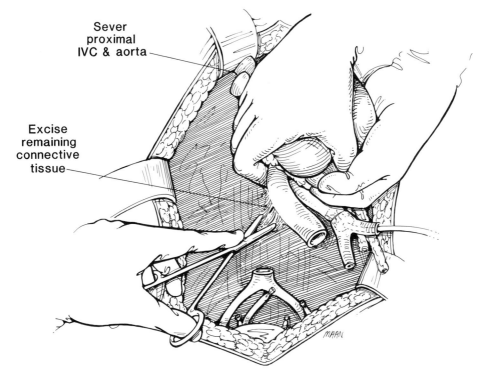

Sever
proximal
IVC & aorta

Excise
remaining
connective
tissue

Excision of kidneys and major vessels

Figure 6–11

ment of aorta and vena cava are removed to a basin with iced saline slush. Excess fibroareolar tissue is removed in the basin. The proximal end of the aorta is sewn together if the kidneys are to be placed on perfusion. If the kidneys are to be placed in iced storage, they can be separated by dividing anterior and posterior walls of the aorta. The arteries and veins are counted and identified. The left renal vein is divided at its origin with the vena cava. The right renal vein may be lengthened by dividing the vena cava transversely as depicted and the edges oversewn (Figs. 6–12 and 6–13).

LIVING RELATED DONOR NEPHRECTOMY

We prefer to use the left kidney because of the greater length of the renal vein. The patient is positioned on the right side after intubation in such a manner that the tip of

the 12th rib overlies the kidney rest. The patient is secured with tape. The table is then flexed and the kidney rest is raised. Incision is made from the tip of the 12th rib to the lateral border of the rectus sheath (Fig. 6–14).

The incision is deepened through the layers of the abdominal wall including the skin, subcutaneous tissues, the oblique and transversus muscles, and the transversalis fascia. The peritoneum is not entered. The peritoneum and its contents are bluntly dissected and retracted both anteriorly and medially. Gerota's fascia is now incised. The kidney is gently dissected free by blunt finger dissection (Fig. 6–15A).

The dissection of hilum of the kidney is begun by following the renal vein anteriorly. Both the adrenal vein and the gonadal vein are identified, isolated, divided, and ligated. The dissection is carried anteriorly until the vena cava is encountered (Fig. 6–15B).

The dissection is then begun posteriorly along the renal artery. The dissection is car-

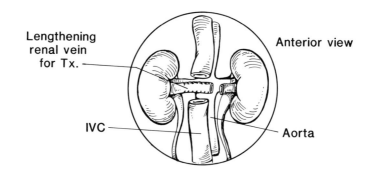

Lengthening renal vein for Tx.

Anterior view

IVC

Aorta

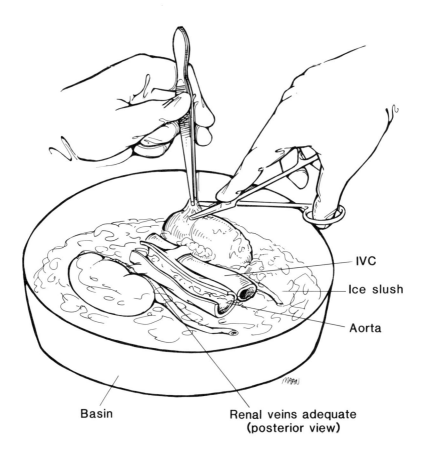

IVC

Ice slush

Aorta

Basin

Renal veins adequate (posterior view)

Removal of excess tissue

Figure 6–12

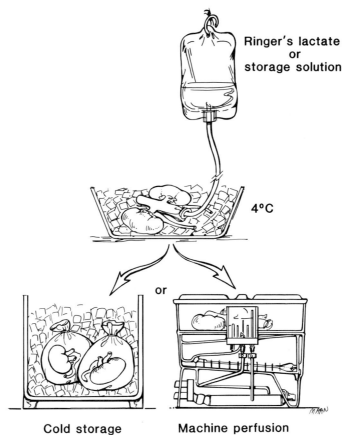

Ringer's lactate
or
storage solution

4°C

or

Figure 6–13   Cold storage   Machine perfusion

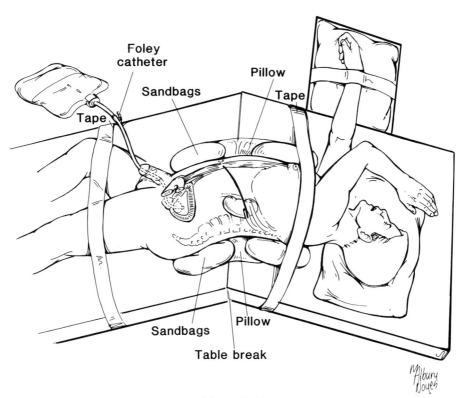

Foley
catheter

Pillow

Sandbags

Tape

Tape

Tape

Sandbags

Pillow

Table break

Figure 6–14

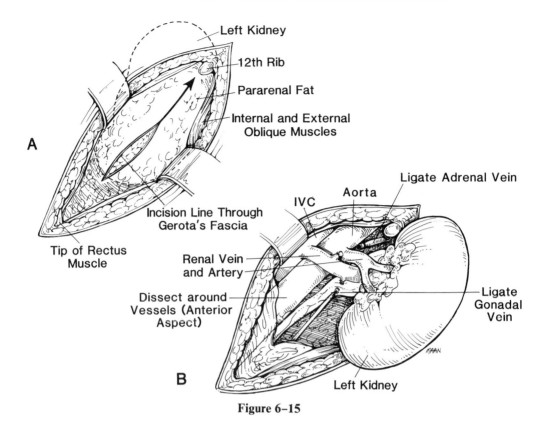

Figure 6–15

ried along the renal artery to the junction of the renal artery and the aorta. A lumbar vein may be encountered, which will necessitate a division and ligation (Fig. 6–16).

The ureter is dissected to the point where it crosses the iliac vessels. Care is taken to preserve a fibroareolar arcade of tissue surrounding the ureter. The ureter is ligated at this point and divided (Fig. 6–17).

Both the renal artery and vein are clamped with vascular clamps and divided. The kidney is removed to a side table, where it is perfused with cold flush solution. The stumps of both vessels are oversewn with 5-0 prolene cardiovascular sutures. The wound is closed in layers (Fig. 6–18a, b).

RENAL TRANSPLANT TECHNIQUE

The incision is made in the groin region, starting at the pubic tubercle and extending laterally to a point approximately 1 inch above the iliac crest. The fascia of the external oblique and the rectus sheath is divided with a scalpel. The rectus muscle and the muscles of the anterior abdominal wall

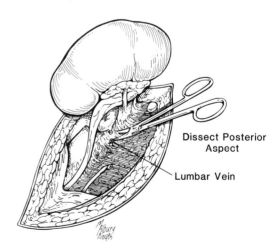

Figure 6–16

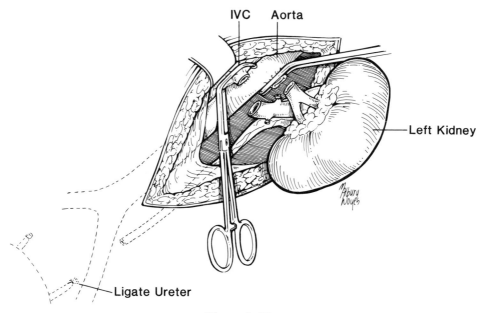

IVC   Aorta

Left Kidney

Ligate Ureter

Figure 6–17

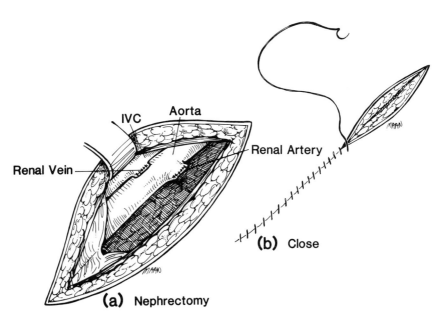

IVC   Aorta

Renal Artery

Renal Vein

(b) Close

(a) Nephrectomy

Figure 6–18

are incised along the course of the incision (Fig. 6–19).

The peritoneum is mobilized off from the iliac vessels by a blunt dissection. The peritoneum is then retracted superiorly and laterally. The iliac vessels and the ureter are visualized. The round ligament or spermatic cord may be divided for better exposure (Fig. 6–20).

The iliac vessels are dissected by both sharp and blunt dissection. The common iliac is encircled with a vessel loop to obtain proximal control (Fig. 6–21).

If the internal iliac is to be used for anastomosis, the dissection is carried downward into the pelvis along the internal iliac artery to the point of its bifurcation. The two branches of the bifurcation are tied distally. A bulldog clamp is applied to the proximal internal iliac artery. The artery is then divided just above the bifurcation. The external iliac vein is mobilized by sharp and blunt dissection.

A large Satinsky clamp is placed on the external iliac vein. A venotomy of length sufficient to match the donor renal vein is made (Fig. 6–22).

Stay stitches are placed on either side in the midportion of the venotomy to hold the vein edges apart for anastomosis. The renal vein is then anastomosed to the external iliac vein end-to-side with a 5-0 prolene cardiovascular suture (Fig. 6–23).

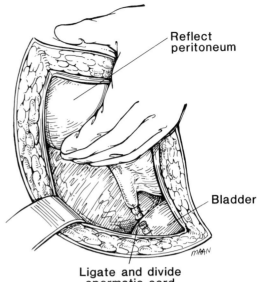

Transplant Site

Figure 6–20

The renal artery anastomosis may be end-to-end to the internal iliac or end-to-side to the external iliac artery. When the renal artery is anastomosed to the internal iliac artery, both the donor renal artery and

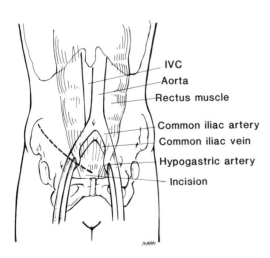

Anatomy and incision site

Figure 6–19

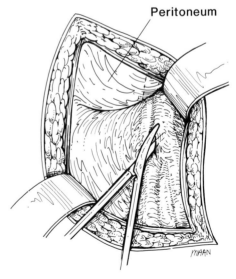

Dissecting Out
Iliac Vessels

Figure 6–21

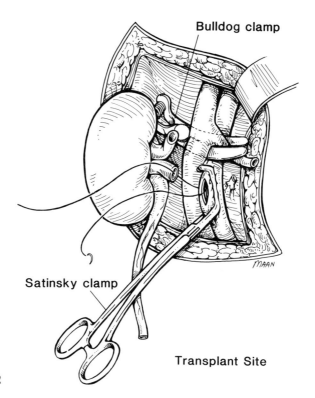

Bulldog clamp

Satinsky clamp

Transplant Site

Figure 6–22

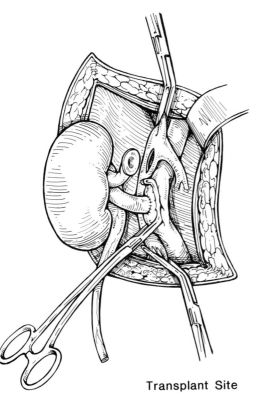

Transplant Site

Figure 6–23

the internal iliac artery are cut obliquely. This will prevent later scar formation from causing a stenosis at the point of anastomosis.

A continuous suture technique is made with 6-0 prolene suture; interrupted suture technique may also be used. We prefer to suture one side continuously while using interrupted sutures for the opposite side of the anastomosis.

When the anastomosis is between the renal artery and the external iliac artery, an oval patch of the aorta is usually included at the orifice of the renal artery. Clamps are applied to both the proximal and distal external iliac artery. The arteriotomy is made in the external iliac artery to match the donor renal artery (see Fig. 6–23). When the renal artery is anastomosed to the external iliac artery, a continuous suture of 5-0 prolene is used to anastomose the oval patch of the aorta to the external iliac artery.

After arterial and venous anastomoses are completed, the Satinsky clamp is removed followed by the removal of the arterial clamps. The operator momentarily observes the kidney as it fills with blood and changes color from gray to pink. The arterial anastomosis can be palpated to ensure patency (Fig. 6–24A, B).

Next the urethral neocystostomy is fashioned. The peritoneum is dissected from the urinary bladder. The bladder is distended with betadine solution prior to beginning the operation. The dome of the bladder is opened vertically. The edges of the opened bladder are retracted to allow visualization of the trigone region. Two 1-cm incisions are made horizontally in the

bladder mucosa on the lateral wall of the urinary bladder just above the urethral orifice. The second incision is made 2 cm anterior to the first. A right angle is used to make a tunnel beneath the mucosa between the two incisions. The right angle is then forced through the muscular wall of the urinary bladder at the level of the operative incision. The ureters are grasped between the jaws of the clamp and pulled through. At a right angle the ureter is then pulled submucosal through the lower opening in the bladder mucosa. The ureter now can be

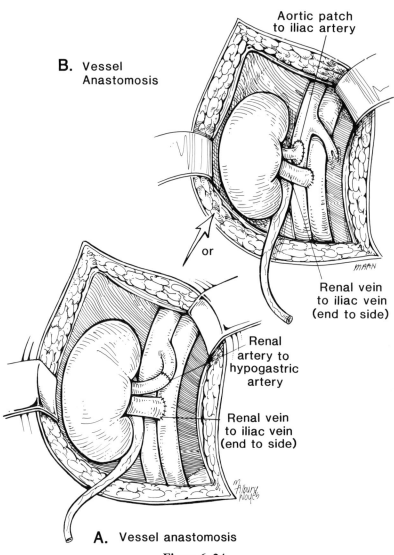

B. Vessel Anastomosis

Aortic patch to iliac artery

Renal vein to iliac vein (end to side)

or

Renal artery to hypogastric artery

Renal vein to iliac vein (end to side)

A. Vessel anastomosis

Figure 6–24

anastomosed to the bladder mucosa with interrupted sutures. The bladder incision is closed in three layers using absorbable suture (Fig. 6–25a through e).

An alternative method of ureteroneocystostomy is a ureter-to-bladder onlay patch. An oblique incision is made in the muscular layer of the urinary bladder down to the mucosa. The mucosa is allowed to balloon through the incision. An ellipse of bladder mucosa is excised with scissors from the most medial portion of the bladder incision. The end of the ureter is cut obliquely and anastomosed to the mucosa of the urinary bladder with interrupted absorbable sutures. The muscularis is then closed over the ureter to form a submucosal tunnel with absorbable sutures (Fig. 6–26a through e).

After completion of the ureteral neocystostomy the wound is inspected to ensure hemostasis. A suction catheter is placed in the wound and is exited through a stab wound. The abdominal wall is then closed in layers (Fig. 6–27).

The donor kidneys with multiple renal arteries are managed by a variety of techniques:

1. Double renal arteries of near-equal caliber may be joined on their opposing sides to form a common channel. The joint vessels then can be anastomosed to the external or internal iliac artery (Fig. 6–28A).

2. If the two renal arteries' orifices are widely separated on the aorta, the larger of the two renal arteries can be anastomosed end-to-end to the internal iliac artery, and the smaller, end-to-side to the external iliac artery with an aortic patch. Also, both renal arteries with their separate aortic oval patch can be individually anastomosed to the external iliac artery through two separate arteriotomies (Fig. 6–28B)

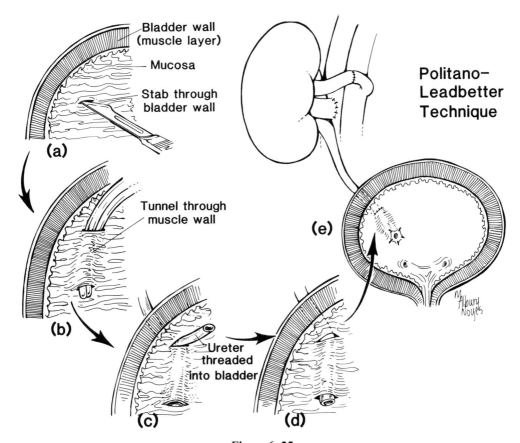

Figure 6–25

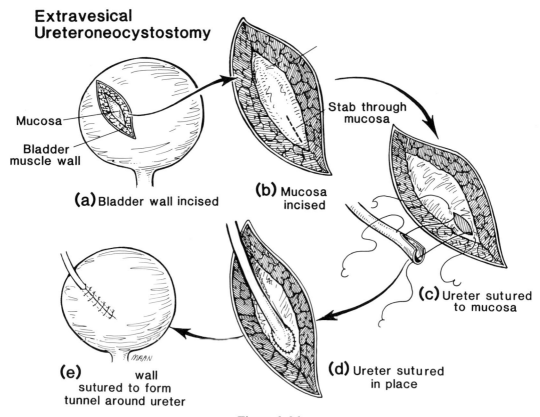

Extravesical Ureteroneocystostomy

Mucosa

Bladder muscle wall

(a) Bladder wall incised

(b) Mucosa incised

Stab through mucosa

(c) Ureter sutured to mucosa

(d) Ureter sutured in place

(e) wall sutured to form tunnel around ureter

Figure 6–26

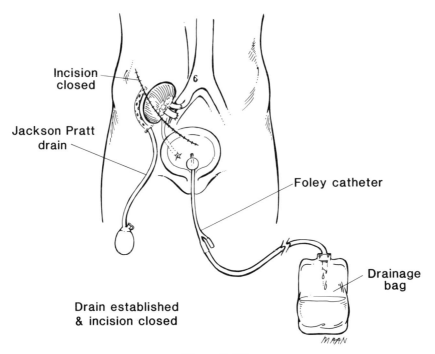

Incision closed

Jackson Pratt drain

Foley catheter

Drainage bag

Drain established & incision closed

Figure 6–27

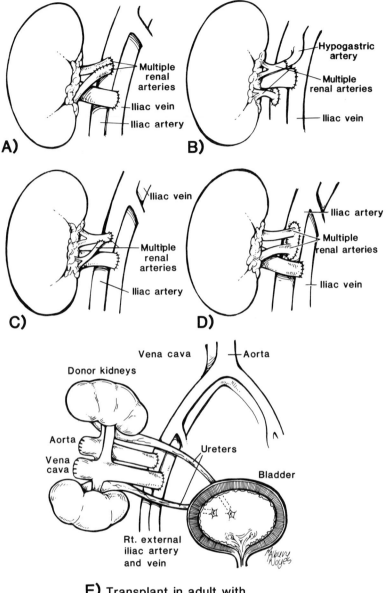

A)

Multiple renal arteries
Iliac vein
Iliac artery

B)

Hypogastric artery
Multiple renal arteries
Iliac vein

C)

Iliac vein
Multiple renal arteries
Iliac artery

D)

Iliac artery
Multiple renal arteries
Iliac vein

E) Transplant in adult with infant kidneys

Vena cava · Aorta
Donor kidneys
Aorta
Vena cava
Ureters
Bladder
Rt. external iliac artery and vein

Figure 6–28

3. Double renal arteries of unequal caliber can be converted to a single donor-recipient anastomosis by anastomosing the smaller artery end-to-side to the larger renal artery. Then the joined renal artery can be anastomosed to the external iliac artery end-to-side or the internal iliac artery end-to-end (Fig. 6–28C)

4. Often there are two renal arteries of approximately the same size and their orifices are located within 1 cm or 2 cm of each other on the aorta. A large oval aortic patch containing both orifices of the renal arteries can be anastomosed end-to-side to the external iliac artery (Fig. 6–28D).

5. Infant kidneys, if removed en bloc, may be transplanted into an adult as a pair using the aorta and the vena cava for arte-

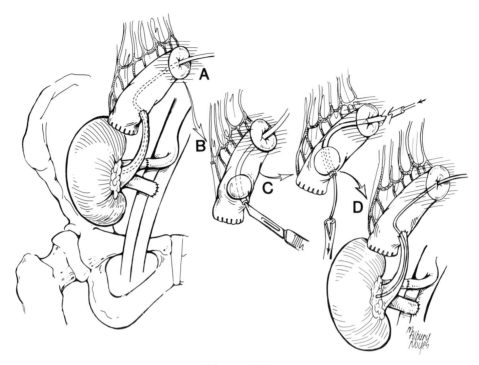

Figure 6–29

rial and venous anastomosis. Of course, it is necessary to implant both ureters in the urinary bladder separately (Fig. 6–28E).

Urethral ileal conduit anastomosis. As used by Sutherland and colleagues at the University of Minnesota, a Foley catheter with a tip amputated is helpful. The catheter is inserted through the abdominal stoma of the ileal conduit. The amputated tip can be palpated through the bowel wall. A 1-cm incision is made over the tip and the tip is forced through the bowel wall. This allows a nipple over which the ureter can be anastomosed to the bowel mucosa. The urethral ileal anastomosis is done with interrupted absorbable sutures. A stint is placed through the Foley catheter into the ureter prior to its removal. The stint is left in place after the Foley catheter is removed. (Fig. 6–29).

PEDIATRIC RENAL TRANSPLANT TECHNIQUE

If the child weighs less than 20 kg, the renal transplant is done transperitoneally through a long midline incision (Fig. 6–30). If greater than 20 kg, the previously described approach is used (Fig. 6–31).

The right colon and small intestine are mobilized and reflected superiorly and to the left. The distal aorta and vena cava and common iliac arteries and veins are thus exposed (Fig. 6–32).

The renal vein is anastomosed end-to-side to the vena cava and the renal artery is anastomosed end-to-side to the aorta or common iliac artery (Figs. 6–32 and 6–33A, B). If two renal arteries are present, one renal artery can be anastomosed to the aorta and the other to the common iliac artery end-to-side. The ureter is brought through a retroperitoneal tunnel. It is tunneled submucosally through the bladder wall and anastomosed to the bladder mucosa through an opened incision in the bladder. The bladder incision is closed in three layers as usual for ureteral neocystostomy. Prior to removing the occluding vascular clamps, 75 to 100 ml of blood is given to compensate for blood required to fill the kidney. Also, 1 mg per kg of sodium bicarbonate is given to offset the acidosis produced by anaerobic metabolism in the

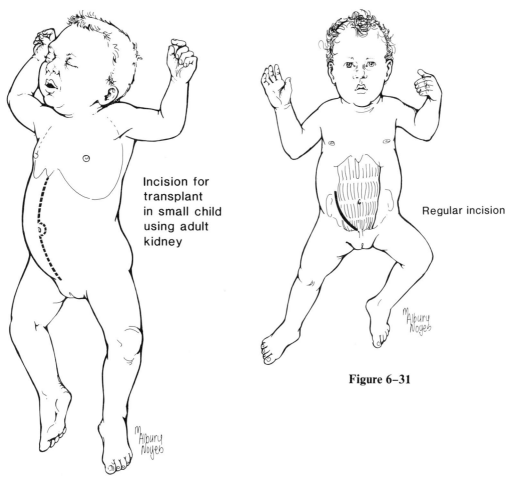

Incision for
transplant
in small child
using adult
kidney

Regular incision

Figure 6–31

Figure 6–30

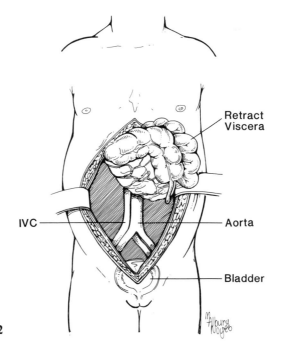

Retract
Viscera

IVC

Aorta

Bladder

Figure 6–32

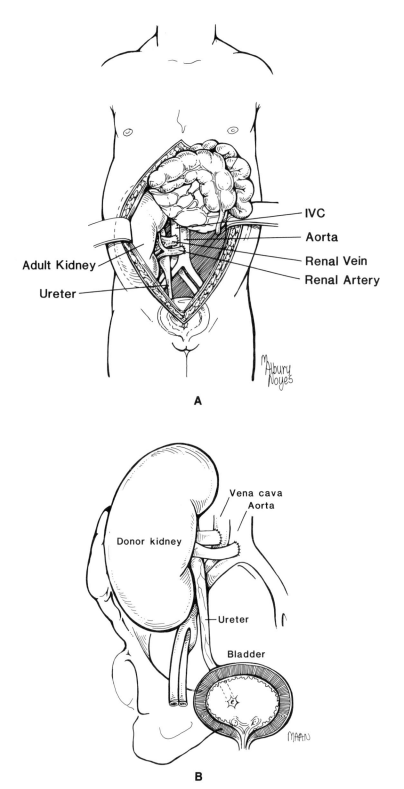

IVC
Aorta
Renal Vein
Renal Artery
Adult Kidney
Ureter

A

Vena cava
Aorta
Donor kidney
Ureter
Bladder

B

Figure 6–33

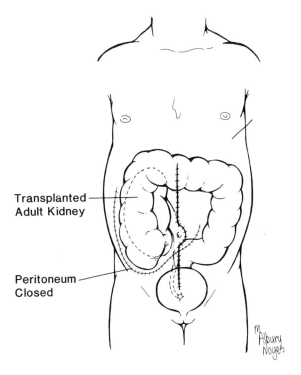

Figure 6–34

lower extremities during the time the aorta is clamped (see Fig. 6–33).

The kidney is then placed in the right retroperitoneal space and the right colon is placed over the kidney. The cecum is fixed to the parietal peritoneum and the posterior peritoneum is repaired to hold the kidney in place (Fig. 6–34).

TRANSPLANT NEPHRECTOMY

Early in the postoperative period the kidney can be easily removed; the wound is simply opened. There is little fixation of the kidney to the surrounding tissues. Any fixation is easily broken by blunt finger dissection. The kidney is then pulled out of the wound, placing the renal vessels on mild traction. Renal artery and vein are both clamped with a small Satinsky clamp at the level of the anastomosis. Care should be taken at this point to palpate the external iliac artery to ensure that it is not clamped. The vascular pedicle is then divided and the kidney removed. The stump of the renal artery and vein is oversewn with a continuous 3-0 prolene suture.

If nephrectomy is later in the postoperative course, the kidney capsule is densely

inherent to the parietal peritoneum and the dissection in this plane is both tedious and dangerous. The peritoneum is easily entered and visceral injury may occur. For this reason a subcapsular technique is used. The skin incision follows the previously transplant incision and is carried through the muscle and fascia until the kidney is encountered (Fig. 6–35).

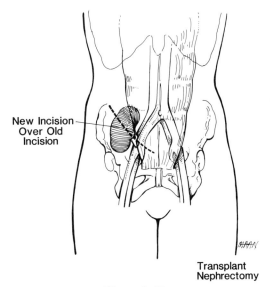

Transplant Nephrectomy

Figure 6–35

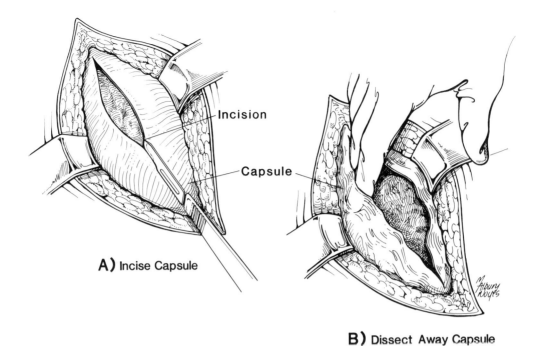

Incision

Capsule

A) Incise Capsule

B) Dissect Away Capsule

Figure 6–36

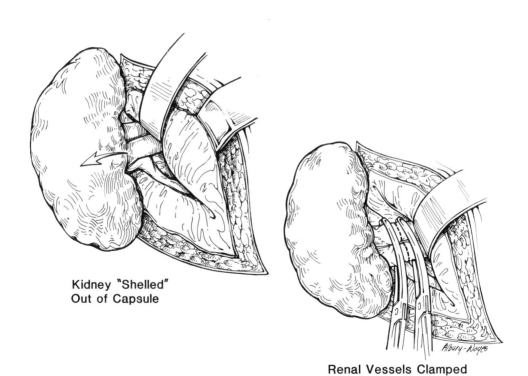

Kidney "Shelled"
Out of Capsule

Renal Vessels Clamped
and Severed

Figure 6–37

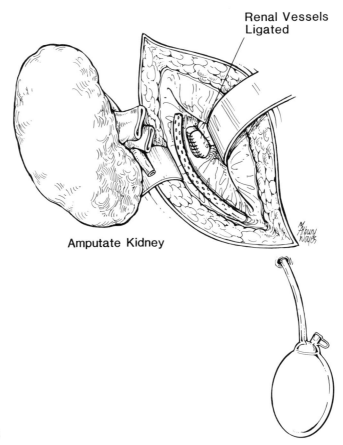

Figure 6-38

The capsule is incised from pole to pole with a scalpel. By finger dissection the renal parenchyma is separated from the capsule down to the hilum by finger dissection (Fig. 6–36).

The kidney is "shelled" out of the capsule. The vascular pedicle, including the renal artery and vein, is identified, but no effort is made to separate the two vessels within the pedicle. The pedicle is clamped with a Kelly clamp. The distal external iliac artery is palpated to ensure that it is not included in the clamp. The pedicle is then divided and the kidney removed (Fig. 6–37).

The vascular pedicle is oversewn with 3-0 prolene and the clamps removed. A suction catheter is placed in the wound and exited through a stab wound. The wound is then closed in layers (Fig. 6–38).

Chapter 7

Clinical Course and Care of the Posttransplant Patient

ELEANOR D. LEDERER
WADI N. SUKI

Although improvements in surgical technique and immunosuppression have been primarily responsible for the increased acceptance of renal transplantation in the treatment of renal failure, the success of any transplantation program is equally dependent upon the quality of postoperative care. The specific needs of transplant patients are best met by a team of physicians, nurses, and other paramedical personnel familiar with the usual course and complications of these individuals. In this chapter we will discuss the approach to the transplant patient during the immediate perioperative and subsequent in-hospital period. Routine daily management strategies as well as anticipation, prophylaxis, and timely treatment of complications occurring during this early period will be reviewed.

IMMEDIATE POSTOPERATIVE PERIOD

Evaluation of the patient in the immediate postoperative period should include examination of the operative record as knowledge of pertinent intraoperative events helps in the anticipation of postsurgical complications. Particularly useful data include the duration and type of preservation,[1-3] the general appearance of the kidney before and after vascular anastomosis, the presence or absence of anomalies of the vasculature or ureter which may have complicated the surgical procedure,[4-7] and whether urine formation began intraoperatively. Certainly it is crucial to know about any intraoperative complications such as hypotension, arrhythmias, bleeding, hypoxia, and hyperkalemia. As the routine postoperative orders are being written after the initial evaluation (Table 7–1), one should keep in mind the documented complications that may occur immediately postoperatively in the transplanted renal failure patient.

Cardiovascular Considerations

Fluid administration at this time is dictated primarily by the volume status as assessed clinically or with the help of a central venous line. Most patients will have reasonable cardiac function and, therefore,

---

Table 7–1 Post-op Orders for Renal Transplant Recipients

1. Stat CBC, SMA-6, glucose, arterial blood gases
2. Serum K+ q 6 hr × 4
3. Notify physician if:
   Urine output less than 50 ml/hr
   CVP: less than 3- or greater than 10.0-cm H_2O
   Systolic BP greater than 180 or less than 110 mmHg
4. NPO
5. I.V. Fluids: _____ at _____ ml/hr
6. Vital signs q 15 min × 2 hr or until stable, then q 30 min × 4 hr, then q 1 hr
7. Intake and output HOURLY
8. Daily weights and record
9. Foley catheter: Call physician for any problems with catheter
10. Head of bed: Elevate 30 degrees
11. Respiratory: Volume respirator at _____
12. Chest x-ray stat and q AM × 3. STAT KUB
13. EKG stat and q AM × 3
14. NG tube to low suction
15. Hemodialysis access _____ arm—no venipuncture or cuff blood pressure
16. CBC with platelet count, SMA-6 q 5 AM—label STAT
17. Arterial blood gases q 4 hr until extubated
18. Medications for pain: _____ IV q _____ hr prn pain
    _____ IM q _____ hr prn pain
    Antibiotics: _____ IV q _____ hr
    Anti-ulcer:
    Immunosuppressives:

right atrial pressure measurement will be an acceptable indicator of volume status. A central venous line is more accurate than physical examination alone in volume status evaluation and thus carries a significant advantage in many of these patients, who may be chronically hypotensive, secondary to autonomic dysfunction, or chronically hypertensive. However, any indwelling catheter also represents a potential source for infection and should be maintained only as long as clinically necessary. Urine output may not be a reliable indicator of volume status. This is self-evident in the case of the initially nonfunctioning kidney. However, even when there is urine formation, the urine output may not reflect volume status in the presence of an osmotic diuresis, nonoliguric acute tubular necrosis, or a salt-wasting state.[8] The patient's weight postoperatively may also be compared with the usual dry weight to aid in determination of volume status. While acute pulmonary edema secondary to volume overload must be avoided, volume depletion during the early critical hours may lead to oliguria and should also be avoided. For significantly depressed hemoglobin concentrations, the fluid of choice is packed red blood cells. Otherwise, isotonic or hypotonic saline in 5 percent dextrose is satisfactory, depending upon volume status, current urine output, and serum sodium level. Generally, achievement of a central venous pressure of 7 to 12 cm of water is adequate to perfuse the newly connected kidney and avoid pulmonary edema.[9] Daily weights and continuous intake and output records should also be routine aids in monitoring the volume status. The postoperative evaluation should be completed with a chest radiograph both as a baseline for future comparison and as an aid to volume status evaluation.

Significant alterations of blood pressure are common and may have quite deleterious results. Hypotension could result in or exacerbate an already established acute tubular necrosis. More frequently, however, these patients emerge from the operating suite quite hypertensive secondary to their underlying disease, fluids received during surgery, and withdrawal of antihypertensive medications. Severe hypertension may endanger the vascular anastomosis, precip-

itate seizures, or cause intracerebral bleeding and should be treated aggressively. In the short term nitroprusside is quite effective, but if the kidney is not functioning, this agent can be used for only 1 to 2 days because of thiocyanate toxicity.[10] Thus, other antihypertensives that can be given parenterally, such as alphamethyldopa and labetalol, should be initiated concomitantly to allow nitroprusside to be withdrawn within a brief period. For the volume overloaded patient, diuresis by means of intravenous diuretics or dialysis is indicated. Less commonly, volume depletion may result in hypertension and should be treated appropriately.

Hematologic Considerations

Frequent hemoglobin determinations are mandatory within the first 24 to 48 hours. The majority of transplant patients are moderately to severely anemic at the time of surgery, and although transplantation surgery is not generally accompanied by significant blood loss, even small decrements in the hemoglobin may result in symptoms. In addition, gastrointestinal bleeding may occur, contributing to the anemia. This may be aggravated by abnormal platelet function of the uremic state[11] or by hypoprothrombinemia induced by malnutrition, antibiotics, or both. If the bleeding time is prolonged the patient may benefit from the administration of DDAVP.[12] If the prothrombin time is prolonged, vitamin K or fresh frozen plasma is indicated. White blood cell count and platelet count should be obtained at this time for baseline determination.

Biochemical Considerations

Abnormalities of serum chemistries are always a concern in the postsurgical renal failure patient. Serum potassium should be followed carefully during the first 24 to 48 hours, especially if the patient is oligoanuric. The stress of surgery, medications, blood administration, mannitol administration, and hematoma reabsorption, coupled with a possible missed dialysis, places these patients at increased risk for the development of life-threatening hyperkalemia.[13] Hyperglycemia is also a common complication, occasionally resulting in massive diuresis and volume depletion. Thus glucose determinations should be included in the routine postoperative orders. Serum BUN and creatinine determinations immediately postoperatively and on a daily basis are necessary to assess graft function.

Infectious Considerations

Routine antibiotic administration in the perioperative period is effective in the prevention of wound infection and relatively safe if used properly. Generally an agent such as a first- or second-generation cephalosporin given immediately prior to the transplant and for no longer than 48 hours postoperatively suffices. Studies have documented that prophylatic antibiotics reduce the incidence of wound infection.[14-19] On the other hand, the risks of unnecessary antibiotic therapy, though uncommon, can be devastating and include infection with resistant organisms; development of mucocutaneous, gastrointestinal, or genitourinary candida infestation; hypoprothrombinemia; unfavorable interaction with immunosuppressives; allergic reactions; and pseudomembranous colitis. Therefore, prophylactic antibiotics should be used only for a defined period of time. Oral nystatin may be given concomitantly to help prevent candida overgrowth. Prothrombin time should be checked and evidence of gastrointestinal bleeding evaluated frequently.

Gastrointestinal Considerations

Gastrointestinal bleeding is a significant early complication of renal transplantation, stemming in part from the use of high dose corticosteroids.[20] Other risk factors for the development of peptic ulcer or other form of gastrointestinal bleeding include cadaveric transplantation, prior history of ulcer, acute tubular necrosis, cytomegalovirus infection, the use of anticoagulants for dialysis or rejection, and hypercalcemia.[21-24] Dyspepsia and reflux symptoms are quite common in the immediate postoperative period and generally respond to simple antacid therapy. Whether every posttransplant patient should be placed on prophylactic antiulcer therapy has not been examined in a controlled clinical trial. In addition, the comparative efficacies of antacids and H_2 receptor antagonists have also not been conclusively determined.[22,25-29] Cimetidine is generally an effective, well-tolerated medication, but in a small percentage of patients may have significant side effects, including altered mental status, hematologic abnormalities, hyponatremia, and interstitial nephritis.[30,31] There is also an increasing body of evidence that cimetidine may have immunomodulatory properties, specifically activation of the natural killer cells, which may increase the incidence of acute rejection.[30-34] Clinical studies[22,25,28,35,36] evaluating the significance of this potential effect have yielded conflicting results. Ranitidine, a newer agent of the same class, has been associated with fewer side effects, and, in vitro, with lesser effect on lymphocytes, and thus may be a better choice.[37] In view of the potential severity of major gastrointestinal bleeding in this period, it is certainly justified to initiate antiulcer therapy on any individual known to have a past history of ulcer disease or other form of upper gastrointestinal bleeding.[22,38] In addition, any patient who complains of abdominal pain, burning dyspepsia, or other suspicious symptomatology should be placed on some form of therapy. Whether truly asymptomatic individuals should take antacids or H_2 receptor antagonists is debatable. A final controversy concerning transplant associated gastrointestinal bleeding is the issue of pretransplant prophylactic anti-ulcer surgery. While some centers routinely recommend such measures, others disagree.[23,24,39,40,41] For patients with severe recurrent problems, refractory to medical management, strong consideration should be given to some form of selective vagotomy or other surgical procedure pretransplantation, depending upon the local surgical experience and expertise. In patients for whom oral antacid therapy is prescribed, periodic measurements of the serum magnesium and serum phosphorus are indicated. Hypermagnesemia can develop in patients with renal insufficiency who are given magnesium-containing antacids. Furthermore, binding of phosphate in the gut may compound the renal phosphate wasting of the transplantation patient and result in hypophosphatemia.

Surgical Considerations

Aside from medical complications, there are also surgical complications to anticipate. Bleeding at the surgical site generally will be readily apparent if of a significant degree, although some bleeding can be retroperitoneal and require ultrasound or CT scanning for detection. It may result from a leak at one of the anastomotic sites, a tear in the kidney or a wound vessel, or generalized oozing secondary to a coagulopathy induced by malnutrition, antibiotics, or the uremic state. Clinically a bluish red discoloration develops at the transplant site and extends back to the flank, causing bulging of that general area and exquisite pain around the kidney and posteriorly.[42] Depending upon the severity there may be evidence of cardiovascular collapse with falling hemoglobin. The treatment is surgical exploration and correction of the coagulopathy if present.

Another uncommon condition, but one which needs to be recognized immediately, is rupture of the transplanted kidney. The literature has reported 152 cases for an overall incidence of about 4.8 percent. A recent review[43] of the topic disclosed the following features: The usual presentation is the sudden onset of severe pain at the transplant site, generally of a constant deep nature. The kidney will be quite tender to palpation, and there will be a sense of fullness in the region. One may also see evidence of hematoma formation or bulging of the flank. This complication does not necessarily result in loss of the kidney as the site of the rupture is frequently confined to one pole and amenable to surgical repair. The cause of kidney rupture is unknown but may be related to swelling with severe rejection. Other potential etiologic factors include prior renal biopsy, ureteral obstruction, uncontrolled hypertension, and infection. Diagnosis may be assisted by the development of a fluid-filled mass on ultrasound. Laparotomy is confirmatory and es-sential for control of hemorrhage and salvation of the kidney.

Anuria, especially its sudden development in a patient who previously had a significant urine output, warrants immediate attention. It is unusual to see absolute anuria with acute tubular necrosis; thus, this finding suggests urologic or vascular obstruction. Urologic obstruction may be secondary to clot, tissue, or swelling at the suture lines. Catheterization of the bladder or irrigation of the existing catheter easily excludes the possibility of lower tract obstruction. However, ureteric obstruction may not respond to this maneuver and may require either ureteral catheterization or, preferably, an emergency ultrasound to diagnose hydronephrosis. If there is no evidence of outflow obstruction, then vascular obstruction, specifically renal artery occlusion or renal vein thrombosis, is the major consideration. There may be an increased incidence of this complication in patients treated with cyclosporine presumably secondary to drug-induced endothelial damage.[42-46] Emergency arteriogram is indicated to exclude this possibility, as delay will result in loss of the kidney to ischemia.

Primary Graft Dysfunction

Up to 60 percent of all transplants will fail to function initially.[47-54] Acute tubular necrosis is the usual cause and may last from a few days to several weeks. Some of the factors predisposing to initial lack of function are hypotension and the use of vasopressors in cadaveric donors, a prolonged cold or warm ischemia time, the type of preservation used, the presence of anatomic anomalies, and the use of pediatric kidneys in adult recipients.[54-63] The incidence of primary graft nonfunction has not been found to be higher in kidneys procured from multiple organ donors.[64] In the recovery room, volume status should be evaluated very carefully, preferably with the aid of a central venous line, and a fluid challenge administered if the central venous pressure is less than 5 cm water (Table 7-2). If, on the other hand, the patient is adequately volume expanded, further administration of fluids is hazardous. Many transplantation physicians recommend the

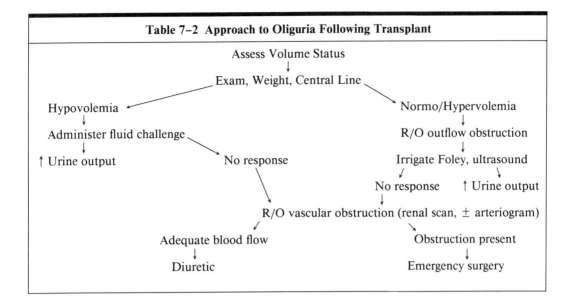

Table 7–2 Approach to Oliguria Following Transplant

use of mannitol in the intra-operative and immediate postoperative period to encourage the development of a good urine output.[65,66,67] However, repeated administration of mannitol in the oligoanuric patient carries the potential for producing pulmonary edema or hyperkalemia.[13,68] Provided the patient is not volume-depleted, bolus furosemide may be used in an attempt to produce renal vasodilatation and to increase urine flow. However, the efficacy of neither of these agents has been firmly established.[69,70] On the other hand there are some preliminary indications that calcium channel blockers may prevent delayed graft function.[71,172]

Another potential cause of initial lack of function is hyperacute rejection. This complication is quite rare with the universal practice of T cell crossmatch prior to transplantation. Additionally, most of the time there will be evidence of its development at the time of the surgery. These patients are frequently quite ill with pain over the transplant, generalized malaise, and a microangiopathic hemolytic anemia.

If an immediately correctable cause of oliguria is not found, these individuals need to be managed like any other oliguric patient, with close attention to daily weights, intakes and outputs, and dialysis as needed.

Since renal function will not be a useful index of adequacy of immunosuppression, it is imperative to monitor other parameters, such as cyclosporine levels, white cell or total lymphocyte counts, and evidence of the development of toxic manifestations of the agents used. Residual urine production by the native kidneys may obscure urine formation by the transplanted kidney, so renal blood flow scan and ultrasound may be valuable noninvasive tools to ascertain the presence of blood flow to the kidney as well as to exclude outflow tract obstruction. The optimal immunosuppressive regimen in the oliguric patient is under debate; there is evidence from some centers that cyclosporine may prolong acute tubular necrosis in this setting.[48,58,72,73]

INTERMEDIATE IN-HOSPITAL PERIOD

Routine Management

The continued inpatient management after transfer out of the intensive care/recovery unit should follow the same principle of careful and frequent patient assessment necessary to anticipate known complications, to make adjustments in immunosuppressives, and to investigate potential problems (Table 7–3).

Table 7–3 In-Hospital Posttransplant Protocol

I. Nursing
   A. Blood pressure and temperature 4 hr while awake
   B. Daily weights
   C. Strict I & O, recorded
   D. Guaiac stools
II. Laboratory
   A. Daily 0500 STAT except in hemodialysis patients, who can have lab drawn on HD
      1. CBC with platelets
      2. SMA-6
      3. Glucose
      4. Spot urine protein/creatinine ratio
      5. Urinalysis
      6. Cyclosporine level
   B. Weekly
      1. SMA-15 ⎫
      2. Mg^{2+} ⎬ Monday and Thursday
      3. 24-hr urine for protein, creatinine, volume
      4. PT; PTT
      5. Urine culture and sensitivity
      6. Renal ultrasound
      7. Renal scan
      8. Chest x-ray
III. Medications
   A. Immunosuppressives
      1. Steroids
      2. Cyclosporine adjusted to level drawn every day
      3. Imuran, to be written after results of CBC known
      4. ATGAM, to be written after results of CBC known
   B. Bactrim, PenVK or Ultracef if asplenic
   C. Mycelex troches 2 troche 3 ×/day between meals
   D. Colace 100 mg, PRN
   E. Alternagel, 30 ml, 1 and 3 hr after meals if kidney nonfunctioning
      Maalox, 30 ml, 1 and 3 hr after meals if kidney functioning
   F. Zantac 150 mg PO q.d.
   G. Acyclovir 200 mg, b.i.d. if HSV + until prednisone dose is 10 mg/day
   H. INH 300 mg, q.d. if PPD +
      Pyridoxine 50 mg, q.d. if PPD +

Daily history should include questions to ensure early detection of infection such as the development of a sore throat, headache, cough, shortness of breath, sputum production, dysuria, nausea, vomiting, diarrhea, and rash. The degree of pain over the transplant site should be evaluated and an attempt made to determine whether the pain is at the surgical incision or is deeper within the graft. Rupture of a kidney or acute rejection can be marked by severe pain over the graft. Other gastrointestinal symptoms including abdominal pain, hematemesis, and melena, should also be elicited.

Daily physical examinations should be reasonably complete and directed primarily toward assessment of volume and blood pressure status, the presence of infection, and the condition of the graft. Mild temperature elevations are not uncommon in the postoperative period, often secondary to atelectasis. However, persistent elevations of temperature greater than 100°F should prompt an investigation for the source. As noted previously control of blood pressure to avoid both severe hypertension and hypotension is important. Daily pulmonary examination is of utmost importance as pneumonia ranks as one of the major killers of transplantation patients. The rest of the examination should include a daily assessment of the transplanted kidney: evaluation of size, degree of swelling, tenderness, erythema, warmth, the presence or absence of a bruit, and the presence or absence of drainage from the surgical incision site. Intake and output records with particular attention to urine output are essential. Increasing urine outputs may signal recovery of kidney function in initially oligoanuric patients or the development of steroid-induced diabetes mellitus. On the other hand, decreasing urine outputs may signify the onset of acute rejection, volume depletion, urinary tract obstruction such as from a blood clot, drug-induced allergic interstitial nephritis, or cyclosporine toxicity.

Daily BUN and creatinine determinations are mandatory in assessment of the response to immunosuppression and volume status. Hemoglobin should be determined on a daily basis, as gastrointestinal bleeding is a significant and common complication in the immediate posttransplant period. White blood cell and platelet counts are mandatory in the daily laboratory assessment if the patient is on cyclophosphamide, azathioprine, or ATGAM. However, even in the individual on cyclosporine alone, the leukocyte count trend may indicate the development of infection, rejection, or other complications. Thrombocytopenia should prompt an evaluation to determine whether severe rejection is present, whether this is a complication of ATGAM therapy, or whether this represents the development of the hemolytic uremic syndrome secondary to cyclosporine. Less frequent liver function, calcium, phosphorus, and magnesium tests are necessary. Chest radiography should be performed at least once a week, or more frequently if indicated clinically, both for help in evaluation of volume status and to detect early pneumonia. As well, renal ultrasound done soon postoperatively is useful as a baseline for future studies for determination of size, the presence of fluid collections, and exclusion of obstruction. The utility of radionuclide scans seems to vary significantly from institution to institution. Where they are used extensively, they can be helpful in follow-up comparisons. They may also be useful in the anuric patient to establish the patency of the engrafted renal artery. However, in severe rejections, there is a significant incidence of false negative scans (i.e., the finding of no blood flow on scan but a patent artery with arteriogra-

phy). Therefore, if a renal scan suggests the absence of blood flow, it is necessary to perform a renal arteriogram in order to confirm an occluded renal artery. There is not yet enough information to comment on the possible usefulness of magnetic resonance imaging.

Complications

Surgical Complications

Surgical complications are discussed in a later chapter.

Renal Complications

Deterioration of kidney functions occurs frequently during the early posttransplant period. The differential is extensive including rejection, infection, vascular obstruction, urinary outflow obstruction, urinary leak, drug-induced renal dysfunction (specifically interstitial nephritis, functional hemodynamic nephropathy, and cyclosporine nephrotoxicity), recurrent renal disease, volume depletion, and CMV infection (Table 7–4).

The peak period for the occurrence of acute rejection is in the first few weeks after transplantation. However, with the advent of cyclosporine, it is not uncommon to see rejection delayed more than 3 months.[74] Unfortunately, there are no absolute diagnostic clinical features to assure the physician that rejection is occurring. Pain and swelling over the transplant, fever, generalized malaise, thrombocytopenia, proteinuria, and a rapidly rising BUN and creatinine if present are very highly suggestive of rejection. Frequently, however, deterioration of kidney function may be the only signal of the onset of rejection. Likewise, fever or proteinuria may be the initial manifestation of rejection and may precede by days the rise in BUN and creatinine. Many transplantation clinicians consider that although the same number of rejections occur with cyclosporine as with azathioprine immunosuppression, the rejections are milder in severity both clinically and chemically.[75] Infection of the kidney, urinary tract, or perirenal area may also be accompained by deterioration of kidney function.[76–78] Outflow or vascular obstruction

Table 7–4 Differential Diagnosis of Poor Renal Transplant Function

I. Medical
  A. Rejection
  B. Pyelonephritis
  C. Recurrent disease
  D. Acute tubular necrosis
    1. Ischemic
    2. Toxic: dye, aminoglycosides
  E. Acute interstitial nephritis
  F. Hemodynamic compromise, volume depletion, congestive heart failure, nonsteroidal anti-inflammatory drugs
  G. Cyclosporine nephrotoxicity
II. Surgical
  A. Urologic
    1. Obstruction
      a. Stone
      b. Edema of anastamotic site
      c. Clot
    2. Lymphocoele
    3. Urinary leak, urinoma
    4. Ureteral necrosis
  B. Vascular
    1. Renal artery stenosis
    2. Renal artery/vein thrombosis

can be excluded by ultrasound and renal blood flow scan. A renal blood flow scan may also detect a urinary leak, perinephritic fluid collections, or obstruction. Drug toxicity is another significantly common cause of transplant dysfunction. Cyclosporine is a potent nephrotoxin, producing evidence of vascular and tubular toxicity.[79–82] Additionally, many drugs interfere with cyclosporine metabolism either to decrease its blood level and predispose to rejection or to increase the level and augment its nephrotoxic potential (Table 7–5).

Dilantin,[83] phenobarbital,[84] and rifampin[85,86] may cause an enhanced metabolism of cyclosporine, resulting in subtherapeutic drug levels; on the other hand, ketoconazole,[87] erythromycin,[88,89] cimetidine,[90] and melphalan[91] may impair the metabolism of cyclosporine, leading to cyclosporine toxicity. Some drugs enhance cyclosporine toxicity through unknown mechanisms. Included in this list are trimethoprim,[92] cotrimoxazole,[93] aminoglycosides,[94] amphotericin B,[95] and cephalosporins.[96] Many drugs may also contribute to deterioration of renal function by causing either acute tubular necrosis or allergic interstitial nephritis (Table 7–6).

Eosinophilia or eosinophiluria may be a

Table 7–5 Drug Interactions with Cyclosporine

Erythromycin Ketoconazole	Inhibit cyclosporine metabolism—elevate levels, enhance toxicity
Phenytoin Rifampin Phenobarbital	Accelerate cyclosporine metabolism—decrease levels, underimmunosuppress
Amphotericin B Aminoglycosides Melphalan Trimethoprim	Synergistic nephrotoxicity

Table 7–6 Drugs Causing Disordered Renal Function

Antibiotics	Chemotherapeutic and
Aminoglycosides	Immunosuppressive Agents
Cephalosporines	Cis-platinum
Sulfonamide, Co-trimoxazole	Methotrexate
Tetracyclines	Mitomycin
Amphotericin B	5-Azacytidine
Polymyxin, Colistin	Nitrosoureas
Bacitracin	Cyclosporine A
Pentamidine	D-penicillamine
Anesthetic Agents	Antihypertensive Agents
Methoxyflurane	Captopril
Enflurane	Enalapril
Contrast Media	Heavy Metals
Diatrizoate	Recreational Drugs
Iothalamate	Heroin
Bunamiodyl	Amphetamines
Iopanoic acid	Miscellaneous
Antiulcer Regimens	Dextrans
Cimetidine	EDTA
Excess of milk-alkali	Radiation
Analgesics and Nonsteroidal	Silicone
Anti-inflammatory Agents	Epsilon-amino caproic acid
Diuretics	

clue to an underlying allergic interstitial nephritis (Table 7–7). In addition, nonsteroidal anti-inflammatory agents cause well-documented decreases in the glomerular filtration rate.[97]

Renal biopsy is used liberally in many institutions for the evaluation of the cause of abnormal renal transplant function when the cause is not obvious on clinical grounds or when the findings on biopsy could radically alter the proposed course of therapy.[98–103] Some of the more common situations in which biopsy may be useful are a prolonged period of nonfunctioning transplant; sudden deterioration of kidney function with no other overt evidence of rejection (i.e., fever, graft tenderness); differentiation of cyclosporine toxicity from acute rejection; exclusion of drug-induced acute interstitial nephritis; and confirmation of severe irreversible rejection when discontinuation of immunosuppressive therapy is contemplated. A newer modality of assessment of renal pathology is

Table 7–7 Drugs Causing Acute Interstitial Nephritis

Penicillins
  Methicillin, ampicillin, carbenicillin, penicillin, nafcillin, oxacillin, amoxicillin
Other Antibiotics
  Sulfonamides, polymyxins, cephalosporins, rifampin, erythromycin, co-trimoxazole, p-aminosalicylate
Nonsteroidal Anti-inflammatory Agents
  Indomethacin, fenoprofen, mefenamic acid, phenylbutazone
Metals
  Gold, bismuth
Diuretics
  Thiazides, furosemide
Miscellaneous
  Allopurinol, antipyrine, azathioprine, captopril, cimetidine, clofibrate, glafenine, phenazone, pheninedione, phenytoin, sulfinpyrazone

fine needle aspiration.[104,105] This procedure carries the advantage of being technically simple and less traumatic. Series in which biopsy and skinny needle aspirate were performed simultaneously suggest good correlation between the two procedures.[106]

Arteriograms are rarely indicated as other procedures yield the same information without subjecting the kidney to a dye load. However, under certain conditions an arteriogram is mandatory, for example, in excluding renal artery thrombosis, renal artery stenosis, renal vein thrombosis, or intrarenal arteriovenous fistula.

Infectious Complications

Like any other immunosuppressed population, these patients frequently develop infections. During the period of maximum immunosuppression, fever is a common occurrence and can signify infection, rejection, or drug reaction. Since infection is one of the major concerns during this time, proper use of antibiotics is of primary importance. Prophylactic antibiotics in the peri-operative period are justified but probably should not be extended beyond 2 days postoperatively, for reasons discussed earlier. It is also advisable to administer prophylactic antibiotics prior to other invasive procedures such as cystoscopy. The only exception to short prophylactic therapy is the asplenic patient, who should probably receive antibiotics on a chronic basis.[173] Other prophylactic measures such as laminar air flow rooms and routine surveillance cultures for the prevention of bacterial infection have not been studied in the renal transplant population. In clinical conditions such as leukopenic acute leukemia, however, the utility of such maneuvers has remained an unresolved issue.[116–121] In the case of unexplained fever, cultures of the blood, sputum, urine, and surgical site drainage if present should be obtained and broad-spectrum antibiotic therapy initiated empirically, treating these patients as other immunosuppressed individuals and covering for Pseudomonas, Staphylococcus, and whatever organisms may be particularly prevalent within the specific hospital environment. Other indications for antimicrobial prophylaxis include acyclovir for recurrent herpes virus, oral topical anticandidal agents, and INH for tuberculosis. Equally important if not more so than specific drug prophylaxis is prevention. Screening of donor and recipient for infection prior to transplant; vaccination with hepatitis B vaccine, pneumococcal vaccine, and influenza vaccine; and simple technical measures such as handwashing, isolation of the patient from individuals with infectious disease, and attention to indwelling catheters are sound basic principles in the care of these patients.

Bacterial Infections. Although renal transplant patients are at high risk for unusual opportunistic infections, they more commonly develop the usual bacterial infections, especially in the first month. These are usually transmitted infections, urinary tract infections, wound infections, line sepsis, and pneumonia. Infection through a contaminated donor is now a well-documented occurrence, particularly in the cadaveric transplant situation.[107–113] Although some reports[111–113] confirm the potentially disastrous consequences of such an occurrence, a later report[112] suggests that adequate microbial coverage may allow salvage of the kidney without risk to the patient. Early-occurring urinary tract infection is often associated with frank pyelonephritis and may be associated with deterioration of renal function.[76] Decline of renal function may be a direct effect of tissue invasion and concomitant bacteremia. However, there is also evidence for a potential immunostimulatory effect resulting in enhanced rejection.[114,115] Because of the high rate of relapse, a 6-week course of therapy is recommended. Wound infections and line sepsis have been discussed previously. Pneumonia is discussed below.

Fungal Infections. The frequency of opportunistic infections in this population has stimulated considerable interest in prophylaxis and treatment. Risk factors for the development of mucocutaneous candida are high-dose steroids, broad-spectrum antibiotics, diabetes mellitus, and generalized immunosuppressed states. When these factors may be present, oral nystatin or clotrimazole is useful in avoiding oral and gastrointestinal candida infection, though their efficacy in the prevention of systemic candida infections is not clear.[122] Ketoconazole may be equally efficacious; however, there have been reports of adverse reactions when used with cyclosporine.[87] It is therefore probably less risky to use the oral topically active agents. If the patient develops oral candida, one should probably culture sputum and urine to determine the extent of total body colonization. Odynophagia should alert the physician to the possibility of esophageal candidiasis. Endoscopy may be useful in evaluation of the extent of infection. Other clues may be skin and retinal lesions.[123] For invasive disease one should initiate amphotericin therapy, despite its well-documented nephrotoxicity. The diagnosis of disseminated candidiasis is primarily clinical, as candida serology may not be a reliable indicator of systemic disease in this patient population.[124]

Other fungal infections have also been reported fairly commonly in this population, including histoplasmosis,[125,126] aspergillosis,[127] cryptococcosis,[128] and others.[129-131] Disseminated fungal infection necessitates withdrawal of immunosuppression. Once the infection has been eradicated clinically, immunosuppression may be reinstituted. However, we have seen relapses, particularly if the patient was unable to tolerate a full course of amphotericin therapy.

Viral Infections. Viral infections are a major cause of morbidity in the posttransplant period, particularly the herpes viruses.[129,130,132-136] Several trials in transplant patients have now confirmed the efficacy of prophylactic oral acyclovir in the prevention of recurrent herpes infections.[137-141] Which populations would benefit best from this therapy is as yet undetermined. Certainly the individual who suffers recurrent oral or genital infection receives definite benefit from chronic acyclovir use. Whether all patients who have preoperatively high herpes simplex virus titers should receive acyclovir and if so for how long is not known. Acyclovir has a documented nephrotoxic effect in high doses but has not as yet been seen in the lower oral doses. Herpes zoster infection may be prevented by pretransplantation immunization with a live attenuated varicella vaccine.[142] Additionally, it is recommended that immunologically naive patients exposed to zoster posttransplantation receive zoster-immune globulin.[130]

Cytomegalovirus (CMV) infections are ubiquitous in this population.[143-146] Presentations are protean and may include unexplained fever, deterioration of renal function, retinitis, pneumonia, enteritis, and hepatitis. They may represent recurrences of prior disease or newly acquired illness. In the normal host CMV is generally a benign, self-limited illness. In the immunocompromised host, however, serious CMV infection carries significant morbidity and mortality either directly secondary to tissue invasion or indirectly secondary to viral-induced immunosuppression and superinfection.[136] Whether CMV positivity alone adversely affects renal function or the outcome of renal transplantation is controversial.[143-150] Ongoing trials with the experimental agent DHPG may provide clinicians with at least one tool to treat this otherwise untreatable infection.[151] Additionally, acyclovir prophylaxis and immune globulin have been demonstrated to provide some protection in the renal transplant and bone marrow transplant populations, where CMV infection is a common problem and has been studied more extensively.[152-156] Primary prevention by refraining from transplanting kidneys from CMV-positive donors into CMV-negative recipients may also be helpful.[143-146,157] Additionally, work is being done to develop an effective vaccine.[158]

Parasitic Infections. Another infectious agent frequently encountered in immunosuppressed patients is *Pneumocystis carinii*. Presentation of this illness is frequently as subtle as a nonproductive cough or dyspnea on exertion. Infiltrates on chest radiograph may occur late, and the only clue to organic pulmonary illness may be hypoxemia. Most patients who develop this infection will respond to withdrawal of immunosuppression and initiation of specific chemotherapy (i.e., trimethoprim/sulfamethoxazole or pentamidine). The incidence of this complication may have diminished in the past few years with the use of lower doses of steroids both in routine posttransplant protocols and in acute rejection protocols. Some centers have advocated the prophylactic use of trimethoprim/sulfamethoxazole.[159] This drug, however, may be associated with clinically significant side effects such as allergic interstitial nephritis, drug fever, and pancytopenia.

Neurologic Complications

Besides meningitis, the major central nervous system complication is seizures. Risk factors for this event are uncontrolled hypertension, electrolyte abnormalities, particularly hypomagnesemia, and cyclosporine.[160-164] Cyclosporine has been shown to induce magnesuria and consequent hypomagnesemia, which may then predispose the patient to the development of seizures.[160,163,164] Additionally, hypertension may occur in association with cyclosporine therapy and predispose to seizures. Cyclosporine use has been associated with other neurologic manifestations including tremor, paresthesias, myoclonus, ataxia, and confusion.[162] We have noted an association between OKT3 and neurotoxicity, specifically headache, meningeal signs, and CSF pleocytosis.

Cardiovascular Complications

The major cardiovascular complications during this time are volume overload, hypertension, and myocardial infarction. Volume overload is a particular hazard in the oliguric patient; however, it may occur in patients with functioning transplants. In an attempt to avoid volume depletion, hypotension, and acute tubular necrosis, the transplant team may prescribe copious amounts of saline and/or mannitol, resulting in volume overload. Intravenous medications, particularly antithymocyte globulin, are frequently administered in a substantial volume of fluid. Another contributory factor is sodium retention induced by high-dose steroids. Careful attention to intake and output records and daily weights can prevent this problem. Volume overload is one of the major factors predisposing to hypertension in this period. Additional risk factors include a prior history of hypertension, cyclosporine and renal artery stenosis.[165] The subject of hypertension in this population is more thoroughly reviewed in another chapter.

Myocardial infarction may also occur during this time. In one series, 5 percent, or 11 of 212, consecutive renal transplant recipients suffered a documented myocardial infarction. In two of these patients it occurred within the first few days after surgery, resulting in one death.[166] The major discriminating factor in this study was a prior history of angina. Pretransplant clinical screening, with cardiac catheterization if indicated may help identify individuals at high risk.[167-169] In our institution as well as in others cardiac catheterization is required prior to transplantation if the patient is diabetic or has clinical features highly suggestive of coronary artery disease. Whether cardiac surgery truly alters the cardiovascular morbidity and mortality posttransplantation has not been examined in controlled clinical trials.

Pulmonary Complications

The most frequent pulmonary complication is the development of bilateral pulmonary infiltrates (Table 7-8).

This may represent either simple volume overload or infection. Volume overload is suggested by weight gain, a strongly positive intake and output record, and other physical evidence of fluid retention such as S3 gallop, jugular venous distention, ascites, and peripheral edema. Absence of fever, though favoring volume overload, cannot be relied upon to make the distinction in an immunocompromised host. A variety of infections—including Staphylococcus, Legionella, tuberculosis, Pneumo-

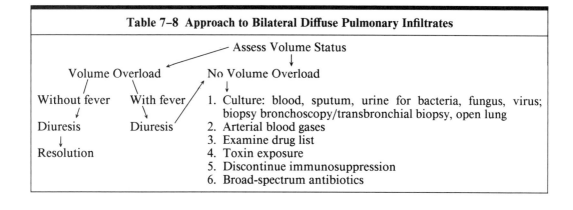

Table 7-8 Approach to Bilateral Diffuse Pulmonary Infiltrates

Assess Volume Status

Volume Overload / No Volume Overload

Without fever / With fever

Diuresis / Diuresis

Resolution

1. Culture: blood, sputum, urine for bacteria, fungus, virus; biopsy bronchoscopy/transbronchial biopsy, open lung
2. Arterial blood gases
3. Examine drug list
4. Toxin exposure
5. Discontinue immunosuppression
6. Broad-spectrum antibiotics

cystis, and many viruses—can produce a similar clinical picture. A nonspecific injury reaction such as seen with severe sepsis or shock, the so-called adult respiratory distress syndrome, can present similarly. Rarely some drugs, for example, cyclophosphamide, may cause bilateral pulmonary injury. Additionally, it is not uncommon for more than one of these factors to coexist. If the cause clinically appears to be simple volume overload, diuresis or ultrafiltration should result in rapid clearing of the chest radiograph as well as in symptomatic relief. Should this not occur, or if the diagnosis is not obvious on clinical grounds, an aggressive approach to diagnosis is mandated. Immunosuppression should be withdrawn. Sputum for Gram stain, special stains, and culture should be obtained. If the patient is unable to produce a sputum specimen, bronchoscopy with transbronchial biopsy as well as bronchial washing can be done. Portions should be sent for Gram, acid-fast fungal, Giemsa, and fluorescent Legionella stains. The examining pathologist should be notified of the specific suspected organisms. Arterial blood gas measurement will help determine the need for supplemental oxygen administration as well as indicate the severity of involvement. The mortality of bilateral pneumonia in this population is 50 percent,[170] underscoring the gravity of this situation. Antibiotic coverage should be started empirically to cover the most likely organisms, including Staphyloccocus, Pseudomonas and Pneumocystis in particular.

Other pulmonary infections such as abscess and empyema are seen less frequently. Pulmonary embolus may also occur during this time, but rarely.

Renal transplantation is but one of the therapeutic options for a patient with end stage renal disease (ESRD). This principle must be kept in mind, particularly when severe life-threatening complications of the transplant or the concomitant immunosuppression occur. Although it is disappointing for both the patient and the transplantation team for an allograft to fail, it is certainly in the patient's best interests to relinquish a transplanted kidney and return to dialysis in the face of a potentially fatal complication rather than to succumb to an infection with normal renal function. We recommend withdrawal of immuno-

suppression in the presence of central nervous system infection, septicemia, and pneumonia, either bilateral or unilateral with hypoxemia. These complications have exceptionally high mortality rates. Additionally disseminated CMV infection is immunosuppressive in and of itself and thus warrants consideration for immunosuppressive discontinuation. Finally, it is advisable to limit the number of major rejection episodes that will be treated over a defined period. Closely repetitive high-dose immunosuppressive regimens render the individual highly vulnerable to opportunistic infection and possibly later neoplastic disease. It is indeed a rare patient who cannot accept a second or third transplant after a time.

OUTPATIENT PERIOD

Routine Management

An uncomplicated posttransplantation course is gratifying both for the patient and for the responsible medical team. Patients almost immediately enjoy an improved sense of well being with resolution of the uremic state. There may be an augmentation of cardiac function, an increase in the hematocrit, and resolution of the uremic neuropathy. Fertility and sexual function are significantly ameliorated in comparison to that of dialysis patients. Additionally, there is a much better rehabilitation potential in the patient with a transplant.

In the initial few months outpatient clinic visits should be quite frequent for several reasons. The incidence of acute rejection is highest in the first 3 months. Frequent clinical and laboratory assessments are necessary to ensure the adequacy of immunosuppression and the absence of toxicity. As well, most patients require changes in other medications such as antihypertensives and antacids. This is also a time of emotional adjustment for most patients. During the frequent clinic visits of the first few months they have the opportunity to air their concerns about losing the kidney and about participating in exercise or other activities that may have been curtailed while they were on dialysis. For many individuals the resumption of a reasonably independent life carries as many fears as joys. Well established family structures may be disrupted by the vast changes in the patient's capabilities. For young adults, marital discord is quite common during this period. The close relationship established with the posttransplant team, physicians, nurses, and other paramedical personnel can be crucial in helping the individual cope with these changes. Frequently all that is needed is a sympathetic ear and reassurance that these feelings and fears are the rule and not the exception. In addition, these early frequent visits to clinic reinforce compliance with the medications and recognition of potential problems by the patients themselves.

The patient should be questioned specifically concerning the presence of potential infection. Fever, cough, sputum production, shortness of breath, headache, dysuria, or suprapubic pain should be included in the history. In addition one should investigate the pattern of urine output, any changes in the amount of urine output, pain over the transplant, or swelling. Finally, the patient should be questioned concerning toxicity of the medications, such as altered mental status, seizures, tremor, mouth sores, flushing around the face and neck, excessive hair growth, changes in body habitus, acne, abdominal pain, melena, or jaundice. Subjective fever may indicate infection, rejection, or drug reaction and should never be dismissed lightly.

Reasonably complete physical examinations should be performed on the patients early in their course because of the intensity of the immunosuppression at this stage. Specifically, one should examine the mouth for the presence of herpetic or candida infection. Gum hypertrophy may be seen with cyclosporine, signifying the need for dental intervention. Pulmonary and cardiac examinations are equally important in detecting early pneumonia or volume overload. The transplanted kidney should be examined to establish firmness, size, tenderness, and the presence or absence of a bruit. Finally edema should be noted, as it may suggest simple volume overload, hypoalbuminemia secondary to the development of the nephrotic syndrome, transplant failure, or thrombophlebitis.

Routine diagnostic laboratory evaluation should include BUN and creatinine deter-

minations with every clinic visit. During this period, rejection is most likely to occur and cyclosporine toxicity may occur with changing body metabolism or changing medication schedules. If the patient is receiving cyclosporine, complete blood count should be performed once or twice a month to monitor the recovery of the hematocrit and to alert one to the development of a gastrointestinal bleed or the hemolytic uremic syndrome associated with cyclosporine. If the patient is receiving azathioprine or cyclophosphamide, complete blood counts should be performed more regularly to monitor white cell count. Hypercalcemia and hypophosphatemia are fairly frequent post-transplantation, and calcium and phosphorus levels should be monitored at least once a week in the early post-transplant period. Liver function tests should also be checked at least once a week in the early months, as abnormalities may alert one to potential cyclosporine toxicity, azathioprine toxicity, or the development of a viral hepatitis. The role of serum or blood cyclosporine levels in the management of the outpatient is a subject of debate. Certainly if the patient experiences deterioration of renal function, liver function abnormalities, or other evidence of toxicity, a cyclosporine level may help confirm the clinical impression. There is emerging evidence that the lower the cyclosporine levels can be maintained, the less the cumulative renal damage that may occur. However, "safe" levels of the drug have not been established, and so the utility of levels is unclear.

Finally, urinalysis should be performed, with particular attention to protein excretion, at least once a week. An increase in protein excretion may signal the onset of rejection, the development of a recurrence of the original disease in the transplant, or the development of a de novo illness. While a 24-hour urine collection is the gold standard, just as much information about protein excretion may be gleaned from measurement of spot urine protein to creatinine ratio and at much greater convenience to the patient.[171] Certainly a urinalysis is indicated for the evaluation of failing renal function, symptoms of dysuria, or hematuria.

Other more specialized studies should be done as indicated. Radiographic examination of the kidney is indicated for the evaluation of failing renal function, hematuria, or pain in the graft itself. Routine yearly ultrasound is performed in some centers to detect early obstruction and to evaluate size. Arteriogram is indicated for the evaluation of new-onset or difficult-to-control hypertension, failing renal function in the absence of obstruction or rejection, or hematuria. Finally, biopsy may be performed as a routine aspect of posttransplantation follow-up of kidney function or in the evaluation of failing renal function or new onset nephrotic syndrome.

Complications

After the first few months, the incidence of acute rejection lessens significantly, and from that point onward, the follow-up is directed toward anticipation of the late complications of renal transplantation. These complications are primarily a result of the chronic steroid and immunosuppressive therapy and are discussed in Chapter 18.

REFERENCES

1. Marshall, VC: Renal preservation. In Morris, PJ (ed): Kidney Transplantation. ed 2, Grune & Stratton, New York, 1984, p 130.
2. Sacks, SA, Petritsch, PH, and Kaufman, JJ: Canine kidney perfusion using a new perfusate. Lancet 1:1024, 1973.
3. Jablonski, P, et al: Recovery of renal function after warm ischemia. Transplantation 35:535, 1983.
4. Pick, JW and Anson, BJ: The renal vascular pedicle: An anatomical study of 430 body-halves. J Urol 44:411, 1940.
5. Vineyard, GC and Tilney, NL: An effective technique for management of transplant kidneys with polar branches. Arch Surg 111:1407, 1976.
6. Salvatierra, O, et al: Urological complications can be prevented or controlled. J Urol 117:421, 1977.
7. Schiff, M and Lytton, B: Secondary ureteropyelostomy in renal transplant recipients. J Urol 126:723, 1981.
8. Kreis, H: Transplanted kidney: Natural history. In Hamburger, J, et al (eds): Renal Transplantation Theory and Practice, ed 2. Williams & Wilkins, Baltimore, 1981.
9. Carlier, M, et al: Maximal hydration during anesthesia increases pulmonary arterial pressures and improves early function of human renal transplants. Transplantation 34:201, 1982.
10. Palmer, RF and Lass, KC: Sodium nitroprusside. N Engl J Med 292:294, 1975.
11. Livio, M, Benigui, A, and Remuzzi, G: Coagulation abnormalities in uremia. Seminars in Nephrology 5:82, 1985.
12. Mannucci, PM, et al: Deamino-8-D-arginine vasopressin shortens the bleeding time in uremia. N Engl J Med 308:8, 1983.
13. Hirshmann, CA, and Edelstein, G: Intraoperative hyperkalemia and cardiac arrests during renal transplantation in an insulin-dependent diabetic patient. Anesthesiology 51:161, 1979.
14. Judson, RT: Wound infection following renal transplantation. Aust NZ J Med 54:223, 1984.
15. Schweitzer, R, Kountz, S, and Belzer, F: Wound complications in recipients of renal transplants. Ann Surg 177:58, 1973.
16. Tilney, N, et al: Factors contributing to the declining mortality rate in renal transplantation. N Engl J Med 299:1321, 1978.
17. Muakkassa, WF, et al: Wound infections in renal transplant patients. J Urol 130:17, 1983.
18. Novick, AC: The value of intraoperative antibiotics in preventing renal transplant wound infections. J Urol 125:151, 1981.
19. Tillegard, A: Renal transplant wound infection: The value of prophylactic antibiotic treatment. Scand J Urol Nephrol 18:215, 1984.
20. Messer, J, et al: Association of adrenocorticosteroid therapy and peptic ulcer disease. N Engl J Med 309:21, 1983.
21. Cohen, EB, et al: Unexpectedly high incidence of cytomegalovirus infection in apparent peptic ulcers in renal transplant recipients. Surgery 97:606, 1985.
22. Garvin, PJ, et al: Peptic ulcer disease following transplantation: The role of cimetidine. Am J Surg 144:545, 1982.
23. Sarosdy, MF, et al: Upper gastrointestinal bleeding following renal transplantation. Urology 26:347, 1985.
24. Haffner, JFW, Jakobsen, A, and Flatmark, AL: Upper gastrointestinal bleeding in renal transplant recipients: The role of prophylactic gastric surgery. World J Surg 7:738, 1983.
25. Grekas, D, et al: Prophylactic treatment with cimetidine after renal transplantation. Nephron 40:213, 1985.
26. Isenberg, JI, et al: Healing of benign gastric ulcer with low dose antacid or cimetidine. N Engl J Med 308:1319, 1983.
27. Ivarsson, LE: Antacids and H2-receptor antagonists in the prophylaxis and treatment

of erosive gastritis: Clinical aspects. Scand J Gastroenterol 105 Suppl:86, 1984.

28. Schiessel, R, et al: Failure of cimetidine to prevent gastroduodenal ulceration and bleeding after renal transplantation. Surgery 90:456, 1981.

29. Walter, S, et al: Effect of cimetidine on upper gastrointestinal bleeding after renal transplantation: A prospective study. Br Med J 289:1175, 1984.

30. Finkelstein, W and Isselbacher, KJ: Cimetidine. N Engl J Med 299:992, 1978.

31. Kaye, WA, et al: Cimetidine induced interstitial nephritis with response to prednisone therapy. Arch Intern Med 143:811, 1983.

32. Avella, J, et al: Effect of histamine H-2 receptor antagonists on delayed hypersensitivity. Lancet 1:624, 1978.

33. Gifford, RRM, Hatfield, SM, and Schmidtke, JR: Cimetidine induced augmentation of human lymphocyte blastogenesis by mitogen, bacterial antigen and alloantigen. Transplantation 29:143, 1980.

34. Zammit, M, and Toledo-Pereyra, LH: Cimetidine for kidney transplantation: Experimental observation. Surgery 86:611, 1979.

35. Ahonen, J, et al: Ranitidine and cimetidine in renal transplantation: A clinical trial. Int J Tissue React 5:373, 1983.

36. Van Roermund, HPC, et al: Cimetidine prophylaxis after renal transplantation. Clin Nephrol 18:39, 1982.

37. Zeldis, JB, Freidman, LS, and Isselbacher, KJ: Ranitidine: A new H2 receptor antagonist. N Engl J Med 309:1360, 1983.

38. Ahonen, J, et al: Peptic ulceration in kidney transplantation. Proc Eur Dial Transplant Assoc 14:396, 1977.

39. Feldman, M and Richardson, CT: Total 24-hour gastric acid secretion in patients with duodenal ulcer. Gastroenterology 90:540, 1986.

40. Vincenti, F, Parfery, PS, and Briggs, W: Skeletal, gastrointestinal, hepatic, and hematologic disorders following kidney transplantation. In Garovoy, MR and Guttmann, RD (eds): Renal Transplantation. Churchill Livingstone, New York, 1986.

41. Briggs, JD: The recipient of a renal transplant. In Morris, PJ (ed): Kidney Transplantation, ed 2. Grune & Stratton, New York, 1984.

42. Vidne, BA, et al: Vascular complications in human renal transplantation. Surgery 79:77, 1976.

43. Thukral, R, Mir, AR, and Jacobson, MP: Renal allograft rupture: A report of three cases and review of the literature. Am J Nephrol 2:15, 1982.

44. Jordan, ML, Cook, GT, and Cardella, CJ: Ten years experience with vascular complications in renal transplantation. J Urol 128:689, 1982.

45. Merion, RM and Calne, RY: Allograft renal vein thrombosis. Transplant Proc 17:1746, 1985.

46. Schlanger, RE, et al: Identification and treatment of cyclosporine-associated allograft thrombosis. Surgery 99:329, 1986.

47. Anderson, CB, Sicard, GA, and Etheredge, EE: Delayed graft function and long term cadaver renal allograft survival. Transplant Proc 11:482, 1979.

48. Canadian Study Group: A randomized clinical trial of cyclosporine in cadaveric renal transplantation. N Engl J Med 309:809, 1983.

49. Brophy, D, Najarian, JS and Kjellstrand, CM: Acute tubular necrosis after renal transplantation. Transplantation 29:245, 1980.

50. Cho, SI, et al: Regional program for kidney preservation and transplantation in New England. Am J Surg 131:428, 1976.

51. Ferguson, RM, et al: Cyclosporin A in renal transplantation: A prospective randomized trial. Surgery 92:175, 1982.

52. Flechner, SM, et al: The effect of cyclosporine on early graft function in human renal transplantation. Transplantation 36:268, 1983.

53. Najarian, JS, et al: A prospective trial of the efficacy of cyclosporine in renal transplantation at the University of Minnesota. Transplant Proc 15:438, 1983.

54. Salmela, K, et al: Rejection and early nonfunction in renal allografts. Transplant Proc 18:77, 1986.

55. Barry, JM, Norman, DJ, and Bennett, WM: Pediatric cadaver kidney transplants into adults. J Urol 134:651, 1985.

56. Bollinger, RR, et al: The impact of donor renal abnormalities in cadaveric transplantation. Transplant Proc 18:459, 1986.

57. Dafoe, DC, Campbell, DA, and Turcotte, JG: Use of single kidneys from donors two to five years of age for transplantation into nonpediatric recipients. Transplant Proc 18:477, 1986.

58. Fedusha, NJ, et al: Analysis of some factors that might affect the outcome for cadaveric kidney transplants in cyclosporine treated patients. Transplant Proc 18:519, 1986.

59. Neumayer, HH, et al: Factors influencing primary kidney graft function. Transplant Proc 18:506, 1986.

60. Ontario Renal Transplant Research Group: Factors contributing to primary non-function of cadaveric kidney transplants. Transplant Proc 18:516, 1986.

61. Sanfilippo, F, et al: The detrimental effects

of delayed graft function in cadaver donor renal transplantation. Transplantation 38:643, 1984.

62. Sarparanta, T, et al: The effect of long cold ischemia time on primary and secondary cadaver renal allografts. Transplant Proc 18:80, 1986.

63. Whelchel, JD, et al: The effect of high dose dopamine in cadaver donor management on delayed graft function and graft survival following renal transplantation. Transplant Proc 18:523, 1986.

64. Toledo-Pereyra, LH: Effect of multiple organ harvesting on subsequent renal function. Transplant Proc 18:434, 1986.

65. Santiago-Delphin, EA: Pharmacological principles. In Toledo-Pereyra, LH (ed): Basic Concepts of Organ Procurement, Perfusion, and Preservation for Transplantation. Academic Press, Orlando, FL, 1982, p 73.

66. Diethelm, AG, et al: Large volume diuresis as a mechanism for immediate maximum renal function after transplantation: Surg Gynecol Obstet 138:869, 1974.

67. Grecn, RD, et al: Pharmacological protection of rabbit kidneys from normothermic ischemia. Transplantation 28:131, 1979.

68. Moreno, M, Murphy, C, and Goldsmith, C: Increase in serum potassium resulting from the administration of hypertonic mannitol and other solutions. J Lab Clin Med 73:291, 1969.

69. Kaplan, MP, et al: Effect of furosemide and/or mannitol on the immediate function of preserved cadaver kidneys: A prospective double blind and randomized study: Preliminary observations. Transplant Proc 18:504, 1986.

70. LaChance, SL and Barry, JM: Effect of furosemide on dialysis requirement following cadaveric kidney transplantation. J Urol 133:950, 1985.

71. Wagner, K, Albrecht, S, and Neumayer, HH: Prevention of delayed graft function in cadaveric kidney transplantation by a calcium antagonist: Preliminary results of two prospective randomized trials. Transplant Proc 18:510, 1986.

72. Bear, R, Walker, F, and Lang, A: Prolonged oliguric renal failure related to cyclosporin A in a renal transplant recipient. Am J Nephrol 3:293, 1983.

73. Siekert, W, et al: Cyclosporine A in kidney-transplanted patients without initial diuresis. Transplant Proc 16:285, 1984.

74. Winchester, JF, et al: Early indicators of renal allograft rejection. Kidney Int 23 (Suppl 14):534, 1983.

75. Salomon, D, and Strom, TB: Diagnosis and treatment of rejection. In Garovoy, MR and Guttman, RD (eds): Renal Transplantation. Churchill Livingstone 1986, p 143.

76. Gillum, DM and Kelleher, SP: Acute pyelonephritis as a cause of late transplant dysfunction. Am J Med 78:156, 1985.

77. Ramsey, DE, Finch, WT, and Birtch, AG: Urinary tract infections in kidney transplant recipients. Arch Surg 114:1022, 1979.

78. Rubin, RH, et al: Usefulness of the antibody-coated bacteria assay in the management of urinary tract infections in the renal transplant patient. Transplantation 27:18, 1979.

79. Mihatsch, MJ, et al: Morphological patterns in cyclosporine-treated renal transplant recipients. Transplant Proc 17 (Suppl 1):101, 1985.

80. Wallace, AC: Histopathology of cyclosporine. Transplant Proc 17 (Suppl 1):117, 1985.

81. Sullivan, BA, Hak, LJ, and Finn, WF: Cyclosporine nephrotoxicity: Studies in laboratory animals. Transplant Proc 17 (Suppl 1):145, 1985.

82. Paller, MS, and Murray, BM: Renal dysfunction in animal models of cyclosporine toxicity. Transplant Proc 17 (Suppl 1):155, 1985.

83. Keown, PA, et al: Interaction between phenytoin and cyclosporine following organ transplantation. Transplantation 38:304, 1984.

84. Burckart, GJ, et al: Cyclosporine clearance in children following organ transplantation. J Clin Pharmacol 24:412, 1984.

85. Langhoff, E, and Madsen, S: Rapid metabolism of cyclosporin and prednisone in kidney transplant patient receiving tuberculostatic treatment. Lancet 2:1031, 1983.

86. Van Buren, D, et al: The antagonistic effect of rifampin upon cyclosporine bioavailability. Transplant Proc 16:1642, 1984.

87. Ferguson, RM, et al: Ketoconazole, cyclosporine, metabolism, and renal transplantation. Lancet 2:882, 1982.

88. Gonwa, TA, et al: Erythromycin and cyclosporine. Transplantation 41:797, 1986.

89. Martell, R, et al: The effects of erythromycin in patients treated with cyclosporin. Annals Intern Med 104:660, 1986.

90. Freeman, DJ, et al: Ann R Coll Physicians Surg Can 17:301, 1984.

91. Morgenstern, GR, et al: Cyclosporin interaction with ketoconazole and melphalan. Lancet 2:1342, 1982.

92. Wallwork, J, et al: Cyclosporin and intravenous sulphadimidine and trimethoprim therapy. Lancet 1:366, 1983.

93. Thompson, JF, et al: Nephrotoxicity of trimethoprim and cotrimoxazole in renal al-

lograft recipients treated with cyclosporine. Transplantation 36:204, 1983.

94. Hows, JM, et al: Serum levels of cyclosporin A and nephrotoxicity in bone marrow transplant patients. Lancet 2:145, 1981.
95. Kennedy, MS, et al: Acute renal toxicity with combined use of amphotericin band cyclosporine after marrow transplantation. Transplantation 35:211, 1983.
96. Whiting, PH and Simpson, JG: The enhancement of cyclosporine A induced nephrotoxicity by gentamicin. Biochem Pharmacol 32:2025, 1983.
97. Clive, DM and Stoff, JS: Renal syndromes associated with nonsteroidal anti-inflammatory drugs. N Engl J Med 310:563, 1984.
98. Burdick, JF, et al: Characteristics of early routine renal allograft biopsies. Transplantation 38:679, 1984.
99. Matas, AJ, et al: The value of needle renal allograft biopsy: III. A prospective study. Surgery. 98:922, 1985.
100. Parfrey, PS, et al: The diagnostic and prognostic value of renal allograft biopsy. Transplantation 38:586, 1984.
101. Vangelista, A, et al: Graft biopsy in renal transplantation: Correlation with clinical, immunological, and virological investigation. Kidney Int 23 (Suppl)14:541, 1985.
102. Talseth, T, et al: Prognostic information in biopsies of transplanted kidneys with unsatisfactory response to anti-rejection therapy. Transplant Proc 19:1623, 1987.
103. Mozes, MF, et al: The prognostic value of the post rejection treatment biopsy in renal transplantation. Transplant Proc 19:1625, 1987.
104. Von Willebrand, E and Hayry, P: Reproducibility of the fine needle aspiration biopsy. Transplantation 38:314, 1984.
105. Helderman, JH, et al: Confirmation of the utility of the fine needle aspiration biopsy of the transplanted kidney. Transplant Proc 19:1653, 1987.
106. Belitsky, P, Gupta, R, and Campbell, J: Diagnosis of acute cellular rejection in kidney allograft by fine needle aspiration cytology. Transplant Proc 16:1076, 1984.
107. Nelson, PW, et al: Unsuspected donor pseudomonas infection causing arterial disruption after renal transplantation. Transplantation 37:313, 1984.
108. Majeshi, JA, et al: Transplantation of microbially contaminated cadaver kidneys. Arch Surg 117:221, 1982.
109. Spees, EK, et al: Experiences with cadaver renal allograft contamination before transplantation. Br J Surg 69:482, 1982.
110. Van der Vliet, JA, et al: Transplantation of contaminated organs. Br J Surg 67:596, 1980.
111. Weber, TR, Freier, DT, and Turcotte, DG: Transplantation of infected kidneys. Transplantation 27:63, 1979.
112. Odenheimer, DB, et al: Donor cultures reported positive after transplantation: A clinical dilemma. Transplant Proc 18:465, 1986.
113. Rattazzi, LC: Fatal post transplant infection transmitted with the kidney graft. Dialysis and Transplantation 15:92, 1986.
114. Holmgren, J and Smith, JW: Immunological aspects of urinary tract infections. Prog Allergy 18:289, 1975.
115. Byrd, LH, et al: Association between streptococcus faecalis urinary infections and graft rejection in kidney transplantation. Lancet 2:1167, 1978.
116. Levine, AS, et al: Protected environments and prophylactic antibiotics. N Engl J Med 288:177, 1973.
117. Gurwith, MJ, et al: A prospective controlled investigation of prophylactic trimethoprim/sulfamethoxazole in hospitalized granulocytopenic patients. Am J Med 66:248, 1979.
118. Nauseef, WM and Maki, DG: A study of the value of simple protective isolation in patients with granulocytopenia. N Engl J Med 304:448, 1987.
119. Dekker, AW, et al: Prevention of infection by trimethoprim-sulfamethoxazole plus amphotericin B in patients with acute nonlymphocytic leukaemia. Ann Intern Med 95:555, 1981.
120. Kramer, BS, et al: Role of serial microbiologic surveillance and clinical evaluation in the management of cancer patients with fever and pancytopenia. Am J Med 72:561, 1982.
121. Kauffman, CA, et al: Trimethoprim/sulfamethoxazole prophylaxis in neutropenic patients. Am J Med 74:599, 1983.
122. Bodey, GP and Rosenbaum, B: Effect of prophylactic measures on the microbial flora of patients in protected environment units. Medicine 53:209, 1974.
123. Edwards, JE, et al: Severe candidal infections. Ann Intern Med 89:91, 1978.
124. Felice, G, Yee, B, and Armstrong, D: Immunodiffusion and agglutination tests for candida in patients with neoplastic disease: Inconsistent correlation of results with invasive infections. J Infect Dis 135:349, 1977.
125. Case Records, Case 24, 1984. N Engl J Med 310:1584, 1984.
126. Wheat, LJ, et al: Histoplasmosis in renal allograft recipients. Arch Intern Med 143:703, 1983.

127. McClellan, SL, et al: Severe bleeding diathesis associated with invasive aspergillosis in transplant patients. Transplantation 39:406, 1985.
128. Watson, AJ, Whelton, A, and Russell, RP: Cure of cryptococcemia and preservation of graft function in a renal transplant recipient. Arch Intern Med 144:1877, 1984.
129. Peterson, PK, et al: Infectious diseases in hospitalized renal transplant recipients: A prospective study of a complex and evolving problem. Medicine 61:360, 1982.
130. Peterson, PK, et al: Fever in renal transplant recipients: Causes, prognostic significance and changing patterns at the University of Minnesota Hospital. Am J Med 71:346, 1981.
131. Morales, LA, Gonzalez, ZA, and Santiago-Delpin, EA: Chromoblastomycosis in a renal transplant patient. Nephron 40:238, 1985.
132. Charpentier, B: Viral infections in renal transplant recipients: An evolutionary problem. Adv Nephrol 15:353, 1986.
133. Hogan, TF, et al: Human polyomavirus infections with JC virus and BK virus in renal transplant patients. Ann Intern Med 92:373, 1980.
134. Kalb, RE, and Grossman, ME: Chronic perianal herpes simplex in immunocompromised hosts. Am J Med 80:486, 1986.
135. Rubin, RH, et al: Multicenter seroepidemiologic study of the impact of cytomegalovirus infection on renal transplantation. Transplantation 40:243, 1985.
136. Schooley, RT, et al: Association of herpes virus infections with T-lymphocyte-subset alterations glomerulopathy, and opportunistic infections after renal transplantation. N Engl J Med 308:307, 1983.
137. Balfour, HA, et al: Burroughs Wellcome Collaborative Acyclovir Study Group: Acylcovir halts progression of herpes zoster in immunocompromised patients. N Engl J Med 308:1448, 1983.
138. Griffin, PJA, et al: Oral acyclovir prophylaxis of herpes infections in renal transplant recipients. Transplant Proc 17:84, 1985.
139. Pettersson, E, et al: Prophylactic oral acyclovir after renal transplantation. Transplantation 39:279, 1985.
140. Seale, L, et al: Prevention of herpesvirus infections in renal allograft recipients by low dose oral acyclovir. JAMA 254:3425, 1985.
141. Straus, SE, et al: Suppression of frequently recurring genital herpes. N Engl J Med 310:1545, 1984.
142. Broyer, M and Boudaillez, B: Prevention of varicella infection in renal transplanted children by previous immunization with a live attenuated varicella vaccine. Transplant Proc 17:151, 1985.
143. Hamilton, JD: CMV infection in renal allograft recipients. In Melnick JL (ed): Monographs in Virology, vol 12, 1982, p 31.
144. Peterson, PK, et al: Cytomegalovirus disease in renal allograft recipients: A prospective study of the clinical features, risk factors and impact on renal transplantation. Medicine 59:283, 1980.
145. Fryd, DS, et al: Cytomegalovirus as a risk factor in renal transplantation. Transplantation 30:436, 1980.
146. Luby, JP, et al: Disease due to cytomegalovirus and its long-term consequences in renal transplant recipients. Arch Intern Med 143:1126, 1983.
147. Riaudet, P, et al: Serological status of cytomegalovirus and outcome of renal transplantation. Kidney Int 23 (Suppl)14:550, 1983.
148. Tourkantonis, A, and Lazaridis, A: Interaction between cytomegalovirus infection and renal transplant rejection. Kidney Int (Suppl)14:S46, 1983.
149. Flechner, SM, Novick, AC, and Steinmuller, R: Improved cadaver allograft survival in transfused recipients who remain serologically negative for cytomegalovirus. J Urol 127:644, 1982.
150. Chatterjee, S, et al: Association of immune responses to cytomegalovirus infection with survival of renal allografts. J Urol 124:448, 1980.
151. Collaborative DHPG Treatment Study Group: Treatment of serious cytomegalovirus infections with 9-91, 3-Dihydroxy-2-Propoxymethyl) guanine in patients with AIDS and other immunodeficiencies. N Engl J Med 314:801, 1986.
152. Blacklock, HA, et al: Successful treatment of cytomegalovirus pneumonitis after allogeneic bone marrow transplantation using high titer CMV immunoglobulin (Cytotect). Exp Hematol 13 (Suppl 17):76, 1985.
153. Gluckman, E, et al: Prophylaxis of herpes infections after bone marrow transplantation by oral acyclovir. Lancet 2:706, 1983.
154. Meyers, JD, et al: Prevention of cytomegalovirus infection by cytomegalovirus immune globulin after marrow transplantation. Ann Intern Med 90:442, 1983.
155. Rogers, TR, et al: A trial of intravenous immunoglobulin for prevention of CMV infection after marrow transplantation. Exp Hematol (Suppl 17)13:77, 1985.
156. Winston, DJ, et al: Cytomegalovirus immune plasma in bone marrow transplant recipients. Ann Intern Med 97:11, 1982.
157. Hanshaw, JB: Prevention of cytomegalovi-

rus disease following renal transplantation. Am J Dis Child 131:841, 1977.

158. Glazer, JP, et al: Live cytomegalovirus vaccination of renal transplant candidates. Ann Int Med 91:676, 1979.

159. Hardy, AM, et al: *Pneumocystis carinii* pneumonia in renal-transplant recipients treated with cyclosporin and steroids. J Infect Dis 149:143, 1984.

160. Joss, DV, Barrett, AJ, and Kendra, JR: Hypertension and convulsions in children receiving cyclosporin A. Lancet 1:906, 1982.

161. Nordal, KP, et al: Aluminum overload: A predisposing condition for epileptic seizures in renal-transplant patients treated with cyclosporin. Lancet 2:153, 1985.

162. Atkinson, K, et al: Cyclosporine-associated central nervous system toxicity after allogeneic bone marrow. Transplantation 38:34, 1984.

163. Thompson, CB, et al: Association between cyclosporin neurotoxicity and hypomagnesemia. Lancet 2:1116, 1984.

164. June, CH, et al: Profound hypomagnesemia and renal magnesium wasting associated with the use of cyclosporine for marrow transplantation. Transplantation 39:620, 1985.

165. Curtis, JJ: Hypertension and kidney transplantation. Am J Kid Dis 7:181, 1986.

166. Gunnarsson, R, et al: Acute myocardial infarction in renal transplant recipients: Incidence and prognosis. Eur Heart J 5:218, 1984.

167. Morrow, CE, et al: Predictive value of thallium stress testing for coronary and cardiovascular events in uremic diabetic patients before renal transplantation. Am J Surg 146:331, 1983.

168. Weinrauch, LA, et al: Asymptomatic coronary artery disease: Angiographic assessment of diabetes evaluated for renal transplantation. Circulation 50:1184, 1978.

169. Philipson, JD, et al: Evaluation of cardiovascular risk for renal transplantation in diabetic patients. Am J Med 81:630, 1986.

170. Ramsey, PG, et al: The renal transplant patient with fever and pulmonary infiltrates: Etiology, clinical manifestations, and management. Medicine 59:206, 1980.

171. Ginsberg, JM, et al: Use of single voided urine samples to estimate quantitative proteinuria. N Engl J Med 309:1543, 1983.

172. Agatstein, EH, Farrer, JH, Kaplan, LM, Randazzo, RF, Glassock, RJ, and Kaufman, JJ: The effect of verapamil in reducing the severity of acute tubular necrosis in canine renal autotransplants. Transplantation 44:355, 1987.

173. Zarrabi, MH and Rosner, F: Serious infections in adults following splenectomy for trauma. Arch Intern Med 144:1421, 1984.

Chapter 8

Hypertension, Diabetes, and Cardiovascular Disease

DONALD R. STEINMULLER

PRETRANSPLANTATION HYPERTENSION

Incidence and Etiology

Hypertension is frequently associated with kidney failure. Eighty to 90 percent of patients with end stage renal disease (ESRD) at the onset of dialysis have an elevated blood pressure for their age and sex. Both systolic and diastolic blood pressure are usually elevated. The causes of hypertension associated with renal disease are multifactorial. Table 8-1 outlines the various factors that may play a role in these patients.

The primary disease process may effect some of these factors more than others. Glomerular disease and vascular disease (vasculitis, hemolytic-uremic syndrome, renal artery stenosis) are associated with an increase in salt and water reabsorption in the remaining nephron segments, and these diseases are often associated with salt and water retention and edema. Hypertension may be related predominately to this factor.[1] Renin release is often stimulated by these diseases (especially vascular diseases) and may contribute to the hypertension.[1,2] Some interstitial diseases not associated with salt and water retention may be associated with a certain obligatory salt and water loss. When ESRD develops, however, even these diseases are often associated with hypertension, again due to a combination of factors.

Therapy of Pretransplantation Hypertension

Since hypertension accelerates the progression of kidney disease in both animals[3] and humans,[4,5] control of hypertension is important in order to preserve function in a diseased kidney. This is true no matter what the cause of the kidney disease.[6] Thus, most patients approaching end-stage renal disease have been maintained on antihypertensive drug therapy in order to normalize the blood pressure. The goal blood pressure for renal failure patients is the same as the goal blood pressure for individuals with normal renal function—140/90 or lower.

The drugs used are also similar, but there are special considerations with renal failure. Loop diuretics are often needed before dialysis is instituted to maintain salt and water balance. Often high doses (up to 400 mg of furosemide per day) are needed. Thiazide diuretics are ineffective as diuretics when GFR falls below 30 to 50 percent of normal, although they may still maintain some antihypertensive effect.[7] Beta blockers, alpha blockers, vasodilators, angiotension converting enzyme (ACE) inhibitors, and sympathetic antagonists can all be used with renal failure, although some agents require dosage adjustments[8] and some, such as the ACE inhibitor captopril, may have more risk of toxicity in renal failure.[9]

After the initiation of dialysis, blood pressure control generally improves.[1] This may be due to effective removal of extracellular fluid volume and attainment of dry weight. Also, it is possible that dialyzable pressor substances are removed by the dialysis process, although these factors remain unidentified. The severity of the hypertension can be best assessed by reviewing the blood pressure control and drug requirements after stabilization on dialysis.

The role of pretransplant nephrectomy for the pretransplantation and posttrans-

---

Table 8–1 Etiologic Conditions and Contributing Factors to Hypertension with Renal Failure

Associated primary hypertension
Impairment of the normal pressure-natriuresis response
Extracellular fluid volume excess due to inability of the kidney to maintain sodium balance
Excess or inappropriate activity of the renin, angiotensin, aldosterone system secondary to the kidney disease
Impairment of the normal function of renal vasodilatory hormones—prostaglandins, kinins, kallikrein
Associated abnormalities of renal failure with potential deleterious effect on hypertension—↑PTH, ↑uric acid

plantation control of hypertension is controversial. In the 1960s and early 1970s, bilateral nephrectomy was often performed if a patient's blood pressure remained uncontrolled on maintenance dialysis. It was believed that the diseased kidneys could still be producing excessive renin and aggravate the hypertension on that basis, even with control of fluid balance on dialysis. Studies[1] have documented the benefit of bilateral nephrectomy on blood pressure control. Even if the renin activity were normal or low, some patients had improvement of blood pressure control after bilateral nephrectomy. The mechanism for this is unclear, and nonspecific effects of surgery or dietary changes after nephrectomy may be responsible for this.

The procedure of bilateral nephrectomy has significant morbidity and mortality associated with it. Mortality ranges from 2 to 16 percent;[10-16] diabetics with diabetic nephropathy and patients with polycystic kidney disease have a higher risk. Bleeding and infectious complications are more common in the presence of renal failure and can complicate this procedure. Hyperkalemia can occur within hours after bilateral nephrectomy and can be fatal if not identified and treated promptly and effectively. The loss of all urine output and thus any elimination of potassium, the catabolism associated with the trauma and stress of surgery, and sometimes other factors (such as diabetes or iatrogenic potassium administration) make this clinical setting particularly conducive to the development of severe life-threatening hyperkalemia.

There are also long-term sequelae of bilateral nephrectomy. The loss of erythropoietin production aggravates the anemia of renal failure. Despite ESRD, most dialysis patients have an elevated erythropoietin level, although not as high as expected for the degree of anemia. After bilateral nephrectomy anemia worsens, often increasing the requirements for blood transfusions. Although pretransplantation blood transfusions improve the chance of success for cadaver transplantation (with both conventional and cyclosporine immunosuppressive therapy), blood transfusions, especially in excessively large numbers, have definite risks for patients maintained on dialysis. Hepatitis, AIDS, and other infectious illnesses can be transmitted. Also, repetitive transfusions can cause iron over-

load and hepatic and bone disease associated with hemochromatosis. Transfusions also increase the risk of sensitization in the potential transplant recipient.

After bilateral nephrectomy, dialysis may be more difficult. Dialysis time may need to be increased due to the loss of whatever residual GFR was present in the native kidneys. Dietary restriction of sodium, potassium, protein, and fluid may need to be more severe to make up for amounts excreted in any remaining urine output. The requirement for more aggressive fluid and solute removal during dialysis may also increase symptoms associated with the disequilibrium of dialysis.

On the positive side, pretransplantation bilateral nephrectomy can make post-transplantation management easier. The urine output and any abnormalities (proteinuria, cylinduria, pyuria, hematuria) can be isolated to the transplanted kidney. When the native kidneys remain intact posttransplantation, these parameters are not very useful, since the contribution of native and transplant kidneys is uncertain. Also, pretransplantation nephrectomy may be associated with improved graft survival posttransplantation,[17] although it is difficult to separate this factor from associated factors that can improve graft success, such as pretransplantation transfusion, splenectomy, and patient selection.

Overall, the disadvantages of bilateral nephrectomy as an adjunctive procedure for hypertension control outweigh the benefits unless the blood pressure cannot be managed in any other fashion. Fortunately, better dialysis techniques and drug therapy have enabled nephrologists to control hypertension in almost all renal failure patients. More efficient dialysis and newer techniques of CAPD and hemofiltration reduce the incidence of hypertension refractory to dialysis therapy. The availability of the potent vasodilator minoxidil has reduced the number of dialysis patients refractory to drug therapy. The blood pressure of almost all patients can be controlled by combining minoxidil in appropriate doses with a beta blocker or sympathetic antagonist.[18] One of the latter agents is needed to control the tachycardia associated with the vasodilation produced by minoxidil. Edema due to minoxidil can be controlled with effective fluid removal on dialysis and dietary restriction. Hirsutism, however, may limit its use, particularly in women.

Due to these considerations, pretransplantation bilateral nephrectomy for control of hypertension is rarely performed at the present time.

POSTTRANSPLANTATION HYPERTENSION

Incidence and Etiology

Hypertension is common after renal transplantation, its incidence ranging from 25 to 80 percent.[19-22] A variety of factors may play a role in causing or aggravating posttransplantation hypertension. Table 8–2 outlines those factors.

The two most important clinical features that directly relate to the incidence of hypertension are the degree of renal functional impairment and the presence of the native kidneys. There is a relationship between improved renal function and decreased incidence and severity of hypertension.[35] This is to be expected due to the high incidence of hypertension in association with renal insufficiency in the nontransplant population. Even if the transplanted kidney functions normally, there may be a slight increased tendency to have hypertension. After unilateral nephrectomy, normal kidney donors may have a slightly higher blood pressure in some long-term follow-up studies.[36,37] Other studies[38,39] have not confirmed this, however.

The presence of the native kidneys increases the incidence of posttransplantation hypertension.[20,21,30,31] This may be mediated through the renin-angiotensin system or possibly other mechanisms.

The use of cyclosporine is associated with an increase in blood pressure. This has been documented in nontransplant patients and non–renal transplant patients treated with this agent. The effect on blood pressure in these patients is shown in Table 8–3. The effect is mild in renal transplant recipients, but more significant in heart transplant patients. In renal transplant patients the effect of cyclosporine on blood pressure is difficult to document. Reducing the risk of rejection, may provide less risk of hypertension because of better maintenance of renal function and the prevention of other effects of rejection that may aggravate hypertension. The mechanism responsible for an increase in blood pressure with cyclosporine is not clear. Long-term studies show a decrease in the renin-angiotensin system. Cyclosporine is associated with a decrease in GFR, possibly on a hemodynamic or vascular basis. This could relate to the increase in blood pressure, although the exact pathophysiology has not been elucidated. There are also vascular effects of cyclosporine that may relate to an increase in blood pressure. Some patients have developed an arteriopathy with fibrin deposits similar to the lesions seen with the hemolytic-uremic syndrome.

Both acute and chronic rejection are associated with hypertension in the transplant recipient. This may be related in part to the loss of renal function associated with rejection. However, hypertension may precede the loss of renal function seen with acute rejection. With chronic rejection hypertension may be out of proportion to the

---

Table 8–2 Etiologic Conditions and Contributing Factors to Hypertension Post Renal Transplantation

Associated primary hypertension[21] (recipient and/or donor[23])

Renal insufficiency of the transplanted kidney due to rejection[21,24,25] or other causes resulting in excessive renin activity, abnormal pressure—natriuresis response, and/or abnormal vasodilatory hormone activity[26]

Acute and chronic rejection[21,24,25]

The effect of corticosteroids[27]

Stenosis of the arterial supply of the transplanted kidney[24,28,29]

The presence of the diseased native kidneys[20,22,30-32]

Extracellular fluid volume excess due to inability of the transplanted kidney to maintain sodium balance due to the effect of medications (steroids),[27] or to excessive dietary intake[33]

The effect of cyclosporine[34]

Table 8–3 Effect of Cyclosporine on Blood Pressure			
Type of Patient	BP with Cyclosporine	BP Controls	Reference
Heart transplant	115 (mean)	95 (mean)	40
Renal transplant	143/91	134/86	34

change in renal function. The pathophysiology of hypertension secondary to rejection is probably related to the small vessel ischemia present with both types of rejection. Acute rejection results in ischemia due to edema and the presence of interstitial infiltrates with or without a vascular inflammatory process. Increased salt and water reabsorption in the kidney and retention in the patient are manifestations of this ischemia. It also aggravates the blood pressure elevation. Renin release and other hormonal changes may play a secondary role. In chronic rejection there is vascular sclerosis with obliteration of the vascular lumen and subsequent ischemia leading to similar events.

Stenosis of the arterial supply to the transplanted kidney is a rare cause of posttransplantation hypertension. The incidence of this problem varies from 5 to 50 percent.[24,28,29,41–45] The stenosis usually occurs months to years after the transplantation. The cause of the stenosis may be any one or more of the following:[45]

1. Technical problem due to a poor anastomosis or kinking of the blood vessels
2. Atherosclerosis of the native or transplant vessels
3. Intimal damage to the transplanted artery, occurring at the time of harvesting or preservation
4. Fibrosis around the vessels due to infection or idiopathic causes
5. Stenosis due to fibrinoid deposition in the transplanted artery, possibly secondary to rejection

Angiographic demonstration of the stenosis may help to determine the cause. Digital subtraction angiography after a venous injection is often unsuccessful in visualizing the vessels due to overlap of vessels and poor renal blood flow.[46]

The presence or absence of a bruit over the graft is not a reliable indication of a stenotic lesion. Bruits are present when there is a large blood flow across the anastomosis.[47] Most grafts with normal function and normal blood flow exhibit a systolic bruit. The presence of a diastolic component to the bruit may be more specific for transplant renal artery stenosis, as is the case with renal artery stenosis of the native kidneys. Determination of renin activity or response of hypertension to angiotensin inhibition is not helpful in the diagnosis of transplant renal artery stenosis. Other factors may increase renin activity, resulting in false positive results.[22,48]

Excessive dietary intake of sodium[33] may aggravate underlying posttransplantation hypertension. Increased appetite due to correction of the renal failure and the use of corticosteroids make adherence to dietary restriction more difficult. For some patients who have had problems with dietary excess in the past, this may be a very difficult problem, leading to excess weight gain. Increasing weight also will aggravate posttransplantation hypertension.[35]

Therapy of Posttransplantation Hypertension

Therapeutic goals and techniques are similar to those of other clinical settings associated with hypertension. Goal blood pressure values are similar (140 systolic, below 90 diastolic). Therapy should follow the outline in Table 8–4. Although it is important to assess possible etiologic or aggravating factors, some of these may not warrant intervention. The benefits of cyclosporine outweigh its deleterious effect on blood pressure, and hypertension generally does not affect the decision on dosing or using this agent. Steroid dose may have an effect on blood pressure control,[35] and although steroids cannot be discontinued, alternate-day administration may decrease the incidence of hypertension.[49] Renal artery stenosis may not be worth pursuing unless hypertension is severe or the clinical

Table 8–4 Therapy for Posttransplantation Hypertension
Identify any etiologic conditions or aggravating factors and treat if possible
Rejection
Excessive intake of sodium and fluid
Volume overload
Use of cyclosporine
Renal artery stenosis
If hypertension persists >140/90, treat with medications
Diuretics usually needed
Thiazides may aggravate hyperparathyroidism and hypercalcemia
Loop diuretics often needed
May cause or aggravate ↓K, ↓Mg, ↑blood surgar, ↑cholesterol
Beta Blockers
May mask hypoglycemia in diabetics (cardioselective agents preferable)
May aggravate posttransplantation hyperlipidemia by depressing HDL (pindolol, with intrinsic sympathomimetic activity, may not do this)
Often useful for BP control
May suppress sinus tachycardia that is often present posttransplantation
Effect on kidney function is generally not clinically important
Sympathetic Antagonists
CNS side effects may limit usefulness in patients whose goal is rehabilitation and return to normal life-style
Often effective in controlling BP
No adverse metabolic or lipid effects
Vasodilators (direct and indirect)
May be useful for control of BP without metabolic, lipid, CNS or sexual side effects
ACE inhibitors may be very useful to block the renin angiotensin activity from native or transplant kidney. Can cause renal insufficiency, however, when renal artery stenosis is present[50,51]
Calcium channel blockers, alpha blockers can often be used alone as antihypertensive agents

setting is very suggestive of renovascular disease (sudden onset of hypertension, risk factors for a stenotic lesion, renal insufficiency with ACE inhibition,[50,51] elevated renin activity).

Blood pressure elevation associated with acute rejection may improve dramatically after therapy and resolution of the rejection process. However, intravenous solumedrol (pulse) therapy during rejection may temporarily aggravate underlying hypertension. Antihypertensive therapy must be reasonably aggressive: loop diuretics or fluid removal with dialysis in association with the usual oral antihypertensive agents. Parenteral therapy may be required. Sublingual nifedipine, intravenous aldomet, labetolol, or nitroprusside can be used in these patients.

Hypertension associated with chronic rejection may be very refractory to therapy due to the vascular occlusive disease that is the hallmark of chronic rejection. Often multiple drugs are required. It is best to use a combination of agents that have different mechanisms of action to try to maintain optimum antihypertensive effect with minimal side effects.

If hypertension is refractory or requires several drugs that are not well tolerated, consideration should be given to a search for renal artery stenosis or removal of the native kidneys. If renal artery stenosis is present, it may be amenable to intervention with percutaneous transluminal angioplasty[52] or surgical bypass.[45] The ability to dilate a lesion will depend on its cause and anatomy. Ostial atherosclerotic lesions at end-to-side (renal artery to external iliac) anastomoses may be difficult to dilate and may recur. The incidence of complications of dilatation in transplanted kidneys may be similar to the incidence in native kidneys: however, the presence of a single functioning kidney makes any complication potentially more catastrophic.

Surgical correction of transplant renal artery stenosis is often difficult due to scar tissue from prior surgery and abnormal anatomy. Success rates are much less than rates for correction of native renal artery stenosis.[45,53] Again the presence of only one functioning kidney makes any complication more serious, so these invasive procedures are reserved for severe or uncontrolled hypertension where the benefits outweigh the significant risks of the procedures.

Posttransplantation bilateral native nephrectomy can be considered for patients with difficult-to-control hypertension.[54,55] Embolization of the native kidneys has also been described as successful therapy to reduce posttransplantation hypertension.[56] Some investigators feel that blood pressure response to ACE inhibitors may identify patients who will benefit from nephrectomy.[57] Although sometimes successful,[22] efforts to localize the source of renin release by venous sampling may be difficult to interpret because of unequal renal blood flow in transplant and native kidneys, difficulty in localizing the venous return of the transplanted kidney, and potential drug effects on renin release. Now that pretransplantation nephrectomy is rarely performed for hypertension control, this may be a more important consideration. Better documentation in larger numbers of patients will be needed to determine if response to ACE inhibition is sensitive and specific enough to identify patients in whom to consider nephrectomy. At present, because of the uncertainty of benefit, the procedure is probably warranted only for patients with refractory hypertension.

DIABETES MELLITUS

Clinical Characteristics of Diabetic Nephropathy

Patients with diabetes mellitus who develop renal failure secondary to diabetic nephropathy remain some of the most difficult to manage before and after renal transplantation. For most transplant and dialysis centers, the diabetic population is an ever-increasing source of patients to be considered for these modalities of therapy. Approximately 20 to 25 percent of patients with renal failure have diabetic nephropathy as the cause.[58]

The clinical course of diabetic nephropathy is quite characteristic.[59] Patients who develop diabetic nephropathy generally have had insulin-dependent diabetes for many years. Juvenile-onset diabetics will characteristically develop diabetic nephropathy 15 to 20 years after the onset of the diabetes. Adult-onset diabetic patients have an earlier onset, often 8 to 12 years after clinical manifestations of diabetes begin. This may be due to subclinical diabetes prior to the time the diagnosis of diabetes is established.

The clinical course is characterized by hypertension, proteinuria that generally progresses to the nephrotic range, and renal insufficiency progressing from relatively normal glomerular filtration to end-stage disease over 2 to 5 years.

The other secondary complications of diabetes, especially retinopathy, are generally present when patients develop diabetic nephropathy. Progressive disease secondary to these complications often causes difficult clinical problems. Neuropathy, enteropathy, microvascular disease (with the risk of peripheral ulcer formation, infection, and amputation), and atherosclerosis of major vessels in other organ systems (especially the heart and the central nervous system) are typical features of the patient with long-standing diabetes and diabetic nephropathy.

Management of the Diabetic Patient

Because the patient with diabetes and its secondary complications has a progressive and lethal systemic disease, it is important to identify all the problems that are present for the individual patient and to direct a therapeutic plan that will most successfully stabilize or prevent these complications.

Diabetic Nephropathy

There is increasing evidence that diabetic nephropathy develops because of the deleterious effects of hyperglycemia on the renal glomerulus and microvasculature.[60] Animal studies suggest that hyperglycemia is the causative factor. Correction of hyperglycemia by transplantation of kidneys from diabetic animals to normal animals results in reversal of changes similar to diabetic nephropathy in humans.[61] This has been also described after human transplantation of a kidney from a diabetic patient to a nondiabetic recipient.[62] Human studies after renal transplantation document the recurrence of diabetic changes within the glomerulus[63] and have suggested that better control of blood sugar by frequent blood sugar monitoring and multiple daily injections of insulin may decrease the incidence of this recurrent disease. However, current techniques for maintaining euglycemia, including frequent blood sugar monitoring and multiple daily injections, insulin pump infusions, and pancreas transplantation, may not be as successful as necessary at normalizing the blood sugar. It remains to be determined whether or not such intervention to stabilize or improve secondary diabetic complications including diabetic nephropathy will be successful. Studies to assess the effect of these techniques on early and established diabetic nephropathy are under way. It is the opinion of most diabetologists and nephrologists that if euglycemia can be attained throughout the day and maintained indefinitely, secondary diabetic complications will be eliminated.[64]

Despite the fact that definitive therapy to correct or prevent diabetic complications has not been developed, several factors may accelerate the progression of diabetic nephropathy. Hypertension has been well recognized to accelerate the course of most glomerular disease in both animals and humans. Studies have documented the benefit of hypertension control in patients with early diabetic nephropathy.[4,5] The rate of decline of glomerular filtration rate was significantly slowed when blood pressure control was improved with the addition of antihypertensive agents. Although maintenance of normotension is extremely important in these patients, this goal is often difficult to attain.[65] Diabetic autonomic nephropathy may predispose to postural hypotension. This may be aggravated by the addition of antihypertensive agents. Maintenance of euvolemia is also difficult because renal insufficiency often makes the individual refractory to diuretic therapy. If the patient does respond to aggressive diuretic medication, there is the risk of volume depletion and postural hypotension. In addition, the hypertension in this clinical situation is often moderately severe and may require multiple medications. Other side effects of antihypertensive agents including impotence, central nervous system (CNS) depression, and gastrointestinal symptoms may be aggravated by the presence of diabetic and/or uremic complications.[65]

Prior to institution of dialysis, almost all these patients will require some maintenance diuretic to maintain euvolemia. In addition to diuretic therapy, treatment with the alpha blocker prazosin may be successful in controlling the blood pressure.[65] However, the postural hypotension and syncope associated with this drug may be aggravated by diabetic autonomic neuropathy and volume depletion. Beta blockers are relatively contraindicated in individuals with insulin-dependent diabetes because they may mask the hypoglycemic symptoms secondary to the β-adrenergic effects of catecholamines released during hypoglycemia. However, the use of cardioselective beta blockers (atenolol and metoprolol) can be successfully used, since these cardioselective agents in low doses do not inhibit the diaphoresis associated with hypoglycemia.[4,5] The long-acting atenolol is relatively contraindicated in the presence of advanced renal failure because it is renally excreted and may accumulate to toxic levels. Sympathetic antagonists such as alpha-methyldopa, clonidine, and guanabenz can be successfully used for these patients, although they may cause problems with CNS depression, impotence, or postural hypotension. Single, larger doses at night often minimize these side effects and also help to maintain normotension in the supine position. Vasodilators such as apresoline or the more potent minoxidil may be useful in combination with the other agents mentioned above. The reflex tachycardia associated with these drugs limits their efficacy if not used in conjunction with a beta blocker or a sympathetic antagonist. Captopril or enalapril, the converting enzyme inhibitors, are attractive for use with diabetes because of the lack of significant metabolic or CNS side effects. However, the incidence of complications (proteinuria and granulocytopenia) with captopril is higher in the presence of renal insufficiency, and these complications need to be looked for carefully if this agent is used. The presence of underlying proteinuria may make it more difficult to detect superimposed captopril-induced proteinuria in patients with diabetic nephropathy. Angiotensin-converting enzyme inhibitors can also result in significant increases in the serum potassium due to inhibition of aldosterone production. Patients with diabetic nephropathy are susceptible to impairment of the renin aldosterone axis with subsequent hyporeninemic hypoaldosteronism that can further aggravate hyperkalemia.[66] Renal insufficiency and changes in intracellular uptake of potassium due to insulin lack may further aggravate the risk of hyperkalemia in this clinical setting.

The diabetic patient with end-stage diabetic nephropathy on maintenance dialysis or subsequent to renal transplantation[67] often continues to have hard-to-control problems with hypertension. Fluid balance may be more easily maintained in this situation because of the effectiveness of dialytic therapy or the presence of a functioning allograft. Most of the other considerations mentioned regarding therapy of hypertension in the diabetic patient pertain to the dialysis or transplantation patient. Although the renal transplantation patient may have relatively normal renal function, as assessed by glomerular filtration rate and serum creatinine, well-recognized abnormalities in sodium and potassium excretion in these patients make the transplant recipient with hypertension susceptible to fluid retention or hyperkalemia. Diabetic neuropathy and other diabetic complications, although sometimes stabilized after initiation of dialysis, and often stabilized or improved after renal transplantation, may still create problems when combined with the deleterious effects of antihypertensive agents.

Other therapeutic considerations for individuals with diabetic nephropathy include the following:

1. Dietary restriction of protein, sodium, and potassium is important. Dietary restriction of protein in animals may prevent or slow the progression of renal insufficiency due to a variety of causes, and evidence for the beneficial effect of dietary protein restriction in human renal disease is beginning to appear.

2. Other potential insults to kidney function must be considered. Obstruction may be more common due to the presence of a neurogenic bladder and/or papillary necrosis. Diabetic patients are more susceptible to urinary tract infections and pyelonephritis, a potential source of reversible deterioration of renal function.

3. Nephrotoxic agents such as contrast agents and drugs should be avoided in the diabetic patient.

After renal transplantation, diabetic nephropathy can recur in the allograft.[63] However, this takes a year or longer to manifest microscopically and has been infrequently a cause of significant renal insufficiency in the posttransplantation diabetic patient. Rejection and other technical problems remain the most frequent source of renal dysfunction after transplantation in the diabetic population.

Diabetic Retinopathy

Diabetic retinopathy is almost universally present in individuals who have diabetic nephropathy. The absence of any evidence of diabetic retinopathy raises serious question about the diagnosis of diabetic nephropathy. It is extremely important to assess the status of the retina in individuals who have long-standing diabetes and diabetic nephropathy. Panretinal photocoagulation has been documented to prevent loss of vision in a significant percentage of diabetic patients with proliferative diabetic retinopathy.[68] Background diabetic retinopathy does not require this therapy, but frequent assessment of the clinical stage of diabetic retinopathy is required in order to assess appropriate timing of therapeutic intervention. Patients who have had vitreous hemorrhage or scarring due to proliferative diabetic retinopathy may also be amenable to therapeutic intervention with vitrectomy. Maintenance of vision is a major priority for these patients to try to preserve the marginal quality of life often present. A cooperative effort by the nephrologist and ophthalmologist is required for successful management of these patients.

Diabetic retinopathy may progress after development of end-stage renal failure while an individual is on dialysis or after renal transplantation. The use of anticoagulation with hemodialysis was once considered a possible risk factor for the development of intraocular hemorrhage. However, hypertension,[69] inadequate dialysis, and rapid fluid shifts may be more important risk factors, since better dialysis and control of blood pressure have resulted in lowering the rate of visual loss for both hemodialysis diabetic patients[70] and peritoneal dialysis patients.[71] Several studies, however, have suggested that vision is as well or better maintained after successful renal transplantation than on either form of dialysis[72,73] (Table 8–5).

Diabetic Neuropathy

Diabetic neuropathy is also universally present in individuals who have diabetic nephropathy and reach end-stage renal failure. It is a polyneuropathy similar to the neuropathy associated with uremia. The presence of underlying diabetic neuropathy often results in significant symptoms (paresthesias, numbness, weakness of the distal extremities) at a higher glomerular filtration rate than is the case in uremic patients without diabetes. Often symptoms develop or worsen at a GFR of 15 to 20 ml per min or higher despite the absence of symptoms in patients without diabetes who have this level of renal function. Patients on either hemodialysis or peritoneal dialysis often have continuing symptoms due to neuropathy despite adequate dialysis by other parameters. Successful renal transplantation generally improves and stabilizes symptoms due to diabetic neuropathy more successfully than dialysis.[72] (See Table 8–6.)

Diabetic Enteropathy

Although difficult to assess quantitatively, diabetic enteropathy as a manifestation of diabetic neuropathy is probably present in most patients with diabetic nephropathy and end-stage renal failure. Patients with GFRs of 10 to 20 ml per min often have symptoms of loss of appetite and nausea that persist despite onset of dialysis therapy. This again may be a manifestation of underlying diabetic enteropathy with superimposed uremic complications. These symptoms are almost always significantly improved after successful renal transplantation and may be one of the most significant factors resulting in improvement in the quality of life after transplantation for diabetic patients. These gastrointestinal symptoms may result in significant malnutrition or difficulty in controlling diabetes for patients on dialysis. These symptoms may be aggravated by the procedure of peritoneal dialysis, although this procedure offers the ability to provide some caloric intake by absorption of glucose in the dialysate through the peritoneal membrane.

Diabetic enteropathy may increase the risk of certain complications post–renal transplantation. Bezoars have occurred and may cause problems before or after renal transplantation. The postoperative recovery of gastrointestinal function may be delayed in the diabetic allograft recipient, and

Table 8–5 Progression of Retinopathy with Different Treatment Modalities for Diabetic ESRD			
	Visual Acuity at Follow-up		
Treatment Modality	*Improved*	*Stable*	*Worse*
Hemodialysis (n = 29)		11 (38%)	18 (62%) (a)
Peritoneal dialysis (n = 18)		15 (83%)	3 (17%) (b)
Renal transplantation (n = 45)	2 (4%)	37 (84%)	6 (11%) (c)
(a) versus (b) (p = 0.002)			
(a) versus (c) (p = 0.0001)			
(b) versus (c) (p = 0.73)			

Table 8-6 Progression of Neuropathy After Renal Transplantation and Chronic Dialysis in Diabetic Patients

Initial Neuropathy		Neuropathy at Follow-up	
		Stable or Improved	*Worse*
(a) Renal transplantation	(n = 48)		
Mild or moderate	(n = 15)	15 (100%)	0
Severe	(n = 33)	13 (39%)	20 (61%)
(b) Chronic dialysis	(n = 45)		
Mild or moderate	(n = 43)	20 (44%)	23 (53%)
Severe	(n = 2)	1	1

this may increase the risk of malnutrition, steroid complications, fecal impaction, and other upper and lower gastrointestinal complications.

Microvascular Disease

Patients with diabetes generally have microvascular disease due to the direct effects of diabetes and the increased risk of atherosclerosis of both large and small vessels, which occurs in the presence of abnormal glucose metabolism. Ischemia of the extremities, especially the hands and feet, is a significant risk for these patients.[72,74] Ulcers may develop due to minor trauma or pressure and they may become infected. The degree of infection may be difficult to detect clinically in the diabetic patient, especially after renal transplantation, when the individual is on immunosuppressive medication and generally taking corticosteroids.

Therapy is most successful if these complications are prevented. Individuals with diabetes need to be educated on how to care for their feet and hands. Nail trimming must be done very carefully and routinely to avoid complications secondary to overgrown or ingrown nails. Shoes should be properly fitted to avoid any pressure sores. Any other potential source of pressure sores such as prolonged bedrest, a brace, or a cast, must be identified and avoided if at all possible. If the problem of potential pressure sores is considered, often a therapeutic regimen can be undertaken that will avoid this problem. An individual who has

a fracture and requires a cast needs careful fitting of the cast and frequent cast removal to assess for pressure sores. If a cast can be avoided, that may be the best therapy. If an individual needs to have bed rest, a water mattress or other device to reduce or eliminate pressure points should be used. Most problems occur when individuals providing medical care for these patients neglect to consider this potential complication.

Infection in any lesion needs to be aggressively treated with antimicrobial therapy. Surgical intervention with debridement and drainage may create problems arising from further impairment of the tenuous blood supply to the area. Certainly significant collections of purulent material must be drained; however, aggressive debridement of an ulcer may be best avoided. Careful cleaning and application of antiseptic agents may be useful, but care needs to be taken to avoid further tissue injury. Peripheral ulcers, infection, and amputations are, unfortunately, frequent after renal transplantation. An overall incidence of 17 percent for amputations, often involving the upper extremities, has been reported.[74] This complication is also a potential problem on dialysis. However, if anything there may be an equal or greater risk after transplantation (10 percent incidence in both groups at the Cleveland Clinic Foundation).[72,73]

Atherosclerosis of Large Vessels

Diabetes is a significant risk factor for the development of atherosclerosis, and this may cause significant complications due to disease in the coronary or cerebral circulation. The most frequent cause of death for diabetic patients with end-stage renal failure is cardiovascular.[75] Diagnosing coronary disease may be difficult because these individuals often have significant disease in the absence of symptoms or signs of coronary ischemia.[76] The best technique for the diagnosis of coronary disease is coronary angiography. Because of the high risk of morbidity and mortality due to cardiovascular disease in these patients, we routinely perform coronary angiography in diabetics in preparation for renal transplantation.[76] There is an increased risk of contrast-induced acute renal failure in this population.[77] If the patient is on dialysis, this risk is probably acceptable. Even before the patient is on dialysis, coronary angiography can be performed without significant risk of irreversible renal failure if the procedure is done carefully and a minimum amount of contrast is used.[78] Patients who have significant coronary disease, as defined as the presence of greater than 70 percent stenosis in one or more coronary vessels and/or the presence of left ventricular dysfunction, have a significantly poorer prognosis either on dialysis or after renal transplantation (Table 8–7). Patients who do not have these findings on coronary angiography are at low risk for mortality from a coronary event.[76]

High-risk patients who are amenable to coronary bypass procedures or coronary angioplasty may be identified. Angiography also helps to determine the appropriate follow-up to assess progression of coronary disease in these patients.

Cerebrovascular disease can generally be assessed by using noninvasive ultrasound or Doppler studies combined with digital subtraction venous angiography, and in selected cases, conventional carotid angiography. Again, these studies help to assess prognosis, identify individuals who may benefit from surgical intervention, and help to determine appropriate follow-up to assess disease in this vascular system.

Dialysis Versus Transplantation for the Diabetic Patient with Renal Failure

When comparing patient survival for dialysis and for renal transplantation, several factors must be considered in order to make an appropriate comparison. Patient selection is often a significant factor in determining patient survival after renal transplantation. Dialysis populations tend to be an unselected group with renal failure. Patients who undergo transplantation have been selected for that procedure, and this selection process may eliminate high-risk individuals, especially diabetics with multiple complications secondary to their diabetes. Also, since patients are treated with several therapeutic modalities, combining dialysis and transplantation, it is more appropriate to consider survival while maintained on a specific therapeutic modality rather than survival for individual patients.

	(n)	1 yr (%)	2 yr (%)	5 yr (%)	
Cardiac disease	(87)				
Absent	(49)	96	75	40	p = 0.0002
Present	(38)	76	45	19	
Cardiac patients	(38)*				
Transplantation	(12)	100	67	40	p = 0.05
Transplantation Candidates	(9)	67	44	15	
Nontransplantation Candidates	(17)	65	29	6	

Table 8–7 ESRD Secondary to Diabetic Nephropathy Cumulative Percentage Survival

*From onset of first ESRD treatment

Table 8–8 ESRD Secondary to Diabetic Nephropathy Cumulative Percentage Survival					
	(n)	1 yr (%)	2 yr (%)	5 yr (%)	
Dialysis survival	(75)	89	74	12	p = .04
Transplant survival	(52)	81	67	45	

Thus, the survival time on dialysis while waiting for transplantation should be included as survival on dialysis. If one considers the population of diabetic renal failure patients who do not have significant cardiovascular disease (as defined as greater than 70 percent stenosis of one or more coronary vessels and/or left ventricular dysfunction) and if one performs an analysis of therapeutic modalities based on the Cox Proportional Hazards model, short-term survival is comparable on dialysis with renal transplantation as shown in Table 8–8. However, long-term survival (greater than 2 years) is significantly better with the modality of renal transplantation when compared with dialysis.[75]

Rehabilitation is also better after renal transplantation.[72] (See Table 8–9.) More important, however, the quality of life for diabetic patients with renal failure due to diabetic nephropathy is significantly better after renal transplantation due to improvement in symptoms related to diabetic complications and stabilization of diabetic retinopathy, enteropathy, and neuropathy. Because of the early onset of uremic symptoms when renal failure is combined with the diabetic complications of neuropathy and enteropathy, it is often best to proceed with renal transplantation at a higher glomerular filtration rate to avoid significant complications from these two factors (uremia plus secondary diabetic complications). Often transplantation can proceed prior to the need for dialysis. Earlier dialysis may also be needed to avoid uremic symptoms and complications prior to cadaver or living related transplantation. It is often appropriate to proceed with consideration of dialysis and transplantation in diabetic patients when their glomerular filtration rate is 15 to 20 ml per min or higher. Both peritoneal dialysis and hemodialysis are effective therapies for these patients prior to transplantation.[79] There does not seem to be any significant increased incidence of complications for patients who are transplanted while being maintained on peritoneal dialysis.[80]

Both cadaver and living-related donor transplantation are effective therapies for diabetic patients with renal failure.[79,81] Donor-specific blood transfusions and cyclosporine have significantly improved the success rate with one-haplotype-matched living related donor recipient pairs.[82] Cyclosporine has significantly improved the success rate of cadaver transplantation in diabetic patients.[83] Graft rejection in patients with diabetic nephropathy is similar to that of nondiabetic renal failure patients. However, there is a slight increase in patient mortality that results in a slightly lower overall graft survival for patients with diabetic nephropathy.[81,84]

Pancreas Transplantation

Pancreas transplantation has been employed to correct the hyperglycemia more adequately in insulin-dependent diabetic

Table 8–9 Rehabilitation			
	Transplant	Dialysis	
Employed full or part-time	60%	26%	p < 0.05

patients who have developed diabetic complications. Various surgical techniques have been employed in order to manage the exocrine secretions of the whole gland or the segmental graft. The vascular anastomosis employed has also been variable, but often the iliac vessels are employed as with renal transplantation.

Several centers have used a combined transplant procedure in diabetic patients with end-stage diabetic nephropathy. Combined renal and pancreas transplantation has been performed from a single cadaver donor.[85,86] Technical complications, including vascular thrombosis and fistula formation from the exocrine pancreas, have been significant and have resulted in poorer results for graft survival after pancreas transplantation compared with renal transplantation. Despite the use of cyclosporine, graft success of 50 percent at 1 year has generally not been exceeded after pancreas transplantation.[87]

Other centers have employed transplantation of pancreas grafts after successful renal transplantation.[88] Living related donors have been used, transplanting the distal segment of the pancreas.[87] HLA-identical pancreas transplant have been the most successful, but concerns about glucose intolerance in the donor raise questions concerning the appropriateness of this type of transplantation.

It is hoped that pancreas transplantation may help to stabilize the diabetic complications in other organ systems for individuals with diabetic nephropathy and renal failure. It would also be anticipated that euglycemia after successful pancreas transplantation would eliminate the risk of recurrence of diabetic nephropathy in the renal allograft. Whether this will be a successful adjunctive procedure combined with renal transplantation, or may even prevent the need for renal transplantation, remains to be seen.

CARDIOVASCULAR DISEASE

Cardiovascular disease remains the most frequent cause of morbidity and mortality in the end-stage renal failure population both while maintained on dialysis and after renal transplantation.[89–93] Death due to cardiovascular disease accounts for greater than 50 percent of patient deaths in long-term dialysis and transplantation patients.[94]

Atherosclerotic Cardiovascular Disease

Etiology

Various risk factors present in patients with renal failure before and after onset of dialysis[95] and after renal transplantation affect the high incidence of cardiovascular events in this clinical setting. Almost all patients are hypertensive, as outlined in the previous section, and hypertension has the well-recognized effect of increasing the risk of all types of cardiovascular events. Although there have been significant advances in the treatment of hypertension associated with renal disease, blood pressure control often remains suboptimal and may increase the risk of cardiovascular complications in these patients.

There are well-recognized lipid abnormalities associated with renal failure and after transplantation[96] that also tend to increase the risk profile for the progression of atherosclerosis and cardiovascular events. Renal failure patients tend to have a type 4 hyperlipidemia[98] and changes in HDL lipoproteins.[98,99] This is not completely corrected by dialysis. After renal transplantation there tends to be elevation of the serum cholesterol[100,102] and drug therapy with corticosteroids,[103,104] and propranolol[105] may affect the lipid profile and risk for cardiovascular disease.

A large percentage of patients with renal failure have diabetes as its cause, a well-known risk factor for atherosclerosis. This, combined with the other risk factors of renal failure, results in a very high risk for progression of atherosclerosis as outlined in the section on diabetes.

Often patients with renal failure lead a sedentary life because of the limitations on physical activity imposed by their renal failure. Anemia is often significant, and tolerance for physical activity is poor because of this and other uremic factors. There is a well-recognized association of sedentary life-style with an increased risk of atherosclerotic disease and its complications.

Other risk factors such as smoking and heredity may be present in this population as in others.

Management

Management of cardiovascular disease in the renal failure patient is similar to management of this disease process in other individuals. Successful intervention should be directed to three areas: prevention, diagnosis, and therapy of established disease.

The various risk factors for atherosclerosis should be assessed and risk factors amenable to therapeutic intervention should be corrected. These include control of hypertension, cessation of smoking, and correction of lipid abnormalities through dietary modification or medication alteration whenever possible. Sometimes medication alteration is not feasible, since most patients require ongoing steroid therapy, although with the availability of cyclosporine long-term maintenance dosages can perhaps be reduced to minimize the effect on lipid metabolism. Dietary modification for blood pressure control and lipid reduction are unfortunately often unsuccessful due to difficulties with alteration of patient life-styles after successful transplantation. Smoking cessation may also be difficult to implement.

Diagnosis and Therapy of Established Disease

The use of various diagnostic techniques, including noninvasive studies such as ultrasound, stress testing, and thallium scanning for cardiac ischemia, as well as routine angiographic procedures (digital subtraction venous studies and routine arterial studies), should be considered in this population when appropriate. When performing angiographic procedures after transplantation, there is a concern to avoid contrast-induced renal failure. Patients with successfully functioning renal allografts are not at high risk of developing contrast-induced renal failure. These studies can be employed, when indicated, as long as care is given to avoid high doses of contrast, repetitive procedures, and volume depletion in association with the study.

It must be remembered that patients with renal failure, on dialysis or after renal transplantation, have a high risk of complications related to various invasive diagnostic procedures and therapeutic interventions for the correction of established vascular disease. Coronary bypass procedures have been associated with higher complication rates and mortality in the renal failure patient on dialysis.[106,107] It may be that coronary bypass procedures may be more safely performed after successful renal transplantation. More data are necessary to assess the risk of complications with these procedures.

Cardiomyopathy and Congestive Heart Failure

Significant left ventricular dysfunction has been described in renal failure. Some of this myocardial dysfunction may be secondary to uremic toxins. Hemodialysis is associated with an improvement in ejection fraction in a certain subgroup of patients with congestive heart failure.[108] This improvement in left ventricular contractility may be related to an increase in ionized calcium associated with hemodialysis.[109] Smoking may play a role in this myocardial dysfunction, since nicotine levels are significantly elevated in hemodialysis patients.[110]

Renal transplantation is associated with a further improvement in myocardial function. In a group of 14 patients studied before and after renal transplantation, there was significant improvement in cardiac index, stroke volume, ejection fraction, mean normalized posterior wall velocity, mean velocity of fiber shortening, and mitral valve diastolic closure rate.[111] This suggests that there is a poorly dialyzable uremic toxin that is removed after successful renal transplantation. Besides these effects on myocardial function, other factors accompanying renal failure such as fluid retention, an arteriovenous fistula, anemia, hypertension, and electrolyte abnormalities may play a role in aggravating the abnormality. All these factors may be better controlled after renal transplantation.

Some patients who have severe myocardial disease—atherosclerosis, idiopathic cardiomyopathy, or the combination of factors present with uremia and renal transplantation—may develop progressive myocardial dysfunction and failure and be unresponsive to medical management. These may be some of the most difficult patients to treat. Since both dialysis and renal transplantation can result in significant improvement in myocardial function, it may be difficult or impossible to identify the minority of patients before transplantation who will not respond and who will have progressive disease.

REFERENCES

1. Vertes, V, et al: Hypertension in end-stage renal disease. N Engl J Med 280:978, 1969.
2. Wiedmann, P, et al: Plasma renin activity and blood pressure in terminal renal failure. N Engl J Med 285:757, 1971.
3. Iversen, BM and Ofstad, J: Influence of hypertension on the course of experimental hypertension in rats (abstr). Kidney Int 18:142, 1980.
4. Parving, HH, et al: Early aggressive antihypertensive treatment reduces rate of decline in kidney function in diabetic nephropathy. Lancet 1:1175, 1983.
5. Mogensen, CE: Long-term antihypertensive treatment inhibiting progression of diabetic nephropathy. Br Med J 285:685, 1982.
6. Pohl, JE, Thurston, H, and Swales, JD: Hypertension with renal impairment: Influence of intensive therapy. Q J Med 43:369, 1974.
7. Jones, B and Nanra, RS: Double-blind trial of antihypertensive effect of chlorothiazide in severe renal failure. Lancet 1258, 1979.
8. Bennett, WM, et al: Drug prescribing in renal failure: Dosing guideline for adults. Am J Kid Dis 3:155, 1983.
9. Shindo, K, et al: Captopril-associated granulocytopenia in hypertension after renal transplantation. Clin Nephrol 22:314, 1984.
10. Aronian, JM, et al: Bilateral nephrectomy in chronic hemodialysis and renal transplant patients. Am J Surg 126:635, 1973.
11. Wilkinson, R, et al: Plasma renin and exchangeable sodium in the hypertension of chronic renal failure: The effect of bilateral nephrectomy. Q J Med 39:377, 1970.
12. Talley, TE, et al: Bilateral nephrectomy and splenectomy in renal failure. Urology 4:378, 1974.
13. Matas, AJ, et al: Lethal complications of bilateral nephrectomy and splenectomy in hemodialyzed patients. Am J Surg 129:616, 1975.
14. Viner, NA, et al: Bilateral nephrectomy: An analysis of 100 consecutive cases. J Urol 113:291, 1975.
15. Calman, KC, et al: Bilateral nephrectomy prior to renal transplantation. Br J Surg 63:512, 1976.
16. Yarimizu, SH, et al: Mortality and morbidity in pretransplant bilateral nephrectomy: Analysis of 305 cases. Urology 12:55, 1978.
17. Barnes, BA, et al: The 13th report of the human renal transplant registry. Transplant Proc 9:9, 1977.
18. Pettinger, WA and Mitchell, HC: Minoxidil: An alternative to nephrectomy for refractory hypertension. N Engl J Med 289:167, 1973.
19. Cole, GA, et al: Hypertension following cadaveric renal transplantation. Postgrad Med J 48:399, 1972.
20. Cohen, SL: Hypertension in renal transplant recipients: Role of bilateral nephrectomy. Br Med J 3:78, 1973.
21. Curtis, JJ, et al: Hypertension after successful renal transplantation. Am J Med 79:193, 1985.
22. Pollini, J, et al: Late hypertension following renal allotransplantation. Clin Nephrol 11:202, 1979.
23. Curtis, JJ, et al: Remission of essential hypertension after renal transplantation. N Engl J Med 309:1009, 1983.
24. Bennett, WM, et al: Posttransplant hypertension: Studies of the cortical blood flow and the renal pressor system. Kidney Int 6:99, 1974.
25. Starzl, TE, et al: Long-term survival after renal transplantation in humans: (with special reference to histocompatibility matching, thymectomy, homograft, glomerulonephritis, heterologous ALG, and recipient malignancy). Ann Surg 172:437, 1970.
26. O'Connor, DT, et al: Urinary kallikrein excretion after renal transplantation: Relationship to hypertension, graft source, and renal function. Am J Med 73:475, 1982.
27. Popovtzer, MM, et al: Variations in arterial blood pressure after kidney transplantation: Relation to renal function, plasma renin activity, and the dose of prednisone. Circulation 47:1297, 1973.
28. Smellie, WAB, Vinik, M, and Hume, DM: Angiographic investigation of hypertension complicating human renal transplantation. Surg Gynecol Obstet 128:963, 1969.
29. Morris, PJ, et al: Renal artery stenosis in

renal transplantation. Med J Aust 1:1255, 1971.

30. Murray, JE, Merrill, JP, and Harrison, JH: Kidney transplantation between seven pairs of identical twins. Ann Surg 148:343, 1958.

31. Grunfeld, JP, et al: Permanent hypertension after homotransplantation in man. Clin Sci 48:391, 1975.

32. Linas, SL, et al: Role of the renin-angiotensin system in post-transplantation hypertension in patients with multiple kidneys. N Engl J Med 298:1440, 1978.

33. Kalbfleisch, JH, et al: Habitual excessive dietary salt intake and blood pressure levels in renal transplant recipients. Am J Med 73:205, 1982.

34. Theil, G, et al: Is cyclosporine A-induced nephrotoxicity in recipients of renal allografts progressive? Transplant Proc 17:169, 1985.

35. Jacquot, C, et al: Long-term blood pressure changes in renal homotransplantation. Arch Intern Med 138:233, 1978.

36. Hakim, RM, Goldszer, RC, and Brenner, BM: Hypertension and proteinuria; Long-term sequelae of uninephrectomy in humans. Kidney Int 25:930, 1984.

37. Miller, IJ, et al: Impact of renal donation. Am J Med 79:201, 1985.

38. Hoitsma, AJ, et al: Long-term follow-up of living kidney donors. Neth J Med 28:226, 1985.

39. Anderson, CF, et al: The risks of unilateral nephrectomy: Status of kidney donors 10 to 20 years postoperatively. Mayo Clin Proc 60:367, 1985.

40. Morien, M, Tomlanovich, S, and Myers, BD: Cyclosporine induces chronic nephropathy in human recipients of cardiac allografts. Transplant Proc 17:185, 1985.

41. Lindfors, O, et al: Renal artery stenosis in hypertensive renal transplant recipients. J Urol 118:240, 1978.

42. Schact, RA, et al: Renal artery stenosis after renal transplantation. Am J Surg 131:653, 1976.

43. LaCombe, M: Arterial stenosis complicating renal allotransplantation in man. Ann Surg 181:283, 1975.

44. Ricotta, JJ, et al: Renal artery stenosis following transplantation: Etiology, diagnosis and prevention. Surgery 84:595, 1978.

45. Dickerman, RM, et al: Surgical correction of post transplant renovascular hypertension. Ann Surg 192:639, 1980.

46. Rath, M, et al: Digital subtraction angiography in the diagnosis of arterial complications after renal transplantation. Eur J Radiol 4:34, 1984.

47. Braun, WE: The renal-allograft bruits: An indicator of good function. N Engl J Med 286:1350, 1972.

48. Zawada, ET, et al: Saralasin acetate test in renal transplant hypertension. Arch Intern Med 144:65, 1984.

49. Curtis, JJ, et al: Prevalence of hypertension in a renal transplant population on alternate-day steroid therapy. Clin Nephrol 5:123, 1976.

50. Van Der Woude, FJ, et al: Effect of captopril on blood pressure and renal function in patients with transplant renal artery stenosis. Nephron 39:184, 1985.

51. Hricik, DE, et al: Captopril-induced functional renal insufficiency in patients with bilateral renal artery stenosis or renal artery stenosis in a solitary kidney. N Engl J Med 308:373, 1983.

52. Gerlock, AJ, at al: Renal transplant arterial stenosis: Percutaneous transluminal angioplasty. AJR 140:325, 1983.

53. Novick, AC, et al: Diminished operative morbidity and mortality in renal revascularization. JAMA 246:749, 1981.

54. Castaneda, MJ, et al: Selective post-transplantation bilateral native nephrectomy: Indications and results. Arch Surg 118:1194, 1983.

55. Curtis, JJ, et al: Surgical therapy for persistent hypertension after renal transplantation. Transplantation 31:125, 1981.

56. Thompson, JF, et al: Control of hypertension after renal transplant by embolization of host kidneys. Lancet 2:424, 1984.

57. Curtis, JJ, et al: Benefits of removal of native kidneys in hypertension after renal transplantation. Lancet 2:739, 1985.

58. Eggers, PW, Connerton, R, and McMullan, M: The Medicare experience with end stage renal disease: Trends in incidence, prevalence and survival. Health Care Financing Review 5:69, 1984.

59. Krolewski, AS, et al: The changing natural history of nephropathy in type 1 diabetes. Am J Med 78:785, 1985.

60. Viberti, GC, et al: Long-term correction of hyperglycaemia and progression of renal failure in insulin dependent diabetes. Br Med J 286:598, 1983.

61. Lee, CS, et al: Renal transplantation in diabetes mellitus in rats. J Exp Med 139:793, 1974.

62. Abouna, GM, et al: Reversal of diabetic nephropathy in human cadaveric kidneys after transplantation into non-diabetic recipients. Lancet 2:1274, 1983.

63. Mauer, SM, et al: The development of lesions in the glomerular basement membrane and mesangium after transplantation of normal kidneys to diabetic patients. Diabetes 32:948, 1983.

64. Peterson, CM, et al: The role of self blood glucose monitoring and glucose control in preventing diabetic sequelae. In Friedman, EA and L'Esperance, FA (eds): Diabetic Renal-Retinal Syndrome. Grune & Stratton, New York, 1982.

65. Lipson, LG: Special problems in treatment of hypertension in the patient with diabetes mellitus. Arch Intern Med 144:1829, 1984.

66. Christlieb, AR, et al: Aldosterone responsiveness in patients with diabetes mellitus. Diabetes 77:732, 1978.

67. Chou, LM, et al: Hypertension jeopardizes diabetic patients following renal transplant. Trans Am Soc Artif Inter Organs 30:473, 1984.

68. The diabetic retinopathy study research group: Preliminary report on effects of photocoagulation therapy. Am. J Ophthalmol 81:383, 1976.

69. Knowler, WC, Bennett, PH, and Ballintine, EJ: Increased incidence of retinopathy in diabetics with elevated blood pressure. N Engl J Med 302:645, 1980.

70. Shapiro, FL and Comty, CM: Hemodialysis in diabetics 1981 (update). In Friedman, EA and L'Eperance, FA (eds): Diabetic Renal-Retinal Syndrome. Grune & Stratton, New York, p. 309, 1982.

71. Amain, P, et al: Continuous ambulatory peritoneal dialysis in diabetics with end stage renal disease. In Friedman, EA and L'Esperance, FA (eds): Diabetic Renal Retinal Syndrome. Grune & Stratton, New York, p. 331, 1982.

72. Khauli, RB, et al: Comparison of renal transplantation and dialysis in the rehabilitation of diabetic end stage renal disease patients. Urology 27: 521, 1986.

73. Kjellstrand, C, Comty, C, and Shapiro, F: A comparison of dialysis and transplantation in insulin dependent diabetic patients. In Friedman, EA and L'Esperance, FA (eds): Diabetic Renal-Retinal Syndrome. Grune & Stratton, New York, p. 405, 1982.

74. Peters, C, et al: Patient and graft survival in amputated versus nonamputated diabetic primary renal allograft recipients. Transplantation 32:498, 1981.

75. Khauli, RB, et al: A critical look at survival of diabetics with end-stage renal disease: Transplantation versus dialysis therapy. Transplantation 41:598, 1986.

76. Braun, WE, et al: The course of coronary artery disease in diabetics with and without renal allografts. Transplant Proc 15:1114, 1983.

77. Harkonen, S and Kjellstrand, CM: Exacerbation of diabetic renal failure following intravenous pyelography. A J Med 63:939, 1977.

78. Richards, C, et al: Effect of coronary angiography on renal function in diabetic nephropathy (abstr). Kid Int 19:135, 1981.

79. Friedman, EA: Improving the course of diabetic nephropathy. Contrib Nephrol 44:173, 1985.

80. Steinmuller, DR, et al: Renal transplantation of patients on chronic peritoneal dialysis. Am J Kid Dis 6:436, 1984.

81. Sutherland, DER, et al: Improved patient and primary renal allograft survival in uremic diabetic recipients. Transplantation 34:319, 1982.

82. Salvatierra, O, et al: Improved transplant survival in diabetic recipients with donor specific blood transfusions. In Friedman EA and L'Esperance FA (eds): Diabetic Renal Retinal Syndrome. Grune & Stratton, New York, p. 405, 1982.

83. Opelz, G: Personal communication.

84. Khauli, RB, et al: Improved results of cadaver renal transplantation in the diabetic patient. J Urol 130:867, 1983.

85. Land, W, et al: Improved results in combined segmental pancreatic and renal transplantation in diabetic patients under cyclosporine therapy. Transplant Proc 17:317, 1985.

86. Traeger, J, et al: Cyclosporine in double simultaneous pancreas plus kidney transplantation. Transplant Proc 17:326, 1985.

87. Sutherland, DER and Kendall, D: Clinical pancreas and islet transplant registry report. Transplant Proc 17:307, 1985.

88. Sollinger, HW, et al: Results of segmental and pancreaticosplenic transplantation with pancreaticocystostomy. Transplant Proc 17:360, 1985.

89. Linder, A, et al: Accelerated atherosclerosis in prolonged maintenance hemodialysis. N Engl J Med 290: 697, 1974.

90. Wing, AJ, et al: Combined report on regular dialysis and transplantation in Europe. Proc Eur Dial Transplant Assoc Eur Ren Assoc 15:4, 1978.

91. Braun, WE, et al: Coronary arteriography and coronary artery disease in 99 diabetic and nondiabetic patients on chronic hemodialysis or renal transplantation programs. Transplant Proc 13:128, 1981.

92. Ikram, H, et al: Cardiovascular changes in chronic hemodialysis patients. Kidney Int 24:371, 1983.

93. Rostand, SG, Kirk, KA, and Rutsky, EA: Dialysis-associated ischemic heart disease: Insights from coronary angiography. Kidney Int 25:653, 1984.

94. Nicholls, AJ, et al: Accelerated atherosclerosis in long-term dialysis and renal-transplant patients: Fact or fiction? Lancet vol. 276, 1980.

95. Rostand, SG, Kirk, KA, and Rutsky, EA:

Relationship of coronary risk factors to hemodialysis-associated ischemic heart disease. Kidney Int 22:304, 1982.

96. Chan, MK, et al: Lipid abnormalities in uremia, dialysis and transplantation. Kidney Int 19:625, 1981.

97. Haas, LB, Brunzell, JD, and Sherrard, DJ: Atherosclerotic risk factors in a chronic dialysis population (abstr). Kidney Int 16:888, 1979.

98. Goldberg, AP, et al: Racial differences in plasma high-density lipoproteins in patients receiving hemodialysis. N Engl J Med 308:1245, 1983.

99. Jung, K, et al: Abnormalities in the composition of serum high density lipoprotein in renal transplant recipients. Clin Nephrol 17:191, 1982.

100. Bagdade, JD, Casaretto, A, and Albers, J: Effects of chronic uremia, hemodialysis and renal transplantation on plasma lipids and lipoproteins in man. J Lab Clin Med 87:37, 1976.

101. Casaretto, A, et al: Hyperlipidaemia after successful renal transplantation. Lancet 1:481, 1974.

102. Lazarus, JM, et al: Cardiovascular disease in uremic patients on hemodialysis. Kidney Int S3:S167, 1975.

103. Ponticelli, C, et al: Lipid disorders in renal transplant recipients. Nephron 20:189, 1978.

104. Chan MK, et al: The role of multiple pharmacotherapy in the pathogenesis of hyperlipidemia after renal transplantation. Clin Nephrol 15:309, 1981.

105. Jackson, JM, and Lee, HA: The role of propranolol therapy and proteinuria in the etiology of post renal transplantation hyperlipidemia. Clin Nephrol 18:95, 1982.

106. Buszta, C, et al: Open heart procedures in patients with end-stage renal disease. Presented at National Kidney Foundation Meeting, Washington, DC, 1981.

107. Francis, GS, et al: Coronary-artery surgery in patients with end-stage renal disease. Ann Intern Med 92:449, 1980.

108. Hung, J, et al: Uremic cardiomyopathy: Effect of hemodialysis on left ventricular function in end-stage renal failure. N Engl J Med 302:547, 1980.

109. Henrich, WL, Hunt, JM, and Nixon, JV: Increased ionized calcium and left ventricular contractility during hemodialysis. N Engl J Med 310:19, 1984.

110. Perry, RJ, et al: Elevated nicotine levels in patients undergoing hemodialysis. Am J Med 76:241, 1984.

111. Lai, KN, Barnden, L, and Mathew, TH: Effect of renal transplantation on left ventricular function in hemodialysis patients. Clin Nephrol 18:74, 1982.

Chapter 9

Transplantation in Children

J. THOMAS ROSENTHAL

Etiology
Selection Criteria
Mental Status
Psychological Assessment
Pretransplantation Evaluation
Other Pretransplantation Operations
Donor Operation
Recipient Operation
Perioperative Management
Immunosuppression
Results

The treatment of the child with ESRD is difficult and demanding for patients, their families, nurses, and physicians. Chronic dialysis and transplantation together are the treatment options for infants and children. In 1970 Reinhart[1] stated, "When the cost to the child in terms of physical and emotional discomfort is considered, I seriously doubt the value of chronic dialysis or renal transplant for these patients." Because of improvements since then in both dialysis and transplantation, few would now question whether to treat most children with renal failure. He went on to say, "Progress of dialysis and renal transplantation should be carefully evaluated not in terms of gross survival but in parameters of meaningful growth and development—living." This is still true. Most nephrologists and surgeons agree that when successful, transplantation offers the best potential for normal growth, development, and rehabilitation. Harmon and Ingelfinger[2] stated that "Dialysis is a way station en route to transplantation. However, for an increasing number of children with failed grafts, lack of donor, or increased sensitization, chronic dialysis is a long-term therapy."

Most aspects of transplantation in children are no different from those in adults. These include the role of tissue typing on outcome, basic surgical techniques of the transplant operation, the use of immunosuppression, and the risk of excessive immunosuppression resulting in infection or malignancy. Certain aspects of transplantation in children are specific to the age group. These include, for example, some technical considerations of the operation brought about by size discrepancy between recipient and kidney in the very small child or infant, higher incidence of lower urinary tract anomalies necessitating special intervention, greater difficulties dealing with the stress of chronic disease, and differences in immunosuppressive regimens because of differences in absorption and side effects of the drugs, to list a few. The rest of this chapter will discuss pediatric renal transplantation, focusing on aspects that are special and important in children.

ETIOLOGY

It is important, whenever possible, to know the etiology of renal failure. Figure 9–1 shows the etiology of end-stage renal disease in pediatric recipients at the University of Minnesota.[3] Certain of the causes are hereditary, the knowledge of which will be useful in screening family members and to avoid any potential living related donors (LRDs) who may also be affected. Cystic diseases are one example where both an au-

tosomal dominant and recessive pattern of polycystic kidney disease have been identified. Cystinosis is another entity leading to chronic renal failure (CRF) and transplantation where a late-onset form has been observed in multiple offspring in the same family.

Another important reason to know the etiology of renal failure is that several diseases are known to recur frequently in the individual with a transplant. Focal-sclerosis glomerulonephritis and oxalosis are two examples. In a recent review, the recurrence rate of focal-sclerosis was found to be 23 percent. This accounted for 11 percent of all graft loss.[4] The risk of development of recurrent disease was found to be highest in those children who had the original disease for less than 36 months and those who had mesangial proliferation in addition to focal sclerosis in the native kidneys.[5] Oxalosis has been considered a contraindication to transplantation because of

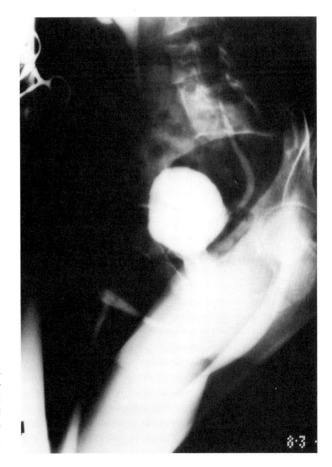

Figure 9–1. Cystogram from a child with posterior urethral valves and urethral stricture secondary to fulgeration of the valves who developed chronic renal failure. Cystogram shows gross reflux, indwelling suprapubic catheter, and a long urethral stricture.

its rapid recurrence in the graft.[6] However, a careful conditioning program that reduces the recurrence rate and has led to long-term survival, in what is an otherwise untreatable disease, has been developed.[7,8] The essence of the strategy is an early after-transplant conditioning program of pyridoxine, phosphate, magnesium, and diuretics to avoid oxalate deposition in the allograft. Scheinman[8] reported transplantation in 11 such children. Seven have satisfactory graft function; six have no evidence of recurrent oxalate deposition in the kidney. One case has been reported in which a child with type I primary oxalalosis, who had failed one cadaveric renal transplant due to oxalate deposition in the kidney, was treated by transplantation with both a liver and kidney.[9] Although the patient subsequently died of sepsis, there was evidence that the liver transplantation had replaced the missing enzyme to a useful extent.

Other disorders that either recurred in grafts or had an adverse effect on graft survival are systemic lupus erythematosus (SLE) and Henoch-Schoenlein purpura, although the number of affected patients who have been transplanted is small. Waiting until the diseases are quiescent before transplantation has been recommended.

Hemalytic-uremic syndrome (HUS) is an uncommon cause of CRF and has not been thought to recur in the graft, probably because the syndrome mimics other causes of graft loss such as acute vascular rejection.[10] Hebert reported 14 children undergoing renal transplantation for HUS with definite recurrence of HUS in 7 and possible recurrence in 3.[11] Although cyclosporine, which has been implicated in the de novo development of HUS,[12,13] was used in some of these patients, other patients developed recurrence in the absence of cyclosporine.

In children most of the time the etiology of renal failure is known. The diagnosis was not discerned in only 3.7 percent of the EDTA registry,[14] while 10 to 15 percent of adult patients did not have a specific diagnosis.[15] Congenital nephropathy accounts for 66 percent of cases of ESRD in children; obstructive uropathy accounts for 21 percent of all cases.[16] In adult patients glomerulonephritis, pyelonephritis, cystic diseases, and multisystem diseases account for 70 percent of cases.[15] Wilms tumor and nephroblastoma account for 2 to 6 percent of cases.[17] Fewer children are rendered anephric by treatment for bilateral Wilms tumor or neuroblastoma because of the effectiveness of chemotherapy. However, children who do end up without kidneys are candidates for renal transplantation. Penn reported 20 children transplanted for Wilms tumor after a 1-year disease-free interval with no development of recurrent disease.[18]

An important difference between adults and children is the large percentage of children with obstructive uropathy. It may be thought that improvement in urologic care, especially the treatment of reflux, may reduce the incidence of ESRD in children due to obstructive uropathy. The actual percentage of patients coming to transplantation with obstruction and other anomalies of the lower urinary tract may increase with improved care, since many children with severe lower urinary tract disorders now survive to reach puberty, where many of these children died in the past. It is important to be aware of the obstructive uropathy group so that careful urologic evaluation of the lower urinary tract can be carried out prior to transplantation so that the graft does not fail due to inadequate bladder function (Figs. 9–1 and 9–2). Posterior urethral valves, reflux with infection, prune belly syndrome can lead to renal failure. Neuropathic bladder secondary to myelodysplasia, while not mentioned as an etiology of ESRD in any review prior to 1984, was the cause of renal failure in three children transplanted in Pittsburgh in the past 5 years.

SELECTION CRITERIA

Absolute contraindications for transplantation in children include any associated medical conditions that would preclude survival from the operation, such as severe heart disease, active serious infection, existing malignancy within 1 year, and inability to comply with immunosuppressive drugs after transplantation. All other children with ESRD should be considered. There are two areas of controversy. One is whether any age or size consideration should play a role in accepting or turning down a patient for transplantation. Size is probably the more important of the two,

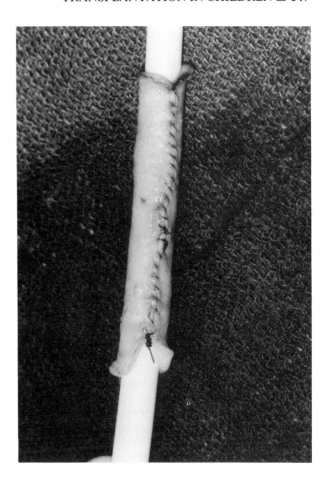

Figure 9–2. Long tube graft urethral replacement for repair of long urethral stricture in the same patient.

since one of the problems in transplanting the very young patient is graft loss secondary to vascular thromboses related to the small size of the vessels. The results from several series, reported between 1970 and 1980 of transplantation in children of less than 2 years old or of less than 10 kg weight, were generally poor.[19,20] Moel and Butt[21] reported 10 infants receiving cadaveric grafts. Only two of these infants had graft survival at 2 years posttransplantation, and only three patients survived 2 years. There were three technical failures. Lum reported five infants transplanted between 1970 and 1980, with two grafts functioning and three deaths. The three deaths occurred from technical causes.[22] In contrast, the results of transplants from living related donors were more successful. Rizzoni[23] in 1980 reported graft survival in three of four children less than age 5 receiving living related donor grafts. Cadaver donor graft survival was 33 percent in first

grafts. Similarly, in 1982 Miller[24] reported the result of adult living related donor kidneys placed intraperitoneally in small children weighing between 5400 and 8800 grams. Ten received LRD grafts. Two died and two others lost grafts to chronic rejection at greater than 2 years. Two infants in that series had received cadaveric transplants and did well. These results taken together suggest that the chances for success were significantly greater when using LRD transplants in tiny infants and children. Fine[25] went so far in assessing the results of cadaveric transplantation in infants by saying, "In terms of gross survival, these results are dismal, and one could question the choice of transplantation for this age group."

More recently, several series showing improved results using cadaveric grafts have appeared. Trompter[26] reported 12 cadaver grafts in infants weighing 8 to 15 kg. Seven grafts functioned longer than 1 year, and overall patient survival was 75 percent. Brodel[27] reported 11 cadaveric transplants in seven patients. There were three vascular thromboses. However, there was only one death. The other six patients are alive with functioning grafts. Arbus[28] reported 39 cadaver grafts in 28 children under six years. Ten recipients weighed less than 10 kg. Nineteen patients had functioning grafts. Mortality was 22 percent. Twelve cadaver transplants were done in eight tiny children over a 4-year period in Pittsburgh. Three continue with functioning grafts 1 to 4 years posttransplantation. Three patients died in the perioperative period. While these results, on the whole, are an improvement over what was obtained 10 years ago with cadaveric transplants in small children, they do not compare favorably with the graft survival or mortality in older children or adults or in infants using LRDs. All centers reporting transplants in recipients under 6 years of age comment on the great time and effort involved in their procedures and recommend these grafts be done only in specialized centers experienced in treating these children. Technically successful cadaveric transplantation in a neonate has not been reported.[29]

Unfortunately, the infant or small child is the one whose renal failure is the most likely to produce negative effects on growth and development. The growth and development abnormalities in children with renal failure have been well described and are among the worst sequelae of CRF in children.[30] Correction of growth failure, to allow full human potential, is one of the main goals of therapy of children with CRF. The worst growth failure seems to occur in children whose renal failure develops in the first year of life.[31] There seems to be no single factor occurring in renal failure that accounts for the growth failure. Hormone changes, metabolic disturbances, and nutritional deficiencies have been implicated.[32] Chronic acidosis, potassium depletion, renal osteodystrophy, abnormalities in somatomedin secretion, malnutrition from low caloric intake, and chronic anemia are some proposed mechanisms.[33]

Some have shown the potential for normal growth and development in nondialyzed children with CRF.[34] Thirty-four children from age 1 month to 12 years, presenting with renal insufficiency, were carefully managed with correction of acidosis, electrolyte imbalance, and caloric insufficiency. Normal growth velocity was achieved in a large percentage despite marked decrease in GFR. Several infants with GFR less than 5 ml per min, however, failed to thrive despite all therapy.

A number of neurologic disorders in CFR have been demonstrated. These include dialysis disequilibrium and dementia, and hypertensive encephalopathy. In addition, there is evidence of a severe effect of CRF on brain development in infants. A progressive and profound neurologic abnormality in infants who developed renal failure in the first year of life has been identified.[35,36,37] This has been shown to consist of developmental delay, microcephaly, myoclonus, dysarrthria, seizures, and coma. This encephalopathy appeared to be independent of dialysis. The implication was that the developing brain was especially sensitive to the consequences of uremia. Whether or not the mental defects are due to uremia or malnutrition that can accompany it is unclear. The consequences of uremia on development were studied.[31] Twelve children who had had CRF since infancy underwent early dialysis (mean 18 months) and early transplantation (mean 28 months). By age 1 year six had head circumferences at least two SD below the mean. Eight children functioned subnormally, and five were moderately to severely retarded. Crittendon[37] reported on 66 children ages 6 months to 20 years with renal failure. Children less than 2 years scored the lowest on IQ testing. Consequently, it is clear that the growth and development potential for children developing ESRD in infancy is severe and significant.

An earlier impetus for transplantation was failure of access sites for chronic dialysis. With improvements in peritoneal dialysis in small children this is seldom a pressing reason for transplantation. The emergence of continuous ambulatory peritoneal dialysis (CAPD) has made it possible to dialyze even tiny children who used to be difficult if not impossible to dialyze with hemodialysis. Several studies have shown that children managed with CAPD have better growth and development than those managed by hemodialysis.[39] More recent reports, while continuing to show the superiority of peritoneal dialysis over hemodialysis, have shown growth rates that were retarded (less than fifth percentile)[40] and maintained the same growth velocity during the time on dialysis. Potter[41] followed 51 children maintained on CAPD. There were some advantages of CAPD over hemodialysis in terms of better maintenance of metabolic and electrolyte levels. However, there was a high complication rate and approximately 10 percent mortality rate. This indicated the need for further evaluation of CAPD.

Whether or not transplantation or earlier institution of dialysis, or more careful metabolic and nutritional support can prevent the neurologic damage and allow more normal growth and development is unresolved. But the answer to this question will determine the optimum therapy for infants with CRF.[42]

One successful technique for dealing with ESRD in infants was reported by Kohaut.[43] Three infants presented with ESRD within the first month of life. They were managed on CAPD for 12 to 14 months. During that time an aggressive nutritional support program, including enteral tube feeding, was instituted in two patients. All three received parental living donor grafts at age 13 to 15 months. Although the sizes of the children at the time of transplantation, were not given, all three were within 2 standard deviations (SD) for height and 1 SD for weight and head circumference. Whether there is an early time that transplantation should be carried out to achieve optimal development and to prevent growth and mental retardation or allow catch-up growth if growth arrest has occurred is unclear.

Therefore, based on the entire available data, including results of transplantation, results of nutritional therapy, and the results of dialysis in tiny children, the optimum strategy for treatment of tiny children and infants with ESRD remains undetermined. Transplantation should be carried out as early in the child's course as is technically possible. Based on the data available, if a suitable LRD is available, satisfactory results can be obtained with transplantation at an early age. Whether this should be carried out as soon as the diagnosis of ESRD is made or after an appropriate interval of maintenance on CAPD and nutritional support to give the child a

chance to grow and achieve a size that will lend itself more easily to technically feasible transplantation remains to be seen. If no LRD is available, then the most prudent recommendation is to try to achieve growth by a combination of CAPD and aggressive nutritional support. If growth occurs, then cadaveric transplantation can be carried out when the child is larger. If while monitoring the child carefully with head circumference, neurologic examination, and growth charts there is evidence that the child is failing to thrive, then a cadaveric graft should be carried out. Potential morbidity and mortality remains high in this group. Why tiny children with cadaveric grafts have done so poorly in comparison with those with living related grafts is unclear. The technical complications should be no greater than with living related grafts, except that the living related transplants can be planned and scheduled, which may make them safer. The immunosuppression may be more difficult to manage, since higher doses are required for cadaveric graft maintenance, and small changes in dosing may be fatal to a cadaveric graft. Patients who receive a cadaveric graft are often metabolically and nutritionally in poor condition, putting them at much higher risk of serious infection. There may be significant selection factors in choosing which infants receive cadaveric and which receive LRD grafts. Thus, it remains to be seen whether results for healthier infants treated with cadaver grafts will improve and more closely approximate the results of living related grafts, much like the gradual evening out of results between LRD grafts and cadaver grafts in another high-risk recipient population—those with diabetes. In the first significant reports from Minnesota on transplantation of diabetics, graft survival with cadaver grafts was 22 percent, with LRD 75 percent.[44] In subsequent series, the difference has been much less.[45]

MENTAL STATUS

The question of treatment of ESRD in children with moderate to severe retardation is not clearly answered. Whether to treat or not to treat severely retarded children with CRF is more a matter of values and judgment. Consequently, once it has been determined that mental changes are not acutely caused by uremia, careful discussion with patients' families is necessary to provide them with adequate information to determine treatment options, including no treatment. It has been argued that parental involvement is mandatory in order to provide ESRD treatment for infants and children.[46] Removal of a child from parental care is unlikely to allow adequate treatment.

PSYCHOLOGICAL ASSESSMENT

The severe impact of chronic disease and CRF in particular on the social and psychological functioning of children has been well described. Depression, withdrawal, poor body image, loss of control, and underlying aggression all occur and are most exacerbated during adolescence, since this is the time of maximal difficulty in psychological adaptation even in healthy children.[47] One manifestation of the effect of chronic illness and transplantation is the noncompliance with medication.[48] Inability to comply with the posttransplantation immunosuppressive regimen is considered by most to be a contraindication to transplantation, because noncompliance is a significant cause of graft loss, especially in adolescent recipients. Unfortunately, this diagnosis is usually made after transplantation, not before. Psychosocial evaluation by social workers and psychiatrists, as well as by others involved in the transplant team, is essential to try to develop the ability to predict and intercede in these cases.[49,50] Poor family support, poor family function, low self-esteem, complex medical course, low income, adolescence, female sex, and a history of noncompliance have been shown to be predictors of noncompliance.[51] Of these, the history of noncompliance is the only risk factor occurring frequently enough to contraindicate retransplantation. Unfortunately, intervention programs have proved to be only partially successful. Beck[52] described an intensive educational program in pediatric renal transplant families. Forty-three percent of patients were initially noncompliant with medications; 19 percent were noncompliant even after intensive education. Com-

pliance was found to be best when there was direct parental involvement with the child's daily medication and when medication calendars were voluntarily maintained. Compliance was less likely if parents did not come to the clinic with their children. It was concluded that knowledge was important, but not necessarily the determining factor; motivation was the most important factor in achieving patient compliance with immunosuppressive regimens. For adolescents, regimens that minimize changes in body image are the most useful in preventing noncompliance and potential graft loss. Otherwise it seems that, for the present, the potential for noncompliance, and hence graft loss, is one of the increased risk factors in renal transplants in children, especially adolescent girls.

PRETRANSPLANTATION EVALUATION

Careful history and physical examination by nephrologist and transplant surgeon is necessary. Nine pages of forms are reproduced in a recent article,[53] showing the detailed examination that is carried out for the child who is a potential transplantation candidate. In essence the evaluation is similar to that in adults.

Lower urinary tract must be carefully examined to ensure adequacy. In children whose renal failure is secondary to nonurologic causes, a history of normal voiding and a normal voiding cystourethrogram are adequate evaluation. Children whose history suggests any voiding dysfunction or whose renal failure is caused by obstructive uropathy may need more intense investigation (Figs. 9–3 and 9–4). This may include cystoscopy and urodynamic investigation. The critical mistake is to fail to detect an abnormality in lower urinary tract function prior to transplantation; this may prove critical to the outcome of the transplant. The criteria for a functioning bladder include ability to store an adequate volume of urine at low pressure without leaking and ability to empty entirely at an appropriate time.[54] In the past serious urinary tract anomalies were often considered contraindications to transplantation. Recent important advances in pediatric urology have dramatically improved the care of

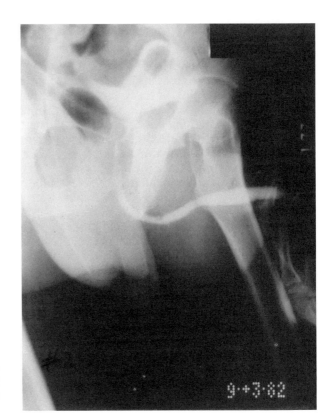

Figure 9–3. Postoperative voiding cystourethrogram after stricture repair and closure of the suprapubic tract in preparation for transplantation.

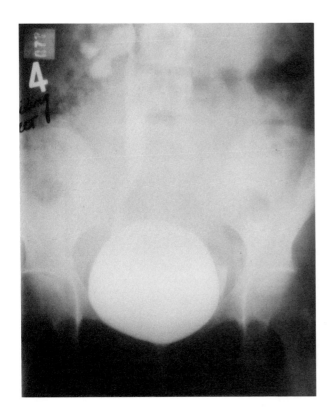

Figure 9–4. Voiding cystourethrogram from a child developing CRF secondary to reflux and chronic pyelonephritis. Transplantation was carried out without bilateral nephrectomy or repair of the reflux without sequelae.

all children with lower urinary tract abnormalities, and, as a consequence, have also extended the possibility of transplantation in this group. In the late 1970s a series of reports demonstrated the possibility of carrying out renal transplant in the face of selected lower tract abnormalities. Butt[55] reported two patients and Firlet[56] reported five patients with posterior urethral valves and CRF who were successfully transplanted with reresection of the valves. Likewise, patients who had undergone supravesical diversion for lower urinary tract anomalies and who consequently had defunctionalized bladders underwent successful transplantation with the allograft ureter placed into the bladder.[57] The ability of such defunctionalized bladders to recover and function normally was demonstrated in a number of clinical and experimental studies.[58–60] The potential adequacy of these bladders could be tested prior to transplantation by a variety of techniques including placement of a tiny suprapubic catheter and cycling the bladder intermittently with saline to simulate normal bladder filling and emptying.[61]

The timing of reresection of valves is important. Children who are making no urine or who have had supravesical diversion may have a higher risk of urethral stricture if the valves are fulgerated in the absence of urine flow.[62] In this situation resection shortly after transplantation can be done. It is obviously important to be aware of the valves if they are going to be resected posttransplantation so that the Foley catheter can be left indwelling until the valve resection.

More recently, patients with more severe

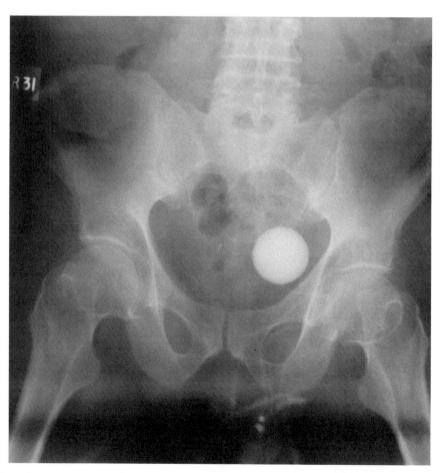

Figure 9–5. Roentgenogram of the pelvis in a patient with neurogenic bladder and an artificial urinary sphincter. Cuff is around the bulbous urethra.

types of abnormalities such as neurogenic bladder, exstrophy of the bladder, prune belly syndrome, microcystis and megacystis have had successful transplants after rehabilitation of the lower urinary tract or after placement of a conduit for diversion. These cases require careful urodynamic evaluation, which may include simultaneous cine voiding and pressure measurements and sphincter electromyography.[63-65] In any case the evaluation of such children is probably best carried out by a pediatric urologist with special interest in these problems. In most cases now a functional lower urinary tract can be created by combination of clean intermittent catheterization, pharmacologic agents, bladder augmentation with bowel, and artificial urinary sphincter so that supravesical diversion is seldom necessary.[66-73] (Fig. 9-5). Complex urinary reconstructions should be carried out in advance of transplantation. Gonzalez[74] carried out undiversion in 13 children with CRF in advance of transplantation, resulting in sterilization of the urinary tract in 12 patients, and noted significant psychosocial benefits to the children. In the occasional case where it is not possible to salvage lower urinary tract function, transplantation can be carried out into an intestinal conduit. Because of dissatisfaction with the long-term results of ileal conduits in children,[75,76] and on the basis of clinical and experimental evidence,[77,78] antirefluxing colonic conduits have become the preference in children, using either sigmoid colon or ileocecal segments. These conduits should be placed several months prior to transplantation or at the time of transplantation.[79]

OTHER PRETRANSPLANTATION OPERATIONS

Splenectomy is seldom performed. There was evidence in the past of improved graft survival in patients who had had adjunctive splenectomy.[80] A high risk of sepsis and mortality has been identified in these patients, obviating any potential gain in immunosuppression from the operation.[81] Most studies fail to demonstrate any graft survival advantage in patients who have had splenectomy.[82]

Bilateral nephrectomy, either prior to or at the time of transplantation, is seldom performed. In Pittsburgh only 2 children out of 75 undergoing transplantation required bilateral nephrectomy. Even in children with minimal GFR, when the native kidneys continue to excrete water and make erythropoietin and vitamin D, subsequent dialysis management is significantly easier and safer. Because of improved antihypertensive drugs it is seldom necessary to remove kidneys for hypertension. Even significant levels of reflux do not seem to predispose to unusually high risk of septic complications after transplantation.[83] Cystic disease does not necessitate nephrectomy unless a specific septic focus is present. If there is a specific septic focus in one or the other kidney, severe uncontrolled hypertension, or severe symptomatic proteinuria, unilateral or bilateral nephrectomy can be carried out. Another indication for bilateral nephrectomy was proposed by Mahan[84] in children with congenital nephrotic syndrome, whose chronic protein loss creates severe malnutrition and increases operative mortality.[84] Infants in their program with that syndrome undergo elective bilateral nephrectomy prior to transplantation.

If bilateral nephrectomy is considered and a retroperitoneal transplant is to be done, the bilateral nephrectomy can be done prior to transplantation with minimal morbidity through small posterior or subcostal incisions. If an intraperitoneal graft is contemplated, then bilateral nephrectomy can be performed through the midline transplantation incision at the time of transplant.

One consequence of being able to transplant most children with obstructive and congenital urinary tract anomalies is that transplantation has to be considered as part of the continuum of urologic care. As an example, newborns with severe azotemia secondary to posterior urethral valves and evidence of bilateral renal dysplasia may be better managed with percutaneous nephrostomy drainage, to see if any renal function will be restored, than with high cutaneous ureterostomy, which has been the standard treatment in this situation. If transplantation is likely to be necessary, the cutaneous ureterostomies have to be taken down, whereas the percutaneous tubes can merely be removed. Likewise, it is indicated to fix severe reflux, even when such repair may not salvage renal function, in order to refunctionalize the bladder and avoid bilateral nephrectomy.

The prospective renal donor should be screened for hepatitis, HTLV-3, and cytomegalovirus (CMV). The effect of CMV on subsequent graft survival and morbidity has been controversial, though the bulk of evidence indicates that placement of a seropositive donor kidney into a seronegative recipient results in more morbidity and decreased graft survival.[85,86] This has important implications in pediatric renal transplants, since there is a higher frequency of seronegativity in younger persons. In a multicenter seroepidemiologic study of CMV infection on renal transplants it was concluded that CMV has an important adverse effect on morbidity and graft survival in kidneys from cadaver donors.[87] In another study of cadaver renal transplant patients treated with cyclosporine, of 19 patients who were seronegative and received seropositive grafts, 11 seroconverted within the first 3 months after transplant, with 10 being hospitalized due to complications related to primary CMV disease.[88] A significantly smaller percentage of patients receiving positive-to-positive or negative-to-negative combinations developed symptomatic CMV or seroconverted. Consequently, while it is not an absolute contraindication to carry out transplantation from a CMV-positive donor to a CMV-negative recipient, these data should be considered. It is more difficult to screen cadaver donors than LRD prior to transplantation, but it is possible.

DONOR OPERATION

Whether children under the age of consent should serve as living related donors is an ethical question. If such children undergo living related donation, the operation is done in one of several standard ways and is no different from the operation done in adult live donors.

Like the issue in the recipient, the major unresolved controversy in cadaver donation in children is the use of kidneys from very small donors or anencephalic donors. It has been felt in the past that small kidneys transplanted into large recipients would fail to provide satisfactory GFR. Numerous series, both experimental and clinical,[89,90] have since demonstrated progressive compensatory hypertrophy resulting in rapid adaptation to the size of the recipient (Fig. 9–6A,B). Some multicenter studies have shown decreased graft survival when kidneys from pediatric donors were used than when adult kidneys were used.[91] An approximately 10 percent difference in graft survival with kidneys from donors 0 to 9 years old versus those from donors older than 9 years was reported. Most single-center studies have not shown any effect on graft survival using kidneys from donors older than 2 to 3 years old.[92,93] Barry reported 77 cadaver transplants in adults receiving single kidneys from donors 16 months to 16 years old with similar graft survival to the other recipients.[94] Results of use of single kidneys from donors less than 2 years of age have been mixed.[95] No graft survivors in recipients who received single cadaver grafts from donors less than 2 years of age were reported from one center.[96] Difficulty in performing the vascular anastomoses using small donor vessels can attribute for much of these poor results. Although the complication rate in Barry's series showed an incidence of vascular and ureteral problems no different from those in their other patients, Sheldon[97] reported a 22 percent vascular complication rate in 41 grafts in recipients transplanted with kidneys from donors less than 2 years old. To obviate the potential risk of vascular complication and graft loss, some have used kidneys from tiny donors en bloc, using the aorta and vena cava for the vascular anastomoses, thus increasing the size of the vessels to be anastomosed.[98,99] While this has the disadvantage of reducing the total number of kidneys available, the potential benefit of reducing the complication rate outweighs the disadvantages. Many of these tiny donors were simply not accepted as donor candidates in the past. With the increasing need for livers for small children, this is now less likely to occur. Only rarely is it necessary to sacrifice the kidneys for the liver in these donors.[100,101] Thirty-three kidneys from donors less than 2½ years old were either discarded or shipped out of the country. This represented 6 percent of all such kidneys from the members of the

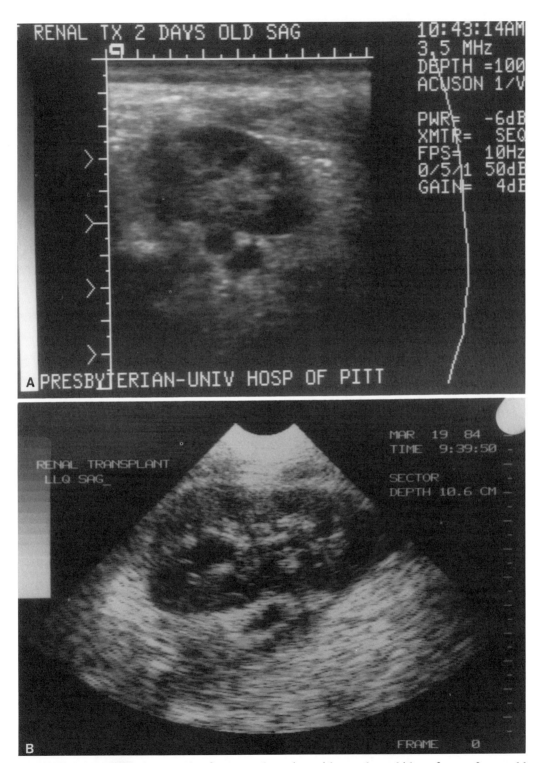

Figure 9–6. Transplant ultrasounds after transplantation with a cadaver kidney from a 2-year-old donor into a 16-year-old recipient showing 2-cm growth from 1 day (*A*) to 2 weeks (*B*) after transplant.

South East Organ Procurement Foundation.[102] Twenty en bloc cadaver transplants were done in Pittsburgh over a 5-year period in donors less than 3 years of age. Many of these kidneys were from pediatric liver donors. There were no vascular complications in the recipients. Three ureters developed obstructions, which is higher than the rate when adult kidneys are used. Nonetheless, with the shortage of cadaveric grafts available it is important that as many as possible of these tiny donor kidneys be used, either singly or en bloc.

The use of anencephalic donors is more controversial. While some reports show successful use of kidneys from anencephalic infants, there are several problems with their use.[103]

1. The small size may create increased technical problems.

2. The extreme circumstances surrounding the availability of these donors make some reluctant to ask for donation from the family.

3. There may be a higher incidence of renal anomalies in these deformed infants.[104]

4. Problems have arisen over the ability legally to establish brain death despite the inevitable lethality of anencephaly. This occurred in a recently reported case.[105,106]

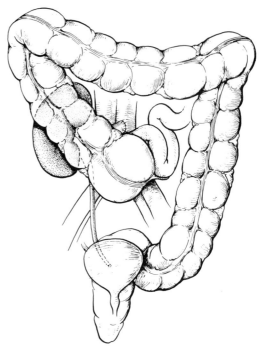

Figure 9–7. Diagram of placement of large kidney into the aorta and vena cava intraperitoneally behind the cecum.

RECIPIENT OPERATION

Unlike the adult operation, where little consideration has to be paid to any size discrepancy between donor organ and recipient, in the child attention must be paid to any difference in size between the donor organ and recipient. Most children of about 30 kg or more can be transplanted with the same technique used in adults regardless of the size of the kidney. Anastomoses are carried out from the renal artery to the external iliac artery in an end-to-side fashion, or to the internal iliac artery in an end-to-end fashion, and between the renal vein and the external iliac vein. The kidney is placed in a pocket retroperitoneally in the iliac fossa. In the child between 15 and 30 kg, a small kidney may be similarly placed using a retroperitoneal approach, while a large kidney with large discrepancy between donor and recipient size may have to be placed intraperitoneally (Fig. 9–7). With the tiny infant less than 15 kg, especially with an adult kid-

ney, an intraperitoneal approach should be used. This has been well described by Miller.[24,107,108] Anastomosis in this case occurs between the renal artery and the aorta in an end-to-side fashion and between the renal vein and the vena cava in an end-to-side fashion. The kidney is placed behind the cecum. There are instances in even tiny children, with tiny kidneys, where an extraperitoneal approach has been successfully used.[29] The advantage of the extraperitoneal approach is that immediate peritoneal dialysis can be carried out if the graft does not function immediately. The advantage of the intraperitoneal approach is that larger vessels more nearly equal in size to the donor vessels can be used to minimize vascular complications. Also, a large kidney can more easily be accommodated without risk of kinking the vessels when placed intraperitoneally. In the LRD, where the warm and cold ischemia times are small, the need for dialysis is much less likely to occur. Hence, the intraperitoneal approach is advantageous.

There are multiple techniques for en bloc transplant using both kidneys with aorta and vena cava.[109] One of these is to oversew the caudad ends of the aorta and vena cava and anastomose them end-to-side into the iliac vessels. Another is to interpose the donor aorta or vena cava either as a complete cylinder or as a patch into the recipient vessels to minimize any potential for clot developing in the closed-off end[101](Fig. 9–8).

Anastamosis of the ureter to the bladder can be carried out using a variety of tech-niques. The need for antirefluxing mechanism is unproven in transplants. However, if the situation is extrapolated from other children with reflux, there are definitely circumstances, such as when there is associated infection in which the occurrence of reflux is detrimental to renal function. Therefore, it seems prudent whenever possible to construct an antirefluxing mechanism when doing transplantation in children. There are several ways to do this,

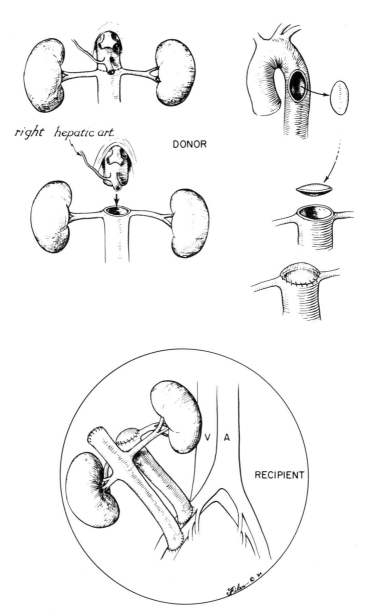

Figure 9–8. Diagram of one method of placement of paired pediatric kidneys where the superior mesenteric artery may have been used for liver transplant.

including creation of a submucosal tunnel intravesically, as described by Politano and Leadbetter.[110] Another is by means of a nipple mechanism created intravesically.[111] An old technique that has obtained new interest because it is simple, quick, and effective is an extravesical approach described by Lich[112] and updated by others. This technique has been used in the last 150 cadaveric transplants in Pittsburgh with a 2.3 percent complication rate, comparable with that obtained using other techniques. The prevention of ureteral complications begins in the donor operation, in which great care has to be taken to avoid damage to the delicate ureteral blood supply and to lower pole renal arteries, which may supply the ureter directly, and continues in the recipient operation, in which the ureter must be handled with great delicacy. When this occurs, the type of bladder repair is probably not so important.

The ureter can, if necessary, be anastamosed into an intestinal segment.[114] Most prefer to create the conduit prior to the transplantation, and the butt end is placed near the iliac vessels for ease in locating at the time of transplantation. This has been done five times in Pittsburgh, with no acute technical difficulties or complications and no adverse effect on graft survival. One patient sustained a late ureteral-ileal stricture that required repair 7 years after transplantation. Others have preferred to create the conduit at the time of transplantation, figuring it easier to then decide the proper placement of kidney and conduit. For diversion in children most surgeons now use a nonrefluxing bowel segment such as the ileocecal segment or sigmoid colon, which may have fewer long-term complications than refluxing ileal segments.[115]

PERIOPERATIVE MANAGEMENT

Careful intraoperative management of the small recipient is required. Central venous pressure and temperature must be monitored closely. When there is a large size disparity between child and donor organ, there is a high risk of vascular thrombosis if good flow through the organ is not maintained as the vascular clamps are released. Such a large kidney can siphon off a significant portion of the circulating blood volume. Recommendations for handling this problem include volume loading to a CVP of 12 to 20 cm water, slow release of the vascular clamps and intravenous bicarbonate to neutralize the acidosis resulting from ischemia in the lower extremities.[107,116] Studies have shown that raising central pressure when measured by pulmonary wedge pressure is effective in reducing the incidence of initial nonfunction. Since few children have significant cardiovascular disease, the measurement of central venous pressure in most instances is adequate. Others have measured central to peripheral temperature monitoring as a noninvasive indicator of adequacy of tissue perfusion.[26,117] Other adjunctive recipient measures that have been used in adults and children to try to lower the incidence of initial graft nonfunction have included low-dose dopamine, mannitol, or furosemide, or loading with colloid at the time of release of the vascular clamps.[118] Since there are so many factors that may determine rate of nonfunction, it is difficult to prove the efficacy of any of these adjuncts. Care must be taken in using high doses of mannitol, since it can exert a cardiac depressant effect and lower the blood pressure.[119] Flushing the Collins solution out of ice-stored kidneys prior to transplantation has been recommended to avoid washing potassium from the kidneys into the circulation. In adults this amount is probably not significant, but may be so in small children.

The consequence of initial nonfunction may be severe, since the children have been volume-loaded and have a propensity for volume-related hypertension. If an intraperitoneal operation has been carried out they may be difficult to dialyze acutely, since the peritoneum is not usable and an acute dialysis catheter may be difficult to obtain. Patient management is also difficult if the graft functions, since the kidney may put out huge quantities of water and electrolytes for several hours after the transplantation. In small children these amounts may equal their blood volume hourly. While similar events often occur in adult transplants, the margin for error in fluid and electrolytes is much smaller in children, and the consequences of mistakes often more dramatic. Seizures and encephalopathy can develop acutely, if sodium, potassium, bicarbonate, glucose, magnesium, calcium, and phosphorous are not closely watched. Measurement of urine concentrations of these substances is a helpful guide to replacement. If water balance is not maintained, hypotension and vascular thrombosis can occur.

Since many children arrive for transplantation having been managed with peritoneal dialysis (PD), there is the question of what to do with the PD catheter at the time of transplantation. If the transplant has been intra-abdominal, then the catheter is of little use postoperatively and can be removed. Since there may be low-grade tunnel infection, it seems prudent to remove the catheter after the transplant dressing has been applied unless it is directly in the way of the incision. If the transplant operation has been extraperitoneal, then there is merit in leaving the PD catheter for eventual use if necessary in the perioperative period. The catheter can be removed a month or so later if the graft is functioning and is past the time of high risk, and when immunosuppression is lower. This has been shown to be a safe and effective means of managing PD catheters after transplantation.[120,121]

IMMUNOSUPPRESSION

There is no evidence of any particular propensity for children to develop tolerance. Therefore the same need for immunosuppression exists in children as adults. All the agents that have been used in adult transplantation have been used in pediatric transplantation, including azathioprine, steroid, and antilymphocyte globulin.[122–124] Between 1961 and 1981 there was a slow progression of improvement in graft survival using these agents in conjunction with aggressive tissue matching.

Two new agents have come into use in the last few years. These are cyclosporine and the monoclonal antibody, OKT-3. The monoclonal antibody was used in Oregon in four children with steroid-resistant rejection. Spectacular reversal of rejection occurred in two with no serious side effects.[125]

Since 1979 cyclosporine has been widely used in a large number of patients.[126–130] Studies on cyclosporine in children have shown it to be safe in the short term.[131,132]

Most studies have shown graft survival superior to conventional immunosuppression, and excluding the tiny children, results are comparable with results in adults treated with cyclosporine. The same problems with cyclosporine that apply in adult transplantation are applicable in children: short- and long-term nephrotoxicity, figuring the appropriate dosage schedule and the most efficacious combination to use with cyclosporine, whether steroid is necessary, whether donor-specific transfusions and conventional immunosuppression are better than no transfusions and cyclosporine in one-haplotype LRD grafts. The answers to some of these questions are particularly relevant to the use of cyclosporine in children, where the lifetimes of the patient and graft are expected to be longer than in adults. It is difficult to determine whether steroids and cyclosporine give better graft survival than cyclosporine alone by comparing different centers' studies, since too many other variables may be affecting outcome. In children this is an important consideration, since high steroid doses cause serious side effects and significant growth impairment. Protocols using cyclosporine and steroid combinations employ doses of steroid that are significantly less than most azathioprine/steroid combinations by a factor of 3 to 4 (Table 9–1).

While acute cyclosporine nephrotoxicity is reversible and dose-related, long-term nephrotoxicity remains a concern. The most convincing studies have been in heart transplantation series, where other renal toxic factors may be present.[133,134] Protocols that use lower doses of cyclosporine are advantageous in children. Since synergism between cyclosporine and azathioprine has been demonstrated, one regimen that is attractive for children includes cyclosporine, azathioprine, and prednisone, all in lower doses than regimens not including one of the drugs.[135,136] Graft survival similar to those treated with double- and single-drug regimens has been shown with this combination with minimal morbidity.

As graft and patient survivals become more similar from one immunosuppression regimen to another, morbidity may be the determining factor in choosing one over another. Similar graft survival has been shown in one-haplotype LRD transplants whether donor-specific transfusions

Table 9–1 Two Representative Immunosuppression Protocols

	Double-Drug Therapy
Cyclosporine	14 mg/kg/d: 2 divided doses by mouth
	Taper after 1 week depending on renal function and cyclosporine levels (whole blood HPLC 150–200)
Prednisone	2 mg/kg/d
	Taper to 0.3 mg/kg/d by 1 month
	Triple-Drug Therapy
Cyclosporine	10 mg/kg/d: 2 divided doses by mouth
	Taper after 1 week depending on renal function and cyclosporine levels (whole blood HPLC 100)
Prednisone	2 mg/kg/d
	Taper to 0.25 mg by 1 month
Azathioprine	1 mg/kg/d
	Titrate to WBC

are used or cyclosporine without transfusion is used.[137,138] This has important consequences in treatment of children. In infants especially it may be critical to achieve success with a one-haplotype match living related graft; if so, it is unacceptable to risk even the 10 to 20 percent sensitization risk of donor-specific transfusions, even though there may be long-term sequelae of having such children on long-term cyclosporine, required to achieve similar graft survival.

Although steroid clearly inhibits growth,[139] and it seems intuitively obvious that the lower the steroid dose in children, the better the growth should be, low steroid doses alone may not help growth impairment. Ellis[140] reported eight children managed with cyclosporine/steroid followed longer than 1 year with low steroids (average dose 0.24 mg per kg per day) and satisfactory renal function 1 year after transplantation. Seven of these failed to have any catch-up growth. Others have reported catch-up growth using cyclosporine and low-dose steroid[141,142] (Fig. 9–9). Age may be a determining factor in achieving catch-up growth after transplantation regardless of steroids or renal function. Ingelfinger[143] reported 11 children less than age 7 who achieved good growth acceleration after renal transplantation and 76 children older than age 7 who showed no catch-up growth after transplantation, although there were no statistics. It was concluded in that study that bone age of less than 12 years, steroid dose of less than 1 mg per kg per day, good renal function, and patient age of less than 7 years were important determinants of growth after transplantation. Likewise, alternate-day steroid therapy, although it may ameliorate some of the undesirable effects of steroid usage, may not improve growth[144] and may be associated with significant risk of rejection. Another approach has been to withdraw steroids after satisfactory engraftment, such as Flechner[145] carried out in one-haplotype LRD grafts. Steroids were withdrawn in patients who manifested low donor-specific mixed lymphocyte reactions 6 months after transplantation without adverse consequences. They similarly treated 26 full-house-match LRD transplants with cyclosporine and steroid and withdrew all steroid in 14 patients.[146] Overall there were only two patients (8 percent) who ever were treated for rejection episodes. In the short term there was little effect of cyclosporine nephrotoxicity. Whether the long-term toxicity of cyclosporine would balance the long-term benefit of steroid withdrawal in children is as yet undetermined.

One significant difference between use of cyclosporine in children and its use in adults is its more rapid metabolism in children, which results in more rapid clearance of the drug.[147,148] Higher dose of drug or more frequent doses per day (three or four instead of the usual one or two) are needed to achieve therapeutic trough levels.[149] Careful monitoring of serum or blood levels by radioimmunoassay or high-pressure liquid chromatography is essential in the

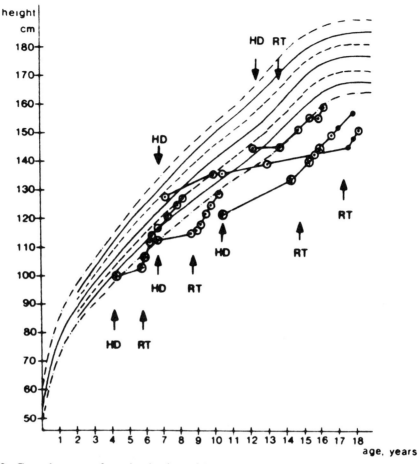

Figure 9–9. Growth curves from institution of hemodialysis through renal transplantation in five boys immunosuppressed with cyclosporine. (From Klare, JF, et al,[141] with permission.)

early posttransplantation period in children to avoid serious rejection due to inadequate drug. Dosing of the drug on a per-body surface area has also been recommended to achieve satisfactory levels.[148] Even then, monitoring of levels is essential.

RESULTS

As a rule interpreting survival data for transplantation has to be done carefully, especially when trying to compare results from one center with those of another and one immunosuppression regimen to another. Numerous variables have been identified as important determinants of patient and graft survival.[150] Thus, wide differences in high risk factors may be present in one series but not another, and this may ac-

count for large differences in survival. The recipient population should be identified. In pediatric studies two important stratifications are LRD and cadaver donor grafts and the age and/or size of the recipient population. Some studies lump LRD and cadaver grafts together and state survival figures. Some studies stratify by age only less than 1 year of age to identify high-risk children, while other studies consider less than age 6 years to be a high-risk factor. Attention has to be paid to whether patient or graft survival is being discussed, which is not always clear. Few centers now report graft survival numbers that exclude graft loss due to patient death, but this has been done in the past. Few centers report anything less than 1-year survival, but 2- and 5-year survival may be more important in assessing results in chidren. Also important are the number of patients at risk for various intervals when actuarial survival is stated.

In earlier reports of transplantation and dialysis results, mortality was similar for living related transplants and hemodialysis in children and slightly worse for children receiving cadaveric transplants.[151] Recent improvements have narrowed the gap for cadaveric grafts. There is often wide variation in graft survival from center to center[2,41,131,152-161] (Table 9-2). Results of transplants in children from large centers have been reported many times over the years.[17,20,22,84,153-156] Their respective cumulative results have recently reported documented results over time: one from the University of Minnesota involving 304 primary cadaveric renal transplants in children over 17 years[3] (Fig. 9-10) and another from the University of California at San Francisco with 203 transplants over 20 years.[157] Immunosuppression regimens varied over time in each center. Patient survival with full-house-match living related grafts was 100 percent in Minnesota and with one-haplotype-match living related

grafts 95 percent over the entire 17-year period. All LRD patients in San Francisco over the last 8 years were alive. Survival in those patients receiving cadaveric grafts in the most recent years reviewed was 95 percent in San Francisco and 90 percent in Minnesota. Graft survival varies over time and varies widely with donor source and recipient age. The primary cause of graft loss over all times reviewed in both series was rejection. The primary cause of death was from infections secondary to excessive immunosuppression in both series.

The impact of cyclosporine has been shown in a large multicenter study.[152] Single-center studies have also shown the effect of cyclosporine in children.[131] Cyclosporine and steroid were used in 18 pediatric recipients, 10 cadaveric and 8 living related, with 100 percent patient survival and 83 percent (n = 15) overall graft survival. Tejani[158] reported 2-year patient and graft survival in 19 patients (11 cadaveric and 8 living related) of 89 percent (n = 17) and 78 percent (n = 15).[158] Nine of these patients were off all steroid.

The effect of HLA and DR matching has

	Number of Patients	% Graft Survival	% Patient Survival	Type
Table 9-2 Representative Graft Survivals from Several Centers Showing Variation That Can Exist in Reported Figures*				
Author	**Number of Patients**	**% Graft Survival**	**% Patient Survival**	**Type**
Fine (1978)[160]	42	39	78	CAD
Fine (1978)[160]	26	73		LRD
Broyer (1983)[152]	256	65	87	CAD
Potter (1986)[157]	99	79	93	LRD
Potter (1986)[157]	103	36	79	CAD
Najarian (1986)[3]	216	70	92	LRD
Najarian (1986)[3]	78	54	84	CAD
Pittsburgh (1986)	35	72	97	CAD
Conley (1985)[131]	10	100	100	CAD
Conley (1985)[131]	8	80	100	LRD
Arbus (1980)[161]	100	55	85	CAD

*Numbers from Fine, et al[160] are actual 5-year survivals and represent cases done from 1967 to 1972. Numbers from Potter and Najarian are actuarial 5-year survivals and represent transplants done over a 20- and a 17-year period, respectively. Conley and Pittsburgh are 2-year survivals, do not include tiny children, and represent results over only a 5-year period with constant immunosuppression regimen.

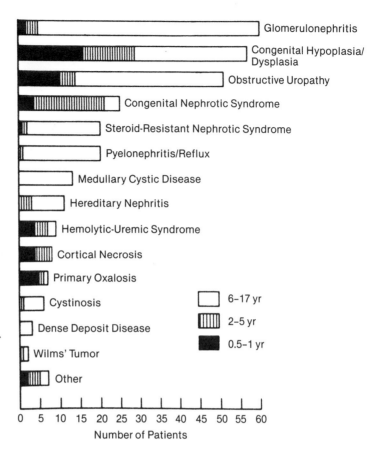

Figure 9–10. The etiology of ESRD and the ages of transplantation in 304 pediatric recipients of primary renal allografts over a 17-year period at the University of Minnesota. (From Najarian, JS, et al,[3] with permission.)

been difficult to prove in single-center studies, but differences between well-matched and poorly matched grafts in large multicenter studies do show up.[159] Presumably these effects would be present with or without cyclosporine.

REFERENCES

1. Reinhart, JAB: The doctor's dilemma. J Pediatr 77:505, 1970.
2. Harmon, WE and Ingelfinger, JR: Dialytic management of end-stage-renal disease. In Tune, BM and Mendoza, SA (eds): Pediatric Nephrology 12:343, 1984.
3. Najarian, JS, et al: The outcome of 304 primary renal transplants in children (1968–1985). Ann Surg 204:246, 1986.
4. Cameron, JS: Glomerulonephritis in renal transplants. Transplantation 34:237, 1982.
5. Strigel, JE, et al: Recurrence of focal segmental sclerosis in children following renal transplantation. Kidney Int (Suppl 19) 29:44, 1986.
6. Chesney, RW and Friedman, AL: The medical management of chronic renal failure. In Tune, BM and Mendoza, SA (eds): Pediatric Nephrology 12:321, 1984.
7. Gilboa, N: Renal transplantation in primary oxaluria. J Pediatr 104:323, 1984.
8. Scheinman, JI, Najarian, JS, and Mauer, SM: Successful strategies for renal transplantation in primary oxalosis. Kidney Int 25:804, 1984.
9. Watts, RWE, et al: Primary hyperoxaluria (Type 1): Attempted treatment by combined hepatic and renal transplantation. QJ Med 57:697, 1985.
10. Fine, RN: Renal transplantation in children. In Morris, PJ (ed): Kidney Transplantation. Grune & Stratton, New York, 1984.
11. Hebert, D, Sibley, RK, and Mauer, SM: Recurrence of hemolytic uremic syndrome in renal transplant recipients. Kidney Int (Suppl 19) 30:51, 1986.
12. Van Buren, D, et al: De novo Hemolytic uremic syndrome in renal transplant recipients immunosuppressed with cyclosporine. Surgery 98:54, 1985.

13. Bonser, RS, Franklin, AD, and McMaster, P: Cyclosporin induced hemolytic uremic syndrome in liver allograft recipient. Lancet 2:1337, 1984.

14. Donckerwolcke, R, et al: Combined report on regular dialysis and transplantation of children in Europe. Proc Eur Dial Transplant Assoc 19:61, 1982.

15. Bryngcr, H, et al: 17th Report. Proc Eur Dial Transplant Assoc 17:2, 1980.

16. Habib, R, Broyer, DM, and Benmaiz, LD: Chronic renal failure in children. Nephron 11:209, 1973.

17. Potter, DE, et al: Treatment of end-stage renal disease in children: A 15-year experience. Kidney Int 18:103, 1980.

18. Penn, IJ: Renal transplantation for Wilm's tumor: Report of 20 cases. J Urol 122:793, 1979.

19. Goodwin, WE, et al: Human renal transplantation: I. Clinical experiences with six cases of renal homotransplantation. J Urol 89:13, 1963.

20. Hodson, EM, et al: Renal transplantation in children ages 1 to 5 years. Pediatrics 61:458, 1970.

21. Moel, DI, and Butt, KMH: Renal transplantation in children less than 2 years of age. J Pediatr 99:535, 1981.

22. Lum, CT, et al: Results of kidney transplantation in the young child. Transplantation 34:167, 1982.

23. Rizzoni, G, et al: Renal transplantation in children less than 5 years of age. Arch Dis Child 55:532, 1980.

24. Miller, LC, et al: Transplantation of the adult kidney into the very small child. J Pediatr 100:675, 1982.

25. Fine, RN: Renal transplantation for children: The only realistic choice. J Ped Kidney International (Suppl 17) 28:15, 1985.

26. Trompter, RS, et al: Renal transplantation in very young children. Lancet 1:373, 1983.

27. Brodehl, J, et al: Kidney transplantation in infants and young children. Transplant Proc (Suppl 3)18:8, 1986.

28. Arbus, GS, et al: Cadaveric renal transplants in children under 6 years of age. Kidney Int (Suppl 15) 24:S111, 1983.

29. Campbell, DA, et al: Cadaveric renal transplantation in a 2.2-kilogram neonate. Transplantation 98:197, 1984.

30. Betts, P and Magrath, G: Growth pattern and dietary intake of children with chronic renal insufficiency. Br Med J 2:189, 1974.

31. McGraw, ME and Haka-Ikse, K: Neurologic-development sequelae of chronic renal failure in infancy. J Pediatr 106:579, 1985.

32. French, CB and Genel, M: Pathophysiology of growth failure in chronic renal insufficiency. Kidney Int (Suppl 19) 29:59, 1986.

33. Kaskel, FJ, Feld, LG, and Schoeneman, MJ: Renal replacement therapy in infants and children. Adv Pediatr 32:197, 1985.

34. Kleinknect, C, Broyer, M and Huot, D: Growth and development of nondialyzed children with chronic rcnal failure. Kidney Int 24S:40, 1983.

35. Baluarte, HR, et al: Encephalopathy in children with chronic renal failure. Proc Clin Dial Transplant Forum 7:95, 1977.

36. Bale, JF, Siegler, RL, and Bray, P: Encephalopathy in young children with moderate chronic renal failure. Am J Dis Child 134:581, 1980.

37. Rotundo, A, et al: Progressive encephalopathy in children with chronic renal insufficiency in infancy. Kidney Int 21:486, 1982.

38. Crittenden, MR, et al: Intellectual development of children with renal insufficiency and end stage disease. Int J Pediatr Nephrol 6:275, 1985.

39. Fennell, RS, et al: Growth in children with various therapies for end-stage-renal-disease. Am J Dis Child 138:23, 1984.

40. Fine, RN and Salusky, IB: CAPD/CCPD in children: Four years experience. Kidney Int (Suppl 19) 29:7, 1986.

41. Potter, DE, et al: Comparison of continuous ambulatory peritoneal dialysis and hemodialysis in children. Kidney Int (Suppl 19) 29:11, 1986.

42. Holiday, MA: Nutrition therapy in renal disease. Kidney Int (Suppl 19) 29:3, 1986.

43. Kohaut, EC, et al: Living-related donor renal transplantation in children presenting with end-stage-renal-disease in the first month of life. Transplantation 40:725, 1985.

44. Najarian, JS, et al: Ten year experience with renal transplantation in juvenile onset diabetics. Ann Surg 190:487, 1979.

45. Starzl, TE, et al: Cadaveric renal transplantation in diabetics in the 1980's: With special reference of cyclosporine. Diab Neph 2:9, 1983.

46. Fine, RN: Renal transplantation in children. J Ped 100:754, 1982.

47. Bouras, M and Raimbault, G: The psychosocial consequences of renal disease and its treatment in children and adolescents: A follow-up study. In Brodehl, J and Ehrich, JHH (eds): Pediatric Nephrology. Springer-Verlag, New York, 1984.

48. Korsch, BM, Fine, RN, and Negrete, VF: Noncompliance in children with renal transplants. Pediatrics 61:876, 1978.

49. Korsch, BM, Negrcte, VF and Gartner, JE:

Kidney transplantation in children: Psychosocial follow-up study on child and family. J Pediatr 83:399, 1973.

50. Korsch, BM: Current issues in comprehensive care for children with chronic illnesses. In Brodehl, J and Ehrich, JHH (eds): Pediatric Nephrology. Springer-Verlag, New York, 1984.

51. Sampson, TF: The child in renal failure. J Am Acad Child Psychiatry 14:462, 1975.

52. Beck, DE, et al: Evaluation of an educational program on compliance regimens in pediatric patients with renal transplants. J Pediatr 96:1094, 1980.

53. Lum, CT, Wassner, SJ, and Martin, DE: Current thinking in transplantation in infants and children. Pediatr Clin North Am 32:1203, 1985.

54. McGuire, EJ: Clinical Evaluation and Treatment of Neurogenic Vesical Dysfunction. Williams & Wilkins, Baltimore, 1984.

55. Butt, KMH, et al: Renal transplantation in patients with posterior urethral valves. J Urol 116:708, 1976.

56. Firlet, CF: Use of defunctionalized bladders in pediatric renal transplantation. J Urol 116:634, 1976.

57. Krieger, JN, Stubenbord, WT, and Vaughan, ED: Transplantation in children with end stage renal disease of urologic origin. J Urol 124:508, 1980.

58. Hendren, WH: Urinary tract refunctionalization after prior diversion in children. Ann Surg 180:494, 1974.

59. Warshaw, BL, et al: Renal transplantation in children with obstructive uropathy. J Urol 123:737, 1980.

60. Schmaelzle, JF, Cass, AS, and Hinman, F: Effect of disuse and restoration of function on vesical capacity. J Urol 101:700, 1969.

61. Marshall, FF, et al: The urological evaluation and management of patients with congenital lower urinary tract anomalies prior to renal transplants. J Urol 127:1078, 1982.

62. Crooks, KK: Urethral strictures following transurethral fulguration of posterior urethral valves. J Urol 127:1153, 1982.

63. McGuire, EJ, and Woodside, JR: Diagnostic advantages of fluoroscopic monitoring during urodynamic evaluation. J Urol 125:830, 1981.

64. Bauer, SB, et al: Urinary undiversion in myelodysplasia: Criteria for selection and predictive value of urodynamic evaluation. J Urol 125:89, 1980.

65. Bauer, SB, et al: Predictive value of urodynamic evaluation of newborns with myelodysplasia. JAMA 252:192, 1984.

66. Lapides, J, et al: Further observations on self-catheterization. J Urol 116:169, 1976.

67. Light, JK, and Scott, FB: Total reconstruction of the lower urinary tract using bowel and the artificial sphincter. J Urol 131:953, 1984.

68. Light, JK, and Engelmann, UH: Reconstruction of the lower urinary tract: Observations on bowel dynamics and the artificial urinary sphincter. J Urol 133:594, 1985.

69. Light, JK: The artificial urinary sphincter in children. Urol Clin North Am 12:103, 1985.

70. Linder, A, Leach, GE, and Raz, S: Augmentation cystoplasty in the treatment of neurogenic bladder dysfunction. J Urol 129:491, 1983.

71. Mitchell, ME: The role of bladder augmentation in undiversion. J Pediatr Surg 16:790, 1981.

72. Mitchell, ME, and Rink, RC: Urinary diversion and undiversion. Urol Clin North Am 12:111, 1985.

73. Rink, RC, and Mitchell, ME: Surgical correction of urinary incontinence. J Pediatr Surg 19:637, 1986.

74. Gonzalez, R, et al: Undiversion in children with renal failure. J Pediatr Surg 19:632, 1984.

75. Schwarz, GR, and Jeffs, RD: Ileal conduit urinary diversion in children: Computer analysis of followup from 2 to 16 years. J Urol 114:285, 1975.

76. Shapiro, SR, Lebowitz, R, and Colodny, AH: Fate of 90 children with ileal conduit urinary diversion a decade later: Analysis of complications, pyelography, renal function and bacteriology. J Urol 114:289, 1975.

77. Richie, JP, and Skinner, DG: Urinary diversion: The physiologic rationale for nonrefluxing colonic conduits. Br J Urol 47:269, 1975.

78. Elder, DD, Moisey, CU and Rees, RWM: A long-term follow-up of the colonic conduit operation in children. Br J Urol 51:462, 1979.

79. Levey, RH, et al: Unique surgical and immunological features of renal transplantation in children. J Pediatr Surg 13:576, 1978.

80. Fryd, DS, et al: Results of a prospective randomized study on the effect of splenectomy versus no splenectomy in renal transplant patients. Transplant Proc 13:48, 1981.

81. Peters, T, et al: Splenectomy and death in renal transplant patients. Arch Surg 118:795, 1983.

82. Sutherland, DER, et al: Long term effects

of splenectomy versus no splenectomy in renal transplant patients: Reanalysis of a randomized prospective study. Transplantation 38:619, 1984.

83. Pontin, AR, and Jacobson, JE: Renal transplantation in primary reflux nephropathy without nephro-ureterectomy. S Afr Med J 12:593, 1985.

84. Mahan, JD, et al: Congenital nephrotic syndrome: Evolution of medical management and results of renal transplantation. J Pediatr 105:549, 1984.

85. Fryd, DS, et al: Cytomegalovirus as a risk factor in renal transplantation. Transplantation 30:436, 1980.

86. Smiley, ML, et al: The role of pretransplant immunity in protection from cytomegalovirus disease following renal transplantation. Transplantation 40:157, 1985.

87. Irvin, B, et al: Morbid outcome of cytomegalovirus-negative transplant recipients receiving cytomegalovirus-positive kidneys. Transplant Proc (in press).

88. Rubin, RH, et al: Multicenter seroepidemiologic study of the impact of cytomegalovirus infection on renal transplantation. Transplantation 40:243, 1985.

89. Baden, JP, Wolf, GM, and Sellers, RD: The growth and development of allotransplanted neonatal canine kidneys. J Surg Res 14:213, 1973.

90. Provoost, AP, et al: Influence of the recipient's size upon renal function following kidney transplantation: An experimental and clinical investigation. J Pediatr Surg 19:63, 1984.

91. Ploeg, RJ, et al: Young cadaver donors for kidney procurement: Graft survival and surgical damage. Transplant Proc 18:485, 1986.

92. Dafoe, DC, Campbell, DA, and Turcotte, JG: Use of single kidneys from donors two to five years of age for transplantation into nonpediatric recipients. Transplant Proc 18:477, 1986.

93. Salvatierra, O, and Belzer, FO: Pediatric cadaver kidneys: Their use in renal transplantation. Arch Surg 110:181, 1975.

94. Barry, JM, Norman, DJ, and Bennett, WM: Pediatric cadaver kidney transplants into adults. J Urol 134:651, 1985.

95. Glass, NR, et al: Results of renal transplantation using pediatric cadaver donors. Surgery 85:504, 1979.

96. Wengerter, K, Matas, AJ, et al: Transplantation of pediatric donor kidneys to adult recipients. Ann Surg 204:172, 1986.

97. Sheldon, CA, et al: Surgically significant complications in pediatric renal transplantation (abstr). N.E. Section, American Urologic Association, Toronto, Canada, 1986.

98. Schneider, JR, et al: Long-term success with double pediatric cadaver donor renal transplants. Ann Surg 197:439, 1983.

99. Andersen, OS, Jonasson, O, and Merkel, FK: En bloc transplantation of pediatric kidneys into adult patients. Arch Surg 35:108, 1974.

100. Rosenthal, JT, et al: Principles of multiple organ procurement from cadaver donors. Ann Surg 198:617, 1983.

101. Taylor, RJ, Rosenthal, JT, and Hakala, TR: Combined cadaveric hepatic and renal organ procurement in infants: Technique for salvage of all organs. Arch Surg 120:1084, 1985.

102. Williams, GM, et al: Reasons why kidneys removed for transplantation are not transplanted in the United States. Transplantation 38:691, 1984.

103. Ohshima, S, et al: Kidney transplantation from an anencephalic baby: A case report. J Urol 132:546, 1984.

104. Naeye, R, Pa, H, and Blanc, WA: Organ and body growth in anencephaly. Arch Pathol Lab Med 91:140, 1971.

105. New York Times: Law thwarts effort to donate infants' organs. Sept 9, 1986.

106. Bailey, LL, et al: Cardiac allotransplantation in newborns as therapy for hypoplastic left heart syndrome. N Engl J Med 315:949, 1986.

107. Miller, LC, et al: Renal transplantation of the adult kidney into the very small child: Technical considerations. Am J Surg 145:243, 1983.

108. Starzl, TE, et al: A technique for use of adult renal homografts in children. Surg Gynecol Obstet 119:106, 1964.

109. Vroemen, JPAM, et al: Surgical experience with neonatal grafts. Transplant Proc 18:482, 1986.

110. Politano, V and Leadbetter, WF: An operative technique for the correction of vesicoureteral reflux. J Urol 79:932, 1958.

111. Pacquin, AJ: Ureterovesical anastomosis: The description and evaluation of a technique. J Urol 82:573, 1959.

112. Lich, R, Hoverton, LW, and Davis, LA: Recurrent urosepsis in children. J Urol 86:554, 1961.

113. Barry, JM: Parallel incision, unstented extravesical ureteroneocystostomy: Follow up of 203 kidney transplants. J Urol 134:249, 1985.

114. Firlet, CF, and Merkel, FA: The application of ileal conduits in pediatric renal transplantation. J Urol 118:647, 1977.

115. Williams, JL, et al: Colon conduit in pediatric renal transplantation. J Urol 125:515, 1980.

116. Sheldon, CA, et al: Improving survival in

the very young renal transplant recipient. J Pediatr Surg 20:622, 1985.

117. Haycock, GB: Intraoperative and immediate postoperative care in the management of the paediatric transplant recipient. In Brodehl, J and Ehrich, JHH (eds): Pediatric Nephrology. Springer-Verlag, New York, 1983.

118. Belzer, FO, Hoffman, RM, and Southard, JH: Organ preservation. Surg Clin North Am 58:261, 1978.

119. Cote, CJ, Greehow, DE, and Marshall, BE: The hypotensive response to rapid intravenous administration of hypertonic solutions in man and in the rabbit. Anesthesiology 50:30, 1979.

120. Patel, S, Rosenthal, JT, and Hakala, TR: Management of the peritoneal dialysis catheter after renal transplantation. Transplantation 36:589, 1983.

121. Scharer, K, and Fine, RN: Renal transplantation in children treated by continuous ambulatory peritoneal dialysis. In Fine, RN, Scharer, K, and Muhls, O (eds): CAPD in Children. Springer-Verlag, New York, 1985.

122. Najarian, JS, et al: Renal transplantation in infants and children. Ann Surg. 174:583, 1971.

123. Leichter, HE, et al: Short-course antithymocyte globulin for treatment of renal transplant rejection in children. Transplantation 41:133, 1986.

124. de Mol van Otterloo, JCA, et al: Long-term results of cadaveric kidney transplantation in children. Transplant Proc 19:1523, 1987.

125. Leone, MR, et al: Monoclonal antibody for reversal of acute renal allograft rejection in pediatric patients. Transplantation 40:574, 1985.

126. Starzl, TE, et al: Variable convalescence and therapy after cadaveric renal transplantation under cyclosporin A and steroids. Surg Gynecol Obstet 154:819, 1982.

127. Rosenthal, JT, et al: Cadaveric renal transplantation under cyclosporine steroid therapy. Surg Gynecol Obstet 157:309, 1983.

128. Rosenthal, JT, et al: Second cadaver kidney transplants: Improved graft survival in secondary kidney transplants using cyclosporin A. J Urol 131:17, 1984.

129. Calne, RY, White, DJG, and Roles, K: Cyclosporine A initially as the only immunosuppressant in 34 recipients of cadaveric organs. Lancet 2:1033, 1979.

130. Merion, RM, et al: Cyclosporine: 5 years experience in cadaveric renal transplantation. N Engl J Med 310:148, 1984.

131. Conley, SB, et al: Use of cyclosporine in pediatric renal transplant recipients. J Pediatr 106:45, 1985.

132. Starzl, TE, et al: Liver and kidney transplantation in children receiving cyclosporin A and steroids. J Pediatr 100:681, 1982.

133. Myers, BD, et al: Cyclosporin-associated chronic nephrotoxicity. N Engl J Med 311:699, 1984.

134. Strom, TB and Loertscher, R: Cyclosporine-induced nephrotoxicity. N Eng J Med 311:728, 1984.

135. Canafax, DM, et al: Combination immunosuppression: Three drugs (azathioprine, cyclosporine, and prednisone) for mismatched related and four drugs (antilymphocyte globulin, azathioprine, cyclosporine, prednisone) for cadaver renal allograft recipients. Transplant Proc 17:2671, 1985.

136. Sommer, BG, Henry, ML, and Ferguson, RM: Sequential conventional immunotherapy with maintenance cyclosporine following renal transplantation. Transplant Proc 18:69, 1986.

137. Potter, DE, et al: Effect of donor-specific transfusions on renal transplantation in children. Pediatrics 76:402, 1985.

138. Flechner, SM, et al: Successful transplantation of cyclosporine treated haploidentical living related donor recipients. Transplantation 37:73, 1984.

139. Travis, LB, et al: Growth and glucocorticoids in children with kidney disease. Kidney Int 14:365, 1978.

140. Ellis, D, et al: Renal function and somatic growth in pediatric cadaveric renal transplantation with cyclosporine-prednisone immunosuppression. Am J Dis Child 139:1161, 1985.

141. Klare, B, et al: Cyclosporine in renal transplantation in children. Lancet, 1:692, 1984.

142. Knight, JF, Roy, LP, and Sheil, AGR, Catch-up growth in children with renal transplants immunosuppressed with cyclosporine alone. Lancet, 1:160, 1985.

143. Ingelfinger, JR, et al: Growth acceleration following renal transplantation in children less than 7 years of age. Pediatrics 68:255, 1981.

144. Feldhoff, C, et al: A comparison of alternate day and daily steroid therapy in children following renal transplantation. Int J Pediatr Nephrol 5:11, 1984.

145. Flechner, SM, et al: Long-term results of cyclosporine therapy in recipients of mismatched living related kidneys. Transplant Proc 18:44, 1986.

146. Flechner, SM, Van Buren, CT, and Kerman, RH: Does cyclosporine improve results of HLA-identical renal transplantation? Transplant Proc 19:1486, 1987.

147. Ptachcinski, RJ, et al: Cyclosporine pharmacokinetics in children following cadav-

eric renal transplantation. Transplant Proc (in press).

148. Hoyer, PF, et al: Dosage of cyclosporin A in children with renal transplants. Clin Nephrol 22:68, 1984.

149. Neiberger, RE, Weiss, RA, and Matas, AJ: Elimination of cyclosporine following oral administration to children with renal transplants. Transplant Proc (in press).

150. Sanfilippo, F, et al: The detrimental effect of delayed graft function in cadaver donor renal transplantation. Transplantation 38:643, 1984.

151. Avner, ED, et al: Mortality of chronic hemodialysis and renal transplantation in pediatric end-stage-renal-disease. Pediatrics 67:412, 1981.

152. Broyer, M, Gagnadoux, MF, and Niaudet, P: Kidney transplantation in children: Results and late sequelae. In Brodehl, J and Ehrich, JHH (eds): Pediatric Nephrology. Springer-Verlag, New York, 1984.

153. Hodson, EM, et al: Renal transplantation in children ages 1 to 5 years. Pediatrics 61:458, 1978.

154. Sheldon, CA, Najarian, JS, and Mauer, SM: Pediatric renal transplantation. Surg Clin North Am 65:1589, 1985.

155. So, SKS, et al: Improved results of multiple renal transplantation in children. Surgery 98:729, 1985.

156. So, SKS, et al: Current results in pediatric renal transplantation at the University of Minnesota. Kidney Int (Suppl. 19) 29:25, 1986.

157. Potter, DE, et al: Twenty years of renal transplantation in children. Pediatrics 77:465, 1986.

158. Tejani, A, et al: Cyclosporine experience in renal transplantation in children. Kidney Int (Suppl. 19) 29:35, 1986.

159. Sanfilippo, F, et al: Benefits of HLA-A and HLA-B matching on graft and patient outcome after cadaver-donor renal transplantation. N Engl J Med 311:358, 1984.

160. Fine, RN, et al: Long-term results of renal transplantation in children. Pediatrics 61:641, 1978.

161. Arbus, GS, et al: Transplantation and complications of chronic renal failure. Can Med Assoc J 122:659, 1980.

Chapter 10

Nutrition

MARK E. ROSENBERG
THOMAS H. HOSTETTER

The role of nutrition in renal transplantation is an often neglected area from both research and clinical standpoints. A wide variety of disciplines would be involved in defining this role, and a range of clinical situations occurring over a large time span would need to be considered in such a definition. Patients undergoing transplantation have sustained variable periods of chronic renal insufficiency and failure, often undergoing dialysis treatment. Hence, they have been subjected to the metabolic and nutritional sequelae that chronic renal failure and its treatment engender. Further nutritional demands are imposed in the acute posttransplantation period by the combined catabolic stresses of surgery and high-dose corticosteroid treatment. The chronic posttransplantation period is often marked by a variety of nutritional problems, some of which are special to transplantation, such as hyperlipidemia and steroid-induced diabetes, and others common to renal disease in general, such as hypertension and hyperphosphatemia. This chapter will highlight some of these issues and present rational plans of management.

PRETRANSPLANTATION PERIOD

To gain insight into the nutritional issues of the immediate posttransplantation period, it is important to understand some aspects of the metabolic derangements of chronic renal failure (CRF).

Carbohydrate

Over 50 percent of patients with CRF demonstrate glucose intolerance.[1] The major mechanism is impaired peripheral tissue uptake of glucose, particularly by skeletal muscle, due to insulin resistance.[2] The causes for this insulin resistance are multifactorial and include the presence of insulin antagonists, receptor and post-receptor abnormalities, and defects in the transmembrane transport system.[3,4] In part the glucose intolerance may be attributed to the increased glucagon and growth hormone levels of CRF. Generally, carbohydrate intolerance is improved by dialysis. Diabetics exhibit a similar increased peripheral resistance to insulin.[5] However, it is important to note that insulin requirements of diabetics may actually lessen due to decreased renal extraction and catabolism of insulin. Often these effects outweigh the development of insulin resistance, and diabetics can suffer hypoglycemic episodes if their insulin dosage is not appropriately adjusted with advancing uremia.

Lipid

Lipid abnormalities occur in 50 to 70 percent of patients with chronic renal failure.[6-8] Hypertriglyceridemia is the most common finding.[7] It is usually accompanied by increases in VLDL-triglyceride and VLDL-cholesterol and a decrease in HDL-cholesterol.[8] This pattern is associated with an increased risk of atherosclerosis. The primary defect resides in a decrease in lipoprotein lipase activity in extrahepatic tissues, leading to accumulation at normal rates of production, although some patients exhibit an increase in triglyceride production.[9,10] In addition, several drugs commonly used in uremics may aggravate these abnormalities. These include diuretics and anabolic steroids. Dialysis does not reverse the hypertriglyceridemia. Indeed, glucose absorption during peritoneal dialysis may aggravate the lipid disorder.[11] These lipid abnormalities often antedate end-stage renal disease by many years, suggesting they are more a manifestation of the uremic state than related to dialysis per se. Again, steroid therapy posttransplantation may aggravate the hyperlipidemia. This complication will be discussed further in a later section.

Protein

Protein malnutrition can be a significant problem in patients with chronic renal failure. Its etiology is often multifactorial. Decreased protein intake can result from both the anorexia of uremia and overzealous protein restriction by physicians. As well, intestinal absorption of amino acids and small peptides may be impaired.[12] Increased protein loss can occur both in the urine as a result of the proteinuria of renal disease and in dialysis fluid in patients undergoing peritoneal dialysis. Complicating these increased losses, protein requirements may be raised because of increased muscle catabolism.[13] Finally, protein synthesis is also often impaired.

Characteristically, plasma amino acid levels are altered in uremia.[14,15] These abnormalities include a decreased tyrosine/phenylalanine ratio due to impaired hydroxylation of phenylalanine, a decreased valine/glycine ratio, and an increase in hydroxyproline, citrulline, and 1,3-methylhistidine. Serine is also often low due to its diminished production from glycine by the diseased kidney. Thus, nonessential amino acids tend to be increased while essential amino acids with some exceptions are reduced in plasma. The severity of these abnormalities is often correlated with the degree of renal insufficiency and tend to worsen when protein intake is inadequate. In addition, the distribution of amino acids between cells and extracellular fluid is often abnormal; thus, the plasma abnormalities differ from those in the intracellular compartment.[15] Decrements occur in the intracellular pools of several essential amino acids including valine, threonine, histadine, and lysine. Of the nonessential amino acids, those of the urea cycle, citrulline, ornathine, and arginine, are elevated in uremic muscle, as is aspartic acid. Some but not all of these abnormalities are reversible by both dietary manipulation and dialysis therapy.

Although these abnormalities of amino acid distribution are undoubtedly related to the defects in protein turnover, a precise mechanism relating the observed abnormalities is not available. However, recent studies by Mitch and colleagues[16] suggest that acidosis contributes to muscle proteolysis since alkali therapy reduces muscle breakdown in experimental uremia. Parathyroid hormone and glucagon have also been incriminated as contributors to muscle dissolution in uremia.[17,18]

Vitamins and Minerals

Abnormalities in the metabolism of calcium, phosphorus, vitamin D, and aluminum are universal in chronic renal failure, and full discussion is beyond the scope of this chapter. Suffice it to say that renal osteodystrophy is often a significant problem in these patients, and hypercalcemia secondary to chronic hyperparathyroidism may occur, especially in the posttransplantation period. Uremic patients may rarely be deficient in pyridoxine, folic acid, and other water-soluble vitamins, if they have been on a very restricted diet or receiving dialysis without vitamin supplements.[19] Attempts to contol hyperkalemia can lead to avoidance of fruits and vegetables and the vitamins they contain. Iron deficiency may result from blood loss through the GI tract, frequent blood sampling, and loss during hemodialysis.

Thus, the patient with chronic renal failure presents with a number of special metabolic problems that should be evaluated carefully prior to transplantation. Secondary consequences of these problems include accelerated atherosclerosis, altered immune responsiveness, bone disease, and anemia. All of these will greatly affect the peritransplantation management of these patients.

ACUTE POSTTRANSPLANTATION PERIOD

Severe protein catabolism may occur in the acute posttransplantation period.[20–23] It is a particularly demanding period in that it combines the stress of surgery with the use of high-dose corticosteroids in patients who already may be protein-malnourished. Resulting morbidity may be greatly increased due to such factors as poor wound healing, gastrointestinal ulceration, osteopenia, myopathy, and increased skin fragility. Abnormal immunoresponsiveness may also occur and lead to increased susceptibility to infection. This section will deal with the combined effects of these stresses in the transplantation setting. For a detailed discussion of the individual metabolic effects of surgery or corticosteroids, the reader is referred elsewhere.[24,25]

Various measures of nitrogen metabolism have been used.[26] The urea nitrogen appearance rate is a measure of the waste nitrogen produced. When the BUN is stable, this parameter is equivalent to the urinary urea nitrogen excretion. When the BUN is changing, which is generally the case in the posttransplantation period, changes in urea nitrogen accumulation, either positive or negative, must be accounted for by multiplying the change in blood urea nitrogen concentration by the urea distribution space, which is approximately equal to total body water, or 60 percent of the body weight. The urea nitrogen appearance is the sum of urea excretion and urea accumulation (positive or negative). The protein catabolic rate is another often-used parameter and is directly calculable from the urea nitrogen appearance rate. Nitrogen balance is calculated by the difference between nitrogen intake and the urea nitrogen appearance rate minus the nonurea nitrogen excretion, estimated as

0.031 g of nitrogen per kg per day. The goal of nutritional therapy is to minimize the urea nitrogen appearance and protein catabolic rate with the result that patients achieve neutral or positive nitrogen balance.

Hoy and associates[20] found that the protein catabolic rate was elevated in transplant recipients on maintenance steroids. It rose over the first few days posttransplantation, then stabilized at an elevated level during the 3 weeks in which these patients were followed. Therapy for rejection with yet higher doses of steroids was associated with a further increase in the protein catabolic rate, and this effect persisted for at least 4 days after treatment was completed. Protein intake did not affect the protein catabolic rate; protein restriction did not decrease it; and higher protein intake did not accelerate this measure of protein catabolism. Since the protein catabolic rate did not change, those on lower protein intakes were inevitably in negative nitrogen balance.

Cogan and colleagues[21] studied nitrogen intake and net urea generation rate in patients undergoing hemodialysis for acute tubular necrosis post renal transplant. All patients were on maintenance steroids, initially 120 mg per day and tapering to 70 to 90 mg per day. Seven patients were maintained on moderately restricted protein (0.7 g per kg per day) and caloric (20 kcal per kg per day) intake. They had high urea generation and protein catabolic rates and were in significantly negative nitrogen balance. Eight similarly treated patients were placed on a high-protein (1.3 g per kg per day) and calorie (43 kcal per kg per day) diet. Their protein catabolic rates were similar to those of the first group, but they were in protein balance without an increase in urea nitrogen generation. These investigators concluded that despite high urea nitrogen generation rates, protein balance could be achieved by increasing protein intake, a regimen that did not require an increase in the number of dialysis treatments.

Liddle and coworkers[22] first observed that dietary modification could alter the nitrogen balance and cushingoid side effects in the posttransplantation period. He demonstrated that patients on a high-protein, low-carbohydrate diet had a lower incidence of the facial obesity, striae, and buffalo hump characteristic of high-dose steroids. Whittier and colleagues[23] also examined the effects of a high-protein, low-carbohydrate diet on nitrogen balance and the incidence of steroid side effects in the immediate posttransplant period. A high-protein (range 1.4 to 3.0 g per kg per day), low-carbohydrate diet converted the negative nitrogen balance to positive during the 28 days of the study. Those on an isocaloric diet but ingesting an average of 1 g per kg per day of protein remained in negative nitrogen balance. As can be seen in Figure 10–1, the nitrogen balance varied directly and proportionally with the protein intake. Again in this study cushingoid side effects,

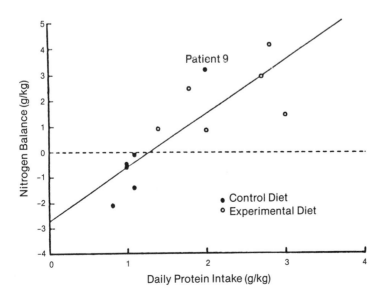

Figure 10–1. Dietary treatment in the acute posttransplant period. Nitrogen balance varied directly and linearly with protein intake (r value, 0.83). The point at which the nitrogen balance is zero is 1.3 g of protein per kg of body weight per day. (From Whittier, FC, et al,[23] with permission.)

especially the typical facial changes, did not develop in those on the high-protein, low-carbohydrate diet, suggesting that one or both of these factors was important in ameliorating steroid side effects.

Protein malnutrition has definite depressant effects on the immune system. This effect raises the question whether there may be a hidden beneficial effect of protein malnutrition in delaying or preventing rejection. Toledo-Pererya and associates[27] examined the effects of peritransplantation nutrition on the acute allograft rejection response in a group of dogs receiving minimal immunosuppression posttransplantation. Dogs malnourished both preoperatively and postoperatively had a significantly delayed time to rejection compared with control animals maintained on a regular diet preoperatively and postoperatively. Animals treated with total parenteral nutrition in the postoperative period did not have accelerated rejection compared with controls. Thus, aggressive nutritional support postoperatively did not heighten the immune response and accelerate rejection. Although pretransplantation malnutrition prolonged the time to acute rejection, other short- and long-term adverse effects of malnutrition were not investigated and would certainly outweigh any beneficial effects.

In summary, increased protein catabolism and negative nitrogen balance often occur posttransplantation due to the combination of pre-existing malnourishment plus the catabolic effects of surgery and steroids. Neutral and even positive nitrogen balance can be restored by increasing protein intake to at least 1.3 g per kg per day.[23] This may result in some increase in blood urea nitrogen, potassium, and phosphorus but at least in one study does not necessarily increase dialysis requirements.[21] This higher protein intake when combined with a carbohydrate intake reduced to approximately 1 g per kg per day may lessen steroid side effects.[22,23] These manipulations should be accompanied by adequate caloric intake (30 to 35 calories per kg per day) for expression of the beneficial effects of this higher protein intake. This prescription necessitates the use of a fairly high-fat diet, but it should be emphasized that this distribution would only be maintained for the first 3 to 4 weeks posttransplantation. As discussed below, after this initial period, carbohydrate intake should be increased and the fat intake decreased to avoid hyperlipidemia.

CHRONIC POSTTRANSPLANTATION PERIOD

The most common causes for late failure of renal allografts are chronic rejection and recurrent de novo glomerulonephritis.[28] Experimental and clinical evidence indicate that after some critical reduction in functioning renal mass, chronic renal insufficiency predictably progresses to end-stage renal failure.[29,30] Although the predictability and tempo of this process have not been extensively examined in the late-failing renal allograft, it seems likely that the available observations and pathophysiologic evidence obtained in other chronic renal diseases are applicable to this type. Numerous factors have been proposed to explain the progressive tendency of renal disease. Included among them are persistence of the initiating insult, systemic and glomerular capillary hypertension, crystal deposition in the renal parenchyma as a result of abnormal calcium and phosphorus metabolism, serum lipid abnormalities, altered coagulative and platelet interactions with the glomerular capillary network, and late secondary immune attack.

Dietary protein restriction reduces renal injury and progression in virtually all models of experimental renal injury, and increasing clinical data suggest such a beneficial effect in a variety of chronic renal diseases. Although this beneficial effect has been recognized in experimental models for over 50 years, its mechanisms like those of the progression of renal failure are unsettled.[30] Effects on both the kidney and systemic factors known to influence renal function have been proposed to explain the salutary effects of dietary protein restriction. We will now turn to a discussion of how dietary protein restriction may interact with proposed mechanisms favoring progressive renal disease. It should be noted that these mechanisms are at varying degrees of clinical and experimental support, and furthermore, their individual applicability to chronically failing renal allografts remains largely unsettled. However, the prevailing view that many if not all chronic renal diseases have final common pathways of destruction makes it extremely likely that these effects of dietary protein and mechanisms of renal damage are in large part applicable to the problem of late allograft loss (Figure 10–2).

Progression of Experimental Renal Damage and Dietary Protein

Hemodynamic Mechanisms of Progression

Systemic Hypertension. Arterial hypertension is a common problem in the post-transplantation course, especially in the setting of renal insufficiency. Studies of diabetic nephropathy suggest that blood pressure control may reduce the rate of loss of renal function.[31,32] Few studies have systematically explored the influence of dietary protein on systemic arterial pressure in experimental models of hypertension; even less information is available on clinical material, and none in the chronic transplantation population. Reduced dietary protein has been effective in lowering systemic arterial pressure in mineralocorticoid-induced hypertension in rats, so-called DOC-salt hypertension.[33] However, in other forms of experimental hyperten-

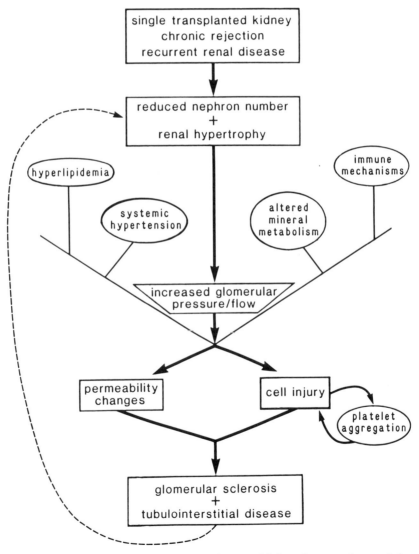

Figure 10–2. Proposed scheme for progressive renal failure in transplant recipients.

sion, dietary protein restriction has not reduced systemic pressure. Notably the systemic hypertension that develops in rats following surgical reduction of renal mass persists even with severe dietary protein restriction,[34,35] and hypertension in the spontaneously hypertensive rat or Dahl salt-sensitive rat is uninfluenced by reduced protein intake.[36,37] Finally, in at least one preliminary study of two-kidney, one-clip renal-vascular hypertension in the rat, a reduced dietary protein intake was associated with a higher systemic pressure.[38] Taken together, these experimental studies suggest no consistent effect of dietary protein on arterial pressure. Most important, in several models in which protein restriction diminishes renal injury, there has been no concomitant diminution in hypertension. This indicates that the beneficial effects of protein restriction do not necessarily depend on an antihypertensive action. Findings in the experimental setting are consistent with recent clinical studies of protein restriction. Rosman and associates[39] found no effect of dietary protein restriction on arterial pressure in their study of the effects of this dietary manipulation on the course of chronic renal disease. The study lasted 1½ years and included 149 patients with a variety of renal diseases. Nevertheless, slowing of the progression to renal failure was observed. Similarly, studies by Rosenberg and coworkers[40] of the short-term effects of dietary protein restriction in patients with renal insufficiency demonstrated no effect on blood pressure, again despite improvement in several measures of renal function.

Intrarenal Hemodynamics. While systemic arterial pressure is not consistently influenced by dietary protein, intrarenal hemodynamics are regularly affected by the level of dietary protein.[34,35] In this regard, dietary protein restriction appears almost unique in altering hemodynamics and protecting against experimental renal injury.

Consequent to loss of functional renal mass, animals ingesting a normal diet with unrestricted protein experience functional and structural enlargement of residual renal tissue.[41] Single nephron GFR of the remaining nephrons rises substantially and in direct proportion to the nephron mass lost; that is, the greater the loss, the greater the compensatory increase in filtration by the remnant units.[41] The neurohumoral and cellular mechanisms underlying this remarkable increase in function and structure are incompletely formulated. However, it seems clear that elevations in glomerular capillary pressure and plasma flow due to reduced renal vascular resistances cause the compensatory increase in single nephron filtration rate in remaining glomeruli.[34]

One of the primary determinants of the degree of functional and structural augmentation in remnant nephrons is dietary protein intake. Numerous studies in experimental animals have demonstrated that a high protein intake augments weight of the kidney and produces cellular evidence of enhanced growth.[30] On the other hand, lowering dietary protein below standard levels will reduce kidney size even in animals with intact kidneys. Besides altered growth, functional changes can be produced in experimental animals and humans with intact kidneys by altering dietary protein. For example, GFR and renal blood flow both increase with either acute or chronic protein loading.[42,43] Finally, the institution of a low-protein diet when renal mass is markedly reduced changes the functional and morphologic evidence of renal enlargement that normally occurs in residual nephrons following loss of renal mass.[30,34]

The finding of blunted functional and structural changes induced by low-protein diets following nephron mass reduction and the observation that dietary protein restriction diminished renal injury have led to the hypothesis that the deleterious effects of normal or increased dietary protein in the setting of renal damage are due to the adaptive increases in pressure and flow in the kidney. In this regard, studies in the remnant kidney rat model of renal insufficiency have demonstrated that a low-protein diet diminishes both intrarenal pressures and evidence of renal injury.[34,35,44] This correlation among glomerular capillary hypertension, glomerular injury, and the reversal of the cycle by dietary protein restriction has also been found in other models of renal injury. Finally, by imposing protein restriction after established compensatory renal hypertrophy and hyperfusion have occurred and by studying several nondietary manipulations of renal diseases, it has been possible to incriminate increased glomerular capillary pressure as the injurious force.[35,45] Based on these correlations, the hypothesis that protein restriction diminishes progressive renal injury by reducing intraglomerular pressure has been championed.[30] Although not specifically addressed in models of transplantation, it is conceivable that similar adaptive hemodynamic changes occur both as a result of the initial decrease in renal mass due to the solitary transplanted kidney and to damage to it as the result of chronic rejection or recurrent glomerulonephritis (see Fig. 10–2).

Immune Mechanisms

As noted above, protein restriction can influence immune mediated injury; clinical and experimental studies point to defects in virtually all areas of immune function with protein or protein-calorie malnutrition.[46] Cell-mediated immune function appears to suffer more than humoral ones, but there are also defects in antibody response and the complement system.

Recent data have emphasized the functional importance of the tubular interstitial infiltrate seen in most chronic renal diseases including chronic rejection. Studies by Agus and colleagues[47] of a model of antitubular basement membrane antibody-induced interstitial nephritis have demonstrated that the course of this disease can be modified by restricting dietary protein. These investigators demonstrated that this immune-mediated, interstitial injury was diminished despite continued high titers of the tubular basement membrane antibody. They hypothesize that the beneficial effect was due to the suppressive effects of relatively severe dietary protein restriction on effector T cell immunity. Although the level of dietary protein restriction employed in these studies was relatively severe, they nevertheless raised the possibility that the beneficial effects of dietary protein restriction can be consequent to influences on the cellular immune system.

Although frank immunosuppression by severe protein restriction is not clinically feasible, modulation of intrarenal inflammation by dietary manipulation has been achieved experimentally by Nath and colleagues.[48] Dietary protein intake entails an acid load to which the kidney responds by excreting acid, in large part through augmented renal ammoniagenesis. Recent studies have demonstrated that reduction in dietary acid load reduces intrarenal ammonia levels and mitigates tubulointerstitial disease in an experimental model of chronic renal insufficiency. The mechanism of this effect is believed to be a reduction in the ammonia-mediated triggering of complement component C3. Thus, one beneficial effect of dietary protein restriction in chronic renal disease may involve a diminution in acid load and in consequence in the intrarenal level of proinflammatory ammonia.[48]

Lipids and Coagulation

Although dietary protein restriction in the strict sense necessitates no change in dietary lipid intake, in practice there are often alterations in the nature and quantity of lipids eaten when dietary protein is restricted. A number of experimental progressive renal diseases including various forms of glomerulonephritis, the glomerular sclerosis of aging, and that induced by renal ablation can be importantly influenced by manipulating the quantity and quality of dietary lipid.[49] It has been difficult to formulate a general mechanism of the effects of manipulating dietary lipids, since studies of experimental lupus nephritis suggest a salutary response to reducing arachidonic acid metabolites, while investigations of the rat remnant kidney model suggest that augmenting these metabolites is beneficial.[50,51] It seems quite likely that these discrepancies derive not only from differences in the models being studied but also in the stage of the disease at which lipid metabolism is altered. Secondary, adaptive, or inflammatory sequelae may be more or less developed at different times in different models and consequently respond in different fashion to lipid perturbations.

Lipid intake may influence renal function through several mediators including the prostaglandin system.[51] At least two mechanisms can explain how prostaglandins influence progressive renal disease. First, direct vasoactive effects of prostaglandins may determine renal hemodynamic function and hence be mediators of some of the intrarenal hemodynamic changes that have been reviewed earlier. Although higher-protein diets have been associated with increased prostaglandin excretion in normal animals, a link between the beneficial effects of dietary protein restriction and reduced or altered renal prostaglandins has yet to be established.[52] A second mechanism that has been advanced to explain the effects of changes in dietary lipids has involved the role of prostaglandins in the clotting system in general and platelet-endothelial cell interactions in particular.[53] Several agents, such as dipyridamole, thromboxane synthetase inhibitors, and heparin, which are capable of interfering with platelet function and/or coagulation proteins, also ameliorate the progressive nature of experimental renal disease. These studies have inspired the view that local platelet activation and coagulation within the glomerular capillary loop perpetuates progressive renal injury.[53] In this scheme prostaglandin species such as thromboxane that enhance the platelet-dependent elements of capillary thrombosis would be critical in the perpetuation of progressive glomerular sclerosis. As with the hemodynamic effects of prostaglandins, the relationship between dietary protein restriction and microvascular thrombosis is uncertain. However, in the obstructed kidney, high-protein diets are associated with increased renal vasoconstriction, which can be blunted by specific thromboxane inhibitors.[54] Thus, production of vasoconstrictive and/or procoagulant prostaglandin species, especially thromboxane, may be diminished by dietary protein restriction, and perhaps this leads to reduced glomerular capillary thrombosis.

Hyperlipidemia is a common problem in the posttransplantation period. Although this abnormality probably contributes to large-vessel damage, its role in progressive glomerular capillary obliteration has only recently been suggested. Moorhead and associates[55] have postulated that circulating lipoproteins may induce renal tubular and microvasculature injury. Kasiske and coworkers[56] have demonstrated in preliminary data that clofibrate-induced reduction of the serum cholesterol level of rats ingesting a standard diet lessened proteinuria and the prevalence of sclerotic glomeruli. The effects were achieved without altering the degree of hypertension or serum triglyceride levels. The role of protein intake in the hyperlipidemia of renal disease is unknown, as is the detailed mechanism whereby hypercholesterolemia contributes

to the glomerular pathology. However, it seems reasonable to speculate that mechanisms analogous to those causing large-vessel disease, including direct endothelial injury and insinuation of cholesterol, its protein carrier, or other noxious agents into the capillary wall and mesangium, may contribute to progressive renal insufficiency.

In summary, changes in lipid metabolism can influence the course of several experimental renal diseases, and plasma lipids are altered not only in clinical renal insufficiency but in a large proportion of posttransplantation patients. Functionally and pathologically important components of these alterations may include effects on circulating lipid levels and intrarenal prostaglandin metabolism. Practical approaches to the problem are discussed below.

Mineral Metabolism

As with lipids, a reduction in protein ingestion usually entails reduction in phosphorus intake. Because dietary phosphate restriction mitigates the progressive renal disease seen after subtotal nephrectomy or experimental glomerulonephritis in the rat, the possibility arises that the therapeutic benefits of protein restriction might derive from concomitant phosphorus restriction. However, studies in which dietary protein, but not phosphorus, has been varied have indicated that dietary protein restriction without coincident phosphate restriction can be beneficial.[57] On the other hand, phosphate depletion without simultaneous protein restriction is also capable of reducing progressive experimental renal disease.[58] Thus each of these dietary manipulations seems capable of independently diminishing progressive renal damage. The mechanism whereby phosphate restriction reduces renal injury is as yet uncertain. Three possibilities exist. First, phosphate restriction, at least in certain circumstances, has been associated with reduction in glomerular filtration rate; hence, advantages relating to diminution of hyperperfusion in residual nephrons may be achieved by phosphate restriction.[59] Second, with severe phosphate restriction, defects in the inflammatory response due to dysfunction of leukocytes may be expected. Third, it has been suggested that suppression of the intrarenal deposition of calcium phospate crystals, which can be demonstrated histologically, may be an important mechanism whereby phosphate restriction slows the progression of chronic renal disease.[60] These mechanisms are not mutually exclusive and may all be at play in yielding the beneficial effect of protein restriction. Nevertheless, it should be noted that salutary effects in experimental models have usually required frank depletion of phosphate. Hence, the clinical applicability of this specific dietary manipulation is uncertain. Indeed, the only available controlled clinical study of phosphate restriction independent of protein manipulation found no beneficial effect on progression injury.[61] Whatever the effect on progression of renal insufficiency to renal failure, dietary phosphate restriction is warranted in patients with renal insufficiency for the prevention of hyperparathyroidism and renal osteodystrophy. Clinical approaches to this goal are discussed below.

Progression of Clinical Renal Disease and Dietary Protein

In the clinical setting, treatment by dietary protein restriction was originally used in the later stages of renal failure to reduce symptomatic uremic toxicity. For the reasons outlined above, recent interest has turned to treatment of early asymptomatic renal insufficiency to prevent progression.

Several studies have attempted to address the safety and efficacy of this approach. Three strategies have been commonly employed. Most commonly dietary protein has been held to the minimum daily protein requirements, approximately 0.55 to 0.60 g per kg per day, or for the 70-kg person, approximately 40 g per day.[62] At least three quarters of this should be high biologic value protein in order to supply enough essential amino acids. Any excess losses such as to proteinuria have usually been supplemented. The second option has been more severe portein restriction, usually 20 to 25 g per day of mixed-quality protein plus an essential amino acid supplement. The advantage of this regimen is that the total amount of protein ingested can be further reduced, but amino acid supplementation allows for a greater range of food options, since patients are not restricted to

foods composed of proteins of high biologic value. The third approach has been a similarly severe degree of protein restriction supplemented by the keto analogs of the essential amino acids. These substances are the carbon skeletons of the essential amino acids without the nitrogen. The original rationale for their use was that the nitrogen formed by the endogenous intestinal degradation of urea could be used to aminate the carbon skeletons. Though further studies have not born out this mechanism, the keto analogs do have protein-sparing effects that may be due to an inhibition of protein degradation.[63] Phosphorus intake has also been reduced in most of these regimens.

Maschio and colleagues[64] prescribed a diet containing approximately 0.6 g per kg per day of protein, most of which was high biologic value protein, to patients with varying levels of renal function. A total of 53 patients with creatinines ranging from 1.5 to 6.7 were studied and their rates of progression were compared with a control population of 30 patients eating an unrestricted diet. The patients on the low-protein diet all showed decreased progression compared with the control group. In a later study, using a similar degree of protein restriction, Oldrizzi and coworkers[65] examined the role of the underlying renal disease and whether it affected the response to this low-protein diet. The creatinine levels of the patients varied between 1.5 and 4.5 mg per dl. The three disease categories were glomerulonephritis, polycystic kidney disease, and pyelonephritis. All three patient groups experienced a slower rate of progression compared with the control group. Those with pyelonephritis had the most benefit. As this form of renal disease is mainly interstitial, it may be the most comparable to chronic transplant rejection. Major problems with these studies were their unrandomized design and the control group's tendency to deteriorate more rapidly than untreated patients previously reported in the literature.

A more recent prospective randomized trial of early protein restriction was conducted by Rosman and colleagues[39] in the Netherlands. A total of 228 patients were studied and 149 followed for at least 18 months. The experimental diet consisted of 0.4 and 0.6 g per kg per day of protein while the control patients ate their usual diets. Patients were stratified according to their renal function, age, and sex. Of the two groups whose creatinine clearances were initially between 30 and 60 ml per min per 1.73 m², the protein-restricted group had a reduced rate of progression by a factor of 3. Likewise for the patients whose creatinine clearances were initially less than 30 ml per min, the protein-restricted group had a reduced rate of progression by a factor of 5. Progression in this study was analyzed by changes in the reciprocal of the serum creatinine versus time. In contrast to the study of Maschio, older patients and those with chronic glomerulonephritis responded better than those with polycystic disease or interstitial nephritis.[39]

Beneficial results of protein restriction have also been shown in studies employing very low protein intake combined with essential amino acid supplements. Alvestrand and associates[66] tested 17 patients whose initial serum creatinines averaged

8.3 mg per dl, for an average of 355 days. All patients had a well-defined rate of progression prior to therapy. All but three patients showed substantial slowing of progression.

Although uncontrolled, one of the more convincing studies of the use of protein restriction in renal failure was performed by Mitch and colleagues.[67] They prescribed a dietary regimen that consisted of 20 to 30 g of mixed-quality protein with a keto acid-amino acid supplement. Ten of 17 patients who had a well-defined rate of progression prior to dietary change showed clinically important slowing of progression when followed for an average of 20 months. Seven of the 17 began treatment before the creatinine had reached 8 mg per dl. Their results are shown in Figure 10–3. As can be seen in six of the seven followed for an average of 22 months, the creatinine has remained at or below the level at the start of treat-

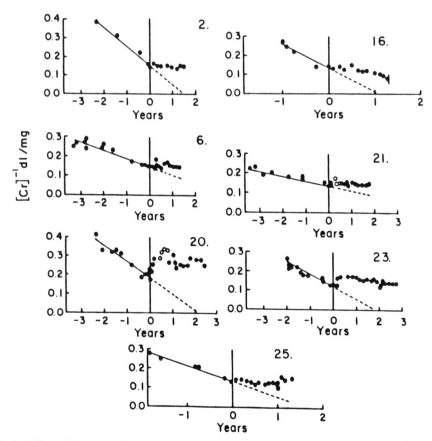

Figure 10–3. Effect of therapy with a protein-restricted diet and keto acid-amino acid supplement on progression of chronic renal failure in patients with serum creatinine levels <8 mg per dl prior to the start of treatment. The vertical lines represent the onset of treatment. All except patient 16 had slowing of their progression. (From Mitch, WE, et al,[67] with permission.)

ment. Though formal comparisons with the other strategies for protein restriction are wanting, preliminary studies by Walser and coworkers[68] suggest that at least in the late stage of renal insufficiency, keto analogues may be more effective than amino acid supplements. The reasons are obscure.

These and other studies are highly suggestive that some type of a low-protein diet is beneficial in slowing progression of renal failure. Dietary protein restriction may safely be implemented in transplant recipients in the chronic posttransplantation period. The dietary prescription consists of 0.55 to 0.60 g per kg day of protein, 75 percent of which should be high biologic value protein. Eggs and milk protein have the highest biologic value, followed by animal products, then cereals (rice, wheat, corn), legumes, and roots. Urinary protein losses should be supplemented. An alternative to this regimen is one containing 20 to 25 g per day of mixed biologic value protein supplemented by essential amino acids, for example Aminess. Keto acid analogues are currently not commercially available for use in the United States. Careful monitoring of the patient's overall nutritional status is mandatory. Parameters followed should include dietary histories, patient weight, anthropometric measurements, serum protein levels (albumin and transferrin for example), lymphocyte counts, and periodic estimate of nitrogen balance and urea nitrogen appearance rates as described above. A multi-vitamin supplement should be taken with these diets.

Posttransplantation Hyperlipidemia

After infection, atherosclerosis-induced vascular disease is the most common cause of death in transplantation patients.[69] Ghosh and associates[70] first noted a high prevalence of hyperlipidemia among transplant recipients. Their initial observations have been confirmed by others.[71,76] The hallmark of posttransplantation hyperlipidemia is concomitant elevations of plasma triglyceride and cholesterol levels. A number of factors may be responsible including steroid therapy, renal dysfunction, basal hyperinsulinism with glucose intolerance, antihypertensive drug therapy (particularly with diuretics), and obesity.

Over two thirds of transplantation recipients may have hyperlipidemia depending on when lipid profiles are examined.[70-76] The incidence of hyperlipidemia declines with time after transplantation but increases with patient age, with those recipients over age 40 having a higher incidence.[73] Types IV, IIA, and IIB are the most common lipoprotein abnormalities found.[71-73] Most studies have shown a correlation between lipid levels and prednisone dosage. Curtis and colleagues showed that recipients on alternate-day steroids had lower cholesterol and triglyceride levels than patients maintained on equal-dose daily steroids, further implicating steroids as a major factor contributing to the hyperlipidemia.[76]

Dietary modification may successfully control the hyperlipidemia. Ponticelli[72] (Fig. 10–4) demonstrated that the institution of a hypocaloric diet normalized cholesterol and triglyceride levels in a subset of transplant recipients, the majority of whom were overweight. Dissler and coworkers[74] also studied the role of diet in both the pathogenesis and control of posttransplantation hyperlipidemia. A total of 21 patients were studied, their diets being modified to decrease daily cholesterol intake to 300 mg or less, to increase polyunsaturated fat intake by the ingestion of 2 tablespoonfuls of sunflower seed oil per day, and to use margarine with a high polyunsaturated fat content. Other changes included the allowance of only one egg a week, carbohydrate restriction with the elimination of simple sugars from the diet, no protein restriction, and prohibition of alcohol intake. Dietary recall over the year of the study showed that in relation to baseline, significant decreases in daily carbohydrates and cholesterol intake and increase in the polyunsaturated to saturated fat ratio were noted. Prior to the study four patients had hypercholesterolemia alone, one had hypertriglyceridemia and the remainder had elevations in both. At the end of the year triglyceride levels had fallen. Although the triglyceride change was not statistically significant, there was a significant decrease in cholesterol concentration. The authors considered that their nonresponders had poorer compliance than the responders.[74] Of note, a high incidence of obesity was present in their patients, with only 10 percent being within ideal body weight. When

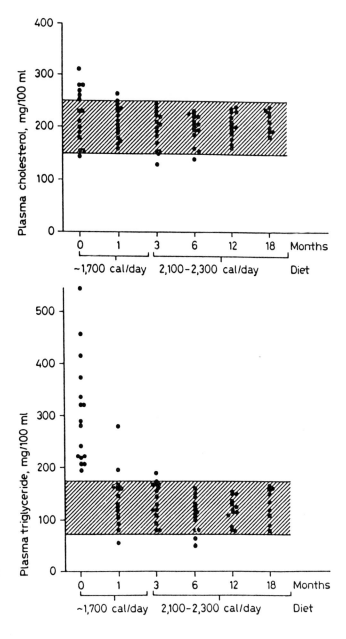

Figure 10-4. The effect of a hypocaloric diet on plasma cholesterol and triglyceride levels in 16 patients post renal transplant. The plasma lipid concentrations returned to normal and remained stable during the period of observation (6 to 18 months). (From Ponticelli C, et al,[72] with permission.)

details of their posttransplantation weight gain were examined retrospectively, the major weight gain was found to occur within the first 12 months after transplantation (Fig. 10–5). This may well be due to the hyperphagic effects of both larger doses of corticosteroids and the patients' new-found sense of well-being. This trend suggests that this period may be an important target interval for dietary counseling.

Shen and associates[75] also showed significant improvement of posttransplantation hyperlipidemia with dietary therapy. After 3 months eight of nine patients with initially elevated serum cholesterol and triglyceride levels had normal values when treated with a diet consisting of less than 500 mg of cholesterol, less than 35 percent of calories from fat, less than 50 percent of calories from carbohydrate, and a polyunsaturated to saturated fat ratio greater than 1. Three patients with only elevated cholesterol levels had a decrease in them, but they remained elevated above normal. Triglyceride increased in one patient and remained normal in two. In 11 patients who

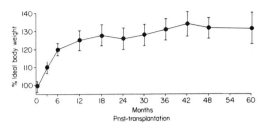

Figure 10–5. Weight gain in 21 transplant recipients charted as the percentage of ideal body weight. Almost all the increase occurs in the first 12 months, emphasizing the importance of early control of obesity. (From Disler PB, et al,[74] with permission.)

did not undergo dietary treatment, cholesterol and triglycerides remained elevated.

Posttransplantation hyperlipidemia is a significant problem and is multifactorial in origin. It is most likely a significant factor in development of atherosclerosis in these patients. Modifications in steroid administration and diet may help ameliorate these lipid abnormalities. Dietary therapy should consist of caloric restriction for patients who are overweight. Cholesterol intake should be less than 300 mg per day and the ratio of polyunsaturated to saturated fat should be 2 to 1. Drug therapy may be required; however, no studies regarding the use of lipid-lowering drugs in the posttransplantation period are available. It should be remembered that clofibrate administration to patients with renal failure is to be avoided, since it can be associated with muscle and liver toxicity.

Diet and Other Posttransplantation Complications

Posttransplantation Diabetes

Starzl and colleagues[77] first recognized the emergence of carbohydrate intolerance in renal transplant recipients whose immunosuppressive treatment included steroids. Its incidence has varied from 3.4 to 46 percent, this wide range perhaps reflecting different diagnostic criteria and immunosuppressive protocols used in various studies.[78] Most studies have implicated steroids as a major etiological factor. Other factors include renal insufficiency, the use

of diuretics, antithymocyte globulin, and hereditary predisposition.

The natural history of posttransplantation diabetes is not well charted, but most studies have found poor survival in those who develop diabetes compared with the nondiabetics.[78,79] This poor survival is consistent with the data on patients with juvenile-onset diabetes who receive transplants, their prognosis being poorer than that of nondiabetic controls. Preventative therapy should be directed to reducing steroid dosage where appropriate, limiting the use of diuretics in patients who demonstrate glucose intolerance, and encouraging weight reduction. Often insulin or oral hypoglycemic agents are necessary.

Hypertension

Hypertension is relatively common posttransplantation and may be due to a variety of factors including corticosteroid and cyclosporine therapy, renal artery stenosis, the presence of the recipient's own diseased kidneys, acute or chronic rejection, and recurrence of primary renal disease.[80] In most cases plasma renin concentration is low. Aggressive drug treatment of the hypertension is in order, for it may be a factor in causing renal disease to progress. The most important dietary modification is sodium restriction to a level of 2 to 3 g per day. When indicated, more severe sodium restriction can be instituted.

Cyclosporine and Hyperkalemia

Hyperkalemia may develop during the course of treatment with cyclosporine. In one study in which renal transplant recipients were randomly assigned to treatment with either cyclosporine or azathioprine, 23 percent of those receiving cyclosporine had hyperkalemia sufficient to warrant treatment, whereas only 6 percent receiving azathioprine needed such treatment.[81] Cyclosporine can cause a suppression of plasma renin activity and a tubular insensitivity to aldosterone, both of which may impair potassium excretion.[82] Patients receiving cyclosporine should avoid high dietary potassium intake, potassium-containing medications, and potassium-sparing diuretics except under careful medical supervision. This is especially true for patients with diabetes mellitus in whom potassium regulation may be further impaired by deficient insulin secretion. Furosemide therapy will promote increased potassium excretion.

Renal Osteodystrophy

Phosphorus restriction is prudent once the glomerular filtration rate is less than 50 ml per min in order to prevent hyperparathyroidism.[83] Such restriction may also have the beneficial effect of slowing the progression of renal failure. Phosphorus, because of its high content in protein, can be reduced by dietary protein restriction. Further reduction (to 600 to 800 mg per day) can be achieved by restricting such high-phosphorus foods as diary products, meat, legumes, chocolate, and nuts. Therapy should be guided by the serum phosphorus level. Phosphate binders such as aluminum hydroxide are often needed to reduce frankly elevated phosphorus levels. Once the phosphorus level is reduced, both dietary phosphorus restriction and calcium carbonate should be used to maintain the normal level, as chronic oral aluminum therapy may be a factor in causing aluminum bone disease and other chronic aluminum toxicities. Once the phosphorus level is controlled, calcium intake should be at least 1000 mg per day. This prescription usually necessitates supplementation with calcium carbonate tablets. For persistent hypocalcemia vitamin D should be given in the form of the active compound 1,25, dihydroxy vitamin D_3.

CONCLUSIONS

Many factors are involved in planning nutritional therapy in renal transplantation patients. Their pretransplantation course should be taken into careful consideration, as they often approach the transplantation with a variety of metabolic problems. These include protein malnutrition, carbohydrate intolerance, hyperlipidemia, and hyperphosphatemia. The acute post-transplantation period is often a time of increased protein catabolism and negative nitrogen balance, a result of the combined effects of surgery and high-dose steroid treatment. Increasing evidence suggests that a high-protein diet during this period may greatly improve overall protein balance and that a low-carbohydrate diet adequate in calories may protect against some of the side effects of steroids. The chronic posttransplantation period is characterized by a number of different problems. Patients often develop hyperlipidemia, glucose intolerance or frank diabetes, obesity, and hypertension. Dietary therapy should be redirected at reducing cholesterol intake, increasing the proportion of polyunsaturated fats, controlling dietary sodium, and reducing caloric intake in obese patients. Increasing evidence suggests that dietary protein restriction carried out under close supervision to avoid negative nitrogen balance may slow the progression of renal insufficiency once it is established.

REFERENCES

1. Westervelt, FB, Jr and Schreiner, GE: The carbohydrate intolerance of uremic patients. Ann Intern Med 57:266, 1962.
2. DeFronzo, RA, et al: Insulin resistance in uremia. J Clin Invest 67:563, 1981.
3. DeFronzo, RA and Alvestrand, A: Glucose intolerance in uremia: Site and mechanism. Am J Clin Nutr 33:1438, 1980.
4. Smith, D and DeFronzo, RA: Insulin resistance in uremia mediated by post-binding defects. Kidney Int 22:54, 1982.
5. Rubenstein, AH, Maki, ME, and Horowitz, DL: Insulin and the kidney. Nephron 15:306, 1975.
6. Chan, MK, Varghese, Z, and Moorhead, JF: Lipid abnormalities in uremia, dialysis, and transplantation. Kidney Int 19:625, 1981.
7. Bagdade, JD, Porte, D, and Bierman, EL: Hypertriglyceridemia: A metabolic consequence of chronic renal failure. N Engl J Med 279:181, 1968.
8. Cramp, DG, et al: Plasma lipoprotein patterns in patients receiving dialysis therapy for chronic renal failure. Clin Chim Acta 76:233, 1977.
9. Saudie, E, et al: Impaired plasma triglyceride clearance as a feature of both uremic and post transplant triglyceridemia. Kidney Int 18:774, 1980.
10. Goldberg, AP, et al: Increase in lipoprotein lipase during clofibrate treatment of hypertriglyceridemia in patients on hemodialysis. N Engl J Med 301:1073, 1979.
11. Cattran, DC, et al: Defective triglyceride removal in lipemia associated with peritoneal and hemodialysis. Ann Intern Med 85:29, 1976.

12. Sterner, G, Lindberg, T, and Denneberg, T: In vivo and in vitro absorption of amino acids and dipeptides in small intestine of uremic rats. Nephron 31:273, 1982.

13. Mitch, WE and Clark, AS. Muscle protein turnover in uremia. Kidney Int 24:S2, 1983.

14. Chami, J, et al: Pharmacokinetics of essential amino acids in chronic dialysis patients. Am J Clin Nutr 33:1652, 1980.

15. Furst, P, Alvestrand, A, and Bergstrom, J: Effect of nutrition and catabolic stress on intracellular amino acid pools in uremia. Am J Clin Nutr 33:1387, 1980.

16. May, RC and Mitch, WE: Alkalai therapy suppresses the muscle proteolysis stimulated by chronic renal failure in rats (abstr). Kidney Int 29:323, 1986.

17. Salter, JM, et al: Metabolic effects of glucagon in human subjects. Metabolism 9:753, 1960.

18. Landau, RL and Kappas, A: Anabolic hormones in hyperparathyroidism: With observations on the general catabolic influence of parathyroid hormone in man. Ann Intern Med 62:1223, 1965.

19. Kopple, JD and Swenseid, ME: Vitamin nutrition in patients undergoing maintenance hemodialysis. Kidney Int (suppl 2)7:579, 1975.

20. Hoy, WE, et al: Protein catabolism during the postoperative course after renal transplantation. Am J Kidney Dis 5:186, 1985.

21. Cogan, MG, et al: Prevention of prednisone-induced negative nitrogen balance; effect of dietary modification on urea generation rate in patients on hemodialysis receiving high-dose glucocorticoids. Ann Intern Med 95:158, 1981.

22. Liddle, VR, et al: Diet in transplantation. Dial Transplant 5:20, 1977.

23. Whittier, FC, et al: Nutrition in renal transplantation. Am J Kidney Dis 6:405, 1985.

24. Gann, DS: Endocrine and metabolic responses to injury. In Schwartz, SI (ed): Principles of Surgery, McGraw-Hill, New York, 1983, p 1.

25. Haynes, RC, Murad, F: Adrenocortical steroids. In Gilman, AG, et al (eds): The Pharmacological Basis of Therapeutics. MacMillan, New York, 1985, p 1463.

26. Mitch, WE and Walser, M: Nutritional therapy of the uremic patient. In Brenner, BM and Rector, FC (eds): The Kidney. WB Saunders, Philadelphia, 1983, p 1769.

27. Toledo-Pereyra, LH, Zammit, M, and Mittal, VK: Total parenteral nutrition in renal transplantation: Experimental observations. Am Surg 49:396, 1983.

28. Petersen, VP, et al: Late failure of human renal transplants. Medicine 54:45, 1975.

29. Mitch, WE, et al: A simple method of estimating progression of chronic renal failure. Lancet 2:1326, 1976.

30. Brenner, BM, Meyer, TW, and Hostetter, TH: Dietary protein and the progressive nature of kidney disease: The role of hemodynamically mediated glomerular injury in the pathogenesis of progressive glomerular sclerosis in aging, renal ablation, and intrinsic renal disease. N Engl J Med 307:652, 1982.

31. Baldwin, DS and Neugarten, J: Blood pressure control and progression of chronic renal insufficiency. In Mitch, WE (ed): The Progressive Nature of Renal Disease. Churchill-Livingstone, New York, 1985, p 81.

32. Morgensen, CE: Long-term antihypertensive treatment inhibiting progression of diabetic nephropathy. Br Med J 285:685, 1982.

33. Dworkin, LD, et al: Hemodynamic basis for glomerular injury in rats with desoxycorticosterone-salt hypertension. J Clin Invest 73:1448, 1984.

34. Hostetter, TH, et al: Hyperfiltration in remnant nephrons: A potentially adverse response to renal ablation. Am J Physiol 241:F85, 1981.

35. Nath, KA and Hostetter, TH: Low protein diet reduces the progression of advanced renal injury by decreasing glomerular capillary pressure (abstr). Clin Res 33:494A, 1985.

36. Dworkin, LD and Feiner, HD: Evidence for hemodynamically mediated glomerular injury in uninephrectomized spontaneously hypertensive rats. Kidny Int 25:243, 1984.

37. Raij, L, Azar S, and Keane, WF: Role of salt induced hypertension and dietary protein in the progression of glomerular damage in glomerulonephritis. Kidney Int 27:249, 1985.

38. Hostetter, TH, Paller, MS, and Ferris, TF: Hypertension, dietary protein, and renal injury: Critical role of glomerular versus systemic pressure (abstr). Clin Res 33:607A, 1985.

39. Rosman, JB, et al: Prospective randomized trial of early dietary protein restriction in chronic renal failure. Lancet 2:1291, 1984.

40. Rosenberg, ME, et al: Glomerular and hormonal responses to dietary protein intake in human renal disease. Am J Physiol: 253 (Renal Fluid and Electrolyte Physiol) f 1083, 1987.

41. Hayslett, JP: Functional adaptation to reduction in renal mass. Physiol Rev 59:137, 1979.

42. Hostetter, TH: Renal hemodynamic response to a meat meal in humans. Am J Physiol 250:F613, 1986.

43. Pullman, TN, et al: The influence of dietary protein intake on specific renal functions in normal man. J Lab Clin Med 44:320, 1954.

44. Olson, JL, et al: Altered glomerular permselectivity and progressive sclerosis following extreme ablation of renal mass. Kidney Int 22:112, 1983.

45. Anderson, S, et al: Control of glomerular hypertension limits glomerular injury in rats with reduced renal mass. J Clin Invest 76:612, 1985.

46. Gross, RL, and Newberne, PM: Role of nutrition in immunologic function. Physiol Rev 60:188, 1980.

47. Agus, D, et al: The inhibitory role of dietary protein restriction on the development and expression of immune anti-TBM disease producing tubulointerstitial disease in rats. Kidney Int 27:240, 1985.

48. Nath, KA, Hostetter, MK, and Hostetter, TH: Pathophysiology of chronic tubulointerstitial disease in rats: Interactions of dietary acid load, ammonia, and complement component C3. J Clin Invest 76:667, 1985.

49. Klahr, S, Buerkert, J, and Purkerson, ML: Role of dietary factors in the progression of chronic renal disease. Kidney Int 24:579, 1983.

50. Hurd, ER, et al: Prevention of glomerulonephritis and prolonged survival in New Zealand Black/New Zealand White F1 hybrid mice fed an essential fatty acid-deficient diet. J Clin Invest 67:476, 1981.

51. Barcelli, YO and Pollak, VE: Prostaglandins and progressive renal insufficiency. In Mitch, WE (ed): The Progressive Nature of Renal Disease. Churchill-Livingstone, New York, 1985, p 65.

52. Paller, MS and Hostetter, TH: Dietary protein increases plasma renin activity and reduces pressor reactivity to angiotensin II. Am J Phys (in press).

53. Klahr, S, Heifets, M, and Purkerson, ML: The influence of anticoagulation on the progression of experimental renal disease. In Mitch, WE (ed): The Progressive Nature of Renal Disease. Churchill-Livingstone, New York, 1985, p 45.

54. Ichikawa, I, et al: Dietary protein intake conditions the degree of renal vasoconstriction in acute renal failure caused by ureteral obstruction. Am J Physiol 249:F54, 1985.

55. Moorhead, JF, et al: Lipid nephrotoxicity in chronic progressive glomerular and tubulointerstitial disease. Lancet 2:1309, 1982.

56. Kasiske, BL, et al: The lipid lowering agent clofibric acid ameliorates renal injury in the 5/6 nephrectomy model of chronic renal failure (abstr). Clin Res 33:448A, 1985.

57. Neugarten, J, et al: Amelioration of experimental glomerulonephritis by dietary protein restriction. Kidney Int 24:595, 1983.

58. Lumlertgul, D, et al: Phosphate depletion arrests progression of chronic renal failure independent of protein intake. Kidney Int 29:658, 1986.

59. Schmidt, RW: Effects of phosphate depletion on acid-base status in dogs. Metabolism 27:943, 1978.

60. Alfrey, AC and Tomford, RC: The case for tubulointerstitial factors, In Narins, R (ed): Controversies in Nephrology and Hypertension. Churchill-Livingstone, New York, 1984.

61. Barrientos, A, et al: Role of the control of phosphate in the progression of chronic renal failure. Miner Electrolyte Metab 7:127, 1982.

62. Scrimshaw, NW: An analysis of past and present recommended daily allowances for protein in health and disease. N Engl J Med 294:136, 198, 1976.

63. Sapir, DG, et al: Nitrogen sparing induced by a mixture of essential amino acids given chiefly as their keto-analogues during prolonged starvation in obese subjects. J Clin Invest 54:974, 1974.

64. Maschio, G, et al: Effects of dietary protein and phosphorus restriction on the progression of early renal failure. Kidney Int 22:371, 1982.

65. Oldrizzi, L, Rugiu, C, and Valvo, E: Progression of renal failure in patients with renal disease of diverse etiology on protein-restricted diet. Kidney Int 27:553, 1985.

66. Alvestrand, A, et al: Clinical results of long-term treatment with a low protein diet and a new amino acid preparation in patients with chronic uremia. Clin Nephrol 19:67, 1983.

67. Mitch, WE, et al: The effect of a keto acid-amino acid supplement to a restricted diet on the progression of chronic renal failure. N Engl J Med 311:623, 1984.

68. Walser, M, Ward, L, and Van Duyn, MA: Comparison of the effects on the progression of chronic renal failure in man of keto acid supplements vs amino acid supplement (abstr). Clin Res 34:730A, 1986.

69. Bryngar, H, Brunner, FP, and Chantler, C: Combined report on regular dialysis and transplantation in Europe. Proc Eur Dial Transplant Assoc 17:2, 1980.

70. Ghosh, P, et al: Plasma lipids following renal transplantation. Transplantation 15:521, 1973.

71. Ibels, LS, Alfrey, AC, and Weil III, R: Hyperlipidemia in adult, pediatric and diabetic renal transplant recipients. Am J Med 64:634, 1978.

72. Ponticelli, C, et al: Lipid disorders in renal

transplant recipients. Nephron 20:189, 1978.

73. Nicholas, ML, Alexandre, GPJ, and van Ypersele de Strihou, C: The evolution of hyperlipidemia late after renal transplantation. Proc Eur Dial Transplant Assoc 16:339, 1979.

74. Disler, PB, et al: The role of diet in the pathogenesis and control of hyperlipidemia after renal transplantation. Clin Neph 16:29, 1981.

75. Shen, SY, et al: Patient profile and effect of dietary therapy on post-transplant hyperlipidemia. Kidney Int (Suppl) 24:S147, 1983.

76. Curtis, JL, et al: Effect of alternate-day prednisone on plasma lipids in renal transplant recipients. Kidney Int 22:42, 1982.

77. Starzl, TE, et al: Factors in successful renal transplantation. Surgery 56:296, 1964.

78. Friedman, EA, et al: Post-transplant diabetes in kidney transplant recipients. Am J Nephrol 5:196, 1985.

79. Ruiz, JO, et al: Steroid diabetes in renal transplant recipients: Pathogenetic factors and prognosis. Surgery 73:759, 1973.

80. Curtis, JJ: Hypertension and kidney transplantation. Am J Kidney Dis 7:181, 1986.

81. Najarian, JS, et al: Comparison of cyclosporine versus azathioprine-antilymphocyte globulin in renal transplantation. Transplant Proc 15:2463, 1983.

82. Bantle, JP, et al: Effects of cyclosporine on the renin-angiotensin-aldosterone system and potassium excretion in renal transplant recipients. Arch Intern Med 145:505, 1985.

83. Coburn, JW and Slatopolsky, E: Vitamin D, parathyroid hormone and renal osteodystrophy. In Brenner, BM and Rector, FC (eds): The Kidney. WB Saunders, Philadelphia, 1985, p 1657.

Chapter 11

Immunosuppression

MITCHELL L. HENRY
RONALD M. FERGUSON

Historically, the technical capability for renal transplantation preceded the development of adequate immunosuppressive medication to allow prolonged graft survival. In the early 1950s several renal transplants were undertaken with technical success, but early rejection resulted in early failure. Long-term technical success was demonstrated with successful renal transplantation between identical twins reported by Murray and coworkers[1] in 1955.

In 1956 Billingham and colleagues,[2] in

Medawar's lab, demonstrated in a series of experiments that graft rejection was an immunologic phenomenon. In searching for a substitute for total lymphoid irradiation, Schwartz and associates[3] found that 6-mercaptopurine (6-MP) prevented rabbits from producing antibodies to the stimulating antigen, a heterologous protein. Following this, Calne and Murray[4] demonstrated that azathioprine, a 6-MP derivative, could provide prolonged graft survival in dogs; this was an improvement over previous studies with 6-MP. The first use of azathioprine in clinical organ transplantation was reported in 1962 by Murray and associates[5] using cadaver donors. One of four recipients treated with azathioprine (Imuran) demonstrated prolonged function. Goodwin and colleagues[6] demonstrated the immunosuppressive effects of prednisone by the successful reversal of a rejection episode in a patient with a renal allograft that had been initially treated with cyclophosphamide. In 1963, Murray and coworkers[7] presented a series of patients treated with azathioprine and added steroids for grafts undergoing rejection. Sixty-four percent of grafts functioned and 36 percent had current function at the time of the report. Starzl and associates[8] described the combined use of azathioprine and prednisone in recipients of living donors, not only for established rejection episodes, but "before and after transplantation." Ninety percent of these patients suffered a first rejection episode, but only 1 of 10 had a second episode. In 1967 Starzl and associates[9] first noted the clinical use of antilymphocyte globulin and touted it only as an adjuvant along with azathioprine and prednisone. He reported 100 percent patient and graft survival in patients receiving this combination, although only with short follow-up. Najarian and his colleagues[10] have also reported success with this drug regimen, using their antilymphocyte globulin preparation with notably longer periods of follow-up. Relatively low-dose steroids (20 mg per day) in combination with azathioprine were used successfully by McGeown and colleagues[11] in 1980 with a decreased incidence of steroid-induced complications.

In 1976 Borel[12] reported experimental results with cyclosporine and offered hope for the use of "selective immunosuppressive" therapy through this drug. The first clinical studies in 1978 by Calne and coworkers[13] reported the efficacy of the drug but suggested that the nephrotoxicity might limit its use. Starzl and his group[14] identified that the use of lower-dose cyclosporine (17.5 mg per kg per day) in combination with steroid use provided good results (94 percent graft and patient survival for first cadaver transplants, with follow-up through 4.5 months), and was safe. Following this, many studies were spawned. These demonstrated the clinical efficacy and safety of cyclosporine use, not only in renal transplantation, but in other solid organ transplantation. Many varying protocols have been used in attempts to optimize the advantages of cyclosporine.

The following discussion will be limited primarily to the use of chemical immunosuppression by drugs that are used widely in clinical application. A heavy emphasis will be placed on a variety of clinical protocols from centers using cyclosporine as the primary immunosuppressant, with respect to their successes as well as the drawbacks. Finally, we will provide speculation as to the modes and methods of immunosuppression and immunomanipulation that lie in the future of transplantation.

CORTICOSTEROIDS

History

One of the earliest reports of the efficacy of corticosteroids was that by Zukoski and colleagues[15] in 1965. He demonstrated that the use of prednisolone in canine renal allografts could provide markedly prolonged allograft survival. Reduction of the prednisolone dose resulted in transient rejection episodes, which were reversed by resuming the original dose. Goodwin and coworkers[6] demonstrated the interventional use of prednisone by treating a patient with renal allograft rejection with high doses of prednisone with subsequent improvement in graft function. Prednisone was used in a multidrug regimen reported by Murray and associates[7] in 1963, and he was able to demonstrate improved graft survival rates compared with historical controls. In 1963, Starzl and associates[8] reported the addition of prednisone to the posttransplantation immunosuppressive protocol as a prophylactic measure and noted that the drug could be used very effectively to treat rejection episodes. These were the beginnings of various clinical protocols in which corticosteroids were used both prophylactically and interventionally to treat rejection episodes.

Pharmacology

While corticosteroids have been used clinically in renal transplantation for nearly 25 years, their exact immunosuppressive mechanism of action has yet to be totally understood. When used as a therapeutic intervention for acute rejection episodes, improvement in renal function can be noted very quickly—in a matter of hours. This has led many investigators to note that its mechanism in treating acute rejection may be based at least in part on its anti-inflammatory capabilities. This effect may be mediated by prostaglandin inhibition by inducement of lipocortin, a protein that is a potent inhibitor of phospholipase A_2.[16] However, more subtle actions by these drugs have been observed. Corticosteroids do cause lymphopenia early, with changes in the lymphocyte subpopulation favoring a depletion of T helper relative to T suppressor cells.[17] Prednisone has also been shown to inhibit the production of a variety of lymphokines, in particular interleukin-1, interleukin-2 and alpha- and gamma-interferon.[18] This can interrupt the activation and proliferation of both cytotoxic and helper T cells in the immune cascade, preventing further immunologic injury to the allograft.

Many side effects of corticosteroids are thought to be dose-dependent. These include impairment of wound healing, increased incidence of infectious episodes, avascular necrosis of long bones, upper GI tract ulceration, hypertension, steroid-induced diabetes, and cataract formation.

Clinical Uses

The use of corticosteroids in both a prophylactic and interventional manner has been imprinted in clinical renal transplantation. The most important question about the use of steroids has been what dosing

regimen will allow optimal immunosuppression without adverse side effects, primarily infectious complications. When prednisone was first introduced into immunosuppressive protocols, the use of high doses was common. However, as the side effects of corticosteroids were more fully appreciated, different dosing schedules were employed. Several studies have addressed the differences in outcomes of protocols using high-dose versus low-dose steroids. Gore and colleagues[19] summarized nine studies comparing these varying dosing schedules. Table 11–1 summarizes the mean doses of the high versus low dose protocols. Notably, McGeown and associates,[11,20] from Belfast, reported that no significant difference in graft survival could be shown in patients who received 20 mg of prednisone daily posttransplantation (low-dose protocol). However, they demonstrated marked decreases in the number of complications that could be attributed directly to the use of lower-dose prednisone. Others (Chan,[21] Salaman,[22] Porticelli,[23] Morris,[24] and their coworkers) have shown essentially no difference in graft survival between high-dose and low-dose steroid regimens posttransplantation, with most able to show a decrease in steroid-related complications. A prospective randomized trial of low-dose versus high-dose steroids was undertaken in Australia and reported by d'Apice and associates.[25] They demonstrated that there was significantly poorer graft survival in the low-dose group. However, there was no difference in survival in their study in patients who received low-dose steroids and azathioprine doses that exceeded 1.75 mg per kg per day. They concluded that the combination of low-dose steroids and low-dose azathioprine pro-

Table 11–1 Mean Dose of Prednisolone for Either High-Dose or Low-Dose Steroid Group*		
	High Dose	**Low Dose**
Day 1	120 mg	40 mg
Week 1	85 mg	31 mg
Month 1	46 mg	25 mg
*Cumulative data of nine studies		

vided inadequate immunosuppression in renal transplantation.

Many different regimens have been used for the treatment of acute rejection episodes. Increases in oral prednisone dosages, as well as intramuscular or intravenous methylprednisolone, have been used with efficacy to treat these episodes. However, prospective randomized studies comparing the routes of administration are not available.

ANTILYMPHOCYTE GLOBULIN

History

Heterologous lymphocyte sera can be traced back to Metchnikoff (1899), but was first used experimentally in transplantation in 1963 by Woodruff and colleagues.[26] It has subsequently been demonstrated in a variety of animal models to be a potent immunosuppressant. Antilymphocyte preparations are a group of compounds including polyclonal antilymphocyte globulin (ALG), antilymphocyte sera (ALS), and antithymocyte globulin (ATG), as well as recently developed monoclonal preparations. While early testing used these preparations alone, it became obvious that any of them should be used as an adjuvant along with other immunosuppressive agents. Starzl[9] noted in 1967 that the immunosuppressive effect of these products was not strong enough to warrant clinical use other than as adjuvant agents. This conclusion followed his own extensive studies on canine models. Other investigators[21,27] also demonstrated that combination therapy with other agents would not diminish the effect of the antilymphocyte preparations, and that there was synergism between them to prolong graft survival. The first clinical study then followed in Denver,[9] where ALG was used both prophylactically and for established rejection episodes. It was reported that the prophylactic use was quite successful, at least in early follow-up. Turcotte and co-workers[28] found significant improvement in both patient and graft survival with incompatible living related grafts in those treated with ALG as opposed to those with-

out ALG. Although he could not find any difference in survival of living related allografts using ALG, Sheil and associates[29] showed statistically significant improvement with ALG in cadaveric grafts as opposed to those treated without ALG. Najarian and colleagues,[10] in a study that was not randomized or prospective, believed that their data demonstrated improved graft survival using ALG and that it could reduce the incidence and severity of rejection episodes. One major problem with comparing findings of studies using antilymphocyte preparations is that a wide variety of preparations have been used in many different centers, with varying protocols and potency of drug.

Pharmacology

The production of antilymphocyte preparations hinges on the ability to immunize a laboratory animal with human lymphoid tissue so that antibody is produced. Cultured human lymphoblasts or thymocytes are the most commonly used lymphoid preparations. Many animal species have been used to produce these antihuman immunoglobulins, but those used most commonly today are the horse and rabbit. Heterologous sera are produced and then fractionated, and it has been found that the IgG component is the immunosuppressive one. Several techniques are used to eliminate allergic reactions; these include absorption of plasma with platelets and red blood cell stroma, silica dioxide stabilization, and sephadex chromatography.[10]

Because of local inflammatory action with intramuscular or subcutaneous injections, as well as marked phlebitic reactions with peripheral intravenous injections, administration via either central venous lines or high-flow AV fistulas has been used.

The exact in vivo mechanism of action of ALG is yet to be delineated. However, studies have shown that total lymphocyte count, in particular T cell numbers, markedly decrease with administration of antilymphocyte preparations. Other cell populations, particularly B cells and NK cells, appear not to be affected. This information suggests that the efficacy of ALG is secondary to T cell depletion and its ability to interrupt the effects of these cells on early cell-mediated rejection.

The effects of antilymphocyte preparations are quite varied according to the particular preparation. However, common side effects from the drug include leukopenia, thrombocytopenia, chills, fevers, skin rashes, and arthalgias. The delayed effects of excessive immunosuppression may include infectious complications, particularly cytomegalovirus. Notably, there are no reports describing increased incidence of malignancies in association with antilymphocyte preparations and standard immunosuppression (azathioprine and prednisone).

Clinical Approaches

The two major uses of antilymphocyte preparations include their use in a prophylactic fashion and as antirejection therapy. Many studies have demonstrated improved graft survival using ALG in both these manners. However, it has been very difficult to compare the various results, since different groups were using heterogeneous products.

Several nonrandomized historically based studies[10] have suggested that the use of antilymphocyte preparations was efficacious in reversing established rejection episodes. Several prospective randomized protocols have identified advantages of the use of interventional therapeutic antilymphocyte preparations for the treatment of acute rejection episodes (Table 11-2). These advantages include improved incidence of reversal of rejection episodes, fewer second rejection episodes, and an improvement in long-term survival.

Improvement in long-term graft function with therapeutic ALG has been shown by Nelson[30] in living related transplantation (94 percent versus 74 percent survival), and in cadaveric recipients by Filo[31] (74 percent versus 49 percent), Nowygrod[32] (73 percent versus 46 percent), Howard[33] (82 percent versus 61 percent), Streem[34] (91 percent versus 75 percent), and Hoitsma[35] (78 percent versus 50 percent). Most[31,32–34,36] have shown an increased ease of reversing first rejection episodes with antilymphocyte preparations. Fewer subsequent (second and third) episodes have also been identified by many[30,32–34,36] with this therapy. The final advantage outlined by using ALG for antirejection therapy is that it can markedly decrease the need for the synchronous use of high-dose steroids, avoiding those associated complications.

		First Rejection Reversed with ALG/Steroids	Second Rejection Episode (Incidence), ALG/Steroids	Long-Term Function (1-Year Graft Survival), ALG/Steroids
Shield[36]	LRD	100%/100%	10%/50%	90%/90%
Nelson[30]	LRD	100%/85%	25%/55%	94%/74%
Filo[31]	CAD	91%/62%	52%/53%	74%/49%
	LRD	92%/78%	55%/36%	74%/63%
Nowygrod[32]		84%/75%	36%/80%	73%/46%
Howard*[33]	CAD	100%/75%	35%/26%	75%/66%
	LRD	100%/69%	15%/26%	92%/54%
Streem*[34]	CAD	100%/83%	45%/66%	91%/75%
Light[117]	LRD	82%/53%†	18%/89%	82%/17%
Hoitsma[35]	CAD	75%/50%†	40%/46%	70%/65%

Table 11-2 Reports Comparing ALG with Steroids Regarding Reversal of First Rejection Episodes, Incidence of Second Rejection Episodes, and Long-Term Graft Function

LRD = living related donor; CAD = cadaveric donor
*Used prophylactic ALG posttransplant
†ALG used as rescue therapy

Clear-cut evidence of the efficacy of the prophylactic use of antilymphocyte preparations is somewhat more difficult to show. In 1971 Sheil and colleagues[29] demonstrated statistically significant improvement in graft survival in patients given prophylactic ATG, with the incidence of rejection episodes in the control group being 3 times greater than those receiving ATG. In 1973 Turcotte[28] was unable to demonstrate any statistically significant advantage using ALG; however, he could demonstrate quite good graft survival in patients not receiving ALG (68 percent 1-year graft survival). Wechter,[37] and Cosimi,[38] both showed trends toward increased allograft survival, but they did not reach statistical significance. Others (Taylor,[39] Bell[40]) could not show positive effects of prophylactic ALG treatment. Kreis[41] and Novick[42] showed significant improvement in graft survival in relatively small patient populations, improving graft survival by 26 and 19 percent per year, respectively. Condie[43] reported a prospective multicenter study using Minnesota ALG versus placebo. Significant differences in the ALG groups were demonstrated with improved early function, shortened hospital stay, notably fewer rejection episodes, and improved long-term graft function (at 3 years). This was accomplished without any increases in infections or neoplasms as compared with the control group.

Even in the absence of clear-cut across-the-board evidence that ALG/ATG is beneficial, most of these studies have noted the delayed onset of rejection episodes, reduced incidence of rejection episodes, and a lessened need for high-dose steroids to treat these episodes.

ALG has been used by some in the cyclosporine era in a sequential fashion in order to avoid early postoperative nephrotoxicity (see cyclosporine section). It has also been used to treat steroid-resistant rejection episodes in patients treated with cyclosporine.

MONOCLONAL ANTIBODIES

The production of monoclonal antibodies was undertaken in response to some of the disadvantages of using polyclonal antilymphocyte sera. Antilymphocyte sera were known to have efficacy and toxicity that varied from batch to batch. Antilymphocyte sera preparations lacked specificity to those cells causing the rejection episode. Some acute rejection episodes were resistant to antilymphocyte sera.

Monoclonal antibodies are produced by an immortal cell line that will secrete a monomolecular species of antibody. This is accomplished in vitro by fusing myeloma cells of mouse tissue with antibody-producing cells from an immunized mouse. The chosen hybridoma cell line is then identified from the variety of cells produced, and this cell line is propagated.[44] These antibodies have been targeted against a variety of lymphocyte populations, including those reactive against helper cells (OKT4), cytotoxic/suppressor (OKT8), and all T lymphocytes (OKT3). It is the latter monoclonal antibody that has been used in early clinical testing.

Most clinical studies have used the OKT3 monoclonal antibody to treat established rejection episodes. Goldstein,[45] Norman,[46] Thistlethwaite[47] and their associates have shown a very high incidence of reversal (90 percent, 96 percent, and 100 percent, respectively) of the first acute rejection episodes by this agent. Rejection episodes have been reversed even in the presence of decreasing concurrent therapy with azathioprine and prednisone. However, recurrent rejection episodes occur often (approximately 60 percent of patients).[47,48] Another problem using the monoclonal antibody identified early in these studies has been side effects associated with the first dose of the drug. These include acute pulmonary edema, shaking, chills, and fever. Kreis and colleagues[49] addressed the use of monoclonal antibodies for prophylactic therapy. They have found, in a small patient population, a lower associated incidence of early rejection and total rejection episodes. Further study of this use is needed.

These initial studies conclude that the OKT3 monoclonal antibody has been shown to be effective and safe for reversing established rejection episodes. However, the ultimate use of this drug has not yet been established, particularly as it relates to optimal dosing and the use of other associated immunosuppressive agents. Wider trials with a number of protocols, as well as the use of newer monoclonals, are under way. Notably lacking in these early studies are randomized prospective trials against cyclosporine alone and other polyclonal antibody preparations.

AZATHIOPRINE

History

Azathioprine and 6-mercaptopurine (6-MP, a cleavage product of azathioprine) were first synthesized in the early 1950s by Elion and Hitchings.[50] Schwartz[3] demonstrated that 6-MP blocked an antibody response to heterologous proteins injected into rabbits and specifically that the immunologic deficit remained after the drug had been stopped. This preliminary information spawned further studies of the efficacy of a number of purine and pyrimidine analogues in laboratory animals. In 1960, in the canine renal allograft, Calne[51] and Zukoski and associates[52] showed significant survival prolongation using 6-MP. Calne later showed that azathioprine gave better results in canines than 6-MP. Murray and colleagues[7] used azathioprine first in clinical organ transplantation (with the addition of steroids) and demonstrated some early success with this drug. Starzl[8] also demonstrated success in clinical trials using azathioprine and adjunctive steroids. With the groundwork laid, in the 1960s and 1970s azathioprine was found to be one of the most valuable immunosuppressants in clinical organ transplantation.

Pharmacology

Azathioprine and 6-mercaptopurine are both thiopurines.[50] 6-MP is the sulfate derivative of hypoxanthine, while azathioprine is the nitroimidazole derivative of 6-MP. Azathioprine has been viewed as a slow-release form of 6-MP, which is the metabolic derivative after it is enzymatically split in vivo.[53] However, differences between 6-MP and azathioprine have been found. These differences suggest that they

may be two different compounds and that azathioprine may not be acting simply as a precursor product of 6-MP.[54] As potent antimetabolites, these drugs are thought to be nonspecific inhibitors of immune function acting by interrupting the propagation of rapidly forming tissues, particularly bone marrow. 6-MP has also been shown to have anti-inflammatory properties.[55] It has been shown that the most effective use of the agent takes place prior to the antigenic stimulus, suggesting that the mode of action is directed at the stage of both proliferation and differentiation of immunocompetent cells. It has been shown biochemically that at the subcellular level thiopurines have multiple actions, including inhibition of the synthesis of DNA, RNA, and protein as well as interference with coenzymes and binding of various amino acids.[51] Despite numerous experimental studies designed to outline the effects of azathioprine on the immune system, there is still no well-delineated description of its actual mechanisms of action.

Azathioprine can be administered by both intravenous and oral routes, former in one half the dose of the latter. Most patients will tolerate between 1.5 and 2.5 mg per kg of the drug, and many centers push the dosage until mild bone-marrow toxicity is identified.

Side effects of the drugs are primarily hematologic in origin. Over 50 percent of the patients taking this drug will suffer some degree of leukopenia during its use. Megaloblastic anemia can be seen. Infection can occur as a secondary manifestation of bone-marrow suppression, particularly viral infections such as cytomegalovirus. Nausea and vomiting are common. Animal studies have demonstrated hepatotoxicity in high doses. Cholestasis has been suggested to occur in humans; however, the evidence for this is poorly defined. Alopecia occurs in some patients.

Clinical Uses

The first clinical use of azathioprine was by Murray and associates,[7] who combined azathioprine and corticosteroids. Results showed for the first time a reasonable patient and graft survival outside of identical twin pairs, making clinical renal transplantation a reality. Starzl and colleagues[8] in the same year demonstrated that the combination of azathioprine and prednisone could provide reasonable graft survival. These studies helped secure the clinical use of azathioprine in renal transplantation and highlighted the efficacy of a combination of azathioprine and steroids. This regimen was widely and rapidly adopted. In 1968 Murray and coworkers[56] reported their collected data from the previous 5 years, noting gradual improvement in graft survival from year to year. In the final year reported, they demonstrated an 85 percent 1-year graft survival (mostly living donors). Lucas and associates[57] using azathioprine and prednisone, reported similar 1-year graft function (78 percent) in recipients of living donors. It is important to note that after these early studies very little objective comparison of agents other than azathioprine and prednisone was carried out until the cyclosporine era. However, Starzl[58] compared the use of cyclophosphamide and prednisone with azathioprine and prednisone and found essentially no difference in the two groups. He concluded that cyclophosphamide could easily be substituted for azathioprine if toxicity of the latter drug was a problem.

A variety of innovations and insights continued throughout the 1960s and 1970s, all with a basic regimen of azathioprine and prednisone. Particularly significant were the development of routine HLA typing and matching of donor kidneys to recipient and the importance of both in prolonging graft survival.[59] With the development of antilymphocyte preparations and their clinical uses, azathioprine and prednisone in combination with these preparations became even more commonly used in clinical transplantation. Observations regarding random blood transfusions,[60] as well as those made by Salvatierra and his group with donor-specific transfusions,[61] further served to improve graft outcome. Azathioprine given pretransplantation during donor-specific transfusions has allowed for a significant reduction in the incidence of sensitization of a recipient to a particular living donor.[62] In recent years the use of combination therapy including azathioprine, cyclosporine, and prednisone has

been beneficial in several settings (see cyclosporine section).

CYCLOSPORINE

History

In 1970 two new fungal strains were isolated from soil samples found to produce cyclosporines. Only one, *Tolyprocardium inflatum,* would grow in a submerged culture, allowing large-scale production. Borel[63] demonstrated an immunosuppressive effect of the isolate of this fungus when it was tested along with many other drugs in in vitro and in vivo experimental model settings. By 1974 the culturing technique of the fungus had improved, yielding purified cyclosporine A, which could undergo further pharmacologic testing. In 1975 the official structure was clarified. The first publication by Borel and coworkers[12] on the immunosuppressive effects of this new drug came in 1976. Then in 1977 and 1978 a flurry of animal studies showed a positive effect in prolonging graft survival in a variety of organ transplants. Notably, these were reported by Kostakis,[64] Calne,[65] Green,[66] and their associates in rat, canine, and rabbit models, respectively. In 1978 clinical trials were begun both in bone marrow recipients in an effort to treat graft-versus-host disease[67] and in renal transplant recipients. Calne reported in 1978[13] a pilot study using cyclosporine in renal allografts; this was followed by a wider experience detailed in 1979.[68] While he was able to demonstrate reasonable graft survival, it was at this time the nephrotoxicity of the drug was noted. In addition, three patients in this original series developed lymphomas.

Pharmacology

Cyclosporine is an 11-amino-acid cyclic peptide with a new, previously undescribed amino acid at the C-9 position. It is rich in hydrophobic amino acids, necessitating administration in a lipid-based vehicle. Assays for serum or plasma concentrations of the drug by both radioimmunoassay and high-performance liquid chromatography were developed by Donatsch and colleagues[69] in 1981 and Niederberger and coworkers[70] in 1980, respectively. At least 17 metabolites of the parent compound have been identified.[71] Over 50 percent of the drug is excreted in the bile, and this accounts for its major route of elimination. Renal clearance is minor: approximately 10 percent of the drug is excreted in the urine, only 0.1 percent of which is unchanged.[72]

A great deal of work has been done to elucidate the immunosuppressive action of cyclosporine, at both the cellular and subcellular levels. A more detailed outline of its action will result from studies now under way. Cyclosporine inhibits the release of interleukin-2 (IL-2) from activated T helper cells.[73] This further interferes with the activation and proliferation of both cytotoxic T cells and T helper cells. Although cyclosporine is not thought to affect B cell function directly, it probably does interfere with the function of T cell-dependent B cell activity. There is evidence that suppressor T cells are generally not affected by cyclosporine, and in fact it may enhance suppressor cell activity. Cyclosporine also inhibits the production of IL-1 by macrophages, IL-3 by T cells, B cell growth factor, macrophage-activating factor, and gamma-interferon.[73] Thus, by its early interruption of the immunologic cascade (primarily by IL-2 inhibition) cyclosporine blocks both the precursors of cytotoxic T cells and the elaboration of many vital lymphokines.[74]

The side effects of cyclosporine are for the most part dose-related. Nephrotoxicity, discussed extensively below, appears to be dose-related and may improve with simple dose reduction. Other common side effects include hirsutism, tremors, and hypertension. Metabolic consequences of the drug include hyperkalemia and hyperuricemia. Hepatotoxicity has been identified but is usually related to high dosing regimens. Increased incidence of lymphoproliferative disorders have been noted, especially in early studies with generous dosing schedules. It is interesting to note that perhaps the marked nephrotoxicity of the drug is one of its true saving graces in that without the specific indications to use lower doses of the drug, excessive immunosuppression and subsequent lymphoproliferative disorders might be much more prevalent.

Clinical Uses

With the introduction of cyclosporine into clinical use, a wide variety of clinical protocols were developed in an effort to use cyclosporine to its maximum advantage. Calne[68] and the European multicenter trial[75] used cyclosporine without steroids with reasonably good results. However, the incidence of rejection episodes was high, and because steroids were used to treat these episodes, the number of patients who remained steroid-free was low. Starzl[14] used cyclosporine with prophylactic steroids and found increased survival rates with the combination therapy. This type of protocol was adopted widely by centers in the United States as well as many European centers after the multicenter trial was abandoned.[76]

Some investigators[77-79] have noted that the immediate use of cyclosporine following transplantation was associated with a high incidence of ATN. In addition, primary nonfunction rates were elevated from about 2 percent with standard therapy to 5 to 8 percent with cyclosporine in some reporting institutions.[39,77,81] Some therefore considered that cyclosporine should be held from patients who were not actively diuresing posttransplantation.[68,75,82] Sommer and associates[83] described the sequential use of ALG, cyclosporine, and prednisone in the early posttransplantation period until it is determined that the graft is functioning well (creatinine less than 2.5). The ALG and azathioprine were discontinued, and cyclosporine was started while the prednisone was continued. It was thought that this method prevented significant toxic effects of cyclosporine from potentiating a pre-existing renal injury caused by harvesting, preservation, and reperfusion. This protocol led to extremely good graft survival (87 percent at 1-year) with no increased incidence of viral infections or neoplasms. The ATN rate associated with this protocol was 9 percent, with primary nonfunction of 1.8 percent.

As the nephrotoxic effects of cyclosporine became more troublesome, several centers adopted the so-called triple therapy. This consists of low-dose cyclosporine combined with azathioprine and prednisone. The Minnesota group[84] has used this in the immediate post-transplantation pe-

Table 11–3 Triple Drug Therapy Composed of Cyclosporine, Azathioprine, and Prednisone as a Secondary Rescue Therapy for Patients Failing Primary Immunosuppressive Regimens

	Triple Drug Therapy[87] The Ohio State University
Number treated	99
Months onset posttransplantation x̄ (range)	10.1 (1–29)
Duration of treatment x̄ (range)	7.3 (1–15)
Rejection/nephrotoxic episodes per patient	0.32/1.87
Creatinine change after treatment	
Decrease	79%
Increase	15%
No change	6%
Actuarial 1-year graft survival after treatment began	97%

Indications to begin treatment
1. Early postoperative graft dysfunction
2. Failure of primary azathioprine therapy
3. Chronic cyclosporine toxicity
4. Concomitant cyclosporine toxicity and rejection

riod quite successfully, with graft survival rates of 89 percent at 1 year in cadaver kidney recipients. Slapak[85] and First[86] have also shown good graft survival at 1 year using this regimen in recipients of cadaver kidneys (85 percent and 82 percent, respectively). Our group has used a similar protocol, only secondarily, as rescue therapy of patients failing primary regimens.[87] This approach has led to very good graft survival and notable improvement in renal function over the previous higher cyclosporine dose (Table 11–3). Several groups[79,88–90] have dealt with the cyclosporine nephrotoxicity and fears of long-term use of cyclosporine by routinely converting patients to standard therapy. While renal function does appear to improve, the relatively high incidence of rejection episodes (20 percent to 42 percent) after withdrawal of cyclosporine may be ultimately detrimental to long-term graft survival.

Cyclosporine and Prednisone in First Cadaver Renal Transplants

Overall patient survival in first cadaver transplants treated with cyclosporine has been extremely uniform, with nearly all reports having greater than 90 percent 1-year survival, and many greater than 95 percent 1-year survival (Table 11–4). When graft function is considered, an interesting observation can be made when comparing results from many centers. Several reports have identified statistically significant improved graft survival when cyclosporine is used compared with standard therapy.[75,80,91,92,93] However, there are nearly as many studies that cannot demonstrate significantly improved survival using cyclosporine.[77,78,94–97] When the data are analyzed, it is found that those without significant differences had high graft survival rates using standard therapy and that these protocols included the use of prophylactic and therapeutic ALG. Reports that showed significant differences, however, had average graft survival rates when patients were treated with azathioprine and prednisone without an antilymphocyte preparation. Most centers reporting graft survival in patients with cadaver kidneys treated with cyclosporine are above 70 percent 1-year graft survival, and many are above 80 percent 1-year graft survival (see Table 11–4).

The incidence of rejection episodes is another interesting finding that is highlighted in Table 11–4. Nearly all studies demon-

Table 11–4 Studies Comparing Azathioprine and Prednisone Versus Cyclosporine With and Without Prednisone

	Patient/Graft Survival		ALG Used c̄ AZA	Steroids Used c̄ CSA	Incidence of Rejection, CSA/AZA
	CSA(%)	AZA(%)			
Ohio State[95]	96/87	96/78	Yes	Yes	39%/87%
Minnesota[94]	90/84	91/73	Yes	Yes	34%/60%
Boston (Combined)[78]	96/76	93/74	Yes	Yes	46%/59%
Australian Multicenter[96]	93/70	97/80	Yes	No	83%/97%
Canadian Tri-Hospital[77]	100/73	96/87	Yes	qod†	NA/NA
Canadian Multicenter[81]	86/80	83/64	Occas	qod†	63%/NA
Houston[91]	96/81	89/51	No	Yes	25%/85%*
Boston (Brigham)[93]	95/78	93/53	No	Yes	53%/72%
Birmingham, England[97]	94/77	91/85	No	14 days only	63%/64%
European Multicenter[75]	94/72	92/53	No	No	86%/91%
Pittsburgh[92]	99/90	99/50	No	Yes	NA/NA

NA: not available; CSA: cyclosporine; AZA: Azathioprine; Occas: Occasional.
*Historical percentage—see reference #46
†Qod (every other day)—started on day 14

strate fewer rejection episodes in patients treated with cyclosporine. However, within the cyclosporine group, centers that used either no steroids[75,96] or every-other-day steroids[81] suffered from a high incidence of rejection episodes compared with those using daily prednisone.

The question has arisen as to why one would continue to use cyclosporine with its disadvantages (particularly nephrotoxicity) when in many instances it cannot be demonstrated that it improves graft survival. Two groups, Minnesota[94] and Ohio State,[95] have shown notable advantages with cyclosporine even though significant improvement in graft function cannot be identified (Table 11–5). These advantages include fewer rejection episodes, fewer multiple rejection episodes, and consequently fewer infectious episodes in the patients who were treated with cyclosporine. In addition, the initial hospital stay and readmission rates were lower, which was reflected by a significantly decreased cost in both initial hospitalization and readmissions.

Transplant Dysfunction

The majority of patients treated with cyclosporine as the primary immunosuppressive agent suffer from transplantation dysfunction in the early postoperative period.

Ferguson[98] has determined that renal dysfunction occurs in 81 percent of renal transplantation recipients in the first 6 months posttransplantation. Nephrotoxicity was identified as the cause of the dysfunction in 3 times as many patients as was rejection (74 percent versus 26 percent). Other series have noted similarly high nephrotoxicity-to-rejection rates.[73,94] This has led our group to a management strategy that includes frequent outpatient monitoring of renal function. Patients are begun on 10 mg per kg of cyclosporine posttransplantation, monitored for early toxicity, and discharged. Outpatient blood work is monitored, and when transplant dysfunction is noted (an increase of creatinine 25 percent above baseline), judicious outpatient dose reductions of cyclosporine are instituted (in 0.5-ml or 50-mg increments). This is based on the assumption that early transplantation dysfunction is a manifestation of cyclosporine nephrotoxicity. If creatinine levels do not return to baseline with dose reduction, the patient is promptly admitted for a percutaneous renal biopsy. If rejection is discovered, the patient is treated with oral prednisone and a gradual taper back to baseline at 3 months. If there is no evidence of rejection on biopsy, cyclosporine dosage reduction continues. If renal function does not improve markedly with these reductions, the cyclosporine is dropped to

Table 11-5 Advantages of Cyclosporine Therapy in the Absence of Demonstrable Improvement in Graft Survival

	Ohio State,[95] CSA/Imuran	Minnesota,[94] CSA/Imuran
Graft survival	87%/78%	84%/73%
Patient survival	96%/96%	90%/91%
% patients readmitted	48%/85%	71%/80%
Initial hospital days	11.6/18.5*	15.6/19.8*
Total hospital days (first 6 months)	20.4/41.7*	21.3/30.3*
Rejection free	61%/13%*	66%/40%*
Multiple rejections	9%/43%*	20%/28%
Overt CMV	4%/26%*	7%/27%*

*Statistically significant.

3 mg per kg and given on a daily or every-other-day basis, and azathioprine is added to the regimen at 1 to 2 mg per kg. If there is no response to the addition of this triple therapy after 30 days, the cyclosporine is discontinued and the patient is maintained on azathioprine and prednisone.

Cyclosporine nephrotoxicity has led many groups to modify posttransplantation protocols. In an effort to reduce the incidence of nephrotoxicity, drug regimens using triple therapy consisting of azathioprine, low-dose cyclosporine, and prednisone have been used with good success. Sequential ALG, prednisone, and azathioprine followed by cyclosporine and prednisone have reduced the early postoperative problems associated with cyclosporine use and high ATN rates, and primary nonfunction as well as early nephrotoxicity.

Costs

In this day of austerity in health care financing, holding the line on costs in transplantation has become an even more important issue. Several studies[91,94,95] have demonstrated shorter hospital stays by those patients treated with cyclosporine as opposed to those of patients treated with standard therapy. Because fewer rejection episodes and the need for less aggressive immunosuppression associated with rejection lead to fewer infection episodes, readmissions have been significantly lower as well. These factors have been directly translated into increased savings both during the initial hospitalization and in the readmissions. While the expense of the drug itself is well known, these advantages make it an attractive immunosuppressant from the point of view of total costs. Other factors that may make it even more cost advantageous are that most centers are using lower starting doses in their protocols, which leads directly to decreased total drug consumption and yearly drug costs. There also is a trend toward using combination therapy and even lower associated cyclosporine doses. Converting patients from cyclosporine to azathioprine and prednisone posttransplantation may also reduce overall costs as long as no marked increases in rejection episodes after conversion necessitate further in-hospital therapy.

High-Risk Groups

Simmons[99] outlined a group of patients treated with standard therapy (cyclosporine and prednisone) who were thought to be at high risk for renal transplantation. Among these patients were those over age 45 years and patients suffering from diabetes. Sommer[100] described the poor results of renal transplantation in the older patient receiving cadaver kidneys treated with standard therapy (43 percent 2-year graft survival, 52 percent 2-year patient survival) in 1981. A second report by Sommer[101] and other reports [102-104] have shown that with the cautious use of cyclosporine and prednisone, patient and graft survivals in older patients parallel those of the younger age groups. He also notes that the older renal transplantation recipient may be less immunologically

responsive and that the selective immunosuppression with cyclosporine not only allows improved graft survival, but results in
fewer rejection episodes in this group.
Sutherland and associates[105] and others[106]
have demonstrated a clear improvement in
cadaveric allograft survival in diabetic patients treated with cyclosporine and prednisone compared with azathioprine, ALG,
and prednisone. Data from the United
States Transplant Registry[103] have shown
that the increased risk of graft loss in the
diabetic patient has been virtually eliminated by the use of cyclosporine in these
patients.

Retransplantation

There is a difficult group of patients who
have previously lost an allograft to rejection and have received a second or third
transplant. Historically, when treated with
azathioprine and prednisone, patients who
have had retransplants have done notably
worse than those receiving first grafts.[107]
Most recent studies that have compared the
results of second and third transplants
against their historical controls (treated
with azathioprine and prednisone) have
noted improved graft survival when cyclosporine is used.[91,98,103,106,108] In fact, many
groups have graft survival rates in the 70

percent range at 1 year for retransplants
treated with cyclosporine.[91,97,103,105]

Transfusions and Matching

A somewhat more controversial subject
regarding cyclosporine is the need for preoperative blood transfusion and HLA
matching. Clear evidence of improved graft
survival has been demonstrated in patients
receiving standard therapy and well-
matched kidneys.[59] Well-defined improvements have also been noted in patients
treated with standard therapy who have received random transfusions prior to transplantation in the cadaver-recipient population[60,109] and donor-specific transfusions
in the living-related recipient population.[61]
However, several single-center groups
using cyclosporine have been unable to
identify improved graft survival with random transfusions[91,98,110] (Table 11–6). Compiled data from the European multicenter
trial,[75] Scandinavian trial,[111] and HCFA[103]
have shown no benefit either. Opelz,[112]
Cats,[113] and the Canadian multicenter
trial[114] present data to the contrary showing
statistically significant improvement with
the transfusion effect of recipients on cyclosporine. It is also interesting to note that
many single-center studies have been unable to find statistically significant differ-

Table 11–6 Comparison of Studies of Renal Allograft Recipients Treated with Cyclosporine When Graft Survival Is Correlated with Transfusions and DR Matching

	Transfusions (1 Yr Graft Survival)				DR Mismatch (1 Yr Graft Survival)			
	0	21	Overall		0	1	2	
European Multicenter[75]	87	73	72	NS	64	75	72	NS
Houston[91]	70	80	81	NS	88	—	83	NS
Opelz[112]	62	75	74	SS	72	68	63	SS*
Scandinavian Multicenter†[111]	72	76	75	NS	77	70	83	NS
Ohio State[97]	90	82	85	NS	75	82	84	NS
Cats (Terasaki)†[113]	65	77	76	SS	79	72	70	NS
Pittsburgh[108,115]	—	—	—		66	71	59	NS
Gardner and associates[110] (Portsmouth)	86	67	74	p = .03	—	—	—	

NS: Not significant; SS: statistically significant.
*Approximate percentages, transfused patients only.
†6-month survival statistics.

ences in graft survival of renal allograft recipients treated with cyclosporine when HLA matching is examined.[91,98,110,115] On the other hand, several reports from large populations in multicenter studies using cyclosporine have found matching, particularly at the DR locus, to have a positive effect on graft survival. Although it is often difficult to sort out the differences between single-institution and multicenter studies, it should be noted that graft survival in some of the poorest groups in those single-institution studies exceed those of the best groups in the multicenter studies on both of these variables (see Table 11-6). This may simply emphasize that with improving graft survival, it is more difficult to identify the effects of particular variables on graft survival and that only well-designed long-term studies with large numbers of patients will give the ultimate answer.

Living Related Transplantation

Most of the early clear-cut advantages of cyclosporine were identified in cadaveric transplantation. Its use in living related donor transplantation had yet to be proven. Haploidentical living related renal transplant recipients treated with standard therapy have benefited markedly with the advent of donor-specific transfusions.[61] With the exceptional graft survival with these protocols, could cyclosporine use provide any additional benefit? A prospective trial at our institution[116] evaluated the differences between donor-specific transfusions coupled with azathioprine and prednisone, or cyclosporine and prednisone, or cyclosporine and prednisone without donor-specific transfusions. The protocol including donor-specific transfusions followed by cyclosporine was found to be notably poor (74 percent 1-year graft survival), compared with the other two arms, and because of this was discontinued. There appeared to be no statistically significant differences between donor-sepcific transfusions and conventional therapy versus cyclosporine and prednisone without donor-specific transfusions. However, without the need for such transfusions there were no potential donor losses from presensitization. Although long-term follow-up is necessary, it appears that in the haploidentical living related donor group, cyclosporine and prednisone

without donor-specific transfusions can yield high graft survival rates without the possibility of presensitizing the donor to the recipient with transfusions.

HLA-identical recipients have enjoyed very successful graft survival rates (≥ 95 percent at 1 year) with standard therapy. Most groups in the cyclosporine era continue to use azathioprine and prednisone for identically matched donor-recipient pairs, as the patient and graft survival rates are so high that it is believed there would be no benefit gained from cyclosporine use. The Houston group[91] has used cyclosporine with HLA-identical kidneys, primarily because they believe these patients do not require prophylactic steroids and have fewer rejection episodes than those treated with azathioprine and steroids.

THE FUTURE

Pharmacologic immunosuppression has advanced sufficiently to allow successful transplantation beyond the expectation of any immunologic theory. However, the blocking of alloresponsiveness in vivo induced by the presence of donor MHC antigens still remains the goal of any immunotherapeutic protocol in clinical transplantation. Current immunosuppressive agents are nonspecific in nature and therefore not only inhibit alloresponses to MHC antigens, but also block primarily T cell responsiveness to any stimulating antigen. This global effect of all immunosuppressives available is necessary but not ideal. The ultimate immunosuppression for organ allografting would specifically inhibit only immunoresponsiveness to donor MHC antigens and create within the recipient a conditioned state of acquired specific unresponsiveness to donor antigens. The role of pharmacologic immunosuppression in inducing such an antigen-specific unresponsive state in man is only now being explored and represents an exciting frontier in transplantation immunology. It is clear that part of the future of solid organ transplantation will be centered on immunoengineering techniques applied to a recipient to induce a state of lasting antigen-specific unresponsiveness. These techniques are not now available. However, with the expansion of our knowledge and understanding of in vivo alloresponsiveness and basic mechanisms of rejection, such techniques may emerge and have a profound effect on clinical organ transplantation.

REFERENCES

1. Murray, JE, Merril, JP, and Harrison, JH: Renal homotransplantation in identical twins. Surg Forum 6:432, 1955.
2. Billingham, RE, Brent, L, and Medawar, PB: The antigenic stimulus in transplantation immunity. Nature 178:514, 1956.
3. Schwartz, R, Eisner, A, and Dameshek, W: The effect of 6-mercaptopurine on primary and secondary immune responses. J Clin Invest 38:1394, 1959.
4. Calne, RY and Murray, JG: Inhibition of the rejection of renal homografts in dogs by Burroughs Welcome 57-322. Surg Forum 12:118, 1961.
5. Murray, JE, et al: Kidney transplantation in modified recipients. Ann Surg 156:337, 1962.
6. Goodwin, WE, et al: Human renal transplantation. J Urol 89:13, 1963.
7. Murray, JE, et al: Prolonged survival of human-kidney homografts by immunosuppressive drug therapy. N Engl J Med 268:1315, 1963.
8. Starzl, TE, Marchioro, TL, and Waddell, WR: The reversal of rejection in human renal homografts with subsequent development of homograft tolerance. Surg Gynecol Obstet 117:385, 1963.
9. Starzl, TE, et al: The use of heterologous antilymphoid agents in canine renal and liver homotransplantation and in human renal homotransplantation. Surg Gynecol Obstet 124:301, 1967.
10. Najarian, JS, et al: Seven years experience with antilymphoblast globulin for renal transplantation from cadaver donors. Ann Surg 184:352, 1976.
11. McGeown, MG, et al: Advantage of low dose steroid from the day after renal transplantation. Transplantation 29:287, 1980.
12. Borel, JF: Comparative study in vitro and in vivo drug effects on cell mediated cytotoxicity. Immunology 31:631, 1976.
13. Calne, RY, et al: Cyclosporin A in patients receiving renal allografts from cadaver donors. Lancet 2:1323, 1978.
14. Starzl, T, et al: The use of cyclosporin A and prednisone in cadaver kidney transplantation. Surg Gynecol Obstet 151:17, 1980.
15. Zukoski, CF, et al: Prolonged acceptance of a canine renal allograft achieved with prednisolone. Transplantation 3:380, 1965.
16. Flower, RJ: Background and discovery of lipocortins. Agents Actions 17(3/4):255, 1985.
17. Fauci, AS: Mechanisms of the immunosuppressive and anti-inflammatory effects of glucocorticosteroids. J Immunopharmacol 1:1, 1978.
18. Dupont, E: Influence of in vivo immunosuppressive drugs on production of lymphokines. Transplantation 39:143, 1985.
19. Gore, SM and Oldhem, JA: Randomized trials of high- versus low-dose steroids in renal transplantation. Transplantation 41:319–332.
20. McGeown, MG, et al: One hundred kidney transplants at the Belfast City Hospital. Lancet 2:648, 1977.
21. Chan, L, et al: Prospective trial of high-dose versus low-dose prednisolone in renal transplantation patients. Transplant Proc 12:323, 1980.
22. Salaman, JR, Griffin, PJA, and Price, K: High or low dose steroids for immunosuppression. Transplant Proc 15:1086, 1983.
23. Ponticelli, C, et al: A search for optimising corticosteroid administration to renal transplant patients. Kidney Int (suppl 14) 23:85, 1983.
24. Morris, PJ, et al: Low dose prednisolone in renal transplantation. Lancet 8271:525, 1982.
25. d'Apice, AJF, et al: A prospective randomized trial of low-dose versus high-dose steroids in cadaveric renal transplantation. Transplantation 37:373, 1984.
26. Woodruff, MFA and Anderson, NF: Effect of lymphocyte depletion by thoracic duct fistula and administration of antilymphocyte serum on the survival of skin homografts in rats. Nature 200:702, 1963.
27. Weil, R and Simmons, RL: Combined immunosuppression for canine renal allograft prolongation. Ann Surg 167:239, 1968.
28. Turcotte, JG, et al: Antithymocyte globulin in renal transplant recipients. Arch Surg 106:484, 1973.
29. Sheil, AGR, et al: Antilymphocyte globulin in patients with renal allografts from cadaver donors. Lancet 2:227, 1973.
30. Nelson, PW, et al: Antithymocyte globulin as the primary treatment for renal allograft rejection. Transplantation 36:587, 1983.
31. Filo, RS, Smith, EJ, and Leapman, SB: Reversal of acute renal allograft rejection with adjunctive ATG therapy. Transplant Proc 13:482, 1981.
32. Nowygrod, R, Appel, G, and Hardy, MA: Use of ATG for reversal of acute allograft rejection. Transplant Proc 13:469, 1981.

33. Howard, RJ, et al: The use of antilymphoblast globulin in the treatment of renal allograft rejection. Transplant Proc 13:473, 1981.

34. Streem, SB, et al: Low-dose maintenance prednisone and antilymphoblast globulin for the treatment of acute rejection. Transplantation 35:420, 1983.

35. Hoitsma, AJ, et al: Treatment of acute rejection of cadaveric renal allografts with rabbit antithymocyte globulin. Transplantation 33:12, 1981.

36. Shield, CF, et al: Use of antithymocyte globulin for reversal of acute allograft rejection. Transplantation 28:461, 1979.

37. Wechter, WJ, et al: Antithymocyte globulin (ATGAM) in renal allograft recipients. Transplantation 28:294, 1979.

38. Cosimi, AB: The clinical value of antilymphocyte antibodies. Transplant Proc 13:462, 1981.

39. Taylor, HE, Achman, CFD, and Horowitz, I: Canadian clinical trial of antilymphocyte globulin in human cadaver renal transplantation. Can Med Assoc J 115:1205, 1976.

40. Bell, PRF, et al: Medical research council trial of antilymphocyte globulin in renal transplantation. Transplantation 35:539, 1983.

41. Kreis, H, et al: Antithymocyte globulin in cadaver kidney transplantation: A randomized trial based on T cell monitoring. Kidney Int 9:438, 1981.

42. Novick, AC, et al: A controlled randomized double-blind study of antilymphoblast globulin in cadaver renal transplantation. Transplantation 35:175, 1983.

43. Condie, RM, et al: Efficacy of Minnesota ALG in renal transplantation. Transplant Proc 17:1304, 1985.

44. Russell, PS, Colvin, RB, and Cosimi, AB: Monoclonal antibodies for the diagnosis and treatment of transplant rejection. Annu Rev Med 35:63, 1984.

45. Goldstein, G, et al: Orthoclone OKT3 treatment of acute renal allograft rejection. Transplant Proc 17:129, 1985.

46. Norman, DJ, et al: Reversal of acute allograft rejection with monoclonal antibody. Transplant Proc 17:39, 1985.

47. Thistlethwaite, JR, et al: Evolving use of OKT3 monoclonal antibody for treatment of renal allograft rejection. Transplantation 38:695, 1984.

48. Kahan, BD, et al: Cyclosporine immunosuppression mitigates immunologic risk factors in renal allotransplantation. Transplant Proc (suppl) 15:2469, 1983.

49. Kreis, H, et al: Prophylactic treatment of allograft recipients with a monoclonal anti-T₃+ cell antibody. Transplant Proc 17:1315, 1985.

50. Elion, GB, Hitchings, GH, and Vander Werff, H: Antagonists of nucleic acid derivative. J Biol Chem 192:505, 1951.

51. Calne, RY: The rejection of renal homografts: Inhibition in dogs by 6-mercaptopurine. Lancet 1:417, 1960.

52. Zukoski, CF, Lee, HM, and Hume, DH: The prolongation of functional survival of canine renal homograft by 6-mercaptopurine. Surg Forum 11:470, 1960.

53. Elion, GB, et al: A summary of investigations with BW 57-322. Cancer Chemother Rep 14:93, 1961.

54. Bieber, S, et al: Suppression of the immune response by drugs in combination. Proc Soc Exp Biol Med 111:334, 1962.

55. Page, AR, Condie, RM, and Good, RA: Effect of 6-MP on inflammation. Am J Pathol 40:519, 1962.

56. Murray, JE, et al: Five years' experience in renal transplantation with immunosuppressive drugs. Ann Surg 168:416, 1968.

57. Lucas, ZJ, et al: Renal allotransplantation in humans. Arch Surg 100:113, 1970.

58. Starzl, TE, et al: Cyclophosphamide and whole organ transplantation in human beings. Surg Gynecol Obstet 133:981, 1971.

59. Ting, A and Morris, PJ: Powerful effect of HLA-DR match on survival of cadaveric renal allografts. Lancet 2:282, 1980.

60. Opelz, G, et al: Effect of blood transfusions on subsequent kidney transplants. Transplant Proc 5:253, 1973.

61. Salvatierra, OJ, et al: Deliberate donor specific blood transfusions prior to living related renal transplantation. Ann Surg 192:543, 1980.

62. Anderson, CB, Sicard, GA, and Etheredge, EE: Pretreatment of renal allograft recipients with azathioprine and donor-specific blood products. Surgery 92:315, 1982.

63. Borel, JF: The history of Cyclosporin A and its significance. In White, DJG, (ed): Cyclosporin A. Elsevier Biomedical Press: Amsterdam, 1982, p 5.

64. Kostakis, AJ, White, DJG, and Calne, RY: Prolongation of cat heart allograft survival by cyclosporin A. IRCS Med Sci 5:280, 1977.

65. Calne, RY and White, DJG: Cyclosporin A: A powerful immunosuppressant in dogs with renal allografts. IRCS Med Sci 5:595, 1977.

66. Green, CJ and Allison, AC: Extensive prolongation of rabbit kidney allograft survival after short-term cyclosporin A treatment. Lancet 1:1182, 1978.

67. Powles, RL, et al: Cyclosporin A for the

treatment of graft-versus-host disease in man. Lancet 2:1327, 1978.

68. Calne, RY, et al: Cyclosporine A initially as the only immunosuppressant in 34 recipients of cadaveric organs. Lancet 2:1033, 1979.

69. Donatsch, P, et al: A radioimmunoassay to measure cyclosporin A in plasma and serum samples. J Immunoassay 2:19, 1981.

70. Niederberger, W, et al: High-performance liquid chromatographic determination of cyclosporin A in human plasma and urine. J Chromatogr 182:454, 1980.

71. Kahan, BD, Ried, M, and Newburger, J: Pharmacokinetics of cyclosporine in human renal transplantation. Transplant Proc 15:446, 1983.

72. Beveridge, T, et al: Cyclosporine A: Pharmacokinetics after a single dose in man and serum levels after multiple dosing in recipients of allogeneic bone marrow grafts. Curr Therap Res 30:5, 1981.

73. Kahan, BD: Clinical and experimental studies with cyclosporine in renal transplantation. Surgery 97:125, 1985.

74. Hess, AD, Tutschka, PJ, and Santos, GW: Effect of cyclosporine on the induction of cytotoxic T lymphocytes. Transplant Proc 15:2248, 1983.

75. European Multicentre Trial Group: Cyclosporine in cadaveric renal transplantation: One year follow up of a multicentre trial. Lancet 2:986, 1983.

76. Bunzendahl, H, et al: Cyclosporine and steroids: Effects on the clinical course after renal allotransplantation. Transplant Proc (suppl) 15:2531, 1983.

77. Halloran, P, et al: Randomized comparison between cyclosporine and conventional therapy plus Minnesota antilymphocyte globulin in cadaveric renal transplantation. Transplant Proc (suppl) 15:2513, 1983.

78. Cho, SL, et al: Comparison of kidney transplant survival between patients treated with cyclosporine and those treated with azathioprine and antithymocyte globulin. Am J Surg 147:518, 1984.

79. Wood, RFM, et al: A randomized controlled trial of short term cyclosporine therapy in renal transplantation. Transplant Proc 17:1164, 1985.

80. Squifflet, JP, et al: Cyclosporine in cadaver renal transplantation at a center with good results using conventional treatment. Transplant Proc 17:1212, 1985.

81. Canadian Multicentre Trial Study Group: A randomized clinical trial of cyclosporine in cadaveric renal transplantation. N Eng J Med 309:809, 1983.

82. Morris, PJ, et al: A controlled trial of cyclosporine in renal transplantation with conversion to azathioprine and prednisone after three months. Transplantation 36:273, 1983.

83. Sommer, BG, Henry, ML, and Ferguson, RM: Sequential conventional immunotherapy with maintenance cyclosporine following renal transplantation. Transplant Proc 18:69, 1986.

84. Simmons, RL, et al: New immunosuppressive drug combinations for mismatched related and cadaveric renal transplantation. Transplant Proc 18:76, 1986.

85. Slapak, M, et al: The use of low-dose cyclosporine in combination with azathioprine and steroids in renal transplantation. Transplant Proc 17:1222, 1985.

86. First, MR, et al: The use of low dose cyclosporine, azathioprine, and prednisone in renal transplantation. Transplant Proc 18:132, 1986.

87. Henry, ML, Sommer, BG, Ferguson, RM: Triple drug therapy: An alternative in renal transplantation. Transplant Proc 19:1920, 1987.

88. Rocher, LL, et al: Utility of azathioprine management of renal allograft recipients initially treated with cyclosporine. Transplant Proc 17:1185, 1985.

89. Tegzess, AM, et al: Improvement in renal function after conversion from cyclosporine to prednisone/azathioprine in renal transplant patients. Transplant Proc 17:1191, 1985.

90. Flechner, SM, et al: The fate of patients converted from cyclosporine to azathioprine to improve renal function. Transplant Proc 17:1227, 1985.

91. Kahan, BD, et al: Impact of cyclosporine on renal transplant practice at the University of Texas Medical School at Houston. Am J Kidney Dis 5:288, 1985.

92. Rosenthal, JT, et al: Cadaveric renal transplantation under cyclosporine-steroid therapy. Surg Gynecol Obstet 157:309, 1983.

93. Tilney, NL, et al: Experience with cyclosporine and steroids in clinical renal transplantation. Ann Surg 200:605, 1984.

94. Najarian, JS, et al: A single institution, randomized, prospective trial of cyclosporine versus azathioprine-antilymphocyte globulin for immunosuppression in renal allograft recipients. Ann Surg 201:142, 1985.

95. Henry, ML, Sommer, BG, and Ferguson, RM: Beneficial effects of cyclosporine compared with azathioprine in cadaveric renal transplantation. Am J Surg 150:533, 1985.

96. Sheil, AGR, et al: Australian trial of cyclosporine in cadaveric donor renal transplantation. Transplant Proc 15:2485, 1983.

97. McMaster, P, et al: Cyclosporine in cadaveric renal transplantation: A prospective trial. Transplant Proc 15:2523, 1983.

98. Ferguson, RM and Sommer, BG: Cyclosporine in renal transplantation: A single institution experience. Am J Kidney Dis 5:296, 1985.

99. Simmons, RL, et al: Renal transplantation in high risk patients. Arch Surg 103:290, 1971.

100. Sommer, BG, et al: Renal transplantation in patients over 50 years of age. Transplant Proc 13:33, 1981.

101. Sommer, BG, et al: Renal transplantation in the middle aged and elderly uremic patient: The recent United States experience and results from a single institution. In Oreopoulos, DG (ed): Geriatric Nephrology. Martinus Nijhoff Publishers, The Netherlands, 1986.

102. Ringden, O, et al: Improved outcome in renal transplant recipients above 55 years of age treated with cyclosporine and low doses of steroids. Transplant Proc (suppl) 15:2507, 1983.

103. Hunsicker, LG: Impact of cyclosporine on cadaveric renal transplantation: A summary statement. Am J Kidney Dis 5:335, 1985.

104. Okiye, SE, et al: Primary renal transplantation in patients 50 years of age or older. Transplant Proc 15:1046, 1983.

105. Sutherland, DER, et al: Results of the Minnesota randomized prospective trial of cyclosporine versus azathioprine-antilymphocyte globulin for immunosuppression in renal transplant recipients. Am J Kidney Dis 5:318, 1985.

106. Milford, EL, et al: The clinical experience with cyclosporine and azathioprine at Brigham and Women's Hospital. Am J Kidney Dis 5:313, 1985.

107. Gifford, RM, et al: Duration of first renal allograft survival as indicative of second allograft outcome. Surgery 88:611, 1980.

108. Gordon, RD, et al: Cyclosporine-steroid combination therapy in 84 cadaveric renal transplants. Am J Kidney Dis 5:307, 1985.

109. Opelz, G, et al: Blood transfusions and renal transplantation. Transplant Proc 11:1889, 1979.

110. Gardner, B, et al: Do recipients of a cadaver renal allograft on cyclosporine require prior transfusions? Transplant Proc 17:1032, 1985.

111. Klintmalm, G, et al: The blood transfusion, DR matching, and mixed lymphocyte culture effects are not seen in cyclosporine treated renal recipients. Transplant Proc 17:1026, 1985.

112. Opelz, G: Current relevance of the transfusion effect in renal transplantation. Transplant Proc 17:1015, 1985.

113. Cats, S, et al: Effect of HLA typing and transfusions on cyclosporine-treated renal allograft recipients. N Engl J Med 311:675, 1984.

114. The Canadian Transplant Study Group: Examination of parameters influencing the benefit/detriment ratio of cyclosporine in renal transplantation. Am J Kidney Dis 5:328, 1985.

115. Taylor, RJ, et al: Influence of DR matching in cadaveric renal transplants performed with cyclosporine. Transplantation 38:616, 1984.

116. Sommer, BG and Ferguson, RM: Mismatched, living related donor renal transplantation: A prospective randomized study. Surgery 98:267, 1985.

117. Light, JA, et al: Antilymphocyte globulin reverses "irreversible" allograft rejection. Transplant Proc 13:475, 1981.

Chapter 12

Cancer

ISRAEL PENN*,†

Inadvertent Transplantation of Cancer
Cancers That Arise De Novo After Transplantation
   Incidence
   Types of Neoplasms
   Time of Appearance of Tumors
   Age and Sex of Patients
   Cancers of the Skin and Lips
   Lymphomas
   Kaposi's Sarcoma (KS)
   Carcinomas of the Uterus
   Carcinomas of the Vulva and Perineum
   Treatment of De Novo Cancers
   Etiology of De Novo Cancers

Any condition that causes profound and prolonged suppression of immunity may be complicated by an increased incidence of certain cancers.[1-3] For example, patients with congenital immunodeficiency disorders have a high incidence of non-Hodgkin's lymphomas, leukemias, and some carcinomas. In addition, the acquired immunodeficiency syndrome (AIDS) is associated with a high incidence of Kaposi's sarcoma (KS) and non-Hodgkin's lymphoma (NHL). The immunosuppression associated with renal transplantation not only permits the survival of accidentally transplanted malignant cells but also is associated with an increased incidence of certain cancers that arise de novo after transplantation. This chapter is based on data collected by the Cincinnati Transplant Tumor Registry (CTTR) up till May 1986.

INADVERTENT TRANSPLANTATION OF CANCER

In the pioneering years of transplantation, kidneys were sometimes obtained from cadaveric or living donors who had cancer. Some organs contained malignant cells that were able to survive, multiply, and spread when placed in patients given

---

*Supported in part by Grant Number 6985 from the Veterans Administration.
†The author wishes to thank his many colleagues throughout the world who have generously contributed data concerning their patients to the CTTR.

immunosuppressive therapy. This experience taught surgeons to avoid using donors with cancer with certain exceptions mentioned below. However, occasional cases of accidentally transplanted tumors still occur, usually following the use of cadaver donors who were suspected to have died of cerebral hemorrhage, but were later found to have had unsuspected cancers that had metastasized to the brain and bled.

The CTTR has data on 94 patients who received kidneys from donors with cancer or had been treated for it up to 5 years before donation.[1,2,4,6] Donors with primary neoplasms confined to the brain were excluded from the study. The tumors in the donors arose mostly from the lung (25), kidney (21), colorectum (8), cutaneous melanomas (8), and breast (7).

Transplanted cancers occurred in 39 recipients (41 percent). The tumors were confined to the allografts in 13 recipients; in 3 there was invasion of surrounding structures; and in 23 there were distant metastases. In two recipients with metastatic cancers the immunosuppressive therapy was discontinued, and the tumor burden reduced by graft nephrectomy. This treatment caused progressive regression and ultimately complete disappearance of the malignancies. Two other recipients with metastases apparently had a similar satisfactory outcome following such therapy. In addition, a patient with local spread of a malignant melanoma rejected the residual tumor after graft nephrectomy and cessation of immunosuppressive therapy. Presumably the immune systems of these five patients recovered from their depressed state and rejected the foreign malignant cells. However, in six other patients, the neoplasms failed to regress and the patients died of cancer despite discontinuation of immunosuppression (six patients), graft nephrectomy (four patients), immunotherapy (one patient), local radiotherapy (one patient), and cytotoxic therapy (one patient). In two of these recipients treatment was started too late and they died shortly after diagnosis. Presumably the immune systems of the other four recipients were overwhelmed by widespread cancer leading to the fatal outcome.

Several lessons may be learned from the accumulated experience.[1,2,4,6] One should avoid using kidneys from donors with cancer except those with low-grade carcinomas of the skin or with primary brain cancers, which rarely spread outside the central nervous system. Whenever possible, a biopsy should be obtained to avoid the pitfall of a metastasis from an occult primary tumor, usually in the bronchus, which mimics a primary brain malignancy or hemorrhage. One should also avoid using donors with brain neoplasms treated with ventriculoperitoneal or ventriculovenous shunts, as these open pathways for dissemination of the cancers.

When harvesting kidneys they must be carefully examined. If a suspicious nodule is found, it should be biopsied and a frozen section examination obtained. If cancer is diagnosed, the tumor should be widely excised and the kidney transplanted, as was done successfully in six cases in this series.[6] All such patients must be carefully followed for long periods for signs of recurrence. If the tumor is too large or excision gives inadequate margins, the kidney should not be transplanted.

When a kidney has been transplanted from a cadaver donor in whom a later autopsy reveals a previously unsuspected but widespread malignancy, the surgeon should promptly remove the allograft, as there is at least a 41 percent chance that it contains cancer cells.[1,2,4,6] Should the surgeon decide to leave the graft in place, he or she must re-evaluate the recipient's condition at frequent intervals. If a transplanted malignancy becomes apparent at a later date, the allograft should be removed, immunosuppressive therapy discontinued, and the patient placed on regular dialysis. If the cancer undergoes complete remission, further renal transplantation should be delayed until the patient has been free of malignancy for at least 12 months.

CANCERS THAT ARISE DE NOVO AFTER TRANSPLANTATION

Incidence

From 1968 till May 1986 the CTTR accumulated data on 2653 types of cancer that arose in 2477 kidney transplant recipients.[1-9] Despite the tens of thousands of renal transplant recipients at risk the incidence of cancer at several major transplant centers has ranged from 1 to 16 percent with an average of 4 percent.[9] The great variation in incidence may indicate differences in the intensity of immunosuppressive therapy given at various centers. Another explanation is that some centers report all malignancies, no matter how trivial, while others report only the more florid types of cancers. The true incidence of tumors is greater than the figure of 4 percent cited above, as many centers include individuals treated in the early years of transplantation, when patient survival was often short. The figures also include recipients with brief follow-up times.

Types of Neoplasms

The cancers most frequently seen in the general population, such as carcinomas of the lung, prostate, colon, and rectum, fe-

male breast, and invasive carcinoma of the uterine cervix, are not increased in incidence in transplant recipients.[1−4,7−9] Instead, the CTTR data show that certain malignancies occur with remarkable frequency (Table 12–1). Skin and lip cancers are the most common neoplasms.[7] Their incidence varies with the amount of exposure to sunshine. In areas with limited exposure, there is a fourfold to sevenfold increase, but in regions with abundant sunshine there is an almost 21-fold increase over the already high incidence seen in the local control population.[1,2,7] A study of 934 renal transplant recipients from a single Swedish center indicates that lip cancers arc increased 29-fold in incidence as compared with controls.[10] Two epidemiologic studies show that the incidence of NHL is 28- to 49-fold above that encountered in age-matched controls.[11,12] In situ carcino-

Table 12–1 De Novo Cancers in Renal Allograft Recipients		
Type of Tumors		**No. of Tumors***
Cancers of skin and lips		1041
Lymphomas		324
Carcinomas of uterus		171
Cervix	154	
Body	17	
Carcinomas of the lung		130
Carcinomas of colon and rectum		95
Kaposi's sarcomas		94
Carcinomas of breast		89
Carcinomas of the kidney		80
Host kidney	71	
Allograft kidney	8	
Unknown	1	
Carcinomas of the vulva, perineum, penis or scrotum		74
Carcinomas of the head and neck (excluding thyroid, parathyroid and eye)		71
Leukemias		66
Metastatic carcinomas (primary site unknown)		64
Carcinomas of urinary bladder		55
Carcinomas of liver and bile ducts		41
Carcinomas of thyroid		37
Soft tissue sarcomas		34
Cancers of stomach		33
Testicular carcinomas		28
Carcinomas of prostate gland		28
Ovarian cancers		27
Cancers of the pancreas		19
Brain neoplasms (excluding lymphomas)		12
Miscellaneous neoplasms		40
	Total	2653

*There were 2477 patients, of whom 168 (6.8 percent) had more than one type of neoplasm involving different organ systems. Eight of these patients each had three separate types of cancer.

mas of the uterine cervix have a 14-fold increase over controls.[13] Nonmelanoma skin cancers and in situ carcinomas of the uterine cervix are usually excluded from cancer statistics. If we omit them from the CTTR data, several other cancers show a substantial increase in incidence. Kaposi's sarcoma then makes up 5.2 percent of malignancies in the CTTR, in comparison with its incidence in the general population in the United States (before the AIDS epidemic started), where it comprised only 0.02 to 0.07 percent of all tumors.[3,8] The high incidence of KS in this worldwide collection of patients is comparable with that seen in areas of the world where it occurs with greatest frequency, namely in tropical Africa, where it makes up 3 to 9 percent of all neoplasms.[14] These observations are in keeping with the finding of a 400- to 500-fold increase in the incidence of KS in renal transplant recipients compared with a control population of the same ethnic origin.[15] Carcinomas of the vulva and perineum make up 4 percent of tumors in the CTTR, a much higher incidence than in the general population.[1-3,5] This finding is in keeping with a 100-fold increase in the incidence of carcinomas of the vulva and anus in renal transplantation patients as compared with controls.[10] There are also small increases in the incidence of leukemia, carcinomas of the kidney, and carcinomas of the liver and biliary passages among kidney transplant recipients.[12]

Time of Appearance of Tumors

As the length of follow-up of kidney transplant recipients increased, it has become evident that certain malignancies are diagnosed at fairly distinct intervals after transplantation.[1-5,7-9] In contrast with other known oncogenic stimuli in humans, which often take 15 to 20 years or more before they cause clinical lesions, neoplasms appear a relatively short time after transplantation.[1-9,11,12] Kaposi's sarcoma is the first to appear at an average of 23 (range 2 to 225.5) months after transplantation.[3,8] Lymphomas appear at an average of 37 (range 1 to 190.5) months after transplantation. Other neoplasms (excluding carcinomas of the vulva and perineum) appear at an average of 63 (range 1 to 244.5)

months following transplantation. Carcinomas of the vulva and perineum appear at the longest interval after transplantation at an average of 91 (range 9 to 215) months.

The incidence of malignancies rises as the length of follow-up after transplantation increases.[1-4] A study of 3846 Australian renal transplantation recipients showed an incidence of 3 percent at 1 year, 14 percent at 5 years, and 49 percent at 14 years.[16] These statistics underline the need to follow transplant patients indefinitely.[1-4,7-9]

Age and Sex of Patients

The tumors occurred in a relatively young group of patients; their average age at the time of transplantation was 40 years (range 7 months to 72 years).[1-4,7-9] Forty-nine percent were under 40 years at the time of transplantation. Sixty-four percent were male and 36 percent female, in keeping with the 2 to 1 ratio of male to female patients who undergo renal transplantation.

Cancers of the Skin and Lips

The most commonly encountered tumors were those of the skin and lips.[1-4,7-9,17] They made up 1027 of 2653 (39 percent) of cancers in the CTTR (Table 12–1). Their incidence increased with the duration of follow-up after transplantation, as shown by an Australian study of 3846 renal transplant recipients, of whom 11 percent had neoplasms at 5 years, 29 percent at 10 years, and 43 percent at 14 years.[16]

The skin malignancies seen in transplant patients show some unusual features in comparison with their counterparts in the general population.[1-4,7-9,17] Basal cell carcinomas outnumber squamous cell carcinomas in the general population, but the opposite is true in transplantation patients, in whom squamous cell carcinomas made up 52 percent and basal cell carcinomas 29 percent (Table 12–2). Another 13 percent of patients had both types of cancer. Another difference is the youth of the transplantation patients, whose average age was 30 years younger than those with similar neoplasms in the general population.[7,18] In

Table 12–2 Carcinomas of the Skin and Lips

Type of Malignancy	No. of Patients
Squamous cell carcinomas	535
Basal cell carcinomas	302
Squamous and basal cell carcinomas	136
Malignant melanoma	50*
Unclassified	11
Merkel's cell carcinoma	4†
Malignant sweat gland carcinomas	2‡
Intracystic subaceous gland carcinoma	1
Total	1041

*Eighteen patients also had squamous or basal cell carcinomas.
†One patient also had squamous and basal cell carcinomas.
‡Two patients also had squamous or basal cell carcinomas.

addition, the incidence of multiple skin cancers, which occurred in at least 43 percent of the patients, is remarkably high and is comparable with that seen only in areas of plentiful sunshine exposure.[7] Several individuals each had more than 100 skin cancers. Malignant melanomas comprised 4.8 percent of the skin cancers in this series in contrast with an incidence of 2.7 percent in the general population of the United States.[19] This finding is consistent with an Australian study showing a fivefold higher incidence of malignant melanoma in transplantation patients than in age-matched controls.[16]

Most skin cancers were of low-grade malignancy, but some were very aggressive.[1,2,3,7] Lymph node metastases were present in 76 patients (7.4 percent), 62 of whom had squamous cell carcinomas, 11 of whom had malignant melanomas, and 3 of whom had other tumors. Of the squamous cell carcinomas with lymph node metastases, 43 involved the skin, 11 affected the lips, and 8 were cases with skin and lip involvement. The metastases probably arose from the skin lesions in four patients in the last group, while in the two they arose from the lip lesions, and in two the origin was unclear. Sixty-six patients (6.4 percent) died of their skin cancers, 43 of squamous cell carcinomas, 21 of malignant melanomas, 1 of basal cell carcinoma, and 1 of Merkel's cell tumor. Of the fatalities caused by squamous cell carcinoma, 31 were caused by lesions arising in the skin, 4

by lesions from the lips, and 8 by lesions involving the lips and skin. The skin lesions apparently were responsible for fatal metastases in four patients, the lip lesions in three, and in one it was not clear which lesions caused the lethal outcome. Not included in the above figures are seven patients, all with squamous cell carcinomas, who are alive with metastases; another two patients who probably died of metastases from a squamous cell carcinoma and a malignant melanoma, respectively; and two patients who died of complications of chemotherapy given to treat an advanced squamous cell carcinoma and a Merkel's cell tumor, respectively. All these findings are in keeping with a more than 10-fold increased mortality resulting from squamous cell carcinoma of the skin observed in Australian renal transplant recipients.[11] The behavior of skin malignancies in the present series is in significant contrast with that seen in the general population, in whom they cause only 1 to 2 percent of all cancer deaths, the great majority of which are from malignant melanomas.[20]

Kidney transplant recipients must be taught about prevention of skin cancer.[1,2,7] As exposure to sunlight is a major etiologic factor, patients should be warned to avoid prolonged exposure. If their occupations or hobbies do not permit this, they should wear wide-brimmed hats, sun visors, and protective clothing, and shield the skin with effective sunscreen preparations.

Hyperkeratoses and warts are common

in transplantation patients and usually present in areas exposed to sunlight. Some lesions may be indistinguishable clinically from skin cancers.[1,2,7,17] In such instances one should biopsy any suspicious areas. Lip carcinomas also may create diagnostic problems, as they often are atypical and appear as superficial ulcers without an indurated base and rolled everted edge.[1,2,7] Occasionally two superficial lip cancers may be present simultaneously. One should biopsy all lip ulcers that persist for more than a month, except during the early posttransplantation period, when herpetic ulcers are encountered frequently.

Treatment of skin and lip cancers includes surgical excision, cryosurgery, or radiotherapy.[1,2,7] Topical applications of 5-fluorouracil or other chemotherapeutic agents are useful for extensive areas of Bowen's disease or multiple superficial carcinomas.[1,2,7] In the general population some patients with multiple skin cancers have been treated satisfactorily with topical immunotherapeutic agents such as DNCB, BCG, or PPD. However, transplantation physicians are reluctant to employ these immunopotentiating agents in immunosuppressed patients for fear of precipitating an allograft rejection crisis.

Lymphomas

Lymphomas in renal transplantation patients show several unusual features in contrast with their behavior in the general population.[1-4,8,9,12] They comprise 3 to 4 percent of all neoplasms in the community at large,[20] but make up 324 of 2653 cancers (12 percent) in the CTTR (Table 12–3). If we exclude nonmelanoma skin malignancies and in situ carcinomas of the uterine cervix, the incidence is 18 percent. In contrast lymphomas were exceedingly common in the recipients of extrarenal organs (pancreas, liver, heart, heart-lung, and bone marrow) in whom they comprised 53 of 87 neoplasms (61 percent).

The lymphomas in this series were strikingly different from those seen in the general population.[1-3,9] The majority (92 percent) were NHLs, whereas Hodgkin's disease is the most common lymphoma seen in the same age group in the general population. Morphologically most NHLs were variously described as immunoblastic sarcomas, reticulum cell sarcomas, microgliomas, or large cell lymphomas. Immunologically most arose from B lymphocytes, but a few T-cell lymphomas were described. Whereas extranodal involve-

Table 12–3 Lymphomas in Renal Transplant Recipients	
Type of Lymphoma	**No. of Patients**
Reticulum cell sarcomas*	176†
Unclassified lymphomas	47
B cell lymphomas	42
Lymphosarcomas	13†
Hodgkin's disease	12
Plasma cell lymphomas	12
B cell hyperplasias (? lymphomas)	7
T cell lymphomas (one case of mycosis fungoides)	6
Lymphoreticular malignancies	4
True histiocytic lymphomas	2
Burkitt's lymphoma	1
Histiocytic medullary reticulosis	1
Null cell lymphoma	1
	Total 324

*Also classified as histiocytic lymphoma, microglioma, immunoblastic sarcoma, reticulosarcoma, and large cell lymphoma.

†One patient had a reticulum cell sarcoma that underwent spontaneous regression. Two years later he developed a lymphocytic lymphoma.

ment occurs in 24 to 48 percent of NHL patients in the community at large,[21,22] it was present in 70 percent of NHLs among renal transplant recipients. Furthermore, extranodal disease was confined to a single organ in 68 percent of the transplant patients. The brain was the organ most frequently involved. In the general population about 1 percent of NHLs involve the brain parenchyma,[23] whereas in renal transplantation patients 33 percent affected the central nervous system (CNS), usually the brain. Spinal cord involvement was rare. Frequently the brain lesions were multicentric in distribution. Another unusual feature was that in 73 percent of patients with CNS involvement the lesions were confined to the brain, whereas in the general population brain lesions are frequently associated with lymphomatous involvement of other viscera. A possible explanation for the remarkable brain involvement is that it has poor immunologic reactions, so that lymphoma cells that arise in it or are carried there from other sites grow more readily in this relatively immunologically privileged site than in other regions.[1]

Whenever a transplantation patient presents with neurologic symptoms, a CNS lymphoma should be considered in the differential diagnosis.[1,2] A thorough work-up is necessary to exclude more common causes of neurologic symptoms, including hypertensive encephalopathy, meningitis, brain abscess, and intracranial bleeding. Studies may include electroencephalography, brain scan, computerized axial tomography, examination of the cerebrospinal fluid, cerebral angiography, and nuclear magnetic resonance scanning.

The gastrointestinal tract is frequently involved by NHLs in transplantation patients. A quite common presentation is acute perforation of an intestinal lymphoma with resultant peritonitis.

Conflicting reports have appeared in the literature concerning whether lymphomas are monoclonal or polyclonal in origin.[24-26] However, many of the differences are related to the different techniques used to determine clonality. In addition, questions have been raised as to whether some posttransplantation lymphomas may be nonmalignant virally induced lymphoproliferations rather than true lymphomas. Some authors describe a spectrum of lesions ranging from benign polyclonal B cell lymphoproliferations on the one hand to frankly malignant monoclonal B cell lymphomas on the other, with an intermediate phase in which a polyclonal B cell proliferation undergoes a clonal cytogenetic change with progression to malignant transformation.[24] Disagreements about clonality are not merely academic exercises but may have therapeutic implications.[24-26] Hanto and associates[24] suggested that at least some polyclonal lesions are caused by the Epstein-Barr virus and treated these with the antiviral agent acyclovir. They obtained remissions in four patients with polyclonal lesions so treated, but monoclonal lesions did not respond to acyclovir and were treated by surgery, radiotherapy, or chemotherapy. In addition, immunosuppression was reduced or discontinued in a few patients. Five of their 19 patients survived without recurrence of their tumors. Cleary and colleagues[25] emphasized the need to establish monoclonality because such lesions required antineoplastic therapy (radiation and chemotherapy), perhaps with reduction in immunosuppressive therapy. However, they did not describe the results obtained following treatment of their 10 patients. In contrast, Starzl and coworkers[26] found that the majority of their patients had complete remissions after reduction or cessation of immunosuppressive therapy and that several seemingly monoclonal lesions regressed as readily as polyclonal lymphomas. They did not recommend the use of acyclovir, radiotherapy, or chemotherapy. Following treatment, 11 of their 17 patients were alive and free of cancer. Several deaths in their series occurred in patients who were not appropriately treated because of failure to make a timely diagnosis. The conflicting opinions expressed above indicate the need for additional studies of larger numbers of patients to determine the importance of clonality and to determine the appropriate forms of treatment of various lymphomas.

Kaposi's Sarcoma (KS)

There were 94 patients with this disorder, 64 men and 30 women. The 2 to 1 men-to-women ratio is the same as that seen in transplantation patients having other neoplasms but is much less than the 9 to 1 to 15 to 1 ratio seen with KS in the general population.[8] KS was most common in transplantation patients who were Jewish, black, or of Mediterranean ancestry.[8] Seven of the 94 patients (7 percent) had other cancers, an incidence similar to that seen in the general population.[27] Sixty-two of the 94 patients (66 percent) had "benign" KS involving the skin, conjunctiva, or oropharyngolaryngeal mucosa; and 32 (34 percent) had the "malignant" variety with involvement of the internal organs, mainly the gastrointestinal tract and lungs. Following treatment complete remissions occurred in 31 of the 62 patients (50 percent) with "benign" disease. Seven of these 31 remissions (23 percent) occurred when the *only* treatment was a drastic reduction of immunosuppressive therapy.[1-3,8] The other 24 remissions followed surgery, radiotherapy, or chemotherapy. In the malignant group 5 of the 32 patients (16 percent) had complete remissions after chemotherapy or radiotherapy together with alteration of immunosuppressive therapy. Twenty of the 62 patients with nonvisceral KS died, usually of causes unrelated to the KS, whereas 19 of the 32 patients with visceral KS are dead, the major cause being the neoplasm.

The physician should suspect KS whenever a transplant patient develops reddish-blue macules or plaques in the skin or oropharyngeal mucosa, or has apparently infected granulomas that fail to heal. If the diagnosis is confirmed, a comprehensive work-up is needed to determine whether there is involvement of the internal viscera.[1-3,8] Upper and lower gastrointestinal endoscopy and computerized axial tomography are particularly valuable studies.

Carcinomas of the Uterus

Carcinomas of the cervix occurred in 154 (17 percent) of the 894 women in this series.[1-4] In situ lesions made up at least 80 percent of the cases. These tumors are probably more common than is realized. It is, therefore, advisable that all postadolescent female patients have pelvic examinations and cervical smears done on a regular basis.[1-4]

Carcinomas of the body of the uterus are uncommon. Perhaps this is because most transplantation patients are young, whereas these neoplasms occur mainly in postmenopausal women.[1-5]

Carcinomas of the Vulva and Perineum

Carcinomas of the vulva, perineum, scrotum, penis, perianal skin, and anus occurred in 74 patients, 55 women and 19 men.[1-3,5] In contrast with patients in the general population who have similar lesions, the patients were surprisingly young. The average age of the women at the time of transplantation was 30 (range 15 to 55) years and of the men 38 (range 25 to 60) years. In women there was sometimes a "field effect" with involvement by cancer of the vulva and vagina and/or the cervix of the uterus. Some patients gave a history of condyloma acuminatum or herpes genitalis, suggesting that oncogenic viruses may play an etiologic role in these immunosuppressed patients.[1-3,5]

Small lesions were treated by local excision. More extensive cancers required radical operations such as total vulvectomy and inguinal node dissection, or abdominoperineal resection.[1-3,5]

Treatment of De Novo Cancers

In addition to conventional therapy of the cancers, we must consider the value of reduction or cessation of immunosuppressive therapy.[1-4,7-9] Several inadvertently transplanted cancers regressed when immunosuppressive therapy was discontinued and the cancerous kidney was removed. Does such treatment help patients who develop de novo malignancies? Seven cases of KS and several lymphomas regressed following drastic reduction of immunosuppressive therapy.[3,8,26] Thus far the CTTR has rarely received reports of regression of epithelial tumors with such treatment. Nevertheless, one may try to reduce the immunosuppression in patients with highly malignant or extensive or advanced neoplasms in the hope that the immune system may recover and help to eliminate the tumors. However, such treatment has the risk that the allograft may undergo rejection and the patient will return to dialysis therapy.

In patients who require cytotoxic therapy for treatment of widespread cancers, we must remember that most agents depress the bone marrow.[1,2,9] It is therefore wise to stop or reduce azathioprine dosage during such therapy to avoid severe bone marrow toxicity. As most chemotherapeutic agents have immunosuppressive side effects, satisfactory allograft function may persist for prolonged periods. Treatment with prednisone may be continued, as it is an important constituent of many cancer chemotherapeutic regimens.[1,2,9]

Etiology of De Novo Cancers

This is discussed in detail elsewhere.[2-4,9] The neoplasms probably arise as a result of a complex interplay of multiple factors including depression of immunity; liberation or activation of oncogenic viruses; oncogenic effects of the immunosuppressive agents; synergistic effects of the immunosuppressive drugs with other carcinogens such as sunlight, tobacco, food additives, and radiation therapy; and variations in individual susceptibility to carcinogenic stimuli.

SUMMARY

Although the overall risk for the development of cancer in renal transplantation recipients is small, it is necessary to follow such patients indefinitely. Women patients require regular pelvic examinations and cervical smears in order to detect cervical or vulvar lesions at an early stage. Any untoward symptoms should be thoroughly investigated, keeping in mind the most common tumors: carcinomas of the skin and lips, lymphomas, KS, in situ carcinomas of the uterine cervix, and carcinomas of the vulva and perineum. As other lesions in transplantation patients frequently mimic neoplasms, any suspicious areas should be biopsied, if accessible.

It may be possible to prevent the development of some tumors. Donors with malignancies should not be used with the exceptions mentioned above. Administration of hepatitis B vaccine to dialysis patients may prevent the development of hepatitis and hepatocellular tumors. In addition, avoidance of excessive sunshine exposure, wearing of protective clothing, and the use of sunscreen may prevent skin cancers. It is possible that early eradication of condyloma acuminatum may prevent the development of carcinomas of the vulva and uterine cervix.

In addition to conventional cancer treatment, drastic reduction of immunosuppression may be worthwhile, particularly in patients with KS and lymphomas.

REFERENCES

1. Penn, I: The price of immunotherapy. Curr Probl Surg 18:682, 1981.
2. Penn, I: The occurrence of cancer in immune deficiencies. Curr Probl Cancer 6:1, 1982.
3. Penn, I: The occurrence of malignant tumors in immunosuppressed states. In Klein, E (ed): Acquired Immunodeficiency Syndrome. Progress in Allergy Series, vol 37. Basel, Karger. 1986, p 259.
4. Penn, I: Chemical immunosuppression and human cancer. Cancer 34:1474, 1974.
5. Penn, I: Cancers of the anogenital region in renal transplant recipients: Analysis of 65 cases. Cancer 58:611, 1986.
6. Penn, I: Transmission of cancer with donor organs. Transplant Proc 18:471, 1986.
7. Penn, I: Immunosuppression and skin cancer. Clin Plastic Surg 7:361, 1980.
8. Penn, I: Kaposi's sarcoma in immunosuppressed patients. J Clin Lab Immunol 12:1, 1983.
9. Penn, I: Allograft Transplant Cancer Registry. In Purtilo, DT (ed): Immune Deficiency and Cancer: Epstein-Barr Virus and Lymphoproliferative Malignancies. Plenum Publishing, New York, 1984, p 281.
10. Blohme, I and Brynger, H: Malignant disease in renal transplant patients. Transplantation 39:23, 1985.
11. Kinlen, LJ, et al: Collaborative United Kingdom–Australasian study of cancer in patients treated with immunosuppressive drugs. Br Med J 2:1461, 1979.
12. Kinlen, L: Immunosuppressive therapy and cancer. Cancer Surveys 1:565, 1982.

13. Porreco, R, et al: Gynecologic malignancies in immunosuppressed organ homograft recipients. Obstet Gynecol 45:359, 1975.
14. Templeton, AC: Kaposi's sarcoma. In Andrade, R, et al (eds): Cancer of the Skin: Biology-Diagnosis-Management. WB Saunders, Philadelphia, 1976, p 1183.
15. Harwood, AR, et al: Kaposi's sarcoma in recipients of renal transplants. Am J Med 67:759, 1979.
16. Sheil, AGR, et al: Cancer development in patients progressing to dialysis and renal transplantation. Transplant Proc 17:1685, 1985.
17. Koranda, FC, et al: Cutaneous complications in immunosuppressed renal homograft recipients. JAMA 229:419, 1974.
18. Mullen, DL, et al: Squamous cell carcinomas of the skin and lip in renal homograft recipients. Cancer 37:729, 1976.
19. Sober, AJ: Diagnosis and management of skin cancer. Cancer 51:2448, 1983.
20. Silverberg, E: Cancer Statistics, 1986. CA 36:9, 1986.
21. Freeman, C, Berg, JW, and Cutler, SJ: Occurrence and prognosis of extranodal lymphomas. Cancer 29:252, 1972.
22. Reddy, S, et al: Extranodal non-Hodgkin's lymphoma. Cancer 46:1925, 1980.
23. Herman, TS, et al: Involvement of the central nervous system by non-Hodgkin's lymphoma: The Southwest Oncology Group experience. Cancer 43:390, 1979.
24. Hanto, DW, et al: Epstein-Barr virus (EBV) induced polyclonal B-cell lymphoproliferative diseases occurring after renal transplantation: Clinical, pathologic, and virologic findings and implications for therapy. Ann Surg 193:356, 1983.
25. Cleary, ML, Warnke, R, and Sklar, J: Monoclonality of lymphoproliferative lesions in cardiac-transplant recipients: Clonal analysis based on immunoglobulin-gene rearrangements. N Engl J Med 310:477, 1984.
26. Starzl, TE, et al: Reversibility of lymphomas and lymphoproliferative lesions developing under cyclosporine-steroid therapy. Lancet 1:583, 1984.
27. Safai, B, et al: Association of Kaposi's sarcoma with second primary malignancies: Possible etiopathogenic implications. Cancer 45:1472, 1980.

Chapter 13

Pregnancy

ROBERT A. WELCH
MARK I. EVANS
ROBERT J. SOKOL

It is now well established that many kidney transplant recipients enjoy restoration of normal physiologic function. This renewed vigor results in the normalization of life-styles, resumption of career pursuits, and return of reproductive function. Since the first report in 1963, over 1000 pregnancies have subsequently been reported worldwide in kidney transplant recipients.[1] This chapter reviews current information regarding the effects of kidney transplantation on the reproductive process. A detailed assessment of the risks of pregnancy for the renal transplant recipient and her offspring is also presented.

REPRODUCTIVE EXPECTATIONS AND LIFE EXPECTANCY

Reproductive Expectations

A variety of etiologies necessitate dialysis and subsequent kidney transplantation in these patients. Among these are chronic glomerulonephritis, pyelonephritis, diabetes mellitus, polycystic kidney disease, Good-Pasture's syndrome, medullary cystic disease, cystinosis, obstructive uropathy, hemolytic uremic syndrome, lupus nephritis, oxalosis, ethylene glycol nephropathy, and trauma.[2]

Animal and human models confirm renal failure and uremia to be associated with decreased fertility and poor reproductive function.[3] General sexual dysfunction and loss of libido are common in uremic patients. Additionally, men suffer from impotence and women suffer from anovulatory vaginal bleeding or amenorrhea. Enhanced sexual function while on dialysis therapy appears to be an exception—only 8 percent of men and 6 percent of women experience any improvement.[4] Pregnancy has been infrequently documented in women of childbearing age on renal dialysis, and few of these patients have achieved live births.[5,6]

Fertility appears to be markedly increased in the patient who is successfully transplanted. Some sexual difficulties continue, however, in approximately 48 percent of men and 26 percent of women after renal transplantation.[7] It has been estimated that 1 of every 50 women of childbearing age with a functional renal transplantation attempts pregnancy.[5]

Life Expectancy

Uncertain life expectancy is one of the problems facing the kidney transplant recipient contemplating pregnancy. Recipients of cadaver kidneys are reported worldwide to have a 5-year survival rate of approximately 42 to 51 percent. Those receiving kidneys from related living donors enjoy a somewhat better 5-year survival rate, 61 to 78 percent.[8] The kidney graft itself has a functional post-transplantation 5-year survival of 29 to 35 percent in recipients of cadaver organs and 45 to 66 percent in recipients of living donor kidneys. The transplantation patient is faced, therefore, with the reality that he or she may be forced to undergo future transplants and may not survive long enough to rear children.[9,10] Recent data from the human renal transplant registry indicate that 2 of 64 mothers and 7 of 68 fathers died within a short time after becoming parents.[11] Patients who have completed their families at the time of transplantation should be offered sterilization.

EFFECTS OF KIDNEY TRANSPLANTATION BY SEX

Male Recipients

Despite restoration of satisfactory kidney function, between 22 and 43 percent of male renal transplant recipients continue to suffer from sexual dysfunction.[12-14] Inadvertent sterilization by division of the spermatic cord during the transplantation process was a primary reason for sterilization during earlier kidney transplantation procedures. Every effort is now being made to preserve the spermatic cord, since survival in these patients has become a reality.[15] Despite problems with sexual dysfunction, including loss of libido and impotence, Penn and associates[16] reported that 50 men in their series were responsible for 67 pregnancies.

The use of immunosuppressive medications to inhibit allograft rejection has caused concern among physicians and patients because of the possibility for abnormal sperm formation. Some teratogenic effects have been demonstrated by Rosenkrantz[17] using azathioprine in animal models. This agent induces chromosomal aberrations, and it is theoretically possible that human sperm is affected. The combined experience of several transplantation centers, however, has shown that the rate of congenital anomalies associated with azathioprine is small, and no specific abnormality has been found.[16,18,19,20] Cyclosporine, a new and more potent immunosuppressive agent, has not been well studied in the male kidney transplant recipient. Thus far there have been no reports of teratogenic effects in the offspring of male recipients taking this medication.[21]

Female Recipients

Some female patients fail to take contraceptive precautions because they have the mistaken impression that they are incapable of having children after the kidney transplantation. It is very important that these patients be thoroughly counseled regarding reproductive function even before the transplant operation. After transplantation, menstruation reappears on the average within 6 months.[16] Improved libido, menstruation, and ovulation result from the restoration of better renal function. Should pregnancy not be desired following the kidney transplantation, sterilization should be offered and performed at the time of the transplantation procedure. In patients who wish to become pregnant, the following recommendations have been made regarding the appropriate interval between transplantation and pregnancy[22,23]:

1. Adequate stable graft function for 18 months after transplantation
2. Good general health for 18 months after transplantation
3. No significant hypertension
4. No significant proteinuria
5. No evidence of pelvicalyceal dilatation on a recent intravenous pyelogram
6. Serum creantinine less than 2 mg per dl
7. Stable low dosage of immunosuppressive drugs

OUTCOME OF EARLY PREGNANCY AND ALLOGRAFT FUNCTION

Early Pregnancy

The mean interval from renal transplantation to pregnancy reported by Davison and Lindheimer[22] in reviewing over 700 gestations was 43 months, with a range of 6 weeks to 13 years. If the pregnancy continues past the first trimester, there is up to a 90 percent likelihood of a successful outcome. Although the majority of pregnancies in transplant recipients have apparently successful outcomes, gestation and delivery are not necessarily free of complications.

Approximately 42 percent of all conceptions in renal transplant recipients end in either therapeutic or spontaneous abortions during the first trimester.[22] This contrasts with approximately 15 percent spontaneous first-trimester abortions in normal pregnancy. Among reasons given by transplant recipients for ending pregnancy with therapeutic abortion are unplanned pregnancy, psychosocial problems, uncertainty about long-term maternal prognosis, unstable renal function before pregnancy, deteriorating renal function and/or severe hypertension in pregnancy, and hereditary renal disease.

Hypothetically, there is a higher risk of ectopic pregnancy in transplantation patients because of pelvic adhesions due to previous urologic surgery, peritoneal dialysis, inflammatory disease, and overzealous use of intrauterine contraceptive devices.[24] In actuality, however, the incidence of ectopic pregnancies in renal transplant patients is only 0.5 percent, compared with 1 to 2 percent for the population in general. Differentiating the amenorrhea or vaginal bleeding of an ectopic pregnancy in these patients from that of an intrauterine pregnancy or that associated with deteriorating renal function may be a major problem.

Davison[22] has stated, "The main clinical pitfall is erroneously attributing genuine gynaecological pathology to the transplant because of its location near the pelvis."

Normal Kidney Function in Pregnancy

In the pregnant patient not suffering from renal disease, a rise of 30 to 45 percent in plasma volume gradually occurs during the second trimester and is sustained until term.[25] Approximately 500 to 900 mg of sodium and 6 to 12 liters of water are gradually accumulated. The added salt and water are distributed between the maternal extravascular fluid and the fetoplacental unit. Peripheral vascular resistance decreases secondary to high progesterone levels, resulting in falling blood pressure despite the increase in extracellular volume.

Early in the second trimester the normal kidney responds to these changes in extracellular fluid volume by increasing the glomerular filtration rate (GFR) to a level about 30 to 50 percent above controls.[26] Renal plasma flow accelerates in a similar manner. This elevation in GFR is sustained by the kidney until after delivery, when GFR rapidly falls to nongravid levels.[27,28] The combination of increased renal plasma flow, GFR, and dilutional effects of pregnancy cause the blood urea nitrogen and serum creatinine to be reduced below nonpregnant values.[29]

In addition to renal changes in the handling of sodium and increased GFR, plasma osmolality generally falls to about 270 milliosmols per kg.[30] It is hypothesized that the plasma bicarbonate falls during pregnancy because of progesterone-induced respiratory alkalosis. There is no increase in urinary protein excretion in normal pregnancy. Rates above 200 mg in a 24-hour period should be regarded as abnormal.[26]

Allograft Function in Pregnancy

For the most part it has been shown that renal function in the kidney transplantation patient is similar to that of the normal pregnant woman.[31] Nonetheless, a transient reduction in GFR may occur in the third trimester. Proteinuria has been seen near term in about 40 percent of these patients but usually disappears after delivery. It may be difficult to distinguish proteinuria secondary to underlying kidney disease from subclinical allograft rejection. This phenomenon has also been noted infrequently in normal pregnancies.[20,32,33]

A greater possibility for permanent renal impairment during pregnancy is correlated with compromised renal function prior to conception.[34,35] Hyperkalemic acidosis in two transplant recipients associated with a decline in renal function during pregnancy has been noted by Warren and associates.[36] However, following delivery of normal-term infants, renal function improved and the hyperkalemic acidosis resolved. The authors concluded that these changes were benign when unaccompanied by other evidence of graft deterioration.

The kidney of a 75-year-old woman has been transplanted into a 36-year-old patient with adequate function during a subsequent pregnancy.[37] It appears that the age of the donor kidney is not a factor in the kidney's ability to respond to the physiologic stresses of pregnancy. In the absence of severe maternal disease, hazards appear to be no greater in the pregnant renal transplantation recipient than in the nonpregnant renal transplant recipient.

PRENATAL COMPLICATIONS

Allograft Rejection During Pregnancy

During pregnancy the rate of allograft rejection does not appear to be different from that of the nonpregnant renal allograft recipient.[38] However, when considering the privileged immunologic state of pregnancy, which should benefit the transplant recipient, the rejection rate may be considered unusually high. Several investigators have reduced or stopped immunosuppressive medications during pregnancy without subsequent rejection episodes.[39,40,53]

Among the first signs of the acute allograft rejection phenomenon are fever, oliguria, and elevated serum creatinine and blood urea nitrogen. Percutaneous biopsy of the renal allograft is safe in the nonpregnant patient and may be used for histologic study to confirm the clinical diagnosis of acute rejection.[41] The increased vascularity of pregnancy, however, biases the procedure of choice to an open biopsy. It appears that the rejection phenomenon may be minimized during pregnancy by the continuation of immunosuppressive medications at maintenance levels along with stress doses of corticosteroids into the puerperium.[16,41] Deterioration of the allograft function and acute rejection are considered sufficient reasons to terminate the pregnancy. Approximately 9 percent of women who carry their pregnancies into the third trimester experience serious rejection episodes.[31]

Pregnancy-Induced Hypertension

The apparent rate of pregnancy-induced hypertension (pre-eclampsia) is between 27 and 30 percent in renal transplant recipients.[16,32] Pre-eclampsia is generally seen in 5 percent of the normal pregnant population.[42] In patients without transplantation who have renal parenchymal disease, however, studies of renal biopsies have shown that the clinical diagnosis of superimposed pre-eclampsia may be wrong in up to 50 percent of cases.[43] Therefore, reports of pregnancy-induced hypertension in renal transplantation recipients made on clinical suspicion may be incorrect. Williams and colleagues[44] have reported a case of a primigravid transplant recipient who developed severe pre-eclampsia that rapidly progressed to eclampsia. They have since reported that the patient's subsequent pregnancy was not complicated by hypertension and had an uneventful outcome.[45] This is the only case of eclampsia, to our knowledge, that has been reported in this patient population. However, many other hypertensive syndromes occurring in renal transplant recipients may be as severe.

One of the most difficult challenges facing the clinician caring for the renal transplant recipient is differentiating the patient who is pre-eclamptic from the patient with continued underlying renal disease. Unfortunately, serum uric acid levels and urine protein excretion may not be useful markers for either the onset or severity of pre-eclampsia in transplantation recipients.

Both of these indices may be above the norm at any stage of gestation in otherwise uncomplicated pregnancies of renal transplant recipients.[46]

Risk of Infection

The risk of infection in the pregnant transplant recipient may be especially high because of the combination of immunosuppressive medications and the immunologically depressed state normally seen in pregnancy. Throughout pregnancy these patients should be carefully monitored for the possibility of infection, and particular attention should be paid to the urinary tract.[32] Prophylactic antibiotics before any surgical procedure, including episiotomy, are recommended, since overwhelming infection is a leading cause of death in these patients.

Besides infection with some of the more common bacterial agents, these chronically immunosuppressed patients are susceptible to *Pneumocystis carinii,* cytomegalovirus, and fungal organisms.[47,48] Virtually all of these patients have been reported to experience bacterial and viral infections during pregnancy.[35] Waltzer[23] has cited infection rates as high as 60 percent. Others have found no increase in the rate of infection in transplant patients during pregnancy.[16,33] As stated by Meier and Makowski,[38] "Despite the conflicting opinions, careful observation for infectious complications and aggressive antibiotic therapy are indicated in these patients."

Chronic viral infections in the viral carrier state are an additional risk to the transplantation patient and her offspring as well as those caring for her. Schooley and associates[48] found 35 primary or reactive herpes virus infections in 28 patients during the first 3 months after transplantation. This represents a significant risk for the pregnant graft recipient and her offspring. At least one case of congenital cytomegalovirus infection has been reported in the offspring of the renal transplantation patient.[49] It has also been shown that 50 percent of dialysis patients are positive for hepatitis B surface antigen.[50] Although the exact rate of hepatitis B surface antigenemia in the renal transplantation recipient is unclear, it is likely to be high. These patients are frequently chronic carriers of hepatitis B as a result of their immunosuppressed state, and they present an infectious risk.[51] In caring for these patients, evaluation for hepatitis B antigen and antibody in the serum should be performed routinely. The possibility of future hepatic dysfunction and perhaps even hepatic malignancy should be considered.[50]

GUIDELINES FOR MATERNAL-FETAL SURVEILLANCE

Antepartum Care

The pregnant transplant recipient should be followed in a high-risk obstetric clinic by a team including a perinatologist, a transplantation nephrologist, a neonatologist, and appropriate psychosocial support personnel.[16] Biweekly visits until 28 weeks with weekly visits thereafter are suggested.[38] Underlying maternal disease, especially if the initial cause for renal failure and subsequent transplantation, may demand an increase in the frequency of these visits. Typically, immunosuppressive agents are continued at prepregnancy levels, since pregnancy cannot be allowed to interfere with the integrity of the renal allograft.[16]

Weight and blood pressure are screened at each prenatal visit. Blood urea nitrogen, creatinine and electrolytes to evaluate renal function should be frequently performed. Creatinine clearance and protein excretion should be determined with 24-hour urine samples. In addition, every visit should include a urinalysis and follow-up with culture if the urinalysis is suspicious for infection. Further, anemia should be evaluated and appropriately treated. Clinical evidence of hyperparathyroidism should be sought, and serum calcium and phosphate levels should be evaluated at least every trimester.[39]

Since these patients have commonly received multiple blood transfusions while on dialysis, they should be screened for regular and irregular blood antibodies in each trimester. Hemolytic disease of the newborn is a potential complication in the offspring of these patients. Chronic steroid therapy may also alter glucose metabolism.

A 50-g oral glucose load followed by a 1-hour random blood sugar (plasma value greater than 135 mg per dl considered abnormal) should be performed at the initial visit and again at 28 to 30 weeks gestational age. Follow-up with a 3-hour glucose tolerance test may be necessary to determine the patient's ability to metabolize glucose.

Fetal Surveillance

Ordinary hormone excretion tests (24-hour urine estriol) and plasma hormone levels (estriol or human placental lactogen) have been shown to be of no value in these pregnancies.[38] Weekly nonstress tests (NSTs) beginning as early as 28 weeks gestational age, backed up by contraction stress tests (CSTs) for nonreactive NSTs appears to provide optimal fetal surveillance. Fetal growth may be followed with serial real-time ultrasound exams. Should intrauterine fetal growth retardation be suspected, the antenatal testing sequence (NST and/or CST) may be performed every 3 to 5 days with early delivery for signs of compromised fetal well-being. The fetal biophysical profile (NST plus ultrasound observation of fetal tone, gross body movement, fetal breathing movements, and amniotic fluid volume) may be used to supplement or substitute for the NST/CST sequence. If evidence of severe fetal growth retardation is discovered, the possibility of congenital cytomegalovirus infection should be considered.[49]

CARE AND MANAGEMENT OF COMPLICATIONS IN LABOR

Management of Labor and Delivery

Meticulous attention should be paid to aseptic techniques during the intrapartum period. During labor and for the first 24 hours postpartum, stress doses of corticosteroids (intravenous hydrocortisone 100 mg every 6 hours) should be administered. Prophylactic antibiotics for all surgical procedures related to the peripartum period, including episiotomy, are recommended.[38]

Concern for the transplanted kidney appears to be unwarranted, since it is generally placed high in the false pelvis and does not represent an impediment to vaginal delivery. Besides not producing mechanical dystocia during labor, the kidney apparently is not damaged during vaginal delivery.[46] Although cesarean section may be necessary for purely obstetric reasons, it is apparent that the rate of 25 percent or more in these patients reflects fear of the unknown rather than a belief that vaginal delivery will damage the mother and/or the child.[46]

Pelvic contractures may be the result of osteodystrophy in patients with chronic renal failure (and dialysis) or of prolonged steroid therapy, particularly when initiated before puberty.[46] Sciarra[35] has recommended simultaneous intravenous pyelogram and x-ray pelvimetry at approximately 36 weeks gestation should doubts concerning kidney compression or the adequacy of the maternal pelvis arise. We are not aware, however, of any studies that support this recommendation and would suggest the more standard practice of allowing a trial of labor. If cesarean section becomes necessary for obstetric reasons, in order to avoid the renal allograft and because of difficulty in exposing the lower uterine segment due to previous pelvic infections or urologic complications, a midline abdominal incision followed by a classical uterine incision may become necessary.[38] Route of delivery aside, labor should be closely managed and fetal surveillance should be performed with electronic fetal monitoring supplemented with fetal scalp blood gases when indicated.

Premature Labor and Delivery

Premature delivery occurs in approximately 50 percent of renal transplant recipients.[46] One hypothesis for this high preterm delivery rate is that the long-term steroid therapy given to these patients may weaken connective tissues and contribute to an increase in premature rupture of membranes.[31] Another factor associated with premature labor in these patients is poor renal function.[52] Although spontaneous premature rupture of the membranes and premature labor occur frequently in the renal transplant recipient, many preterm deliveries are performed for medical or obstetrical indications.

Premature Rupture of the Membranes

Management of premature rupture of the membranes or prolonged rupture of the membranes within these patients is controversial. Because of the need for immunosuppressive medications to avoid allograft rejection, it has been recommended that cervical cultures for beta hemolytic streptococci and other pathogens be obtained and labor induced.[38] This aggressive approach, however, may partially contribute to the high rate of respiratory distress syndrome seen in the offspring of renal transplant recipients.

POSTPARTUM CARE

Stress doses of steroids and antibiotic prophylaxis should be continued for 24 hours postpartum. Other areas to be considered in the postpartum period in the kidney transplant recipient include breastfeeding, contraception, and pelvic cancer screening.

Breastfeeding

There are now limited data on breastfeeding in these patients. Briggs and associates[53] have analyzed infants with continued exposure to prednisone and cyclosporine through breast milk and have noted no short-term effects. Flechner and colleagues[54] noted 25 percent suppression of a third-party mixed lymphocyte culture from fetal serum of an infant exposed in utero to cyclosporine. Since cyclosporine was present in maternal breast milk, the authors recommended that breastfeeding of children by cyclosporine-treated mothers be avoided. No information is available concerning continued exposure of the infant to azathioprine. Any decision regarding breastfeeding must be based on the knowledge that continued exposure of the infant to potent immunosuppressive drugs or their metabolites will occur.

Contraception

Postpartum bilateral tubal ligation is the preferred method for patients who request permanent sterilization.[38] Should the patient elect to maintain her fertility, other forms of contraception are available. These include low-dose oral contraceptive pills (OCPs), barrier methods (vaginal sponge, condom, or diaphragm used with a spermicidal foam or jelly), and the intrauterine device (IUD). Although OCPs provide maximum protection against pregnancy, their use in these circumstances may increase the risk for thromboembolic complications. The IUD appears to be a poor choice in these patients because of the risk of overwhelming sepsis if the IUD becomes infected in their chronically immunosuppressed state.[55] It appears that the safest method for contraception in these patients is the barrier method supported by voluntary interruption of pregnancy in failures if acceptable to the patient.

Risk of Pelvic Malignancy

Pelvic malignancy is increased in these patients because of iatrogenic immunosuppression. Reports of up to a 13-fold increase in the rate of squamous cell carcinoma of the cervix are consistent with theories of a viral etiology of cervical cancer.[6,56,57] In addition to squamous cell carcinoma of the cervix, there are reports of other gynecologic tumors arising in these patients. These include endometrial carcinoma,[58] gestational trophoblastic disease,[59] and simultaneous in situ carcinoma of the cervix, vulva, and perineum.[60] A rapidly fatal case of ovarian carcinoma in a kidney transplantation patient on cyclosporine has also been reported recently.[61]

Postpartum and subsequent follow-up should include a pelvic examination and Papanicolaou smear every 6 months in the nonpregnant patient. Colposcopic examination for the presence of cervical lesions should be performed if the Papanicolaou smear is abnormal. We also recommend this surveillance for the pregnant transplant recipient. Colposcopically directed cervical biopsies may be performed in pregnancy if a suspicious lesion is encountered. Intracervical curettage, which is recommended after colposcopic examination in the nonpregnant patient, is not recommended during pregnancy.

THE OFFSPRING

Prognosis for Carrying a Normal Newborn

The renal transplant recipient may be reassured that the likelihood for carrying a normal newborn is high. Present data suggest that there is no increase in cytogenetic abnormalities in the fetus, and genetic amniocentesis is not indicated solely because of transplantation. Premature delivery continues to be the major problem, occurring in 50 percent of pregnancies, and approximately 20 percent of these are noted to be small for gestational age (SGA). This high percentage of SGA babies emphasizes the risk for intrauterine growth retardation in these pregnancies. SGA babies are susceptible to stillbirth, and close fetal surveillance is of additional importance in these pregnancies.

Problems seen in these offspring and suspected to be caused by chronic immunosuppression include thymic atrophy, transient leukopenia and thrombocytopenia, adrenal insufficiency, reduced blood levels of IgG and IgM, chromosome aberrations in lymphocytes, hypoglycemia, and hypocalcemia.[16,35,62-65] Penn, Makowski, and Harris[16] reported that respiratory distress syndrome occurred in 9 percent of newborns in their study, while 5 percent had adrenocortical insufficiency and 5 percent developed septicemia.

Effects of Immunosuppressive Medications

The major concern, regarding the offspring of transplant recipients, centers on the immunosuppressive medications the mother must take during the pregnancy to avoid graft rejection. Fetuses of mice given mercaptopurine during pregnancy have reproductive problems at maturation.[65] The exposed offspring either were sterile or had decreased litter size and greater frequency of fetal wastage than in control animals. It remains unknown whether a similar problem will evolve in humans. Borrell and coworkers[67] initially discovered the anti-lymphocytic properties of cyclosporine. Cyclosporine appears to have selective action against T cells involved in allograft rejection and is administered in high doses in the renal transplant patient.[68] It has been found to be nephrotoxic at these high doses; the consequences for the recipient patient are unknown. The amount that crosses the placenta and that might effect the offspring's kidneys has not been determined. Two cases[54,69] of pregnancy following transplantation in which cyclosporine was used as an immunosuppressant have now been reported. The results, with no nephrotoxicity or hepatotoxicity, appear encouraging; however, fetal serum at birth displayed 25 percent suppression of a third-party mixed lymphocyte cultures in one of these patients. Cyclosporine was found in the fetal cord blood at delivery in both cases, but no medication has been found in the amniotic fluid. It has also been found in maternal milk 4 days into the postpartum period. Because of the apparent lymphocyte depression caused by cyclosporine, breastfeeding cannot be recommended.

SUMMARY

In the future, it may be expected that the kidney transplantation team will frequently be confronted by patients asking for advice concerning their reproductive capacity. Pregnancy may be considered in renal transplantation patients who experience a return of normal renal function for a period of approximately 2 years posttransplantation. If the pregnancy remains viable into the second trimester, the chances for successful outcome approach 90 percent. Long-term follow-up is needed, however, on the offspring of kidney transplant recipients who are on chronic immunosuppressive therapy throughout pregnancy. At present there is no evidence of direct teratogenic effects on the offspring. Little is known about the action of immunosuppressive medications on the fetal gonads or about the future reproductive potential of these children. Breastfeeding is not recommended in patients taking cyclosporine.

Early consultation with members of the transplantation team, a nephrologist, an obstetrician, and a psychologist or psychiatrist before attempting pregnancy may enhance the likelihood for a successful outcome.

REFERENCES

1. Murray, JE, et al: Successful pregnancies after human renal transplantation. N Engl J Med 269:341, 1963.
2. Penn, I: Transplantation. In Hill, GJ (ed): Outpatient Surgery, ed 2. WB Saunders, Philadelphia, 1980, p 1233.
3. Hayslett, JP: Interaction of renal disease in pregnancy. Kidney Int 25:579, 1974.
4. Nissenson, AR: The use of hemodialysis to treat end stage renal failure during pregnancy. Ann Intern Med 94:667, 1981.
5. Confortini, P, et al: Full term pregnancy and successful delivery in a patient on chronic hemodialysis. Proc Eur Dial Transplant Assoc 8:74, 1971.
6. Schreiner, GE: Dialysis and pregnancy (editorial). JAMA 235:1725, 1976.
7. Levy, MB: Sexual adjustment to maintenance hemodialysis and renal transplantation: National survey by questionnaire—preliminary report. Trans Am Soc Artif Intern Organs 19:138, 1973.
8. Advisory Committee to the Renal Transplant Registry: The 13th Report of a Human Renal Transplant Registry. Transplant Proc 9:9, 1977.
9. Makowski, EL and Penn, I: Parenthood following transplantation. In DeAlvarez, RR (ed): The Kidney in Pregnancy. John Wiley & Sons, New York, 1976, p 215.
10. Penn, I, et al: Parenthood in renal homograft recipients. JAMA 216:1755, 1971.
11. Advisory Committee to the Renal Transplant Registry: The 12th Report of a Human Renal Transplant Registry. JAMA 233:7787, 1975.
12. Thomson, T and Mayor, GH: Parenthood after renal transplantation. Southern Med J 72:950, 1979.
13. Abram, AS, et al: Sexual function in patients with chronic renal failure. J Nerv Ment Dis 160:220, 1975.
14. Salvatierra O, Jr, Fortman, JL, and Belzer, FO: Sexual function in males before and after renal transplantation. Urology 5:64, 1975.
15. Penn, I, et al: Testicular complications fol-

lowing renal transplantation. Ann Surg 176:697, 1972.

16. Penn, I, Makowski, EL, and Harris, P: Parenthood following renal transplantation. Kidney Int 18:221, 1980.

17. Rosenkrantz, JG, et al: Azathioprine and pregnancy. Am J Obstet Gynecol 97:387, 1967.

18. Reinisch, JM, et al: Prenatal exposure to prednisone in humans and animals retards intrauterine growth. Science 202:436, 1978.

19. Scott, JR: Fetal growth retardation associated with maternal administration of immunosuppressive drugs. Am J Obstet Gynecol 128:668, 1977.

20. Merkatz, IR, et al: Resumption of hemoreproductive function following renal transplantation. JAMA 216:1749, 1971.

21. First International Congress on Cyclosporine. Transplant Proc 15:2207, 1983.

22. Davison, JM and Lindheimer, MD: Pregnancy in renal transplant recipients. J Reprod Med 27:613, 1982.

23. Waltzer, WC, et al: Pregnancy in renal transplantation. Transplant Proc 12:221, 1980.

24. Scott, JR, Cruikshank, D, and Corry, RJ: Ectopic pregnancy in kidney transplant patients. Obstet Gynecol 52:565, 1978.

25. Hytten, FH and Paintin, DB: Increase in plasma volume during normal pregnancy. J Obstet Gynaecol Br Commonw 70:402, 1963.

26. Dunlop, W: Serial changes in renal haemodynamics during normal human pregnancy. Br J Obstet Gynaecol 88:1, 1981.

27. Davison, JM and Noble, MC: Serial changes in 24-hour creatinine clearance during normal menstrual cycles in the first trimester of pregnancy. Br J Obstet Gynaecol 88:10, 1981.

28. Peppig, L: Clinique des affections renales pendant la grossesse. Med Hygiene 27:181, 1969.

29. Sims, EAH and Krantz, KE: Serial studies of renal function during pregnancy and the puerperium in normal women. J Clin Invest 37:1764, 1958.

30. Durr, JA, Stamoutsos, B, and Lindheimer, MD: Osmolar regulation during pregnancy in the rat. J Clin Invest 68:237, 1981.

31. Rudolph, JE, Schweizer, RT, and Bartus, SA: Pregnancy in renal transplant patients. Transplantation 27:26, 1979.

32. Whetham, JCG, Cardella, C, and Harding, M: Effective pregnancy and graft function and graft survival in renal cadaver transplantations. Am J Obstet Gynecol 145:193, 1983.

33. Rifle, G and Traeger, J: Pregnancy after renal transplantation: An international survey. Transplant Proc 7:723, 1979.

34. Davison, JM, et al: Effect of pregnancy on renal function in kidney transplant recipients (abstr). Clin Exp Hypertens [B] 1:322, 1982.

35. Sciarra, JJ, et al: Pregnancy following renal transplantation. Am J Obstet Gynecol 123:411, 1975.

36. Warren, SE, Mitas, JA, and Evertson, LR: Pregnancy after renal transplantation: Reversible acidosis in renal dysfunction. Southern Med J 74:1139, 1981.

37. Coulam, CD, Zincke, A, and Sterioff, S: Relationship between donor age and outcome of pregnancy in renal allograft population. Transplantation 33:97, 1982.

38. Meier, PR and Makowski, EL: Pregnancy and the patient with a renal transplant. Clin Obstet Gynecol 27:902, 1984.

39. Kaupman, JJ, et al: Successful normal childbirth after kidney homotransplantation. JAMA 200:162, 1967.

40. Davison, JM, Dellagrammatikas, H, and Parkin, JM: Fetal haematopoiesis and azathioprine therapy in pregnant patients with renal transplants. Clin Exp Hypertens [B] 1:209, 1982.

41. Stuart, FP: Selection, preparation, and management of kidney transplant recipients. Med Clin North Am 62:1381, 1978.

42. Pritchard, JA, MacDonald, PC, and Gant, NF: Incidence of pregnancy-induced hypertension. In William Obstetrics, ed 17. Appleton-Century-Crofts, Norwalk, Conn, 1985, p 539.

43. Katz, AI, et al: Pregnancy in women with kidney disease. Kidney Int 18:192, 1980.

44. Williams, PF and Jelen, J: Eclampsia in a patient who had a renal transplant. Br Med J 2:972, 1979.

45. Williams, PF and Jelen, J: Normal pregnancy in renal transplant recipient with history of eclampsia and intrauterine death. Br Med J 285:1535, 1982.

46. Davison, JM: Pregnancy in renal transplant recipients: Clinical perspectives. Contrib Nephrol 37:170, 1984.

47. Washer, GF, Schroter, GPS, and Starzl, GE: Causes of death after kidney transplantation. JAMA 250:49, 1983.

48. Schooley, RT, et al: Association of herpes virus infections with T-lymphocyte-subset alterations, glomerulopathy and opportunistic infections after renal transplantation. N Engl J Med 308:307, 1983.

49. Evans, TJ, McCollum, JPK, and Valdemarsson, II: Congenital cytomegalovirus infection after maternal renal transplantation. Lancet 1:1359, 1975.

50. Chan, MK and Moorehead, JF: Hepatitis B and the dialysis in renal transplantation units. Nephron 27:229, 1981.

51. Schweitzer, IL, et al: Viral hepatitis B in

neonates and infants. Am J Med 55:762, 1973.

52. Felding, CF: Obstetric aspects in women with histories of renal disease. Acta Obstet Gynecol Scand 48:2, 1969.

53. Briggs, GC, et al: Drugs in Pregnancy and Lactation. Williams & Wilkins, Baltimore, 1983.

54. Flechner, SM, et al: The presence of cyclosporine in body tissues and fluids during pregnancy. Am J Kid Dis 5:60, 1985.

55. Ferner, J, et al: Intrauterine contraceptive devices in renal transplant patients. J Reprod Med 26:99, 1981.

56. Penn, I: Malignancies associated with immunosuppressive or cytotoxic therapy. Surgery 83:492, 1978.

57. Porreco, R, et al: Gynecologic malignancies in immunosuppressed organ homograft recipients. Obstet Gynecol 45:359, 1975.

58. Thorra, Y, et al: Endometrial carcinoma and amyloidosis after kidney transplantation. Transplantation 25:91, 1978.

59. Manifold, IH, et al: Pregnancy complicated by gestational trophoblastic disease in a renal transplant recipient. Br Med J 287:1025, 1983.

60. Lechie, GB and Cotton, RE: Simultaneous in situ carcinoma of the cervix, vulva and perineum after immunosuppressive therapy for renal transplantation. Br J Obstet Gynaecol 84:143, 1977.

61. Maung, R, et al: Development of ovarian carcinoma in a cyclosporin A immunosuppressed patient. Obstet Gynecol 66:895, 1985.

62. Leb, DE, Weisskopf, B, and Kanovitz, BS: Chromosome abberations in the child of a kidney transplant recipient. Arch Intern Med 128:441, 1971.

63. Lower, GD, et al: Problems from immunosuppression during pregnancy. Am J Obstet Gynecol 111:1120, 1971.

64. Price, HV, et al: Immunosuppressive drugs and the fetus. Transplantation 21:294, 1976.

65. Korsch, BM, et al: Physical and psychological followup on offspring of renal allograft recipients. Pediatrics 65:275, 1980.

66. Reimers, TJ and Sluss, DM: 6-Mercaptopurine treatment of pregnant mice: Effects on second and third generations. Science 201:65, 1978.

67. Borell, JF, et al: Biological effects of cyclosporine A: A new antilymphocytic agent. Agents Actions 6:468, 1976.

68. Merion, RM, et al: Cyclosporine: 5 years experience in cadaveric renal transplantation. N Engl J Med 310:148, 1984.

69. Lewis, GJ, et al: Successful pregnancy in a renal transplant recipient taking cyclosporin A. Br Med J 286:603, 1983.

Chapter 14

Immunological Monitoring

LUIS H. TOLEDO-PEREYRA

Spontaneous Blastogenesis (SB)
    Pretransplantation Evaluation
    Posttransplantation Evaluation
T-Cell Rosetting Assay
    Pretransplantation Evaluation
    Posttransplantation Evaluation
Mitogen Blastogenesis
    Pretransplantation Evaluation
    Posttransplantation Evaluation
Delayed Hypersensitivity Testing (DHT)
    Pretransplantation Evaluation
    Posttransplantation Evaluation

The term "immunological monitoring" has been used only since the mid-1970s to refer to a variety of tests and techniques used to evaluate immune reactivity and immunocompetence. Assays are usually performed in vitro and may measure cellular or humoral immunity. The goal of immunological monitoring is to develop techniques that will correlate well with in vitro events and have prognostic value for the clinician. As transplant centers have attempted to improve their results, immunological monitoring has become an important part of this effort.

Several international symposia have provided for exchange of information in the growing field of immunological monitoring. At the first International Symposium on Immunological Monitoring, in 1977, in London, Ontario, Canada, efforts were made to standardize tests and terminology so that results could be more easily compared between clinical centers.[1] During the period between the first and second symposia in Noordwijerhout, the Netherlands, in 1980, a rapid evolution and interest in immunological monitoring occurred, with expanded applications to areas such as assessment of immunocompetence of potential transplantation candidates, studies regarding the phenomenon of immunologic adaptation after transplantation, and investigations in the area of host resistance. Continued efforts were made to diagnose and predict graft rejection using a variety of immunological monitoring assays.[2] In 1982, at the Third International Symposium on Immunological Monitoring, in Miami,

Florida, new developments in immunosuppression (cyclosporine) and immunological monitoring technology (monoclonal antibodies) highlighted the meeting.[3] In 1983 the Fourth International Symposium on Immunological Monitoring was held in Houston, Texas.[4] Topics of discussion included pretransplantation conditioning and the immune status, improved monitoring of immunosuppression, posttransplantation accommodation, and diagnosis of rejection. The impact of cyclosporine therapy and the further application of monoclonal antibodies for immunological monitoring on clinical transplantation were also considered. The Fifth International Symposium on Immunological Monitoring was held in 1985 in Montebello, Quebec, Canada.[5] Topics for this meeting included evaluation of cyclosporine as an immunosuppressive drug, detection of presensitization of the recipient, immunological conditioning of the graft recipient, and monitoring of the effector response to the graft.

IMMUNOLOGICAL MONITORING AND THE TRANSPLANTATION EVENT

This chapter will briefly discuss the types of tests used for immunological monitoring for clinical kidney transplantation, both before and after transplantation, and will present their applications before and/or after transplantation, and their correlation with in vivo immunologic events.

Immunological Monitoring Tests

Since allograft rejection is a complex process that includes both cellular and humoral components, for immunologic monitoring to have prognostic value it must include tests that are capable of detecting these responses. Table 14-1 presents various tests that have been used to monitor the immune status of transplant recipients and the abbreviations commonly used for these tests and their applications.

Pretransplantation Monitoring

Immunologic monitoring assays have become an important part of the clinical pretransplantation evaluation. Besides determinations of the histocompatibility antigens at the A, B, C, and DR loci, and blood antigen typing on each patient, the clinician uses immunological assays to evaluate the immune responsiveness of a potential candidate. This includes tests to determine the degree of presensitization that may be present in a potential recipient as a result of previous antigenic exposure from blood transfusions, pregnancy, or a previous transplantation (see Table 14-1).

Posttransplantation Monitoring

Immunological monitoring after renal transplantation has been applied in two areas: to predict and monitor the rejection process and to tailor immunosuppression to individual patient needs. A considerable amount of research effort has been directed toward developing immunological monitoring assays that would be sensitive enough to detect the early changes occurring during rejection episodes. The ideal assay would predict rejection prior to damage of the allograft and deterioration of function. It would prognosticate rejection before clinical symptoms are apparent, giving the clinician extra time to treat the acute and chronic rejection episodes. Var-

Test	Abbreviation	Application Pretransplantation	Posttransplantation
Assessment of Anti-Donor Specific Immunity			
Mixed lymphocyte reaction	MLR	X	X
Lymphocyte-mediated cytotoxicity	LMC	X	X
Cell-mediated lysis	CML	X	X
Antibody-dependent cell mediated cytotoxicity	ADCC	X	X
Complement-dependent cytotoxicity	CDC	X	X
Anti-B-cell antibody	CDC-B	X	X
Erythrocyte antibody inhibition	EAI	X	X
Macrophage/monocyte inhibitory factors	MIF	X	X
Antiendothelial antibodies	—	X	X
Assessment of Nonspecific Immunity			
Fine-needle aspiration biopsy	FNAB	—	X
Spontaneous blastogenesis	SB	X	X
T cell rosetting assay	—	X	X
T cell subsets identification with monoclonal antibodies	—	X	X
Evaluation of Immune System Integrity			
Mitogen-induced blastogenesis	—	X	X
Delayed hypersensitivity testing	DHT	X	X

Table 14-1 Tests Used for Immunological Monitoring

ious tests have been applied in an attempt to develop the ideal prognostic battery of immunological monitoring assays. Both cellular and humoral immunity have been evaluated, since although rejection episodes occurring in the first few days are considered to be cell-mediated, those occurring later may be mainly humoral, mainly cell-mediated, or both.[6]

In the past decade there has been an enthusiastic effort to develop new methods of immunological monitoring for the purposes of predicting the postoperative course of renal transplants. The various assays that have been developed as part of the search for tests that would prognosticate renal allograft rejection have also led to an increased body of knowledge with regard to the immune phenomenon, both before and after transplantation. One of the major problems has been standardization of these assays among centers. In addition, the effects of immunosuppression on the types of samples obtained have often made the determinations difficult. At present clinical symptoms are still the primary confirmation of the rejection process in most clinical transplantation programs. The increased use of cyclosporine for immunosuppression will undoubtedly affect the way in which the immunological monitoring as-

says are used. Already, however, much information regarding the mechanisms of action of cyclosporine after transplantation has been provided by immunological monitoring techniques.

MIXED LYMPHOCYTE REACTION (MLR)

This test is used to measure lymphocyte blastogenesis in response to antigenic stimulation. MLR assays are set up as either one-way or two-way tests[7] (Fig. 14–1). In the one-way test proliferation of recipient lymphocytes is measured in response to stimulation by donor cells that are irradiated or treated with mitomycin C. The standard culture period is 5 days. Proliferation is determined by measuring ^{3}H-thymidine uptake during DNA synthesis. In the two-way MLR the response of donor and recipient lymphocytes to each other is determined and donor cells are not treated. MLR reactivity is frequently used to determine high or low responder status of potential donor-recipient pairs being evaluated for living related transplants. The logistics of cadaver transplantation, however, make it impractical for testing the com-

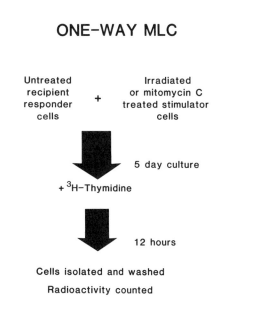

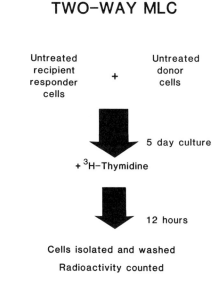

ONE–WAY MLC

TWO–WAY MLC

Figure 14–1. One-way and two-way mixed lymphocyte reaction (MLR). Lymphocyte response to antigenic stimulus is measured by uptake of ^{3}H-thymidine during DNA synthesis.

patibility of donor-recipient pairs in cadaver transplantation.

Pretransplantation Evaluation

Cochrum and associates[8] have observed a correlation between the two-way MLR and graft rejection of cadaver transplants; however, most groups have not noted an association between pretransplantation one-way MLR and rejection.[9,10] It is interesting to note that Terasaki and Opelz[11] found that MLR reactivity of recipient to a third party correlated about as well with graft survival as MLR to the donor. They suggested that MLR in cadaveric recipients is a test of overall immune reactivity as well as donor-specific sensitization. Several groups have also observed a correlation between MLC reactivity and graft rejection in related donors. At our center, as well as in most other transplantation centers, one-way MLC testing is performed on living related transplantation candidates and on potential donors. If the stimulation index is >8, the transplantation candidate is given blood transfusions from the prospective related donor. After completion of the donor-specific blood transfusion protocol, the recipients are transplanted only if a negative cross-match is obtained. In the last year my associates and I have been using cyclosporine to overcome high responder status, and no donor-specific blood transfusions are given. A low responder status is considered if the stimulation index is <8. Low responders are not given transfusions and are transplanted if the cross-match is negative.

Posttransplantation Evaluation

The MLR has been employed after transplantation to assess the development of antidonor or broad-based cellular reactivity. Nonreactivity of the MLR has been seen during both rejection and quiescent periods and appears to have no clinical benefit.[12,13] A possible sequestration of responder cells in the graft during rejection may result in MLR reactivity. Nonreactivity during quiescence has been thought to reflect immune tolerance.[12]

LYMPHOCYTE-MEDIATED CYTOTOXICITY (LMC)

This assay is used to detect the presence of preformed cytotoxic effector killer cells generated in vivo.[1] The LMC is performed with ^{51}Cr-labeled donor target cells and recipient peripheral blood monocytes. This is usually a 4-hour assay, but 12- and 16-hour assays have also been used (Fig. 14–2). In transplantation from living related donors, target cells for ^{51}Cr labeling are obtained from peripheral venous blood samples. With cadaveric donors cryopreservation is used to save cells obtained from spleen and lymph node. Mitogen-activated lymphoblasts are also used as target cells at some centers.

Pretransplantation Evaluation

The LMC is an attractive assay for predicting graft survival, since it can be per-

Lymphocyte – mediated cytotoxicity (LMC)

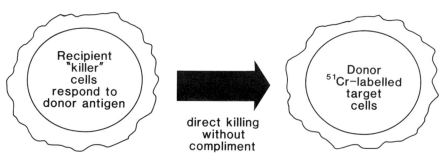

Figure 14–2. In the lymphocyte-mediated cytotoxicity (LMC) test, in vivo generated recipient killer cells sensitized to donor antigens destroy ^{51}Cr-labeled donor target cells directly without complement.

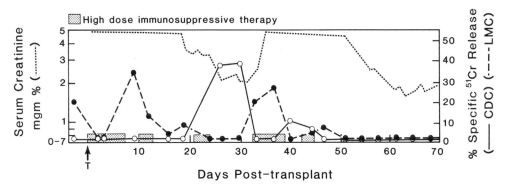

Figure 14–3. In this renal transplant patient, positive LMC was frequently observed in the first 20 days after surgery. The effects of high-dose immunosuppression are evidenced by the negative LMC changes. A plateau in the serum creatinine level and the clinical diagnosis of rejection occurred in association with a rebound in the LMC response. The CDC response appeared to be more variable and was negative during the second rejection episode on day 33. Both assays were negative by day 48 during the quiescent period following rejection. (From Stiller and Sinclair,[71] with permission.)

formed between 4 and 16 hours and is therefore compatible with the logistics of renal transplantation. Many centers have reported on the relationship between pretransplantation LMC and graft failure.[14] This may be dependent on the type of immunosuppression used. When azathioprine and prednisone have been used for maintenance immunosuppression, significant correlations have been noted between a positive LMC cross-match of the recipient against the donor and subsequent graft failure.[12] Kerman and associates,[15] however, have not observed an adverse effect on allograft survival in patients with positive pretransplantation LMC when cyclosporine is used.

Posttransplantation Evaluation

A very good correlation between positive LMC results and acute rejection has been observed.[16,17] The LMC has been found to become positive prior to rejection and therefore may have predictive value (Fig. 14–3). Graft survival has also been reported to be better in patients whose LMC became negative after rejection therapy. A persistently positive LMC is a poor prognostic sign and is associated with irreversible rejection episodes[18] (Fig. 14–4). Some false positive results have been noted, but these may result from technical problems of incubation time and the types of cells used as targets. LMC has been considered

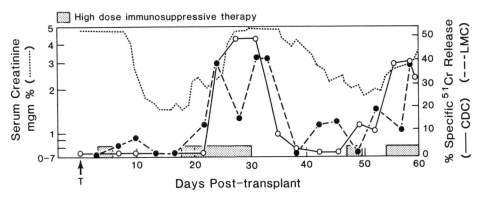

Figure 14–4. An acute irreversible rejection episode in this renal transplant patient on day 18 was associated with positive CDC and LMC levels. However, these elevated levels did not precede the rejection episode. (From Stiller and Sinclair,[71] with permission.)

COMPLEMENT – DEPENDENT CYTOTOXICITY (CDC)

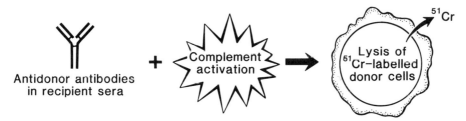

Figure 14–5. In complement-dependent cytotoxicity (CDC), recipient antidonor antibodies and complement cause lysis of ^{51}Cr-labeled donor target cells.

one of the most informative assays for early diagnosis of rejection and prediction of post-treatment outcome.[16]

COMPLEMENT-DEPENDENT CYTOTOXICITY (CDC)

This assay detects recipient antibodies that are able to use and activate complement and to destroy donor target cells[4] (Fig. 14–5). The test is done by incubation of donor lymphocytes in recipient serum at room temperature, followed by addition of complement. Eosin dye exclusion is used as the criterion to calculate the percent killing. Two types of CDC are used for immunological monitoring. The donor-recipient cross-match uses lymphocytes from a prospective donor and sera from the potential recipient. CDC is also used to classify the responder status of a potential recipient by

assessing the cytotoxic response of the recipient's serum to a panel of lymphocytes.

Pretransplantation Evaluation

Donor-Recipient Cross-Match

After it was recognized that donor-specific presensitization of the transplant recipient caused hyperacute or accelerated rejection,[19,20,21] centers began to perform routine serologic lymphocytotoxic tests prior to transplantation. In general, transplants are not performed if the recent serum indicates a positive cytotoxic response.

Cytotoxicity to a Lymphocyte Panel

Another standard test that is used by most transplantation centers is evaluation

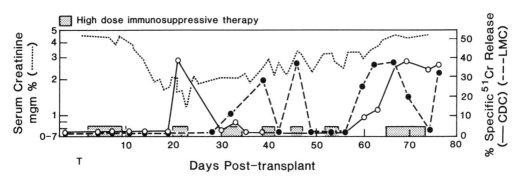

Figure 14–6. Repeated chronic rejection episodes resulted in the loss of this kidney allograft. Antibody-associated rejection around day 20 is seen by a positive CDC at that time. Positive LMC occurred each time the immunosuppression was lifted, and renal function was progressively lost as serum creatinine rose in a stepwise fashion. (From Stiller and Sinclair,[71] with permission.)

of the cytotoxicity of the sera of a potential transplantation patient to a panel of lymphocytes obtained from several individuals. This test was initially developed by Opelz and associates.[22,23] They observed that if patients demonstrated >10 percent cytotoxicity to a randomly selected panel of lymphocytes from normal donors, their survival was lower than those with <10 percent cytotoxicity. As one might expect, the composition of the HLA antigens present in the panel is very important. Some clinical reports indicate that highly sensitized individuals (>50 percent cytotoxicity levels) could make up over half of the potential recipients awaiting transplantation.[24] This is a result of the difficulty in obtaining cross-match negative donors for these sensitized patients. One approach that has been used to decrease the reactivity of a potential candidate's sera is pretransplantation blood transfusion.[25]

Posttransplantation Evaluation

Post-transplantation CDC has been found by Stiller and colleagues[26] to correlate significantly with rejection. In 12 of 15 rejection episodes a positive CDC was associated with rejection. However, this temporal relationship is highly variable, and the clinical usefulness of this assay is lessened (Fig. 14–6).

CELL-MEDIATED LYSIS (CML)

In this test cytotoxic recipient T cells are generated in a 5-to-8-day one-way MLC.[1] They are then placed with ^{51}Cr-labeled donor lymphocyte target cells and lysis is evaluated by release of ^{51}Cr (Fig. 14–7).

Pretransplantation Evaluation

Haisch and coworkers[27] have used CML to pretest potential recipients for their ability to respond to either specific or a third-party donor. They found that 1-year graft survival for the high responder group was 42 percent as compared with 81 percent 1-year graft survival for the low responder group.

Cell Mediated Lysis (CML)

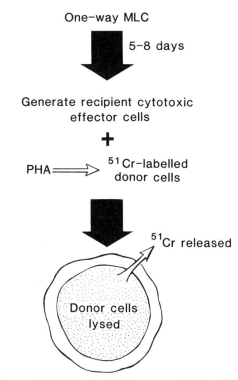

Figure 14–7. In the CML, cytotoxic lymphocytes, generated in vitro in response to donor antigenic stimulation, in a one-way mixed lymphocyte culture (MLC) are combined with ^{51}Cr-labeled donor lymphocytes, which are often activated with phytohemagglutinin. Recipient effector cells then lyse donor target cells.

Posttransplantation Evaluation

There have been few published studies evaluating correlations between clinical posttransplantation status and changes in the CML. However, it appears that a positive CML is associated with the probability of graft rejection and a negative CML is indicative of a quiescent graft.[28]

ANTIBODY-DEPENDENT CELL-MEDIATED CYTOTOXICITY (ADCC)

The ADCC provides a sensitive method of demonstrating the presence of killer cells

ANTIBODY–DEPENDENT CELL–MEDIATED CYTOTOXICITY (ADCC)

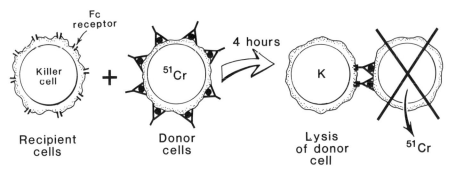

Figure 14–8. In the ADCC assay, nonimmune killer cells interact with the Fc part of the antigen-bound ^{51}Cr-labeled donor target lymphocytes. Presence of these killer cells is evidenced by release of ^{51}Cr after a 4-hour incubation.

in the peripheral circulation of the transplantation recipient.[6] Cytotoxicity requires fixation of IgG to the ^{51}Cr-labeled target cell. Lysis is accomplished by the Fc receptors of the killer cells being targeted toward the IgG on the donor target cells (Fig. 14–8).

Pretransplantation Evaluation

The predictive value of the ADCC has not been clearly established, mainly because so many variations in technique have been used. The purpose of the ADCC is to detect non–complement-binding IgG, which is known to be present in rejecting graft infiltrates.[24] However, the significance of a positive ADCC cross-match before transplantation as an indicator of early graft failure is controversial.[16,29–33]

Posttransplantation Evaluation

Both rejection and quiescence have been reported in association with ADC.[34,35] Some of these discrepancies may be due to technical differences in the assays themselves. Gailiunas and associates[16] reported positive ADCC activity in 41 of 58 (70 percent) of the acute rejection episodes. Kirchoff and colleagues[36] found that donor-specific

ADCC was associated with poor graft prognosis. One-year graft survival was reduced to 30 percent in patients with positive ADCC as compared with 78 percent 1-year graft survival for the entire patient population. Stiller and coworkers[37] noted a strong correlation between positive ADCC and rejection only in patients who had been previously transfused. However, no significant correlation between ADCC and rejection could be established by several other studies.[35,38,39] Recent observations by Dumble and associates[40] have analyzed the relationship between recipient's response to steroid therapy for treatment of rejection and the ADCC response to in vitro steroids. Their results indicate that ADCC resistance to in vitro steroid reflects resistance of rejection to high-dose steroid therapy.

ERYTHROCYTE ANTIBODY (EA) ROSETTE INHIBITION

In the EA rosette inhibition assay, lymphocytes are first separated into T-cell-depleted and T-cell-enriched populations using a nylon-wool adherence method. If anti-B-cell blocking antibodies are present, they will inhibit the rosetting of IgG-coated erythrocytes with B cells or monocytes.[24]

Pretransplantation Evaluation

The results using EA rosette inhibition as a pretransplantation indicator of graft outcome are conflicting. Suthanthiran and colleagues[41] studied 25 cadaver recipients and found a correlation between pretransplantation EA rosette inhibition and poor graft survival. Studies by MacLeod and colleagues[42] however, have documented improved allograft survival in patients with positive pretransplantation EA rosette inhibition. They indicated that the blocking antibodies were not necessarily cytotoxic, nor were they directed against HLA-DR antigens.

Posttransplantation Evaluation

The posttransplantation findings using this test are similar to those obtained using the CDC-B assay. A strong correlation has been observed between the development of positive EA rosette inhibition after transplantation and rejection.[42,43]

ANTI-B CELL ANTIBODIES (CDC-B)

This assay is similar to the standard CDC; however, lymphocytes are separated into T-cell-depleted and T-cell-enriched populations prior to conducting the CDC.[24]

Pretransplantation Evaluation

Many studies have analyzed the implications of a positive cross-match between donor B-lymphocytes and recipient serum.[44–55] Although controversial, results indicate that antibodies directed against donor B cells are not harmful. D'Apice and Tait[47] observed that in 78 patients receiving cadaver renal allografts, 30 had donor-specific B cell cross-matches; however, only 2 of these rejected in the first 6 months. In contrast, 15 of 48 patients negative for anti-B-cell antibodies lost their kidneys. The first reports of a successful transplant in spite of a positive cross-match directed against donor B cells were made by Etten-

ger,[48] Lobo,[49] Morris,[50] and their colleagues. Later studies determined that some of these anti-B-cell antibodies would react between 4° and 22°C (cold-reactive) but not at 37°C (warm-reactive).[51] Winfield and colleagues[52] found that many of the cold-reactive antibodies were autoreactive in character and did not have HLA-A, -B, -C, or -DR specificities. Terasaki and coworkers[53] later determined that only positive B cell cross-matches reactive at 37°C could be correlated with graft survival and could predict early graft failure. Recent studies by Ting[54] have assessed that warm anti-B-cell antibodies are often autoantibodies. Autoreactive IgM antibodies that do not have HLA specificities have been identified in patients who are cross-match-positive.

Posttransplantation Evaluation

Some centers have observed that anti-donor B cell antibodies in the posttransplantation period have been associated with a high degree of graft loss.[28,55–57] The experiences of others, however, have been that although the vast majority of grafts are lost in association with B cell antibodies, nevertheless two thirds of the grafts survive in patients having positive B cell antibodies.[29] Strong B cell cytotoxicity has been found by Ettenger and associates[55] in 22 of 25 patients undergoing allograft rejection. Quiescence was also observed in 13 of 56 patients who developed anti-B-cell antibodies posttransplantation. Soulillou and colleagues[59] observed good long-term function in patients who did not develop anti-B-cell antibodies after transplantation and saw poor graft survival or graft function in those who did. Recently Cardella and Falk[60] have reported that patients with donor-specific B cell antibodies have a significantly worse graft outcome (24 percent) than those without B cell antibodies (75 percent). In addition, in patients with multiple transplants, graft outcome was worse in patients with B cell antibodies (28 percent) than in those without B cell antibodies (37 percent and 44 percent). These differences were not significant because of the small number of patients included in the study. The poor prognosis after development of anti-B-cell antibodies in the posttransplantation period have also been reported by several other centers.[61-63] Studies by Ting and Morris[64] and Luciani and colleagues[65] have not demonstrated this correlation. It is possible that these anti-B-cell antibodies are directed against other (non-HLA-DR) antigens.

ANTIENDOTHELIAL ANTIBODIES

Experience in renal transplantation has shown that the vascular endothelium is the primary target for destruction by the recipient's immune defenses. This is evidenced by deposition of IgG on the vascular endothelium.[66] To detect these antibodies, specific for donor endothelium, indirect immunofluorescence techniques are used on kidney sections, vessel wall preparations, or separated vascular endothelial cells.[67,68]

Pretransplantation Evaluation

Cerilli and associates[68] have correlated early graft rejection with pre-existing antibodies against the endothelial-monocyte antigens. In their renal transplantation patients positive for antivascular endothelium antibody, 63 percent lost their grafts, as compared with only a 14 percent graft loss in negative patients.

Posttransplantation Evaluation

Poor posttransplantation results have been observed in patients when antiendothelial antibodies have been detected in previously negative individuals. Antiendothelial antibodies have also been detected on the endothelium of acutely rejected kidneys from HLA-identical siblings.[69]

MACROPHAGE INHIBITION FACTOR (MIF)

Two methods are commonly used for assaying human MIF.[70] In the one-step direct assay, sensitized lymphocytes are combined with either guinea pig or human monocytes in a capillary tube. After addition of specific antigen, inhibition of macrophage migration is assayed over 24 hours. In the two-step indirect assay, MIF is produced by culture of sensitized lymphocytes with antigen for 24 to 48 hours. Nonimmune guinea pig or human monocytes are then assayed with the cell-free supernatant. In general, a positive MIF response is considered to have occurred when there is a >20 percent inhibition of migration.

Pretransplantation Evaluation

MIF assays are used before transplantation to detect cellular presensitization. Peripheral blood cells are mixed with donor cells, and the release of MIF and its effect on macrophage migration is a gauge of the degree of sensitization of the recipient.[3]

Posttransplantation Evaluation

In general, an association between MIF production and rejection and between inhibition of production and quiescence has been observed.[71] However, a 33 percent incidence of false negative results has also been reported using this test.

T CELL SUBSETS

Monoclonal antibody techniques for identification of T lymphocyte subpopulations has replaced rosetting methods for assessment of T cell numbers. Cells are enumerated using immunofluorescence microscopy or flow cytometry with a fluorescence-activated cell sorter.[72] Several companies have developed commercial preparations for identifying all T cells, T helper cells, T suppressor/cytotoxic cells, B cells, macrophage/monocytes, and natural killer cells (Table 14–2). Many recent studies have focused on correlations between the ratio of helper to suppressor cells in peripheral blood samples and changes after transplantation.

**Table 14–2 Specificities
of Commercial
Monoclonal Antibodies**

Monoclonal Antibody*	Specificity
OKT3, Leu 4	Pan T cell
OKT4, Leu 3a	Helper/inducer T cells
OKT8, Leu 2a	Suppressor/cytotoxic T cells
Leu 7	Natural killer cells, some suppressor/ cytotoxic T-cells
OKT11a, Leu 5	E rosetting

*The OKT series of antibodies is produced by the Ortho Pharmaceutical Corporation, and the Leu series is produced by the Becton Dickinson Company.

Pretransplantation Evaluation

Several studies have analyzed the correlation between pretransplantation OKT4 to OKT8 ratios and graft rejection after renal transplantation.[73,74] In general these have indicated that there is no relationship between high OKT4 to OKT8 ratios (>1.0), or between reduced OKT4 to OKT8 ratios and a decreased rate of acute rejection episodes (Fig. 14–9.)

Posttransplantation Evaluation

In the last 5 years many renal transplantation centers have begun using monoclonal antibodies to monitor changes in T cell subpopulations. Studies have attempted to correlate changes in the ratios of certain T cell subpopulations with clinical events after transplantation.[28] Most centers have observed the normal T helper to T cytotoxic/suppressor ratio (OKT4 to OKT8) to be in the range of 1.9 to 2.0.[28] Many of the preliminary studies in this area demonstrated an association between rejection and an increase in the number of helper cells.[75-79] Certain viral infections have also been seen in association with increased ratios.[80]

At our center, clinical studies of changes

in T cell subsets do not support the hypothesis that renal allograft rejection is accompanied by an increase in the OKT4 helper cell population.[81] Results indicate a marked decrease in the number of helper T cells and an increase in the cytotoxic/suppressor cell populations in kidneys undergoing mild to moderate rejection. A few lymphocytes present were characterized as being from the cytotoxic/suppressor cell subpopulations, with macrophages being the predominant cell type in severely rejecting kidneys. In patients undergoing intractable graft rejection, high levels of cytotoxic/suppressor cells with concurrent low levels of helper cells were maintained throughout the course of their renal transplantation, including transplantation nephrectomy.

The studies of Morris and associates[82] have observed similar findings in patients with intractable graft rejection. In their patients, low OKT4 to OKT8 ratios were exhibited in conjunction with irreversible rejection. These researchers also observed that increased OKT4 to OKT8 ratios occurred without accompanying rejection. They concluded that there was no clear correlation between increased or high OKT4 to OKT8 ratios with renal allograft rejection. Severyn and colleagues[83] were also unable to demonstrate any specific subset pattern with rejection episodes.

Recent clinical results using monoclonal antibodies to monitor changes in T cell subsets are also controversial.[84-89] Some groups have found this type of monitoring valuable because a rise in the OKT4 to OKT8 ratio (>1.0 to 2.0) has been seen just prior to the onset of rejection, in 66 to 100 percent of the rejection episodes. Decreased ratios (<1.0 to 2.0) have also been observed in 20 to 42 percent of the same patient populations in association with rejection episodes. Therefore, although the use of monoclonal antibodies for immunologic monitoring has been enthusiastically applied at major centers, the variety of results obtained lessens their prognostic value with respect to the outcome of graft rejection.

In the cyclosporine era, results of studies assessing the posttransplantation changes in OKT4 to OKT8 ratios and graft rejection have been conflicting. Mazaheri and coworkers[90] observed rises in the OKT4 to OKT8 ratio prior to rejection in patients re-

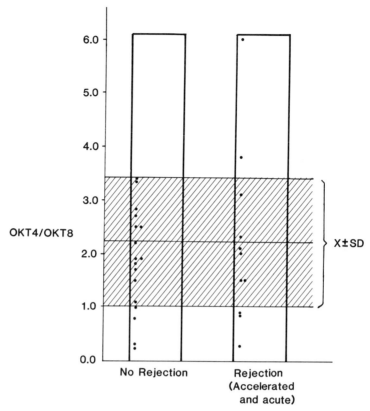

Figure 14–9. In our clinical study, there was no clear association between pretransplant OKT4 to OKT8 ratios and the development of rejection. (From Toledo-Pereyra and Atalla,[73] with permission.)

ceiving cyclosporine immunosuppression. However, Carter and associates[91] found no correlation between rejection and OKT4 to OKT8 ratios. Studies by Daniel and colleagues[92] did not show significant rises in OKT4 to OKT8 ratios during rejection episodes in cyclosporine-treated patients.

FINE-NEEDLE ASPIRATION BIOPSY (FNAB)

This technique was developed as an alternative to peripheral blood sampling or regular biopsy to determine immune status after transplantation.[93–95] A 23- or 25-gauge spinal needle and stylet are inserted percutaneously into the cortical region of the graft, using ultrasound guidance if necessary. After removal of the stylet, the needle is connected to a pistol-grip syringe holder. To obtain a sample the needle tip is moved up and down through a distance of 0.5 to 1.0 cm while suction is applied to the syringe. The small amount of aspirate, 20 to 50 μl, is then suspended in culture medium, and microscopic slides are prepared using a cytocentrifuge. By studying numerous samples, Hayry and colleagues[96] have been able to describe patterns associated with reversible rejection, irreversible rejection, acute tubular necrosis (ATN), and cyclosporine nephrotoxicity. The drawbacks to this technique are that specially trained technicians are necessary and that a significant possibility of sampling errors may exist.

In the hands of experienced individuals, this technique has been useful for diagnosis of rejection and nephrotoxicity.[89–96] Hayry and colleagues[96] have found that early rejection is characterized by lymphocyte and monocyte infiltration. They noted that the appearance of lymphoblasts and macrophages was associated with more severe changes. An increase in the number of macrophages was observed in cases of irreversible rejection. Studies by Wood and associates[97] using monoclonal antibodies have shown increases in the suppressor/cytotoxic T cell population as compared with the T helper population during rejection episodes. It is to be hoped that further work with this assay will provide more information about on-site changes during allograft rejection.

SPONTANEOUS BLASTOGENESIS (SB)

An increase in DNA and RNA synthesis indicating proliferation of recipient lymphocytes has been associated with clinical signs of rejection.[28] However, peripheral lymphocytes from transplantation recipients may also undergo spontaneous blastogenesis in vitro without allogeneic stimulation.[98] The SB assay measures proliferation by determining the rate of ^{3}H-thymidine incorporation by recipient lymphocytes in culture. Usually SB rate is low (680 cpm) prior to transplantation, increases to moderate levels (2300 to 5300 cpm) after transplantation during quiescence, and shows marked elevation during rejection episodes (>10,000 cpm).[99]

Pretransplantation Evaluation

SB assays are performed by some centers prior to transplantation to provide baseline levels for later comparison.

Posttransplantation Evaluation

The relationship between results of this assay and rejection is controversial. Although it has been found to be predictive of rejection,[98] changes in spontaneous blastogenesis may also occur in response to infection.[100]

T-CELL ROSETTING ASSAY

The erythrocyte rosetting (E-rosette) assay has been widely used as a means of identifying T cells. Recently this test has been replaced by T cell characterization methods using monoclonal antibodies directed against cell surface determinants.

Various methods are used to enumerate T lymphocytes that will rosette with sheep erythrocytes after incubation at 4°C.[101]

Pretransplantation Evaluation

It has been demonstrated by Kerman and associates[102] that transplant recipients with high pretransplantation levels of E-rosetting cells have a poorer prognosis.

Posttransplantation Evaluation

Several studies have observed changes in T cell numbers in conjunction with rejection.[103,104] Clinical experience, at our center, indicates that this response was not predictable.[105] Immunological monitoring of the transplant population led us to hypothesize that a decrease in T cell levels was ALG-dependent. Therefore this assay is useful for determining the T cell levels during ALG administration so that dosages may be adjusted. Similar decreases in T cell number have been observed using standardized immunosuppression regimes of steroids and azathioprine alone.[103]

MITOGEN BLASTOGENESIS

Lymphocyte proliferative responses in culture to a variety of mitogens such as phytohemagglutinin and concanavalin A are used as a measure of immune reactivity.[106]

Pretransplantation Evaluation

Using this assay, Thomas and associates[107] reported that normal responsiveness to mitogens was associated with a 44 percent 1-year graft survival rate, whereas an 83 percent graft survival rate was observed in patients exhibiting a low mitogen response.

Posttransplantation Evaluation

PHA- and ConA-induced blastogenesis in the posttransplant period has been evaluated at our center to assess the effectiveness of ALG as an immunosuppressive agent.[105] High daily or alternate-day dosages of ALG corresponded to a decrease in mitogen stimulation in 53 percent of the patients. However, when intermittent (5 to 7 days) ALG was given, no effect was observed on either PHA or ConA stimulation. Other groups have noted either a marked fall in the mitogen reactivity[1] or little effect[108,109] with ALG immunosuppression.

DELAYED HYPERSENSITIVITY TESTING (DHT)

Release of lymphokines by sensitized lymphocytes is assessed by the DHT. Standard techniques involve intradermal injection of a small amount of an allergen such as PPD, *Candida albicans,* streptodornase/streptokinase, or mumps antigen. The subsequent inflammatory response is read at 24 and 48 hours and is graded on the degree of induration that develops.[7]

Pretransplantation Evaluation

Reduced responses to delayed hypersensitivity antigens are frequently observed in the dialysis patient population, but few are totally anergic. However, significantly better graft survival has not been reported in these anergic patients as compared with the rest of the patient population.[110] It is important to consider the transfusion history of the patients when the DHT response is assessed, as transfused patients may have a weaker response than those who have never received a transfusion.[111]

Posttransplantation Evaluation

We are not aware of any published clinical studies evaluating the changes in delayed hypersensitivity during the posttransplantation period.

SUMMARY

The growth of immunological monitoring has been encouraged by the need for a clearer understanding of immunological phenomena and the necessity for a means of detecting changes in immune status. Some progress has been made in achieving these goals and providing more information for the clinician, but there is still a

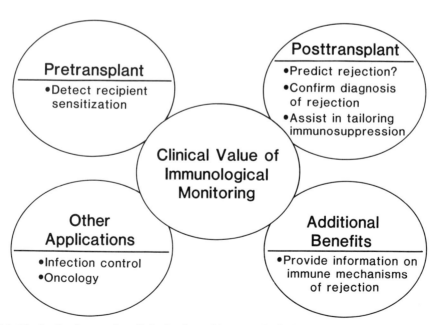

Figure 14–10. In the future, the clinical value of immunological monitoring will depend on the development of accurate methods to provide the physician and surgeon with a more precise view of the patient's immune status.

Table 14–3 Correlation Between Pretransplantation Immunological Monitoring and Graft Outcome

Test	Rejection	Quiescence
Donor-recipient crossmatch	+	−
Cytoxicity to a lymphocyte panel	V (>10%)	V (<10%)
MLR	V	V
LMC	+*	−
CML	High responders	Low responders
ADCC	V	V
EAI	V	V
CDC-B	V†	V
Antiendothelial antibodies	+	−
Mitogen-induced blastogenesis	High responders	Low responders
DHT	NC	NC

+: Positive test result; −: Negative test result; V: Variable results; NC: No correlation.
*Affected by immunosuppression.
†Dependent on specificity of antibodies.

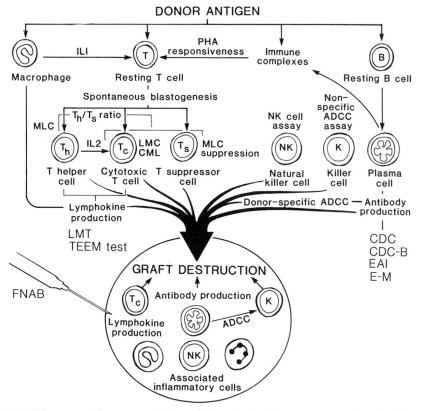

Figure 14–11. Diagrammatic representation of the relationship between various in vitro immunological monitoring techniques and their possible relationship to in vivo mechanisms of graft destruction.

Table 14–4 Correlation Between Posttransplantation Immunological Monitoring and Graft Outcome

Test	Rejection	Quiescence
MLR	V	V
LMC	+	−
CDC	+	−
ADCC	V	V
CDC-B	V*	V*
MIF	Production	Inhibition
T-cell subsets	V	V
FNAB	†	†
Spontaneous blastogenesis	+‡	−
E-rosette-forming cells	V	V

*Depends on specificity of antibodies.
†Experienced individuals able to correlate cellular patterns with quiescence, rejection, or nephrotoxicity.
‡Changes may also be affected by infection or immunosuppression.
V: Variable; +: Positive; −: Negative.

need for methods that will give an even more precise view of the clinical immune picture (Fig. 14–10).

Immunological monitoring before transplantation has been important for detecting recipient presensitization, although results are highly variable with respect to predicting ultimate graft outcome (Table 14–3). It has often been difficult to compare results between centers because of different methodologies and the small numbers of patients in the studies. Future applications of pretransplantation immunologic monitoring will determine the efficacy of the various methods, such as blood transfusions, used to modify the patient's immune response before transplantation.

Posttransplantation applications of immunological monitoring have had the goal of forecasting graft rejection. Experience in this area, however, indicates that no single assay has been able to fulfill these requirements. This may be because of the complexity of the immune response. Nonetheless, immunological monitoring has been important in defining the roles of various cells in allograft rejection. Figure 14–11 indicates in vitro immunological monitoring techniques and their possible relationship to in vivo graft destruction.

Even though it is possible that more in-formation will be obtained from daily immunological monitoring of transplantation patients, the tests are usually time-consuming and expensive, and they often yield variable results (Table 14–4).

One of the potential values of immunological monitoring appears to be the tailoring of immunosuppressive regimes to avoid excessive immunosuppression of the renal transplant recipient.

REFERENCES

1. Thomas, FT, et al: Immunological monitoring as a guide to the management of transplant recipients. Surg Clin North Am 59:253, 1979.
2. Stiller, CR and Keown, PA: Immunologic monitoring: Current perspectives and clinical implications. Transplant Proc 13:1699, 1981.
3. Carpenter, CB: Third international immunologic monitoring symposium: Workshop summary. Transplant Proc 15:1995, 1983.
4. Kerman, R: Foreword. Transplant Proc 16:1403, 1984.
5. Fifth international symposium on immunological monitoring of the transplant patient. Transplant Proc 18: in press, 1986.
6. Suthanthiran, M and Garovoy, MR: Im-

munologic monitoring of the renal transplant recipient. Urol Clin North Am 10:315, 1983.

7. Grieco, MH and Meriney, DK (eds): Immunodiagnosis for Clinicians: Interpretation of Immunoassays. Year Book Medical Publishers, Chicago, 1983.

8. Cochrum K, et al: Mixed lymphocyte culture and cadaver transplantation. Transplant Proc 7:659, 1976.

9. Cullen, P, et al: Mixed lymphocyte reaction and graft survival in 40 cadaveric renal transplantations. Clin Exp Immunol 28:218, 1977.

10. Thomas, F, et al: Pre-transplant immune monitoring of donor-recipient compatibility. Transplant Proc 10:429, 1977.

11. Opelz, G and Terasaki, P: Significance of mixed lymphocyte culture testing in cadaver kidney transplantation. Transplantation 23:375, 1977.

12. Bach, ML, et al: Specific tolerance in human kidney allograft recipients. Cell Immunol 3:161, 1972.

13. Haltler, BG and Miller, J: Changes in mixed lymphocyte culture reactivity as an indicator of kidney rejection. Transplant Proc 4:655, 1972.

14. Carpenter, CB and Morris, PJ: The detection and measurement of pretransplant sensitization. Transplant Proc 10:509, 1978.

15. Kerman, RH, et al: Immunologic monitoring of renal allograft recipients treated with cyclosporine. Transplant Proc 15:2302, 1983.

16. Gailiunas, P, et al: Post-transplant immunologic monitoring of the renal allograft recipient. Transplant Proc 10:609, 1978.

17. Dossetor, JG and Myburgh, JA: Post-transplant immunologic monitoring: Summation. Transplant Proc 10:661, 1978.

18. Stiller, CR, et al: Interpretation of clinical events in the light of measured immune responses. Transplant Proc 13:1628, 1981.

19. Kissmeyer-Nielsen, F, et al: Hyperacute rejection of kidney allografts associated with pre-existing humoral antibodies against donor cells. Lancet 2:662, 1966.

20. Starzl, TE, et al: Schwartzman reaction after human renal homotransplantation. New Eng J Med 278:642, 1968.

21. Patel, R and Terasaki, PI: Significance of the positive crossmatch test in kidney transplantation. New Eng J Med 280:735, 1969.

22. Opelz, G and Terasaki, PI: Histocompatibility in matching utilizing responsiveness as a new dimension. Transplant Proc 4:433, 1972.

23. Opelz, G, Mickey, MR, and Terasaki, PI: HL-A and kidney transplants: Re-examination. Transplantation 17:371, 1974.

24. Carpenter, CB and Milford, EL: Immunological monitoring before transplantation. In Morris, PJ (ed): Kidney Transplantation. Grune & Stratton, London, 1984, p 181.

25. Opelz, G and Terasaki, PI: Prolongation effect of blood transfusions on kidney graft survival. Transplantation 22:380, 1976.

26. Stiller, CR, et al: Immunologic monitoring of the transplant recipient. Transplant Proc 9:1245, 1977.

27. Haisch, CE, et al: Quantitation of immune responsiveness pretransplant by recipient in vitro generation of cytotoxic T effector cells. Transplant Proc 15:1148, 1983.

28. Wood, RFM: Immunological monitoring after renal transplantation. In Morris, PJ (ed): Kidney Transplantation, Grune & Stratton, London, 1984, p 383.

29. Ting, A and Terasaki, PI: Lymphocyte-dependent antibody crossmatching for transplant patients. Lancet 1:304, 1975.

30. Jeannet, M and Vassalli, P: The role of lymphocyte dependent antibody in kidney transplantation. Transplantation 22:493, 1976.

31. Thomas, F, et al: Pretransplant immune monitoring of donor-recipient compatibility. Transplant Proc 10:429, 1978.

32. Myburgh, JA and Smit, JA: Pretransplant lymphocyte-mediated cytotoxicity (LMC) and antibody-dependent cell-mediated cytotoxicity (CDCC) in kidney transplantation. Transplant Proc 10:425, 1978.

33. Keown, P, et al: Recipient presensitization and renal allograft survival. Transplant Proc 10:459, 1978.

34. Grunnet, N and Kristensen, T: Antibody and lymphocyte-mediated immunologic recipient versus donor reactions before and after human renal allotransplantation: A prospective study. Transplant Proc 10:531, 1978.

35. Stiller, CR, et al: Antidonor immune responses in prediction of transplant rejection. New Engl J Med 294:978, 1976.

36. Kirchoff, C, et al: Value of pre- and post-transplant studies of antidonor antibody-dependent cellular cytotoxicity (ADCC). Transplant Proc 13:1565, 1981.

37. Stiller, CR, et al: Diagnostic and prognostic value of donor-specific post-transplant immune responses: Clinical correlates and in vitro variables. Transplant Proc 10:525, 1978.

38. Descamps, B, et al: Complement dependent and lymphocyte dependent antibodies in human allograft recipients. Transplant Proc 7:1, 1975.

39. Jeannet, M, et al: Antibody responses in

kidney transplant recipients and graft survival. Transplant Proc 9:747, 1977.

40. Dumble, LJ, et al: Prediction of renal allograft rejection response to steroids from ADCC response to in vitro steroids. Transplant Proc 15:1145, 1983.

41. Suthanthiran, M, et al: Evidence for close association between B-cell Fc receptors and Ia antigens, and independence from HLA-A, -B locus determined antigens. Transplant Proc 9:1705, 1977.

42. Macleod, AM, et al: Association of Fc receptor blocking antibodies and human renal transplant survival. Transplantation 34:273, 1982.

43. Suthanthiran, M, et al: Detection of anti-donor "Ia" antibodies, a strong correlate of rejection. Transplant Proc 10:605, 1978.

44. Morris, PJ, Ting, A, and Oliver, D: Renal transplantation in the presence of a positive crossmatch. Transplant Proc 10:467, 1978.

45. Soulillou, JP, Peyrat, MA, and Guenel, J: Studies of the antibodies against HLA, Ia-like, Fc, and/or C3 receptors present in pretransplant serum: Anti B-cell antibodies not associated with accelerated graft loss. Transplant Proc 10:475, 1978.

46. Suthanthiran, M, et al: Accelerated graft loss: Association with presensitization to donor B-cell (Ia) antigens. Transplant Proc 10:471, 1978.

47. d'Apice, AJF and Tait, BD: The positive B-cell crossmatch: A marker of active enhancement? Transplant Proc 11:954, 1979.

48. Ettenger, RB, Jordan, SC, and Fine, RN: Cadaver renal transplant outcome in recipients with autolymphocytotoxic antibodies. Transplantation 35:429, 1983.

49. Lobo, PI, Westervelt, FB, and Rudolf, IE: Kidney transplantability across a positive crossmatch. Lancet 1:925, 1977.

50. Morris, PJ, et al: Renal transplantation and a positive serological cross-match. Lancet 1:1288, 1977.

51. Park, MS, et al: Cold reactive antibodies to B lymphocytes and their absorption by platelets and red cells. Transplant Proc 9:1701, 1977.

52. Winfield, JB, et al: Nature of cold-reactive antibodies to lymphocyte surface determinants in systemic lupus erythematosus. Arthritis Rheum 18:1, 1975.

53. Terasaki, PI, et al: Micro droplet testing for HLA-A, -B, -C and -D antigens. Am J Clin Pathol 69:103, 1978.

54. Ting, A: Problems of the strongly sensitized patient. Transplant Proc 15:1198, 1983.

55. Ettenger, RB, et al: Longterm cadaver allograft survival in the recipient with a positive B lymphocyte crossmatch. Transplantation 27:315, 1979.

56. Silberman, H, et al: B-cell antibodies in patients rejecting transplants. Transplant Proc 10:603, 1978.

57. Ting, A and Morris, PJ: Pre- and post-transplant B-cell antibodies in renal transplantation. Transplant Proc 10:393, 1979.

58. Ettenger, RB, et al: Anti-lymphocytotoxins in renal-allograft rejection. New Eng J Med 295:305, 1976.

59. Soulillou, JP, Peyrat, MA and Guenel, J: Association between treatment-resistant kidney-allograft rejection and post-transplant appearance of antibodies to donor B-lymphocyte alloantigens. Lancet 1:354, 1978.

60. Cardella, CJ and Falk, JA: Graft outcome in patients with antibodies reactive with donor T and B cells. Transplant Proc 15:1142, 1983.

61. Deierhoi, MH, Radvany, RM, and Wolf, JS: Correlation of B-cell antibodies and clinical course in DRw-typed renal allograft recipients. Transplant Proc 13:942, 1981.

62. Lepage, V, et al: Anti-B cell lymphocytic antibodies in kidney transplant recipients. Transplantation 25:255, 1978.

63. Mohanakumar, T, et al: Relationship of B cell alloantibodies to renal allograft survival. Transplantation 27:273, 1979.

64. Ting, A and Morris, PJ: Development of donor-specific B lymphocyte antibodies after renal transplantation. Transplantation 28:13, 1979.

65. Luciani, G, et al: Cytotoxic antibodies to B lymphocytes in kidney transplant patients. Transplant Proc 11:1265, 1979.

66. Cerilli, J, Jesseph, J, and Miller, AC: The significance of antivascular endothelium antibody in renal transplantation. Surg Gynecol Obstet 135:246, 1972.

67. Cerilli, J, et al: Antivascular endothelial cell antibody: Its role in transplantation. Surgery 81:132, 1977.

68. Cerilli, J, et al: Immunologic evaluation of renal allograft recipients. Transplant Proc 9:1815, 1977.

69. Moraes, JR and Stastny, P: A new antigen system expressed in human endothelial cells. J Clin Invest 60:449, 1977.

70. Rocklin, RE: Production and assay of macrophage migration inhibitory factor. In Rose, NR and Friedman, H (eds): Manual of Clinical Immunology, ed 2. American Society for Microbiology, Washington, DC, 1980.

71. Stiller, CR and Sinclair, NR StC: Monitoring of rejection. Transplant Proc 11:343, 1979.

72. Russell, PS, Colvin, RB, and Cosimi, AB: Monoclonal antibodies for the diagnosis and treatment of transplant rejection. Annu Rev Med 35:63, 1984.

73. Toledo-Pereyra, LH and Atalla, S: Pretransplant T cell subsets do not predict rejection. Transplant Proc 17:2569, 1985.

74. Helling, TS, Cross, DE, and Shield, CF: Low pretransplant OKT4/OKT8 ratios do not adversely affect patient and allograft survival following renal transplantation. Transplant Proc 17:2550, 1985.

75. Cosimi, AB, et al: Use of monoclonal antibodies to T-cell subsets for immunologic monitoring and treatment in recipients of renal allograft. N Engl J Med 305:308, 1981.

76. Ellis, TM, et al: Immunological monitoring of renal allograft recipients using monoclonal antibodies to human T lymphocyte subpopulations. Transplantation 33:317, 1982.

77. Van Buren, CT, et al: Effect of cyclosporine on immunoregulatory cells of renal allograft recipients. Transplant Proc 15:527, 1983.

78. Binkley, WF, et al: Flow cytometry quantitation of peripheral blood (B) T-cell subsets in human renal allograft recipients. Transplant Proc 15:1163, 1983.

79. Nanni-Costa, A, Vangelista, A, and Frasca, GM: T-cell subsets in renal allograft recipients. Transplant Proc 15:1176, 1983.

80. Carney, WP, et al: Analysis of T lymphocyte subsets in cytomegalovirus mononucleosis. J Immunol 126:2114, 1981.

81. Toledo-Pereyra, LH, et al: Monoclonal antibodies to the cytotoxic-suppressor population of T-cells may identify the high risk transplant patient. Transplant Proc 15:1985, 1983.

82. Morris, PJ, et al: Role of T-cell subset monitoring in renal allograft recipients. N Engl J Med 306:1110, 1982.

83. Severyn, W, et al: The role of immunological monitoring in transplantation. Heart Transplant 1:222, 1982.

84. Schooley, RT, et al: Association of herpes virus infections with T-lymphocyte subset alteration, glomerulopathy and opportunistic infections after renal transplantation. N Engl J Med 308:307, 1983.

85. Colvin, RB, et al: Circulating T-cell subsets in 72 human renal allograft recipients: The OKT4+/OKT8+ cell ratio correlates with reversibility of graft injury and glomerulopathy. Transplant Proc 15:1166, 1983.

86. Chatenoud, L, et al: Interest and limitations of the use of monoclonal anti-T cell antibodies for follow-up of renal transplant patients. Transplantation 36:45, 1983.

87. Smith, WJ, Burdick, JF, and Williams, GM: Immunological monitoring of renal transplant recipients. Transplant Proc 15:1182, 1983.

88. Carter, NP, et al: Monitoring lymphocyte subpopulations in renal allograft recipients. Transplant Proc 15:1157, 1983.

89. Stelzer, GT, et al: Alterations in T-lymphocyte subpopulations associated with renal allograft rejection. Transplantation 37:261, 1984.

90. Mazaheri, R, et al: Lymphocyte subsets in the allograft recipient: Correlation of helper to suppressor ratio with clinical events. Transplant Proc 14:676, 1982.

91. Carter, NP, et al: Monitoring lymphocyte subpopulations in renal allograft recipients. Transplant Proc 15:1157, 1983.

92. Daniel, V, Opelz, G, and Dreikorn, K: Lymphocyte subpopulations in kidney transplant patients with different types of immunosuppression. Transplant Proc 17:2554, 1985.

93. Von Willebrand, E: Fine needle aspiration cytology of human renal transplants. Clin Immunol Immunopathol 17:309, 1980.

94. Von Willebrand, E and Hayry, P: Cyclosporin-A deposits in renal allografts. Lancet 2:189, 1983.

95. Wood, RFM, et al: Monoclonal antibodies and fine needle aspiration cytology in detecting renal allograft rejection. Lancet 2:278, 1982.

96. Hayry, P, et al: Monitoring of organ allograft rejection by transplant aspiration cytology. Ann Clin Res 13:264, 1981.

97. Wood, RFM, et al: Characterization of cellular infiltrates in renal allografts by fine needle aspiration: A simple technique using double labeling with monoclonal antibodies. Transplant Proc 15:1847, 1983.

98. Hersh, EM, et al: In vitro studies of the human response to organ allografts: Appearance and detection of circulating activation lymphocytes. J Immunol 107:571, 1971.

99. Vessela, RL, et al: Correlation of spontaneous leukocyte blastogenesis with human renal allograft rejection. Transplantation 23:277, 1977.

100. Blamey, RW, et al: Measurement of the immune response to an allograft: Amino acid incorporation by peripheral white blood cells in man. Br J Surg 62:863, 1975.

101. Ross, GD and Winchester, RJ: Methods for enumerating lymphocyte populations. In Rose, NR, and Friedman, H (eds): Manual of Clinical Immunology, ed 2.

American Society for Microbiology, Washington, DC, 1980.

102. Kerman, RH, et al: Prognostic significance of the active thymus derived rosette forming cells in renal allograft survival: A preliminary report. Surgery 82:607, 1977.

103. McAlack, RF, et al: Immunologic monitoring parameters in ALG vs. non-ALG treated renal patients. Transplant Proc 11:1431, 1979.

104. Thomas, F, et al: Effective monitoring and modulation of recipient immune reactivity to prevent rejection in early post-transplant period. Transplant Proc 10:537, 1978.

105. Toledo-Pereyra, LH, et al: Immunological monitoring after transplantation. Dial Transplant 10:35, 1981.

106. Chess, L and Schlossman, SF: Methods for the separation of unique human lymphocyte subpopulations. In Rose, NR and Friedman, H (eds): Manual of Clinical Immunology. American Society for Microbiology, Washington, DC, 1980.

107. Thomas, F, et al: Quantitation of pretransplant immune responsiveness by in vitro T cell testing. Transplant Proc 9:49, 1977.

108. Ferguson, R, et al: Functional and anatomic lymphocyte subpopulation redistribution following transplantation. Transplant Proc 4:55, 1977.

109. Schmidtke, JR, et al: The clinical significance of pre- and post-transplant immunological monitoring. Transplant Proc 11:350, 1979.

110. Rolley, R, et al: Monitoring of responsiveness in dialysis-transplant patients by delayed cutaneous hypersensitivity tests. Transplant Proc 10:505, 1978.

111. Klatzman, D, et al: Suppression of lymphocyte reactivity by blood transfusions in uremic patients. Transplantation 35:332, 1983.

Chapter 15

Cadaver Transplantation Results

VIJAY K. MITTAL
LUIS H. TOLEDO-PEREYRA

The success or failure of renal transplants from cadaver donors is determined by numerous variables both before and after transplantation. Some of the factors that influence the outcome of cadaveric renal transplantation include age, sex, and race of the recipient and donor; blood transfusion before transplantation; HLA matching; the method of preservation; the immunosuppressive regimen; initial function of the graft; and the presence of associated diseases such as diabetes mellitus and cardiovascular and pulmonary diseases. The factors affecting graft survival in the living related donor transplants will be discussed in Chapter 20. This chapter will present only cadaveric kidney transplantation results.

DIFFICULTY OF DATA ANALYSIS

Numerous authors have reported on the effects of a particular variable or variables on the outcome of renal transplants at their individual centers. It is often difficult to extrapolate the conclusions of these publications to other transplantation populations owing to the relatively small number of patients included in these studies and the differences in the characteristics of the transplantation populations between centers. We have, therefore, used data from multiple centers compiled into large data bases such as the ones maintained by the University of California at Los Angeles and the European Dialysis and Transplant Association to present the effects of individual factors on the outcome of renal transplantation.

OVERALL TRENDS IN GRAFT AND PATIENT SURVIVAL

In the UCLA registry the 1-year graft survival in cadaveric kidney transplant is 65 percent.[1] A 40 percent 5-year graft survival in cadaveric kidney transplants has been calculated for patients in this data base; the 10-year graft survival rate was approximately 20 percent.[2] The fate of the second or third cadaveric kidney graft is dependent on the source of both the first and second grafts, the cause of graft loss, and duration of the first graft.[1] The 5-year graft survival rate for second and third cadaveric kidneys in the UCLA registry is 30 and 31 percent, respectively.[1] The 10-year graft survival rate for these transplants is 16 percent and 10 percent, respectively.[2] There has been a striking improvement in both patient and graft survival in recent years (Fig. 15–1), which has been attributed to the less vigorous immunosuppressive regimens, less mortality from complications of infection, the better availability of dialysis, and the return of patients with rejected kidneys to regular hemodialysis.

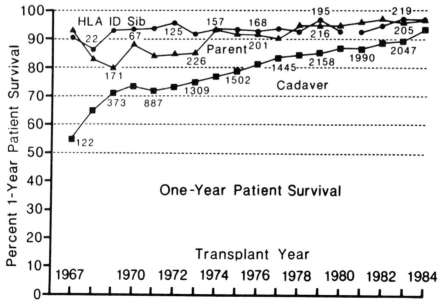

Figure 15–1. A yearly improvement has been observed in 1-year patient survival rates in the UCLA registry. (Used with permission of the UCLA Tissue Typing Laboratory.)

Analysis of the UCLA registry data also indicated that since 1967, only 50 percent of donor transplants throughout the world were cadavers, whereas by 1973, kidneys from cadaver sources increased to 70 percent in the United States. Since then this figure has remained constant. However, in Europe, currently about 85 percent of the renal transplants are from cadaver donors.[1]

FACTORS AFFECTING TRANSPLANTATION RESULTS

Age of the Donor and the Recipient

Conclusions regarding the effect of donor and recipient age on the outcome of the kidney transplant have changed over the years. Clinical analysis of the effect of donor age on graft outcome, conducted in the early years of renal transplantation experience, indicated that kidneys from older donors survived at a lower rate with each successive decade.[3,4] More recent studies,

however, have failed to confirm these conclusions. Several centers have reported similar graft survival for kidneys from donors > 50 years old and < 50 years old.[5,6] Lee and Terasaki[7] have reported that when kidney donors were between 6 and 60 years old, age did not significantly influence the outcome of the transplant (Fig. 15–2). Patient survival was essentially the same for all groups in their analysis, and graft survival was only slightly lower for donor kidneys between 46 and 60 years old.

Early transplantation experience indicated that older patients had higher mortality rates than younger recipients, leading to an exclusion of these patients from renal transplantation.[8] By the early 1970s more transplantation centers were including older patients in their transplantation populations, and results indicated that sepsis, infection, and cardiovascular disease contributed to a higher mortality in patients over 60 years old.[9,10] In more recent studies, however, although the mortality was higher for recipients over 50 years old, the difference from that of younger patients was smaller.[11] Results from Lee and Terasaki[7] indicated that both graft and patient sur-

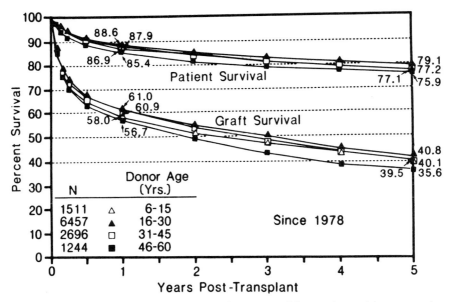

Figure 15–2. Comparative graft and patient survival rates of first cadaver donor transplants with respect to donor age show that kidney donor age between 6 and 60 years old did not significantly influence transplant outcome. (Used with permission of UCLA Tissue Typing Laboratory.)

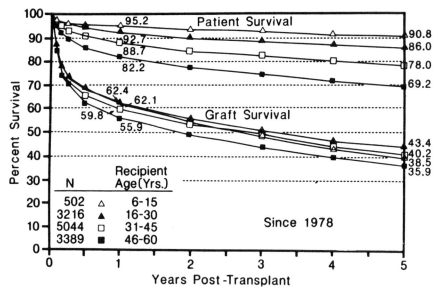

Figure 15–3. Comparative graft and patient survival rates of first cadaver transplants with respect to recipient age show that although no effect of graft survival was observed, patient survival declined with advancing age. (Used with permission of UCLA Tissue Typing Laboratory.)

vival were decreased in very young and in elderly recipients (Fig. 15–3). In their registry data the transplantation outcome in recipients between the ages of 6 and 60 had a relatively constant graft survival, though the patient survival declined with advancing age and almost a 30 percent difference in 5-year patient survival was noted between recipients 11 to 20 years old and more than 60 years old. When 5-year graft survival rates were considered, less divergence was noted.

Sex of the Donor and Recipient

In 1974 Oliver suggested that there may be sex-linked histocompatibility antigens in humans.[12] A few studies have considered the influence of the sex of the donor and recipient on allograft survival.[13,14,15] Studies by Parsons and associates[13] indicated that the sex of the recipient did not significantly affect allograft survival. Previous analysis by Descamps and coworkers[14] has shown that female-to-female transplants do better than male-to-female. However, gender compatibility in male recipients did not appear to be so important. Opelz and Tera-

saki,[15] in a multicenter analysis, could not confirm these observations. They noted that female-to-male grafts actually had somewhat diminished graft survival.

Race of the Donor and Recipient

It has been suggested that black recipients had a significantly lower graft survival rate than caucasian recipients.[16,17,18] Recently Galton and colleagues[19] showed similar results and suggested that other factors such as the center effect were responsible for the apparent poorer survival of grafts in black recipients. In their analysis the graft survival was highest for caucasian-to-caucasian transplants, but there were relatively small differences for all the combinations. Studies by the Southeastern Organ Procurement Foundation[20] have shown no effect of race on graft outcome. At our center the best results were seen in caucasian donor to caucasian recipient transplantation, and the second best results were obtained in caucasian donor to black recipient combinations[21] (Table 15–1). Socioeconomic differences apparently do not effect patient survival rates and similarly may

Table 15–1 Influence of Race on the Outcome of Cadaver Renal Allografts				
			1-Year Survival*	
Group	Racial Combination	N	Graft	Patient
I	White to white	56	43%	43%
II	White to black	43	46%	67%
III	Black to white	12	16%	50%
IV	Black to black	5	20%	60%

*Data from Mittal et al.[21] One hundred sixteen consecutive cadaver renal allografts performed between June 1974 and July 1980 were included in this analysis. When the graft survival results were statistically compared (chi-square), the p value between Group I and Group III was $0.10 > p > 0.05$. No other comparisons of graft survival were statistically significant. When patient survival was compared between the groups, the p value between Group I and Group II was <0.05. All other comparisons were statistically insignificant.

not be responsible for the difference in the graft survival rate. The patient survival results in the interracial transplants were the same, but different graft survival rates were observed.

Associated Diseases

The presence of associated diseases such as cardiovascular and pulmonary disease and diabetes mellitus usually decrease the chances of patient survival and occasionally decrease graft survival. The original disease, causing end-stage renal failure, may also influence graft survival, but there is no convincing evidence to that effect. Analysis of data from the UCLA registry determined the contributions of diabetes, nephrosclerosis, systemic lupus erythematosus, polycystic kidney disease, pyelonephritis, and glomerulonephritis on patient and graft survival (Table 15–2). The lower graft survival rate observed in diabetics as compared with nondiabetics was attributed to a higher mortality in the diabetic group rather than graft loss because of rejection. In the UCLA registry the functional graft survival at 5 years in diabetic recipients is 33 percent, whereas graft survival at 5 years in nondiabetic patients is 40.1 percent.[22]

Time on Dialysis

Overall analysis of data from the European Dialysis and Transplantation Association[23] has shown a better graft survival in patients who were on dialysis for a long time. The better survival may result from the death of poor-risk patients on dialysis before transplantation or from better matching of long-term well-dialyzed patients or from a greater likelihood of transfusions in patients on long-term dialysis.

Table 15–2 Effect of Associated Diseases on Renal Allograft and Patient Survival*		
	5-Year Survival	
Associated Disease	Graft	Patient
Diabetes mellitus	34.7%	62.9%
Nephrosclerosis	34.5%	78.3%
Systemic lupus erythematosus	28.1%	79.6%
Polycystic kidney disease	39.9%	80.4%
Pyelonephritis	40.1%	82.1%
Glomerulonephritis	42.0%	82.8%

*Based on the data of Cats and Galton.[22]

Bilateral Nephrectomy

In a 1975 report of the Human Transplant Registry[24] a small but significant improvement in patient and graft survival was noticed in patients who had bilateral nephrectomy prior to transplantation.[24] The better survival in this group of patients may be attributable to the repeated blood transfusions in nephrectomized patients on dialysis prior to transplantation. A recent retrospective nonrandomized study by Kyriakides and associates[25] of 216 consecutive transplants (129 living related and 87 cadaveric) indicated that 5-year and 2-year actuarial graft survivals were better in patients with bilateral nephrectomy and splenectomy (91 percent and 90 percent, respectively) than with splenectomy alone or in those patients receiving no procedure prior to transplantation. Sanfilippo and colleagues[26] also demonstrated a highly significant increase in graft survival associated with pretransplantation bilateral nephrectomy in 2808 cadaver transplantations. Although the mechanism of improved graft survival with pretransplantation bilateral nephrectomy remains unclear, Kyriakides and coworkers[25] have postulated that removal of the native kidneys may prevent activation of recipients' autoimmune responses after transplantation.

Pretransplantation Blood Transfusion

In the early years of renal transplantation, pretransplantation transfusions were avoided because it was believed that they would induce the development of cytotoxic antibodies in the transplantation candidate, resulting in accelerated rejection upon transplantation.[27,28] Since that time it has been found that pretransplantation transfusions may exert a beneficial rather than deleterious effect on graft survival.[29] The survival rate, until about 1975, was very low and was attributed to withholding transfusion before transplantation. With the gradual widespread adoption of pretransplantation blood transfusion, there was a parallel increase in graft survival. The three main mechanisms postulated for the increase in the graft survival after pretransplantation blood transfusions are first,

induction of cytotoxic antibodies that in turn serve to exclude incompatible donors by advance warning of a positive crossmatch test; second, induction mechanism, wherein the immune system of the transfused patient actively makes a negative immunologic response by induction of either suppressor cells or antibodies that have an enhancing effect; and last, immunization of the patient prior to transplantation with deletion of the reactive clones by immunosuppression posttransplantation.[30–32]

Compilation of the transfusion data in the UCLA Kidney Transplant Registry[33] has indicated that a single blood transfusion prior to transplantation may increase graft survival by 10 percent over that of nontransfused patients. With 5 to 23 pretransplantation transfusions, the 1-year graft survival was reported to be 64 percent. Various kinds of blood transfusion protocols have been used, including whole blood, packed cells, washed packed cells, and frozen blood. Pretransplantation transfusions appear to have greatest effect during the first month posttransplantation. A single transfusion reaches full potential between 1 week and 3 months, and this effect remains remarkably constant over more than 2 years. Fewer transfusions were required to achieve a maximum graft survival in grafts from nonparous females and cadaver kidney transplants under the age of 35 years. The transfusion effect was independent of HLA matching, undiminished by a long period on dialysis, and productive of no significant increase in graft survival in nonparous women. The transfusion prior to transplantation was dependent upon age, and in patients more than 35 years old at the time of transplantation, more than four transfusions significantly increased 1-year graft survival. The transfusion effect can be credited with approximately 20 percent improvement in graft survival in the later half of the 1970s and early 1980s.

When the effects of the number of blood transfusions on subsequent 1-year graft and patient survival were analyzed at our center, in a high-risk patient population during the ALG era, prolongation of graft survival was noted in all transfused patients (59 percent, cumulatively) as compared with nontransfused patients (25 percent)[34] (Figs. 15–4 and 15–5). However, in this series no

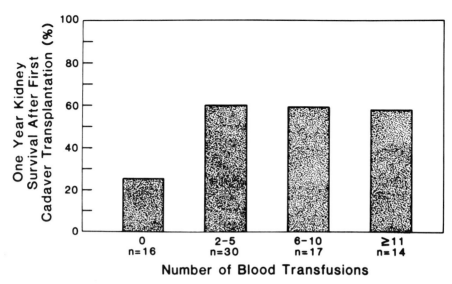

Figure 15–4. Comparative 1-year kidney allograft survival rates in each of the transfusion study groups reveal the positive effect of pretransplant blood transfusions; however, no cumulative effect was observed. (From Zeichner, et al,[34] with permission.)

differences in 1-year graft survival were noted among the various groups receiving increased numbers of blood transfusions. Overall patient survival in this study was 90 percent. Blood transfusions did not affect patient survival. In addition, no pattern of sensitization was demonstrated after multiple blood transfusions and no significant difference was noted in the level of cytotoxic antibodies observed in any group.

Opelz[35] has recently reanalyzed the role of blood transfusions with the application of cyclosporine as an immunosuppressant.

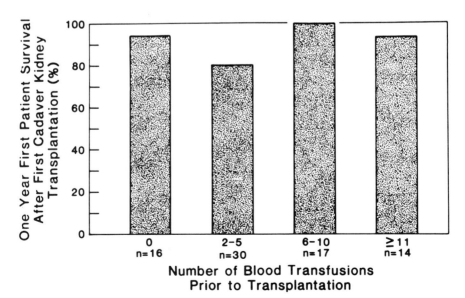

Figure 15–5. When the 1-year patient survival was compared for transfused and nontransfused kidney allograft recipient groups, no effect on patient survival was determined. Overall patient survival was 90 percent. (From Zeichner, et al,[34] with permission.)

This has been a bit difficult, since at present approximately 90 percent of recipients receive transfusions prior to transplantation, and only 10 percent receive transplants without transfusions. The use of cyclosporine appears to have an additive effect to transfusions. Opelz found that survival at day 320 was approximately 75 percent in cyclosporine-treated patients receiving transfusions, as compared with 65 percent in cyclosporine-treated patients without any transfusions. When 2 to 10 and >10 transfusions were given, the survival values were 80 percent and 82 percent, respectively.

Blood Group of the Recipient

Only a few studies have analyzed the effect of recipient blood groups on graft survival. Joysey and associates[36] reported in 1973 that O blood group recipients had a better graft survival than non-O recipients. Cecka[37] pointed out that the effect of HLA matching is influenced by the ABO blood group of the recipient only in non-O recipients.

HLA Matching

Although it is important in living related transplantation, HLA-A and -B matching has only a modest influence on cadaveric graft survival. Matching for HLA-DR, however, appears to have a more important effect on graft survival in cadaveric kidney transplantation.[36] In transplants since 1978, grafts with zero HLA-A,B,DR mismatches had a high 1-year graft survival of 79 percent. One-year graft survival was better for patients with one, two, three, and four HLA-A,B mismatches who were compatible at the DR locus (ranging from 69 to 64 percent, respectively) than for recipients with one DR or two DR mismatches. With two DR mismatches and four HLA-A,B mismatches, 1-year graft survival was decreased to 59 percent (Fig. 15–6). When individual HLA-DR antigens were considered, HLA-DR1 patients had the lowest response among all the HLA-DR types, and these patients made the least cytotoxic antibodies, resulting in the highest kidney transplantation survival rates as compared with HLA-DR7 patients, who had the lowest graft survival.[39]

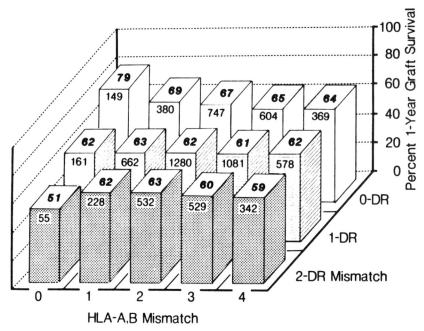

Figure 15–6. One-year graft survival of first cadaver transplant with regard to the number of HLA-A, -B and -DR mismatches. (From Terasaki, et al,[38] with permission of UCLA Tissue Typing Laboratory.)

Status of Donor

The various donor factors identified as affecting the outcome of a cadaveric transplantation include the cause of donor death, donor age, warm ischemia time, cold ischemia time, donor serum creatinine, urinary output prior to harvesting of the donor organ, proteinuria, the condition of the renal artery and the vein, and steroids given to the donor prior to harvesting.[40] In the UCLA registry the cause of death had no significant effect on 1-year graft survival.[40] In that series most of the donor deaths resulted from head injury, traffic accident, or gunshot wound. It was interesting to note that the incidence of nonfunction in kidneys obtained from donors who died of cerebral vascular disease was higher than for kidneys procured from donors who died of head injuries. One-year graft survival of kidneys from donors between age 10 and 49 years old was more than 60 percent. Graft survival decreased with donors younger than 10 years or older than 60 years of age. There was no significant influence of various lengths of warm ischemia time on 1-year graft survival except for a decrease in the group with 11 to 20 min of warm ischemia. Despite no overall effect on graft survival, the incidence of nonfunction was increased if warm ischemia time was more than 10 min. Table 15–3 shows the effects of various other donor variables on graft outcome.[40]

Renal Preservation

After procurement renal allografts are preserved by either cold storage or hypothermic pulsatile perfusion. The debate continues as to which method yields the best immediate and long-term functional results. Preservation by cold storage has obvious advantages compared with machine perfusion, as it is less costly, the logistics are simplified, and technical complications are less frequent. Our recommendation is that either method may be used if kidneys are to be preserved for 24 to 36 hours. However, hypothermic pulsatile perfusion is preferred for extending preservation beyond 36 hours.[41] As will be discussed in the section on delayed graft function, in our experience, ATN increases significantly when kidneys are stored longer than 24 hours or perfused longer than 36 hours. Collins[42] is of the opinion that cold storage has advantages over pulsatile perfusion if the organs are to be preserved for less than 48 hours. However, if the kidneys are to be cold-preserved for more than 48 hours, machine preservation is more successful. A recent trend toward increased use of cold storage can be seen in a recent report of 23,607 transplants in UCLA registry. In 1975, 66 percent of kidneys were machine-perfused; however, by 1982, this number had dropped progressively to 43 percent.[43] This information also points to the fact that cold storage

Table 15–3 Influence of Various Donor Factors on Graft Survival	
Donor Variable	**Effect**
Serum creatinine	No significant effect on graft function and survival if <3.0 mg/dl
Oliguria	Urinary output of 200–3000 mg/dl— no effect
Proteinuria	
Present	44.6% (1-year graft survival) } p <0.1
Absent	55.3% (1-year graft survival)
Polar arteries	45% } p <0.5
Single artery	55%
Steroids to donor	53.2% } NS
No steroids to donor	54.2%
Dopamine to donor	53.8% } NS
No dopamine to donor	52.2%
NS: Not significant, chi-square. *Data from Iguro et al.[40]	

times can safely be extended beyond 24 hours.

The choice of preservation method has also been influenced by the widespread use of cyclosporine. Flechner and colleagues[44] reported twice the incidence of ATN with machine versus storage preservation in recipients treated with cyclosporine, though in their series long-term graft function was not adversely affected. One-year graft survival in machine-preserved kidneys (Waters machine) reported by Iguro and coworkers[40] was 60.5 percent, as compared with storage after flushing with Collins solution, whose 1-year graft survival was 60.6 percent. The incidence of nonfunctioning kidneys after machine preservation was 7.5 percent, significantly lower than 9.5 percent with Collins-stored kidneys. A prospective randomized study by Mozes and associates[45] reported increased incidence of ATN in cold-stored kidneys (54.2 percent) as compared with machine-preserved kidneys (43 percent). The incidence of ATN with machine-preserved kidneys was independent of preservation time. They also reported no difference in the incidence of ATN between cold-stored (4/15, 26 percent) and machine-preserved kidneys (6/14, 42.8 percent, $p > 0.5$) when preservation time was less than 24 hours. With longer preservation times, an increased incidence of ATN with cold-stored kidneys was observed (48/79 or 60.7 percent, versus 33/79 or 41.8 percent for perfusion), but the difference was not significant. They concluded that the two methods of kidney preservation resulted equal 1-year graft and patient survival rates and stressed that if the kidneys are to be cold-stored, the preservation time should be less than 24 hours. In another randomized prospective trial of cold storage versus pulsatile perfusion by Halloran and colleagues[46] from Ontario Renal Transplant Research Group, pulsatile perfusion was associated with a higher probability of increased immediate kidney function (49/88 or 56 percent) whereas cold storage increased the likelihood of delayed graft function (37/86 or 43 percent immediate function) and possible patient morbidity and mortality (6-month patient survival-storage group = 90 percent, perfused group = 98 percent, $p < 0.03$).

The effect of cyclosporine use in relation to length of preservation has been recently assessed by Persijn and coworkers[47] for the Eurotransplant data. The best 2-year graft survival was seen with cold ischemia for less than 24 hours (81 percent). Less than 60 percent 2-year graft survival was observed, however, when cold ischemia times were more than 48 hours. In noncyclosporine transplants no similar difference was observed. No statistically significant difference was seen among the various cold ischemia times.

Transplantation Center Effect

The UCLA Transplant Registry, compiling data from 40 centers in the United States and Europe, has observed a large difference—as great as 40 percent or so—in 1-year graft survival among the various transplant centers.[48] Various factors that influence graft survival among the various centers include immunosuppression, HLA matching, transfusions, and race. The factors influencing the various centers can be divided into pretransplantation and posttransplantation factors. The pretransplantation factors may include criteria for patient selection, the presence of certain original diseases, recipient age, number of transfusions prior to transplantation, and HLA matching. The posttransplantation factors may include posttransplantation patient care, management of rejection, and the immunosuppression regimen for rejection episodes. When the various centers were classified as excellent, good, and fair on the basis of greater than 55 percent, 45 to 55 percent, and less than 45 percent 1-year graft survival, respectively, the following conclusions were reached: More patients were transfused with a greater number of units at excellent and good centers. Tissue typing for HLA-DR was performed at excellent and good centers and a greater number of patients were matched for HLA-DR. Excellent centers also more frequently matched HLA-A,B loci. The use of cyclosporine was more effective at excellent and good centers, resulting in 11 percent and 8 percent increases in graft survival, respectively. At fair centers administration of cyclosporine decreased graft survival by 3 percent, probably owing to the difficulty in diagnosing nephrotoxicity versus rejection at these centers.

Initial Function of the Graft

Most studies have shown that better long-term graft survival is observed in kidneys with good immediate function than in cadaveric grafts, where a delayed function was observed. The delay in the graft function may arise from several factors, which include warm ischemia time, the duration of preservation, and method of preservation. The incidence of ATN after the transplantation and the necessity for posttransplantation dialysis may affect the long-term function of the graft. Studies of data obtained over a 6-year period from the Southeastern Organ Procurement Foundation (SEOPF) indicated a 37.5 percent delayed graft function rate (dialysis in the first posttransplantation week) in 3,454 patients.[49] Patients with delayed graft function had significantly higher overall graft loss, irreversible rejection, and mortality than those with immediate function. Cho and associates[50] also recently concluded that both donor and recipient factors were responsible for ATN, resulting in a significant reduction in transplantation survival. The effect of preservation time on the incidence of ATN and subsequent recovery of normal renal function was recently analyzed at our center.[41] We found that there is generally more ATN in stored kidneys than in kidneys perfused for the same amount of time. ATN was observed to increase in kidneys stored longer than 24 hours and in those perfused longer than 36 hours. The recovery from ATN, however, was not significantly different between short- and long-term preserved organs (Table 15–4).

The recent use of cyclosporine has added caution to the use of long-term renal preservation procedures. The clinician may have difficulty in determining the contribution of cyclosporine nephrotoxicity to impaired renal function when ATN is also present. Therefore, in the immediate postoperative period, when ATN is present, many centers avoid or reduce cyclosporine dosage. When the incidence of ATN was compared at our center between the precyclosporine and the cyclosporine era, no significant difference in the incidence of ATN or the ATN recovery rate was observed when a conservative approach to cyclosporine administration was used (Table 15–5).

Table 15–4 Relationship Between Incidence of ATN and Preservation Time		
	Incidence of ATN/ATN Recovery	
Preservation Time (hr)	Perfused Kidneys (n = 178)	Stored Kidneys (n = 47)
0–12	40%/100%	0%/—
12–24	29%/78%	16%/100%
25–36	36%/76%	78%/80%
36–48	53%/60%	37%/92%
>48	55%/60%	—/—

Technical Factors

Postoperative complications after cadaver kidney transplantation may influence graft as well as patient survival. These are discussed in more detail in Chapter 18. Technical complications including vascular thrombosis and extravasation of the urine may be directly responsible for the graft failure. It has also been pointed out that an end-to-end anastomosis of the renal artery to the internal iliac artery may result in a vascular stenosis and decrease graft survival as compared with an end-to-end anastomosis of the renal artery to the external iliac artery; obtaining a prolonged patency of the vascular anastomosis may result in better graft survival.

Immunosuppression

For many years azathioprine and steroids have been the backbone of posttransplantation immunosuppressive therapy. Recently the use of lower doses of steroids has decreased morbidity and mortality. The other forms of available immunosuppressive therapy include antilymphocyte globulin, which has been used by many centers for years and certainly for treating repeated rejection episodes. The most exciting of the new developments in immunosuppression is cyclosporine, which in most centers has led to improved graft survival figures for the last 4 years or so. This could replace the other immunosuppres-

Table 15–5 Comparison of Incidence of ATN and Subsequent Percentage Recovery of Function in Precyclosporine and Cyclosporine Eras

| | Incidence of ATN/Percent Recovery of ATN Kidneys | | | | | |
| | All kidneys | | ALG Era | | CyA Era | |
	N	%/%	N	%/%	N	%/%
Length of Hypothermic Storage (hr)						
0–12	2	0/—	0	—/—	2	—/—
>12–24	19	16/100	10	30/100	9	0/—
>24–36	7	71/80	2	0/—	5	100/80
>36–48	19	63/92	9	78/86	10	50/100
Length of Hypothermic Pulsatile Perfusion (hr)						
0–12	10	40/100	8	37/100	2	50/100
>12–24	80	29/78	67	28/74	13	31/100
>24–36	53	36/84	39	33/85	14	43/83
>36–48	30	67/70	13	86/64	17	53/78
>48	4	100/100	4	100/100	—	—/—

sive regimens, though the associated nephrotoxicity in the early postoperative period is a major problem. Recently monoclonal antibodies have been used for treating rejection episodes that are resistant to other immunosuppressive therapy. Other forms of immunosuppression, used on a limited basis over the years, include thoracic duct drainage, thymectomy, local graft irradiation, extracorporeal blood transfusion, whole body irradiation, anticoagulants, splenectomy, and other drugs.

Azathioprine and Steroids

Azathioprine and steroids were the standard conventional immunosuppressive regimen for all kidney transplantation centers for almost 20 years. Initially the steroids were used in very high doses. This was associated with a high incidence of morbidity and mortality. Recently, however, the dosage of steroids has been decreased, and the incidence of complications related to steroids also has decreased.[51,52] However, not all trials of low-dose steroids have shown the same graft survival as observed in patients given high doses of steroids.[55] d'Apice observed that low-dose steroids were effective only if the dose of azathioprine was greater than 1.75 mg per kg per day.[54] The patient survival with con-

ventional immunosuppression therapy was 56 percent at 1 year with cadaver donors in 1967, and it increased to 90 percent by 1983; this is a significant improvement. High-dose steroids were given intravenously as bolus for rejection episodes, though recently antilymphocyte globulin is being used with increasing success for steroid-resistant rejection episodes. At our center, with a high-risk transplantation population, the use of a standard azathioprine-prednisolone immunosuppressive regimen was associated with a 1-year actuarial graft survival of 46 percent and a 1-year actuarial patient survival of 60 percent.[55] These results prompted institution of ALG/ATG as the primary immunosuppressive agent, with a concomitant reduction in steroid dosages. Details of the results of these changes will be discussed in the next section.

Antilymphocyte Globulin

Antilymphoblast globulin (ALG) and antithymocyte globulin (ATG) have been used as immunosuppressive agents for over 15 years.[56] There is some controversy as to whether these drugs should be used prophylactically or for the treatment of rejection episodes or both. Initial use of ALG was complicated by a lack of well-controlled studies. In addition, a variety of potencies, dosages, sources, and routes of administration were employed. More recent trials, however, have established the efficacy of ALG/ATG in renal transplantation, and the administration of these drugs has become more standardized.[57,58,59] An overall 10 to 15 percent improvement in graft survival has been observed using ALG/ATG prophylactically, as compared with previously used conventional steroid immunosuppression. Clinical studies indicate that patients receiving prophylactic ALG have fewer, less severe rejection episodes that are more easily reversed.

A significant decrease in the amount of steroids has been accomplished through the prophylactic administration of ALG. Side effects, observed in 5 to 15 percent of the patients, include chills, fever, rash, leukopenia, and thrombocytopenia, although these are easily controlled. No increase in bacterial sepsis has been observed with the switch from conventional steroid therapy to ALG/ATG therapy. However, some centers have reported an increase in cytomegalovirus (CMV) depending on the dosages of other simultaneously administered immunosuppressants.

At our center the switch from conventional steroid therapy to adjunctive prophylactic ALG in a high-risk patient population has resulted in a significant improvement in both graft and patient survival in the past few years[55] (Table 15–6). When we conducted prospective randomized trials comparing the prophylactic and nonprophylactic use of ALG, a trend toward better patient and graft survival was seen in the prophylactic group.[61] With prophylactic ALG the onset of rejection was delayed to an average of more than 3 weeks after transplantation.

The use of ALG/ATG therapy to treat graft rejection has been more readily accepted than the prophylactic use of these drugs. ALG therapy in general has been shown to be superior to conventional steroid treatment of rejection episodes. Several studies have indicated that rejection is more readily reversed by ALG.[62–69] Few groups, however, have used ALG/ATG to treat multiple rejection episodes. Since ALG usually has been used to treat only first rejection episodes, ultimate graft survival is affected by the switch of immunosuppression back to steroids during the course of the transplant.

At our center high morbidity and mortality after transplantation, observed with repetitive treatment of rejection episodes with steroids in high-risk patients, led us to test the use of intermittent ALG alone as alternative immunosuppressive therapy[69] (Table 15–7). Patients were considered to be at high risk if more than two high-risk factors such as age (>45 years), insulin-independent diabetes, cardiovascular and/or pulmonary complications, and no antigen matches were involved. Using ALG in this manner, we were able to treat chronic rejection without an associated increase in steroids, and therefore morbidity and mortality were reduced. ALG administration is also improved by titration of individual rejection courses with adjustment of ALG doses. This alternative approach has allowed for a significant improvement of the posttransplantation course of our high-risk patient population in a safe manner without the risks of steroid administration.

Table 15–6 Comparative Graft and Patient Survival Using Conventional Versus ALG Immunosuppressive Therapy

	1-year Survival					
Immunosuppression	N		Graft		Patient	
Azathioprine + Prednisone	15*	36†	46%*	47%†	60%*	83%†
ALG + azathioprine	15*	31†	75%*	68%†	94%*	87%†

*Data from Toledo-Pereyra et al.[55]
†Data from Novick et al.[60]

Table 15–7 Steroids Versus ALG for Rejection in High-Risk Renal Allograft Recipients*		
Antirejection Treatment	**1-year Actuarial Survival**	
	Graft	*Patient*
Steroids	46%	60%
ALG	75%	94%

*Data from Toledo-Pereyra.[69]

Cyclosporine

Introduced in 1978 for clinical trials, cyclosporine has proved to be an extraordinarily powerful immunosuppressive agent and has been primarily responsible for the recent improvement in graft and patient survival in organ transplantation.[70] Most of the centers around the world have shown that cyclosporine either with or without steroids resulted in an improved graft and patient survival rate when compared with conventional immunosuppressive therapy. However, a number of side effects of cyclosporine have become evident, for example, nephrotoxicity, hepatotoxicity, hypertrichosis, fluid retention, hypertension, gingival hypertrophy, and increased incidence of cutaneous malignancy. By far the most troublesome effect of cyclosporine A is nephrotoxicity, as it is very hard to differentiate between nephrotoxicity and rejection in the early postoperative period. Initial experience with cyclosporine in renal transplantation was reported by Calne and colleagues.[70,71] They found that cyclosporine A was an extremely powerful immunosuppressant and that it could be effective even without concurrent steroid administration. When cyclosporine A was used in kidneys with diuresis, 1-year graft survival increased from 50 to 55 percent to 80 percent in cadaveric renal transplantations. Starzl and coworkers[72] obtained excellent results when cyclosporine A was given with prednisone. One-year graft survival of almost 80 percent was obtained in 66 recipients of 67 cadaveric grafts. Subsequent studies have attempted to assess the efficacy in a randomized prospective manner. In 1983 Hakala and associates[73] reported a prospective randomized study of patients undergoing primary cadaveric kidney transplantation and compared cyclosporine A and steroid therapy with conventional immunosuppressive therapy consisting of azathioprine and prednisolone. One-year graft function was 92 percent with less infection in the cyclosporine group as compared with 56 percent in the conventional immunosuppression group. In 1985 Sutherland and colleagues[74] reported a prospective randomized study comparing a group of patients receiving cyclosporine and prednisolone with a group receiving azathioprine, prednisolone, and ALG. In their study graft survival rates were equivalent between the two groups. Diabetic patients who received grafts from cadaveric donors, however, had significantly increased 1-year graft survival (84 percent versus 66 percent, p <0.04). Infection was lower and the need for hospitalization was also less in the cyclosporine group. In 1985 Johnson and associates[75] reported a 4-year prospective study of cyclosporine in cadaver renal transplantation and showed a 1-year graft survival of 80.2 percent when cyclosporine was used as compared with 65 percent with conventional immunosuppressive therapy. One-year graft survival in patients receiving cyclosporine and steroids was 95.2 percent. In the Eurotransplant data base, between 1981 and 1985, analysis of results of first cadaver transplants has shown a 17 percent higher 2-year graft survival (78 percent) in cyclosporine-treated patients as compared with 61 percent in non-cyclosporine-treated patients.[47] Cyclosporine is a most exciting new treatment that can lead to significant improvement in the graft survival and may prove to be not only a strong immunosuppressive agent with steroid-sparing effects but also one allowing for progress toward the goal of highly specific immunosuppression.

Monoclonal Antibodies

In initial studies with polyclonal antilymphocyte and antithymocyte globulin, improved graft survival and a decreased incidence of rejection episodes were observed. However, because of unavoidable lot-to-lot variability and contamination with non-T-cell-reactive antibodies in these polyclonal preparations, the search has continued to develop an effective monoclonal anti-T-cell antibody. The major disadvantages of ATG and ALG, which monoclonal antibodies should resolve, are the undesired cross-reactive antibodies contained in the polyclonal preparation and the batch-to-batch variability. The initial studies of Cosimi and associates[76] showed that the OKT3 preparation was effective in reversing rejection episodes. However, there was a high rate of recurrence, which required additional immunosuppression. Thistlewaite and colleagues[77] also observed a reduced rejection rate when the daily OKT3 dose was increased and maintenance immunosuppression was begun so as to overlap OKT3 therapy. In their series, only 4 of 30 cadaver renal grafts (13 percent) were lost to rejection. A more recent report by Cosimi[78] evaluated reversal of acute rejection in 32 recipients of cadaver renal allografts. Although there was a consistent pattern of reversal of rejection episodes using OKT3, approximately two thirds had subsequent rejection episodes, which began days or months after discontinuing OKT3 therapy.

In the past few months, Orthoclone OKT3 has been approved for use by all transplant centers. In the controlled clinical trials that preceded this approval, OKT3 was significantly more effective than conventional high-dose steroid therapy in reversing acute renal allograft rejection.[79] In this trial, for a mean of 14 days, 123 patients undergoing acute renal allograft rejection were treated with OKT3 either with concomitant lowering of the dosage of azathioprine and maintenance steroids (n = 63) or with conventional high-dose steroids (n = 60). OKT3 reversed 94 percent of the rejection episodes in the lowered-dose group as compared with a 75 percent reversal rate in the high-dose steroid group. In additional open clinical trials, the rate of reversal of acute rejection using OKT3 was 92 percent in 126 patients. OKT3 has also been used as rescue immunosuppression in cases where steroids and antilymphocyte globulin preparations have failed. In these cases, a 65 percent (n = 225) rejection reversal rate was observed. The manufacturer recommends a reduction in other immunosuppressive agents during the initial days of OKT3 administration to prevent excessive immunosuppression, with a resumption of cyclosporine 3 days prior to cessation of OKT3 treatment.

SUMMARY

Our knowledge regarding the various factors that affect renal allograft outcome has increased in the past two decades of experience in transplanting this organ. Although at various times emphasis has been placed on some factors over others, it is the interaction of the known parameters, plus the contribution of the ones yet to be defined or evaluated, that may lead to the final determination of graft and patient survival. This decade undoubtedly will see a significant contribution to improved results. However, it is to be hoped that attention to other overall donor and recipient variables and the development of more specific immunosuppression options will provide for a reduction in morbidity, mortality, and graft loss in the next decade.

REFERENCES

1. Terasaki, PI, et al: Patient, graft, and functional survival rates: An overview. In Terasaki, PI (ed): Clinical Kidney Transplants. UCLA Tissue Typing Laboratory, Los Angeles, 1985, p 1.
2. Takiff, H, Mickey, MR, and Terasaki, PI: Factors important in 10-year kidney transplant survival. In Terasaki, PI (ed): Clinical Transplants 1986. UCLA Tissue Typing Laboratory, Los Angeles, 1986, p. 157.
3. Darmady, EM: Transplantation and the aging kidney. Lancet 2:1046, 1974.
4. Morling, N, et al: Kidney transplantation and donor age. Tissue Antigens 6:163, 1975.
5. Solheim, BG, et al: Donor age and cumulative kidney graft survival. Tissue Antigens 7:251, 1976.
6. Van der Vliet, JA, et al: Results of renal transplantation using grafts from cadaveric donors over 50 years of age. Scand J Urol Nephrol (Suppl)64:132, 1981.
7. Lee, PC and Terasaki, PI: Effect of age on kidney transplants. In Terasaki, PI (ed): Clinical Kidney Transplants. UCLA Tissue Typing Laboratory, Los Angeles, 1985, p 123.
8. Simmons, RL, et al: Renal transplantation

in high risk recipients. Arch Surg 103:290, 1971.

9. Sommer, BG, et al: Renal transplantation in patients over 50 years of age. Transplant Proc 8:33, 1981.

10. Ost, L, et al: Cadaveric renal transplantation in patients 60 years of age and above. Transplantation 30:339, 1980.

11. Okiye, SE: Primary renal transplantation in patients 50 years of age or older. Transplant Proc 15:1046, 1983.

12. Oliver, RTO: Are there Y-linked histocompatibility antigens in man? Eur J Immunol 4:519, 1974.

13. Parsons, FM, et al: Statistical review. Proc Eur Dial Transplant Assoc 12:3, 1975.

14. Descamps, B, et al: New insights into immunologic selection of human cadaver renal allograft recipients based on immune response capacities. Transplant Proc 10:497, 1978.

15. Opelz, G and Terasaki, PI: Influence of sex on histocompatibility matching in renal transplantation. Lancet 2:419, 1977.

16. Opelz, G, Mickey, MR, and Terasaki, PI: Influence of race on kidney transplant survival. Transplant Proc 9:137, 1977.

17. Oriol, R, LePendu, J, and Chun, C: Influence of the original disease, race, and center on the outcome of kidney transplantation. Transplantation 33:22, 1982.

18. Stuart, FP, et al: Race as a risk factor in cadaver kidney transplantation. Arch Surg 114:416, 1979.

19. Galton, J: Racial effect on kidney transplantation. In Terasaki, PI (ed): Clinical Kidney Transplantation 1985. UCLA Tissue Typing Laboratory, Los Angeles, 1985, p 153.

20. McDonald, JC, et al: Cadaver donor renal transplantation by centers of the South-Eastern Organ Procurement Foundation. Ann Surg 193:1, 1981.

21. Mittal, VK, et al: Influence of race on cadaver kidney transplantation. Dial Transplant 11:960, 1982.

22. Cats, S and Galton, J: Effect of original disease on kidney transplant outcome. In Terasaki, PI (ed): Clinical Kidney Transplants 1985. UCLA Tissue Typing Laboratory, Los Angeles, 1985, p 111.

23. Jacobs, C, et al: In Robinson, B (ed): Proceedings of the European Dialysis and Transplant Association, 14:3, Pittman Med, London, 1977.

24. American College of Surgeons/NIH Organ Transplant Registry. JAMA 233:787, 1975.

25. Kyriakides, GK, et al: Pretransplant bilateral nephrectomy in renal transplantation. Transplant Proc 17:144, 1985.

26. Sanfilippo, F, Vaughn, WK, and Spees, EK: The association of pretransplant native ne-

phrectomy with decreased renal allograft rejection. Transplantation 37:256, 1984.

27. Kissemeyer-Neilsen, F, et al: Hyperacute rejection of kidney allografts associated with preexisting humoral antibodies against donor cells. Lancet 2:662, 1966.

28. Terasaki, PI, Kreisler, M, and Mickey, MR: Presentization and kidney transplant failures. Postgrad Med J 47:89, 1971.

29. Opelz, G, et al: Effect of blood transfusions on subsequent kidney transplants. Transplant Proc 5:253, 1973.

30. Mickey, MR, et al: Transfusion and selection in cadaveric donor kidney grafts. Transplant Proc 15:965, 1983.

31. MacLeod, AM, et al: Possible mechanism of action of transfusion effect in renal transplantation. Lancet 2:468, 1982.

32. Terasaki, PI: The beneficial effect on kidney graft survival attributed to clonal deletion. Transplantation 37:119, 1984.

33. Cecka, M and Cicciarelli, J: The transfusion effect. In Terasaki, PI (ed): Clinical Kidney Transplants 1985. UCLA Tissue Typing Laboratory, Los Angeles, 1985, p 73.

34. Zeichner, WD, et al: Lack of correlation between cadaver kidney transplant survival and the number of pretransplant transfusions. Transplantation 35:500, 1983.

35. Opelz, G: Effect of HLA matching, blood transfusions and presensitization in cyclosporine-treated kidney transplant recipients. Transplant Proc 17:2179, 1985.

36. Joysey, VC, et al: Kidney graft survival and matching for HL-A and ABO antigens. Nature 246:163, 1973.

37. Cecka, M: ABO blood group antigens and kidney transplant. In Terasaki, PI (ed): Clinical Kidney Transplants 1985. UCLA Tissue Typing Laboratory, Los Angeles, 1985, p 179.

38. Madsen, M, et al: HLA-DR matching in cadaveric renal transplantation: An analysis of 201 consecutive transplants performed in Aarhus from 1978 to 1983. Transplant Proc 17:47, 1985.

39. Katz, DV, et al: The immune response and HLA. In Terasaki, PI (ed): Clinical Kidney Transplants 1985. UCLA Tissue Typing Laboratory, Los Angeles, 1985, p 205.

40. Iguro, T, Iwaki, Y, and Terasaki, PI: Donor factors and preservation. In Terasaki, PI (ed): Clinical Kidney Transplants 1985. UCLA Tissue Typing Laboratory, Los Angeles, 1985, p 167.

41. Toledo-Pereyra, LH: Risks of long term preservation (cold ischemia) in renal preservation. Proceedings 18th International Course on Transplantation and Clinical Immunology, Lyon, France, May 1986.

42. Collins, GM: The best method for renal

preservation: Cold storage. Transplant Proc 15:1518, 1985.

43. Perdue, ST, et al: Kidney transplantation trends from UCLA registry data, 1975–1982. Transplantation 36:658, 1983.

44. Flechner, SM, et al: The effect of cyclosporine on early graft function in human renal transplantation. Transplantation 36:268, 1983.

45. Mozes, MF, et al: Comparison of cold storage and machine perfusion in the preservation of cadaver kidneys: A prospective, randomized study. Transplant Proc 17:1474, 1985.

46. Halloran, P, et al: A randomized prospective trial of cold storage versus pulsatile perfusion for cadaver kidney preservation. Transplant Proc 17:1471, 1985.

47. Persijn, GG, et al: Eurotransplant Part II: The Cyclosporine Era 1981–1985. In Terasaki, PI (ed): Clinical Transplants 1986. UCLA Tissue Typing Laboratory, Los Angeles, 1986, p 99.

48. Cicciarelli, J: Transplant center and kidney graft survival. In Terasaki, PI (ed): Clinical Kidney Transplant 1985. UCLA Tissue Typing Laboratory, Los Angeles, 1985, p 93.

49. Sanfilippo, F, et al: The effects of delayed graft function on renal transplantation. Transplant Proc 17:13, 1985.

50. Cho, SI, et al: The influence of acute tubular necrosis on kidney transplant survival. Transplant Proc 17:16, 1985.

51. McGeown, MG, et al: Advantages of low dose steroid from the day after renal transplantation. Transplantation 29:287, 1980.

52. Morris, PJ, et al: Low dose oral prednisolone in renal transplantation. Lancet 1:525, 1982.

53. d'Apice, AJF, et al: A prospective randomized trial of low-dose versus high-dose steroids in cadaveric transplantation. Transplantation 37:373, 1984.

54. d'Apice, AJF: Non-specific immunosuppression: Azathioprine and steroids. In Morris, PJ (ed): Kidney Transplantation, ed 2. Grune & Stratton, London, 1984, p 239.

55. Toledo-Pereyra, LH, et al: Improved results in high risk cadaver kidney transplantation. Proc Dialysis Transplant Forum 10:289, 1980.

56. Starzl, TE, et al: The use of heterologous antilymphoid agents in canine renal and liver homotransplantation. Surg Gynecol Obstet 124:310, 1967.

57. Cosimi, AB: The clinical usefulness of antilymphocyte antibodies. Transplant Proc 15:583, 1983.

58. Hardy, MA: Beneficial effects of heterologous antilymphoid globulins in renal transplantation: One believer's view. Am J Kid Dis 2:79, 1982.

59. Monaco, AP: Antilymphocyte globulin: A clinical transplantation opportunity. Am J Kid Dis 2:67, 1982.

60. Novick, AC, et al: A controlled prospective randomized double blind study of antilymphoblast globulin in cadaver renal transplantation. Transplantation 35:175, 1983.

61. Toledo-Pereyra, LH: Antilymphocyte globulin in kidney transplantation. Proc of the Int Symp on Dialysis and Transplantation, Beijing, China, July 1984.

62. Hardy, MA, et al: Use of ATG in treatment of steroid resistant rejection. Transplantation 29:162, 1980.

63. Filo, RS, Smith, EJ, and Leapman, SB: Reversal of acute renal allograft rejection with adjunctive ATG therapy. Transplant Proc 13:482, 1981.

64. Nowygrod, R, Appel, G, and Hardy, MA: Use of ATG for reversal of acute allograft rejection. Transplant Proc 13:469, 1981.

65. Shield, CF, et al: Use of antithymocyte globulin for reversal of acute allograft rejection. Transplantation 28:461, 1979.

66. Streen, SB, et al: Antilymphoblast globulin for treatment of acute renal allograft rejection. Transplant Proc 15:590, 1983.

67. Toledo-Pereyra, LH, et al: Nonsteroid treatment of rejection in kidney transplantation: A new approach including long term treatment of rejection with antilymphoblast globulin in a high risk population. Transplantation 33:325, 1982.

68. Mittal, VK, et al: Cadaver kidney allograft survival in a high risk black population utilizing antilymphoblast globulin and low steroid therapy. Am J Surg 49:436, 1983.

69. Toledo-Pereyra, LH, et al: Improved results in high risk cadaveric kidney transplantation. Proc Dial Transplant Forum 10:289, 1980.

70. Calne, RY, et al: Cyclosporin A in patients receiving renal allografts from cadaver donors. Lancet 2:1323, 1978.

71. Calne, RY, et al: Cyclosporin A initially as the only immunosuppressant in 34 recipients of cadaveric organs: 32 kidneys, 2 pancreases, and 2 livers. Lancet 2:1033, 1979.

72. Starzl, TE, et al: The use of Cyclosporin A and prednisone in cadaver kidney transplantation. Surg Gynecol Obstet 151:17, 1980.

73. Hakala, TR, et al: Cadaveric renal transplantation with Cyclosporin-A and steroids. Transplant Proc 15:465, 1983.

74. Sutherland, DER, et al: Comparison of cyclosporine and azathioprine for immunosuppression in diabetic and non-diabetic

renal allograft recipients. Transplant Proc 17:1204, 1985.

75. Johnson, RWG, et al: A four-year prospective study of cyclosporine in cadaver renal transplantation. Transplant Proc 17:1197, 1985.

76. Cosimi, AB, et al: Treatment of acute renal allograft rejection with OKT3 monoclonal antibody. Transplantation 32:535, 1981.

77. Thistlewaite, R, et al: Evolving use of OKT3 monoclonal antibody for treatment of renal allograft rejection. Transplantation 38:695, 1984.

78. Cosimi, AB: Treatment of rejection: Antithymocyte globulin versus monoclonal antibodies. Transplant Proc 17:1526, 1985.

79. Ortho Multicenter Transplant Study Group: A randomized clinical trial of OKT3 monoclonal antibody for acute rejection of cadaveric renal transplants. N Engl J Med 313:337, 1985.

SECTION III

REJECTION AND POSTOPERATIVE COMPLICATIONS

Chapter 16

Diagnosis and Management of Rejection

LUIS H. TOLEDO-PEREYRA

The possibility of graft rejection has confronted the clinician since the beginning of clinical renal transplantation, and various means have been used to prevent the host's immune system from mounting a defense against foreign tissue antigens. Early diagnosis and management are important if irreversible graft rejection is to be averted. This chapter discusses the methods now being used for diagnosis of the various types of renal allograft rejection (hyperacute, accelerated, acute, and chronic) and the immunosuppressive strategies employed for reversing these episodes.

HYPERACUTE REJECTION

This type of rejection occurs when the recipient is preimmunized against the histocompatibility antigens of the donor or when there is an ABO incompatibility. Recipient sensitization is usually due to antigen exposure during blood transfusions, pregnancy, or previous organ transplants. The potential for hyperacute rejection is demonstrated before transplantation by the presence of circulating antidonor antibodies in the serum of the recipient with a positive cross-match, which was detailed in Chapter 14. Most instances of hyperacute rejection can be avoided if kidneys are transplanted only when a negative pretransplantation cross-match between recipient sera and donor lymphocytes is obtained.

The hyperacute rejection response begins as preformed antibodies enter the donor kidneys. The antibodies react with the antigenic determinants of endothelial cells of the capillaries of the donor organ. Following activation of complement, polymorphonuclear leukocytes are attracted to the site and destroy endothelial cells. Platelets then attach to the denuded areas of the cap-

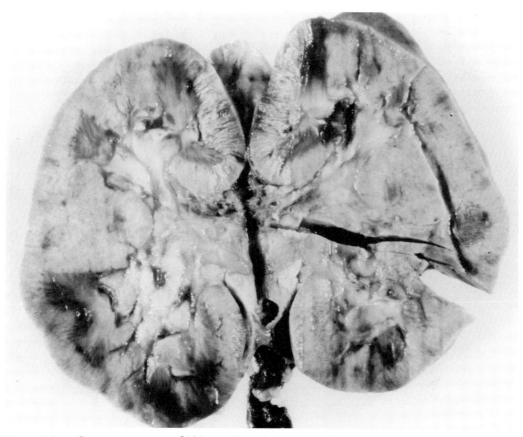

Figure 16–1. Gross appearance of kidney allograft removed after hyperacute rejection shows areas of cortical infarction and necrosis of ureter.

illaries, forming a platelet plug, activating coagulation, and resulting in obstruction of the vessel.[1]

Hyperacute rejection is observed in the renal allograft within minutes of revascularization. There is extensive microthrombosis in glomerular capillaries and juxtaglomerular arterioles. Other vessels such as veins and peritubular capillaries may also thrombose. After the vascular clamps are released, there is a rapid cessation of urine flow, a mottled cyanotic color, and the kidney becomes flaccid (Fig. 16–1), rather than having the normal firm, pink appearance. If the donor-recipient cross-match has been negative and a soft blue kidney is observed immediately after transplantation, the injury may be nonimmunologic in nature.[2] When hyperacute rejection occurs, surgical excision becomes mandatory. Generally no other studies will be required on the operating table to make this decision. When there is considerable doubt, arteriography and renal scan may be performed.[3] Arteriography at this time will show a slowing of or no renal flow, demonstrated by persistence of contrast dye in branches of the transplant arteries. Serious perfusion problems may also be detected by radioactive bolus injection of hippuric acid or technetium. The transplant surgeon then immediately removes the graft.

ACCELERATED REJECTION: DIAGNOSIS AND TREATMENT

Accelerated rejection is defined as a secondary host immune response to the histocompatibility antigens of the graft, occurring between the second and fifth postoperative days. In general, this type of rejection is more resistant than other types of rejection to immunosuppressive agents and is not frequently seen in clinical experience. The accelerated rejection response may be mediated by humoral antibodies and/or primed lymphoblasts. Renal biopsy may be helpful in these cases to differentiate accelerated rejection from oliguria due to acute tubular necrosis. If there is no concurrent infection, suggested treatment consists of methylprednisolone and ALG or ATG, since it is difficult to reverse these rejection episodes with methylprednisolone

alone.[4] Monoclonal antibodies may also be used as an alternative treatment for this type of resistant rejection. If the accelerated rejection is reversed, patients frequently have second and third rejection episodes. Therefore, the likelihood of success is minimal.

ACUTE REJECTION

Acute rejection episodes are observed most frequently in the first 2 weeks after renal transplantation. The frequency, character, and intensity of posttransplantation rejection varies depending on the type of immunosuppression used.[5,6] When azathioprine and prednisolone are given as a basic immunosuppressive regimen, acute rejection episodes frequently appear (75 to 80 percent of cases).[5] If antilymphocyte globulin, prednisolone, and azathioprine are administered prophylactically immediately after transplantation, patients do not frequently experience rejection episodes in the first month after transplant and have only a 60 percent incidence overall.[6] When cyclosporine and prednisolone are given to recipients of cadaver transplantation, the incidence of rejection episodes decreases to between 30 and 35 percent, and the character of the rejection is also changed. Rejection in cyclosporine-treated patients is often mild, rarely as severe as the type of rejection observed when only azathioprine and steroids are given.[6] Monoclonal antibodies are being studied prophylactically for prevention of rejection. More details in the use of immunosuppression have been presented in Chapter 11.

Clinical Symptoms of Acute Rejection

Although acute renal graft rejection is easy to define, it is often difficult to diagnose. Some clinical changes are suggestive of acute rejection; however, none are pathognomonic, and they may have alternative causes[7] (Table 16–1). In general, acute posttransplantation rejection episodes are associated with decreased renal blood flow, increased serum creatinine levels, decreased or halted diuresis, an increase in graft size, increased temperature ($>100°F$),

Table 16-1 Clinical Criteria for Diagnosis of Rejection
Increased serum creatinine ≥0.3–0.5 mg/dl on any day
Decreased urinary output volume (> 25%)
Weight gain (>5 lb)
Kidney swelling
Fever (≥100°F)
Decreased urinary sodium
Proteinuria
Decreased creatinine clearance
Decreased glomerular filtration rate (GRF)

and an increase in arterial blood pressure. However, the last three changes may also be related to complications other than rejection and may be modified by steroid administration. Decreased urinary sodium is observed relative to decreased blood flow. Weight gain in the patient is due to renal failure and exaggerated sodium reabsorption. Proteinuria is observed, but this is also seen during glomerulonephritis, pyelonephritis, and obstructive uropathy. Without proteinuria, however, diagnosis of rejection should be questioned. Decreased creatinine clearance may be a more specific indicator of compromised graft function; however, its use is not practical. Increased serum creatinine concentrations remain the best clinical indicators of rejection.

A rise in the serum creatinine of ≥0.3 to 0.5 mg per dl in a given day is most commonly used to alert the clinician of the potential of an ongoing rejection episode. Various conditions other than rejection, such as ureteral obstruction, lymphocele, arterial stenosis, infection, recurrence of original disease, hyperglycemia, acute tubular necrosis, and drug toxicity, may also cause an elevation of serum creatinine levels.

Because nonrejection causes may elevate serum creatinine, the other concurrent criteria, clinical and laboratory (see Table 16-1), are important in confirming allograft rejection. The use of a rise in serum creatinine alone to diagnose rejection is sometimes not satisfactory, since this change may not occur early enough to be of help in the treatment of rejection.

Other Diagnostic Procedures

Other tests are used to diagnose or predict renal graft rejection episodes. However, not all of these have been applied on a consistent basis. Included in this group are percutaneous renal biopsy, angiography, intravenous pyelography, ultrasound scans, fine-needle aspiration biopsy, fine-needle intrarenal manometry, radionuclide imaging, nuclear magnetic resonance imaging, immunologic monitoring, neopterin determinations, serum-C-reactive protein measurements, urinary exfoliative cytology, fibrinopeptide A and B levels, and beta-2-microglobulin excretion.

Percutaneous Renal Biopsy

The "gold standard" for confirmation of a diagnosis of acute rejection remains the renal biopsy. Since percutaneous renal biopsy is an invasive procedure, not all transplant centers have regularly employed this technique. There are risks of injury to the renal vessels, hemorrhage, and kidney loss; however, various transplant groups have biopsied several hundred transplanted kidneys without any complications.[7] Even so, others remain reluctant and only rarely perform renal biopsies. In general, renal biopsies are used only after an initial rise in serum creatinine is noted, and they have not been used to detect early rejection or to predict a rejection episode. The renal biopsy is very useful in ruling out rejection as an etiology for elevated serum creatinine levels. In patients with prolonged ATN (>2 weeks), we frequently recommend a renal biopsy to determine if the cause of delayed graft function is graft rejection superimposed on acute tubular necrosis (ATN).

On histologic examination, acute rejection is associated with characteristic pathology (Table 16-2), which is discussed in detail in Chapter 17. Briefly, there is a prevalence of interstitial lesions and a marked and diffuse edema and infiltration of round cells, generally in the perivascular region. Peritubular capillaries appear dilated, also with round cell infiltration. Deposits of IgG, IgM, and C3 confined to glomeruli or arterioles and vessels can be seen using immunofluorescence studies.[8]

Mozes and associates[9] have studied the usefulness of percutaneous Tru-cut renal

Table 16–2 Characteristic Pathology Associated with Acute Renal Allograft Rejection*
1. Tubulointerstitial nephritis with widespread edema
2. Focal cortical infiltration by lymphocytes, lymphoblasts, plasma cells, and eosinophils
3. Endothelial swelling of peritubular and glomerular capillaries and arterioles
4. Fibrinoid necrosis of small arteries and arterioles
5. Platelet aggregates and fibrin thrombi in glomerular and peritubular capillaries
6. Foci of tubular necrosis with infiltration of the tubular wall with a mixed cellular infiltrate
*Criteria from Finkelstein et al.[8]

biopsies in the prediction of subsequent acute rejection episodes and graft outcome. Biopsy specimens were obtained at the initiation of treatment for rejection and 10–12 days later. The researchers found that the initial clinical or biopsy grade and the clinical response to treatment were inaccurate parameters for prediction of subsequent acute rejection episodes and graft outcome. Biopsies obtained after the rejection treatment yielded more useful information. Complete resolution of the post-treatment biopsy accurately predicted the absence of subsequent acute rejection episodes in the majority of patients. Incomplete resolution of the post-treatment biopsy was highly sensitive in predicting failure. The post-treatment biopsy, therefore, added useful information in patients who by clinical criteria appear to have complete response to treatment of rejection.

Angiography

This test is useful for providing information regarding vascular perfusion changes in the kidney, for identifying the presence of cortical infarcts, and for assessing the blood flow through the renal artery.[10] It is therefore useful for identifying decreased renal perfusion but is somewhat inadequate to diagnose acute rejection (Fig. 16–2).

Intravenous Pyelography

This technique is helpful in excluding nonimmunologic causes of renal failure such as urinary leak and obstructive uropathy. However, its application during compromised renal function may result in further transient deterioration in renal function.[11]

Ultrasound Scan

This diagnostic tool has assumed a major role in renal transplantation and is often the first investigation used, especially since it is noninvasive. It is more reliable than many other tests to assess renal status post-transplantation and can be performed as frequently as necessary. The superficial position of the renal allograft in the iliac fossa additionally facilitates the use of ultrasound. In addition, ultrasound offers the advantage of exploring perirenal and perivesical spaces. The use of high-frequency transducers allows for satisfactory corticomedullary differentiation and accurate study of the renal sinus. Ultrasonography has been applied by some centers for the diagnosis of renal graft rejection. It is also used to diagnose obstruction, perirenal fluid collection, hematoma, lymphocele, cyclosporine toxicity, and abscess after renal transplantation.[12,13,14]

Fine-Needle Aspiration Biopsy (FNAB)

This technique was first performed by Pasternack[15] in 1968 for monitoring the course of renal transplants. Its development was based on the observation that the rejection process occurs earlier and more strongly within the transplanted allograft than in the peripheral blood or lymphoid organs of the recipient. Therefore, monitoring inflammatory cellular changes in the graft is potentially better than peripheral monitoring. Monocytes are attracted to the site of rejection by lymphokines produced by T cells. The cytotoxic and phagocytic activity of the macrophages is also activated by the lymphokines.

Using the FNAB technique, representa-

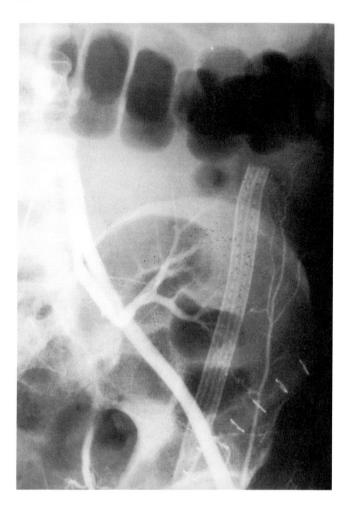

Figure 16–2. In this renal arteriogram of a living related kidney transplant, the end-to-end anastomosis between the transplanted kidney and the left internal iliac artery was widely patent. Rapid tapering of the main arterial branches within the transplanted kidney and nonvisualization of the small arteriolar branches were noted. These findings were compatible with the diagnosis of severe rejection.

tive specimens containing approximately 7 to 50 tubular cells per 100 inflammatory cells are taken[16–20] (Fig. 16–3). The aspirate is evaluated to determine whether there is inflammation; to enumerate the number of blast cells, lymphocytes, monocytes, and macrophages; and to assess the overall morphology of the tubular and endothelial cells, including necrotic changes (Table 16–3). In early acute graft inflammation, blast cells and lymphocytes dominate the cytologic patterns. In advanced severe rejection, the picture is dominated by macrophages and monocytes. In kidneys undergoing ATN, tubular cells appear swollen and other degenerative changes are present in the cytoplasm. In cases of cyclosporine nephrotoxicity, there occur nonspecific changes in the tubular cells, including swelling, vacuolation and increased basophilia. Endothelial cells may also be heavily vacuolated.[16]

A number of studies have shown that the presence of monocytes in the glomerulus of renal allografts and their number increases with the severity of rejection.[17] In studies by Hayry and Von Willebrand,[16] the presence of monocytes in the interstitium and in the glomerulus correlated well with a poor graft prognosis. Egidi and associates[18] have found that patients without clinical evidence of rejection may exhibit different cellular patterns of FNAB according to the immunosuppression used. Activated lymphocytes and monocytes were only rarely seen in azathioprine-treated patients with stable renal function. Patients treated with cyclosporine and steroids exhibited a cell population that consisted mainly of activated lymphocytes and monocytes. This

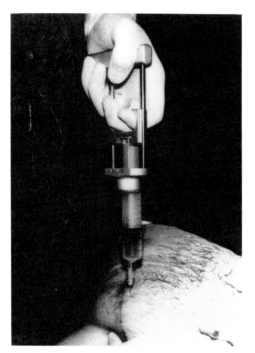

Figure 16–3. Fine-needle aspiration biopsy shows aspiration from the upper pole of a transplanted kidney using a 25-gauge needle and a syringe in a pistol-grip syringe holder. (From Wood,[19] with permission.)

difference has been postulated to be related to cyclosporine nephrotoxicity, which can cause focal inflammation, or to a peculiar immunosuppressive mechanism of cyclosporine, which may modulate the in situ development of lymphoblasts. Patients treated with cyclosporine alone showed an even more marked pattern of cellular activation, which was followed within a few days by clinical rejection.

One of the advantages of fine-needle as-

piration biopsy as a diagnostic tool is that it is easily repeated and can even be performed daily. The major drawback of this technique is that specially trained personnel are needed to read the specimens, and sample adequacy is an important factor in determining the reproducibility of fine-needle aspiration biopsy.[19]

However, in experienced hands, FNAB appears to be a valuable tool for predicting rejection of renal transplants, especially in the early months after transplantation. At that time intragraft events are more easily accessible by this technique. When false-negative results are obtained, at least half of them may be correlated with the histologic lesions of chronic rejection observed using traditional renal biopsies.[20]

Fine-Needle Manometry

It has been observed that intrarenal pressure only rarely accompanies ATN and cyclosporine nephrotoxicity episodes,[21] whereas pressures greater than 40 mmHg are associated with acute rejection.[21] Fine-needle manometry is performed by introducing a 25G spinal needle into the kidney. Ideally, pressures are monitored weekly, more frequently if renal function is declining or absent. If the intrarenal pressure is less than 40 mmHg and renal function is declining, the clinician should suspect cyclosporine nephrotoxicity and reduce the cyclosporine dose. Intrarenal pressures greater than 40 mmHg should lead to suspicion of graft rejection if renal function is also compromised. Antirejection therapy should be initiated in these cases (Table 16–4). Studies by Salaman and Griffin,[21] in 37 patients, indicated that an increase in

---

Table 16–3 Posttransplant Cytologic Patterns Observed with Fine-Needle Aspiration Biopsies*

Early acute graft inflammation	Blast cell, lymphocytes
Advanced severe rejection	Macrophages, monocytes
Acute tubular necrosis	Swollen tubular cells, vacuolation, and other cytoplasmic degenerative changes
Cyclosporine nephrotoxicity	Nonspecific changes in tubular cells; swelling, vacuolation, increased basophilia; endothelial cells may be heavily vacuolated

*Chapter 17 discusses the pathologic changes of rejection.

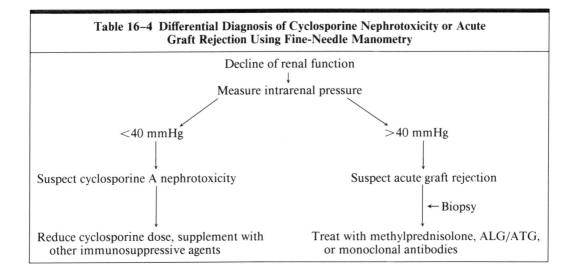

Table 16–4 Differential Diagnosis of Cyclosporine Nephrotoxicity or Acute Graft Rejection Using Fine-Needle Manometry

Decline of renal function

↓

Measure intrarenal pressure

<40 mmHg   >40 mmHg

↓   ↓

Suspect cyclosporine A nephrotoxicity   Suspect acute graft rejection

← Biopsy

↓

Reduce cyclosporine dose, supplement with other immunosuppressive agents   Treat with methylprednisolone, ALG/ATG, or monoclonal antibodies

---

pressure always correlated with rejection. Pressures did not increase, however, in patients with cyclosporine nephrotoxicity.

Immunological Monitoring

In the past decade several standard immunological tests have been proposed to prognosticate renal graft rejection. The details of these applications are discussed in Chapter 14. In general, while changes in vitro often correlate well with compromised renal function, occurring with the onset of rejection, no one test can be consistently used to predict rejection earlier or more accurately than the combination of clinical signs including serum creatinine levels. In addition, the cost of routinely performing many of these tests is prohibitive.

Radionuclide Imaging

Several techniques have been used for diagnosis of rejection and for differentiating rejection from other causes of serum creatinine elevation. ^{131}I-orthoiodohippurate excretion is used to assess renal tubular function. It is accurate, but in general, only well-established rejections can be detected.[22] ^{131}I-hippuran scans are used by some centers to differentiate among acute and chronic rejection, ATN, and obstruction.[23] However, they are not useful to differentiate cyclosporine toxicity from rejection. ^{99m}Tc-DTPA is applied for evaluating renal blood flow and its distribution in the kidney, especially when ATN causes anuria immediately after transplantation. This scan is limited because it may lack sensitivity and specificity.[24,25] [111]In platelet scintigraphy has been used to demonstrate that autologous platelets labeled with[111] In-oxine accumulate in rejecting renal allografts.[26–29] One of the advantages to the use of this isotope is that it is short-lived (28 days). Labeling platelets does not appear to alter function significantly. Imaging with a gamma camera is possible for up to 7 days following a single injection of labeled platelets. Desir and colleagues[29] found that they could diagnose untreated acute renal allograft rejections with a sensitivity of 84 percent and a specificity of 100 percent. False negatives occurred only in patients with mild to moderate cellular rejection, probably because platelet accumulation is not the predominant finding in cellular rejection. Patients with ATN or cyclosporine toxicity had uptake indices in normal range. [111]In platelet scintigraphy was not useful, however, for following the course of the rejection episode. A decrease in the platelet uptake index did not necessarily correlate with a favorable clinical outcome.

Nuclear Magnetic Resonance (NMR)

Proton NMR imaging has been used on a limited basis for evaluating impaired graft function following renal transplantation.[30,31] This technique offers the advantage of providing excellent spatial resolution in a noninvasive manner without the use of radiation or intravenous contrast. During acute rejection episodes an overall loss of signal intensity and a decrease in corticomedullary differentiation was observed. In kidneys undergoing ATN, similar but less consistent findings were seen. Therefore, perhaps further studies in this area are necessary to refine the role of NMR for diagnosing acute rejection episodes (Figs. 16–4, 16–5, and 16–6).

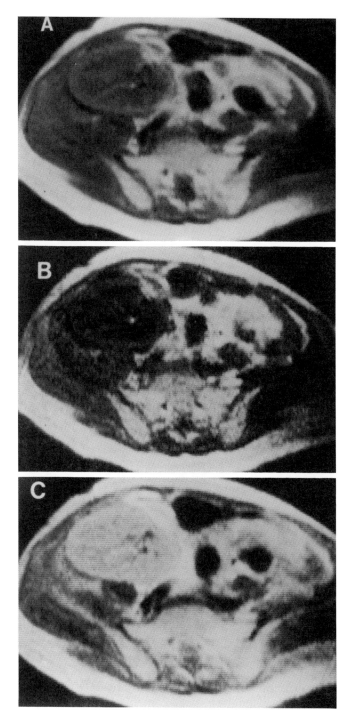

Figure 16–4. Nuclear magnetic imaging of a normal kidney using various pulsing sequences. (*A*) (SE 50/500 msec.) The corticomedullary junction is visualized. The cortex has a higher image intensity than the medulla. (*B*) (IR 30/150 [450] msec.) The spatial resolution is decreased and the contrast is increased. Therefore, the distinction between cortex and medulla is better, even though anatomical details are less well visualized. (*C*) (SE 60/1000 msec.) The corticomedullary junction is not visualized. (From Hau, et al,[30] with permission.)

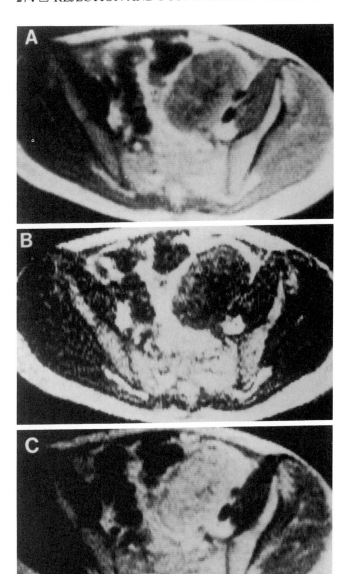

Figure 16–5. These NMR were taken during acute rejection episodes using various pulsing sequences. (*A*) (SE 30/500 msec.) An increase in renal size and loss of corticomedullary junction are demonstrated. (*B*) (IR 30/150 [450] msec.) An increase in renal size and loss of corticomedullary junction are demonstrated. (*C*) (SE 60/1000 msec.) As in the normal kidney in Fig. 16–4*C*, the corticomedullary junction is not visualized. (From Hau, et al,[30] with permission.)

Beta-2 Microglobulin Excretion

This 12,000-dalton class I antigen histocompatibility protein is synthesized by cells bearing these antigens. It is normally found free in serum in low concentrations and is freely filtered by the renal glomerulus. Since synthesis of this protein is relatively constant, the concentration of beta-2 microglobulin in serum reflects the glomerular filtration rate, and concentrations in urine tubular function. Beta-2 microglobulin has therefore been monitored after renal transplantation to determine renal function. Clinical applications of serial beta-2 microglobulin monitoring have determined that there is a good correlation between changes in beta-2 microglobulin levels and changes in serum creatinine. However, whether increases in beta-2 microglobulin always precede increase in serum creatinine and are therefore a more sensitive predictor of rejection remains controversial.[32] In addition, elevations of

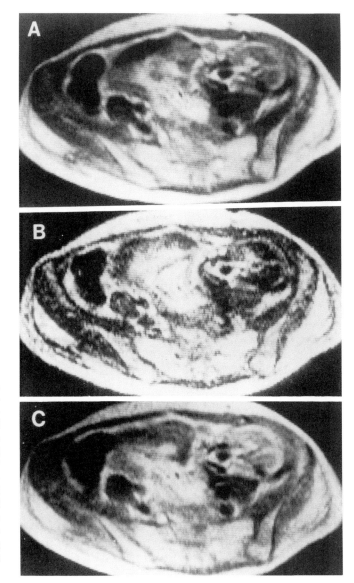

Figure 16–6. NMR studies of a kidney allograft during acute tubular necrosis using various pulsing sequences. (*A*) (SE 30/500 msec.) An increase in differentiation between the cortex and the medulla can be seen. (*B*) (IR 30/150 [450] msec.) Increased differentiation between the cortex and the medulla can be seen. (*C*) (SE 60/1000 msec.) The corticomedullary junction is visible in contradistinction to normal and rejecting kidneys. (From Hau, et al,[30] with permission.)

beta-2 microglobulin have also been observed during viral and bacterial infections and other inflammatory processes.

Several studies have found that changes in serial serum beta-2 microglobulin determinations are more sensitive, more specific, and less affected by acute tubular necrosis and that they significantly precede changes in serum creatinine.[32–35]

Vernon and associates[36] have challenged these findings. They have observed that beta-2 microglobulin levels vary widely on a day-to-day basis. Therefore, it would not be unexpected for random rises in serum beta-2 microglobulin levels to correlate with acute rejection episodes. When beta-2 microglobulin changes were observed with uncomplicated courses and in those with acute rejection without ATN, elevations in beta-2 microglobulin did not precede a change in serum creatinine. Based on these findings, the authors did not recommend use of serum beta-2 microglobulin as the sole monitor of renal function following transplantation. (Table 16–5).

Neopterin

Recently, urinary and serum neopterin levels have been monitored to diagnose re-

Table 16–5 Means and Variance of Serum Creatinine and Serum Beta-2 Microglobulin in Patients with Uncomplicated Posttransplantation Courses, Acute Rejection Episodes Without ATN, or ATN During Immediate Posttransplantation Hospitalization*

| | Uncomplicated | | Acute Rejection Without ATN | | ATN | |
	Mean	*Variance*	*Mean*	*Variance*	*Mean*	*Variance*
β2M (mg/L)	2.6200	0.3440	5.7600	12.6000	14.900	90.90
Δ β2M (mg/L)	−0.0983	0.0316	−0.0028	0.2180	−0.629	1.33
Creatinine (mg/dl)	1.7300	0.2230	2.5800	1.1200	8.370	12.00
Δ Creatinine (mg/dl)	−0.1230	0.0313	−0.0759	0.0246	−0.398	0.10

*From Vernon et al,[36] with permission.

jection prior to the induction of significant cellular damage and the subsequent rise in serum creatinine.[37] Activation of T lymphocytes releases interferon gamma, which in turn activates guanosine-triphosphate-specific cyclohydrolase in macrophages. This leads to the increased synthesis and excretion of neopterin. Studies by Schafer and associates[37] retrospectively evaluated plasma neopterin levels in 172 renal transplant patients. In general, high neopterin levels (500 to 1000 nmol per liter) were observed in patients who had rejection episodes, and reduced plasma neopterin values (100 nmol per liter) were seen in patients with stable graft function. There was a high correlation between changes in plasma neopterin and serum creatinine values; however, viral infection also can cause an elevated neopterin level.

In other studies by Magalini and coworkers[38] on patients receiving cyclosporine, recognition of the strict dependence of urinary neopterin excretion on body weight seemed to increase the validity of using urinary neopterin excretion to diagnose rejection. Urinary neopterin levels were higher in lighter-weight patients, independent of rejection (Table 16–6). Urinary neopterin levels divided by body weight were higher during rejection than during periods of nonrejection in patients with good or poor kidney function. Magalini and colleagues have also studied the behavior of N-acetyl-beta-glucosamine (NAG), an index of tubular damage, in relation to changes in urinary neopterin excretion. With higher cyclosporine blood levels, urinary neopterin excretion diminishes while NAG rises. NAG is a sensitive indicator of nephrotoxicity, while urinary excretion expresses the degree of immunoactivation or immunosuppression. Urinary neopterin can probably best be used as part of a multiparameter analysis. Noel and associates[39] found that urinary neopterin excretion was a less sensitive tool for diagnosis of rejection in patients receiving ATG, since ATG induces an immunologic response.

Table 16–6 Association of Urinary Neopterin Excretion and Body Weight

Body weight	<50 kg	>50 kg
Number of patients	6	17
Determinations	83	179
Urinary neopterin excretion (mean ± SD)	756 ± 459	336 ± 181
Mean body weight (kg ± SD)	30 ± 10	60 ± 10

Serum C-Reactive Protein (CRP)

CRP is synthesized in response to bacterial infection and tissue injury. Its biologic activities include opsonization of bacteria and binding of autogenous material released from necrotic tissue.[40] It is usually produced in nanogram quantities, but synthesis increases as much as 1000-fold within hours after the onset of inflammation.[41] Therefore, serial monitoring of serum CRP levels has the potential of serving as a sensitive indicator of acute tissue injury or inflammation. However, the major problem with using CRP to monitor the posttransplantation course of renal allograft recipients is that one cannot differentiate a rise in CRP due to bacterial infection from that due to tissue injury. In recipients of renal allografts receiving high-dose steroids, the CRP is often elevated prior to episodes of graft rejection.[41–45] It has been difficult to diagnose renal transplant rejection in cyclosporine-treated patients. This suggests that cyclosporine may interfere with the stimulus of the production of IL-1, which induces CRP synthesis.[46] In living related recipients, however, given azathioprine, methylprednisolone, and antilymphoblast globulin as immunosuppression, serum CRP levels were found to be elevated during severe rejection episodes, but not during mild or chronic rejection.[46]

Urinary Exfoliative Cytology

Several investigators have studied the value of exfoliative urinary cytology for the diagnosis of pathologic conditions in renal transplantation.[47–50] The presence of lymphocytes has been considered by some as a sign of an acute rejection episode. Examination of urinary sediment in various studies has favorably compared with results obtained from standard needle biopsies. This technique offers the advantages of being noninvasive, providing rapid evidence of rejection, and aiding in the differentiation of cyclosporine toxicity from rejection. One problem with the method has been difficulty in obtaining a reliable identification of the different cells by means of standard staining techniques. To improve this, computerized flow cytometry techniques have been applied to the analysis of urinary sediment cells. Studies involving flow cytometry indicate that lymphocyturia alone may not be considered as pathognomonic for acute rejection. There was a difference between the T cell subset population in rejecting kidneys and in bacterial urinary tract infections. Rejecting kidneys were found to be positive for OKT3, OKT4, OKT8, and OKT11, whereas during bacterial infection the lymphocyte pattern was characterized by a slight increase in OKT3, a reduction in OKT11, and elevated OKT4 and OKT8.[50]

Fibrinopeptide A (FPA) and Fibrinopeptide B-Beta (FPB-Beta)

The diagnostic significance of urinary FPA and FPB-beta has been recently evaluated by Kano and associates[51] during acute rejection episodes in renal transplantation recipients given cyclosporine as immunosuppression. Both FPA and FPB-beta were found to rise during acute rejection (Fig. 16–7). The authors found that measurement of FPA and FPB-beta was useful for diagnosing rejection during cyclosporine treatment because it is sensitive and noninvasive. Future studies will define the role of FPA and FPB-beta as prognostic indicators of rejection.

Diagnosis of Cyclosporine Nephrotoxicity

Since the initiation of cyclosporine as an immunosuppressive agent, the clinician has had to become aware of the potential for nephrotoxicity resulting from the use of this drug.[52] When cyclosporine toxicity is suspected, it is often difficult to differentiate it from graft rejection[53] (Table 16–7). In some cases, diagnosis of cyclosporine nephrotoxicity may be obvious; in others it may be more subtle; and in some transplant recipients diagnosis may be very difficult. An increase in serum creatinine and blood urea nitrogen and a decrease in the glomerular filtration rate may be apparent at the beginning. Cyclosporine nephrotoxicity may be deduced if the reduction in cyclosporine dosage leads to improvement in renal function. It is also helpful to monitor trough serum cyclosporine levels, especially to identify patients who are clearly

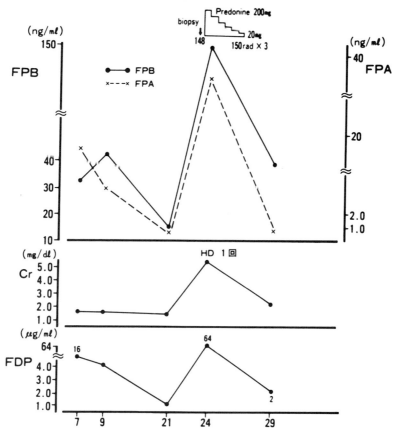

Figure 16–7. Typical elevation in fibrinopeptide A and fibrinopeptide B-beta during rejection episode. Changes in serum creatinine and fibrin-fibrinogen degradation products are also displayed. (From Kano, et al,[51] with permission.)

Table 16–7 Diagnosis and Treatment of Cyclosporine Toxicity
Increased serum creatinine at ≥24 hours posttransplantation
Increased serum cyclosporine 0.5 mg/dl above baseline levels
Increased weight gain (>5 lb)
Decreased urine output (<25%)
Ultrasound findings
Diagnosis of rejection: increased kidney size, enlarging medulla, thickening cortex, and increasing echogenicity of the renal pyramids
Diagnosis of ATN: relatively similar findings
Diagnosis of cyclosporine toxicity: normal ultrasound
Renogram findings
Diagnosis of rejection: delayed accumulation, excretion, and clearance of the isotope
Diagnosis of ATN: similar findings as for rejection, but with normal perfusion
Diagnosis of cyclosporine toxicity: similar to findings with ATN

nephrotoxic or clearly underdosed. Cantarovich[54] has found that sampling at 6 hours after cyclosporine administration rather than at 14 to 16 hours, as is the case at most transplantation centers,[55] may provide a better differentiation between cyclosporine nephrotoxicity and acute rejection episodes. The use of renal biopsies has not been consistent in assisting in differentiation between cyclosporine nephrotoxicity and rejection. If there is an absence of histologic abnormalities on renal biopsy, cyclosporine toxicity should be presumed and the cyclosporine dose should be reduced. A change to alternative immunosuppressive coverage should be considered. Severe rejection will also be apparent from histologic examination. However, when lesions are less severe, it is more difficult to distinguish between rejection and nephrotoxicity.

In retrospective studies at our center, the role of ultrasound in the diagnosis of cyclosporine toxicity after renal transplantation was analyzed in 22 transplantations.[14] We concluded that a normal renal ultrasound and a renal isotope scan consistent with acute tubular necrosis, accompanied by increasing serum creatinine levels at ≥ 24 hours posttransplantation was suggestive of cyclosporine toxicity.

Concurrent ATN and Acute Rejection

In some cases, ATN may occur concurrently with acute rejection. Since the possibility of nephrotoxicity exists, cyclosporine should be administered with caution, if at all, and alternative immunosuppressive approaches should be considered.

MANAGEMENT OF ACUTE REJECTION

Acute rejection episodes after renal transplantation have been handled in a variety of ways using only a few drugs. In the early transplantation experience, rejection was treated by increasing oral steroid dosages or by intravenous bolus methylprednisolone. As polyclonal antilymphocyte globulin preparations such as ALG and ATG became available, they were tested es-

pecially for the treatment of first rejection episodes. Some centers, such as our own, have also used ALG for treatment of multiple rejection episodes. More recently, monoclonal antilymphocyte preparations such as OKT3 have been used to treat acute rejection. Many centers are choosing to use several alternative antirejection protocols, especially in patients whose rejections do not respond to steroid treatment.

Steroid Therapy

Since the earliest days of renal transplantation, methylprednisolone (MP) has been one of the most commonly administered forms of nonspecific antirejection therapy. Either high-dose oral prednisolone (up to 200 mg per day for 3 days, with subsequent tapering) or intravenous bolus methylprednisolone (250 to 1000 mg per day for 3 days) may be given to treat acute rejection. If, after 3 to 5 days, there is no improvement, incomplete response, or another rejection crisis, another course of steroids could be considered. A third course of these drugs, however, is rarely prescribed. At our center, we have opted for ALG/ATG when a second course of immunosuppression is needed to treat rejection episodes.

Immediate side effects of steroid therapy may include increased susceptibility to bacterial and viral infections, gastrointestinal hemorrhage, metabolic abnormalities, such as hyperglycemia, and others (Table 16–8; see Chapter 11). Although MP may be successful in reversing the majority (70 percent) of acute rejection episodes,[56] some rejection remains steroid-resistant, and alternative immunosuppression must be pursued.[57] Also, the morbidity and mortality associated with high steroid dosages has led the clinician to the use of lower dosages and a search for alternatives for antirejection therapy, especially in high-risk patients.

Polyclonal Antilymphocyte Globulin Preparations

The morbidity that often resulted from excessive steroid administration in patients receiving azathioprine and prednisone as maintenance immunosuppression encour-

---

Table 16–8 Potential Side-Effects and Complications of Steroid Administration for Acute Renal Allograft Rejection

---

Sodium retention, fluid retention, congestive heart failure in susceptible patients, potassium loss, hypokalemic alkalosis, hypertension

Muscle weakness, steroid myopathy, loss of muscle mass, osteoporosis, vertebral compression fractures, aseptic necrosis of femoral and humeral heads, pathologic fracture of long bones

Peptic ulcer with possible perforation and hemorrhage, pancreatitis, abdominal distention, ulcerative esophagitis

Impaired wound healing; thin, fragile skin; petechiae and ecchymoses; facial erythema; increased sweating; may suppress reactions to skin tests

Increased intracranial pressure with papilledema, usually after treatment; convulsions; vertigo; headache

Development of cushingoid state; suppression of growth in children; secondary adrenocortical and pituitary unresponsiveness, particularly in times of stress, as in trauma, surgery, or illness; menstrual irregularities; decreased carbohydrate tolerance; manifestations of latent diabetes mellitus; increased requirements for insulin or oral hypoglycemic agents in diabetics

Posterior subcapsular cataracts, increased intraocular pressure, glaucoma, exophthalmos

Negative nitrogen balance arising from protein catabolism

---

aged the use of antilymphoid globulin preparations for the treatment of acute allograft rejection. These have been developed by immunizing horses, rabbits, or goats with human thymocytes, lymphoblasts, or thoracic duct lymphocytes. After each animal develops antibodies to the injection, serum is pooled and unwanted antibodies are removed. Stabilizers are added to the preparation and microbial testing is performed. The polyclonal antiserum (ALG or ATG) is then ready for patient administration.

These drugs have been successfully used at our center and others in two sets of circumstances[57–75]: first as sole antirejection treatment or with steroids, and second, to reverse steroid-resistant rejection episodes.

Disadvantages to the use of ALG/ATG include problems with consistent potency and allergic reactions (Table 16–9). The most common side effects of ALG/ATG administration include fever and chills, erythema, pruritus, local phlebitis, anaphylaxis, arthralgia, thrombocytopenia, and serum sickness.[57,58]

The protocol used at our center for ALG/ATG administration for rejection employs a 10 to 14 day course of ALG or ATG to avert graft loss, while reducing the amount of steroids used[60,69] (Table 16–10). When a

---

Table 16–9 Potential Side Effects and Complications of ALG/ATG Administration

Fever	Hypotension
Chills	Nausea
Leukopenia	Vomiting
Thrombocytopenia	Night sweats
Rash	Pain at infusion site
Pruritus	Peripheral thrombophlebitis
Urticaria	Stomatitis
Wheal and flare	Anaphylaxis
Arthralgia	Dizziness
Chest or back pain	Weakness or faintness
Diarrhea	Edema
Dyspnea	Herpes simplex reactivation
Headache	

Table 16-10 Suggested Protocol for Management of Rejection with ALG

1. No intravenous methylprednisolone
2. No increase in oral steroids
3. No increase in azathioprine levels

First rejection: ALG, 15–20 mg/kg/day for 10 days
Second rejection: ALG, 15–20 mg/kg/day for 10 days
Third rejection: ALG, 15–20 mg/kg/day for 5–10 days with or without total lymph node irradiation
Fourth and subsequent rejection: Periodic intermittent ALG at 10–20 mg/kg/day every 4th to 5th day depending upon creatinine level, patient's response, and general condition

---

rejection episode is identified, there is no increase in methylprednisolone, oral steroids, or azathioprine, and a dose of ALG or ATG (15 to 20 mg per kg per day) is given for 10 to 14 days. We have found that this approach is especially useful in cases of steroid-resistant rejection.[60,69] Some investigators have also used ATG as an adjunct to low-dose steroid therapy.[66] In summary, clinical trials using ALG or ATG to treat rejection have shown that these drugs are effective agents and can be used either as adjunctive or sole therapy to reverse acute rejection episodes in about 80 to 85 percent of the cases (Table 16–11).

Monoclonal Antibodies

Monoclonal antibodies have also been recently tested in clinical trials for the treatment of acute rejection[76-82] (Table 16–12). The use of monoclonal preparations has the potential of being more specific, with less variability from batch to batch, than

available polyclonal ALG/ATG, since they are produced from clones derived from a single cell. Table 16–12 shows the results of the various monoclonal preparations that have been tested as primary antirejection therapy and in cases of steroid-resistant rejection episodes. The monoclonal antibody therapy, especially OKT3, appears to be effective in both of these applications, and in many patients (33 to 84 percent) rejection does not recur.

Initial trials using OKT3 directed against mature human T cells to treat rejection, have shown that it is effective in reversing first acute rejection episodes.[76-79] Maintenance immunosuppression, usually azathioprine and prednisolone, are reduced during OKT3 therapy. In a recent study using OKT3 to treat rejection in 32 patients, 100 percent of the first rejection episodes were reversed.[76]

Side effects of monoclonal therapy have included fever and chills and occasionally bronchospasm, beginning 30 to 40 min after initiation of therapy.[76-79] Other com-

---

Table 16-11 Results of Randomized Trials Comparing Steroids with ATG Plus Steroids for Treatment of Acute Renal Allograft Rejection

Author	Number of Patients in Study	Rejection Reversal (%)		Maintenance Immunosuppression
		Steroids	*Steroids + ATG*	
Filo et al[62]	52	62	91	Aza + Steroids
Howard et al[61]	64	75	100	Aza + Steroids
Nowygrod et al[63]	52	75	84	Aza + Steroids
Streem et al[64]	23	83*	100†	Aza + Steroids ± ALG
Hoitsma et al[75]	100	64	84	Aza + Steroids

*Azathioprine + high-dose prednisone (maintenance immunosuppression).
†Azathioprine + ALG + low-dose prednisone (maintenance immunosuppression).

	Monoclonal	Reversal	
Study	Antibody	Rejection (%)	Recurrence (%)
Cosimi[76]	OKT3	100	66
Kreis and Goldstein[77]	OKT3	94	66
Goldstein et al[78]	OKT3	>90 (60*)	—
Norman et al[79]	OKT3	96 (77*)	58 (40*)
Takahashi et al[80]	CBL 1	(80*)	(30*)
Oei et al[81]	CHAL 1	(64*)	(33*)
Oei et al[81]	CBL 1	(50)	(55)

Table 16–12 Use of Monoclonal Antibodies to Treat Acute Renal Graft Rejection

T cell specificity: OKT3 = pan T cell; CBL 1 = proliferating blast cells; CHAL 1 = T cells, B cells, monocytes.
*Steroid-resistant rejection.

plications are listed in Table 16–13. Some monoclonal antibodies, however, have been given without complications.

Another drawback to monoclonal therapy has been the development of antibodies against the monoclonal preparation, which prevents subsequent use of these drugs.[76,77,78,79] The high rate of recurrence of rejection within days or months after discontinuing OKT3, in as many as two thirds of the treated patients, is also a disadvantage.[76,77]

In prospective randomized multicenter trials reported by Goldstein and associates,[78] OKT3 antirejection therapy was compared with high-dose steroids for treatment of rejection. In OKT3-treated patients, rejection was reversed in 94 percent of the rejection episodes, whereas steroid treatment yielded only a 75 percent rate of reversal of rejection. The subsequent transplant courses were similar in both groups. Graft survival in the OKT3-treated patients was significantly better (approximately 70 percent) as compared with the steroid group (approximately 50 percent).

Kirkman and colleagues[82] have also reported on the initial trial of another monoclonal antibody, anti-T12, which is directed against all post-thymic lymphocytes. Of 19 patients treated for acute renal graft rejection, 7 had a good response, 4 had an equivocal response, and 7 failed to respond.

In summary, when OKT3 is used to reverse first acute rejection episodes, they are successfully treated in almost all cases, usually without the need for high-dose steroids. However, patients remain at risk for subsequent rejection episodes when OKT3 is used. Therefore, refinements in the protocols are required for improving long-term graft survival.

Table 16–13 Potential Side-Effects and Complications of Monoclonal Antibody Administration

Pyrexia
Chills
Dyspnea
Headaches
Chest pain
Vomiting
Wheezing
Nausea
Diarrhea
Tremor
Severe pulmonary edema
Infection
Development of antimurine antibodies

Plasma Exchange and Plasmaleukopheresis Therapy

At a few transplant centers, plasma exchange therapy and plasmaleukopheresis have been used either alone or with standard antirejection therapy to treat steroid-resistant acute rejection episodes.[83-92] They are used in an attempt to lower the levels of anti-HLA antibodies in humorally mediated steroid-resistant rejection episodes. Various plasma exchange protocols have been used (Table 16–14). Some of these trials have indicated a beneficial effect in reversing renal graft rejection, while others have indicated no significant effect. Approximately half of the patients responded well, with reversal of graft rejection and retention of their grafts. In summary, while plasma exchange and plasmaleukopheresis

Table 16–14 Selective Review of Clinical Applications of Plasma Exchange or Plasmaleukopheresis Therapy for Treatment of Renal Allograft Rejection

Author	Uncontrolled Series Plasma Exchange Protocol	Maintenance of Allograft
Cardella et al[83]	2–8 days, 3–4 L exchange	3/5*
Cardella et al[84]	3–10 treatments, 4 L exchange	2/8*
Naik et al[85]	6 treatments, 2.5 L exchange, alternate days	0/6† 2/5‡
Kurland et al[86]	Plasma leukopheresis, 4 L exchange, 6 days + bolus steroids/day × 3	1/1†
Darr et al[87]	5 daily plasmaleukopheresis treatments on alternate days, 1 plasma volume exchange, then 1/week for up to 3 months alternate days	11/20*

Author	Controlled Series Plasma Exchange Protocol	Results
Cardella et al[88]	Bolus steroids + 4 L exchange for 5 days	No difference between 15 plasmapheresis and 22 controls†
Kirubakaran et al[89]	Bolus steroids + 4 L exchange day 1, 2 L on days 2, 3, 4, 5, 6, 7, 11, and 13	8 of 12 patients in treated and control group returned to dialysis†
Gailiunas et al[90]	5 consecutive two-body volume exchanges + bolus steroids for 5 days	8 of 9 patients improved function within 1 week of treatment, but only 2 of 9 patients retained graft function after 3 months
Langley et al[91]	2.5–3.5 L exchanges × 10	18 of 41 patients lost their grafts (9 within 60 days). Graft survival (1 year) (total group = 81%); plasmapheresis group = 70%
Cardella et al[92]	Conventional antirejection therapy (ART) with/ without 5 day intensive plasma exchange	1-year graft survival ART only = 56%, ART + IPE = 74%

*Steroid-resistant rejection episodes.
†First rejection.
‡Postoperative.

Table 16–15 Summary of High-Risk Patients Receiving ALG for the Treatment of Acute and Chronic Rejection

No. of Rejection Episodes	No. of Patients	ALG Dose Mean, g	Range, g	Graft Survival		Cause of Kidney Loss	Patient Survival		Cause of Death
0	1	10.1	10.1	1/1	(100%)	None	1/1	(100%)	None
1	10	24.2	11.8–39.8	4/10	(40%)	3/6 rejection	8/10	(80%)	1/10 unknown, possible aseptic meningitis
						2/6 infection			2/10 uremic encephalopathy and renal failure*
						1/6 acute post-transplant renal failure			
2	4	32.1	29.9–35	3/4	(75%)	1/4 rejection	3/4	(75%)	1/4 uremia†
3	3	36.0	28.7–44	3/3	(100%)	None	3/3	(100%)	None
3 (long-term)	12	68.0	45–122	8/12	(66%)	4/12 rejection	11/12	(92%)	1/12 uremia†
Total	30			19/30	(63%)		26/30	(87%)	

*Patient died after posttransplant rejection and kidney failure, since he refused dialysis as an alternative therapy to overcome failure.

†Patients died while on dialysis without any other evident cause of death such as infection or cardiovascular disease. (From Toledo-Pereyra et al,[69] with permission.)

therapy may present alternatives for the treatment of steroid-resistant rejection in some transplant cases, it appears that many variables remain to be elucidated. It is apparent from the variable results that timing and duration of therapy may play an important part in graft outcome.

CHRONIC REJECTION: DIAGNOSIS AND MANAGEMENT

In chronic rejection a slow progressive destruction of the renal transplant occurs and is difficult to prevent with immunosuppression. In chronic rejection, lesions may be vascular, interstitial, and/or glomerular. Arterial lesions, progressive interstitial fibrosis, and glomerular lesions are observed.

The course of chronic rejection may be diagnosed by any of several means. A gradual and consistent increase in serum creatinine, a decline in glomerular filtration, and other parameters of renal function are observed. Hypertension and steady weight gain associated with retention of salt and water is often one of the first signs of chronic rejection.

The effectiveness of therapy to treat chronic rejection is dependent on the timing of administration and the occurrence of the chronic rejection. Several methods have been used to treat chronic renal allograft rejection.[4,93,94] Some centers have successfully used high-dose steroid pulse therapy during the first few months after transplantation. Others have employed azathioprine to make a substantial reduction in the peripheral white count (to around 4000 per mm³) to achieve long-term graft survival in these patients. Our approach has been to treat chronic rejection with intermittent administration of ALG or ATG, especially in high-risk patients[93] (Table 16–15). This has allowed us to reduce the doses of oral steroids and to decrease patient morbidity and mortality. When cyclosporine is used as the primary immunosuppressive agent, chronic rejection is not too prevalent,[94] but if present it can be more resistant to ALG/ATG manipulation. On the other hand, cyclosporine has been used to rescue some of the non–cyclosporine-treated kidneys that undergo chronic rejection. However, the results are not as good under these conditions.

CONCLUSIONS

The growth of transplantation has been accompanied by better understanding of graft rejection. This has enabled the transplant surgeon or physician to more clearly identify and diagnose the various forms of rejection (Table 16–16). The search continues for the ideal test to prognosticate rejection so that immunosuppression may be instituted earlier in an effort to prevent irreversible graft damage. At present multiple immunosuppressive combinations may

---

Table 16–16 Practical Review of Diagnosis and Treatment of Renal Allograft Rejection

Type of Rejection	Best Diagnostic Test(s)	Best Treatment(s)
Hyperacute rejection	Gross observation	Immediate nephrectomy, future retransplantation
Accelerated rejection	Renal biopsy; serum creatinine	Steroids and/or ALG/ATG or monoclonal antibodies
Acute rejection	Renal biopsy; serum creatinine; ultrasound	Steroids and/or ALG/ATG and/or monoclonal antibodies
Chronic rejection	Renal biopsy; gradual, consistent decline in serum creatinine and GFR	ALG/ATG, monoclonal antibodies

be used to combat rejection episodes and be tailored for each patient's transplantation situation.

CASE STUDIES

Patient 1

This 25-year-old male patient was transplanted with a second cadaver kidney, which functioned well in the immediate posttransplantation period. The patient was given 14 doses of prophylactic ALG, and the serum creatinine at discharge was 2.3 mg per dl. In ultrasound studies taken on day 9 posttransplantation, the kidney measured approximately 10.5 × 6 cm (Fig. 16–8*A,B*). Prominent pyramids were noted with a broad zone of diminished echoes posterior to the kidney. On day 12, by echogram, the approximate size of the kidney was 11.9 × 6.8 cm (Fig. 16–9*A,B*). On echograms taken at 23 days post transplantation (Fig. 16–10*A,B*) the kidney continued to enlarge, measuring 11.2 × 8 cm. Persistent evidence of transplant rejection was observed. The patient was readmitted at 35 days post transplantation with a serum creatinine of 3.0 mg per dl. The site of the kidney transplantation was without signs of infection or tenderness and the physical examination on admission was unremarkable except for a blood pressure of 164/120. Echograms on the day of admission showed a loss of demarcation between the renal pelvis and the cortex, indicating a failing graft. The kidney allograft measured 9.5 × 12.3 cm (Fig. 16–11*A,B*). The patient was given nine doses of horse ALG and was changed to goat ALG for three additional doses because of a reaction to the horse preparation. In spite of the ALG treatment, the serum creatinine rose to 4.3 by 47 days post transplantation at discharge. The patient was admitted on day 55 with a serum creatinine of 4.0 mg per dl and treated with intravenous hydrocortisone sodium succinate followed by three doses of goat ALG. The serum creatinine decreased to 3.3 mg per dl and the patient was discharged and another four doses of goat ALG were given as an outpatient. The patient again developed symptoms of an allergic reaction. The patient was readmitted on day 62 with a temperature of 103°F and a serum creati-

nine of 7.1 mg per dl. Otherwise the physical examination was unremarkable. On day 65 the echograms showed a greatly enlarged kidney (14.4 × 9.4 cm). The cortex had become markedly echogenic; however, prominent pyramids were not detected (Fig. 16–12*A,B*). The serum creatinine continued to rise and the patient showed further symptoms of serum sickness. He was dialyzed and on the sixth day of hospitalization underwent transplant nephrectomy. Figure 16–13 shows the site of the kidney transplantation with the apparent enlarged graft. When the area of the retroperitoneum was opened, the renal allograft was noted to be hugely swollen, measuring at least twice normal size (Fig. 16–14). The kidney allograft was dark blue and extremely friable. After transplant nephrectomy, the patient's condition improved and he was returned to hemodialysis.

Patient 2

This recipient of a cadaver renal allograft maintained excellent graft function for 5 months after transplantation, with serum creatinine values between 1.5 and 1.8 mg per dl. He was given an initial course of prophylactic ALG and was maintained on azathioprine and prednisolone. An echogram was taken of this patient's kidney allograft at 4 months posttransplantation (Fig. 16–15*A*). The renal transplant was well defined in the left iliac fossa, measuring 56 × 112 mm. No abnormalities were detected. At 5 months, his serum creatinine increased to 2.4 and then 2.9 mg per dl and he was admitted for a course of ALG. At this time another renal echogram was performed (Fig. 16–15*B*). The kidney allograft now measured 71 × 130 mm. An increase in cortical echogenicity from the previous study was observed. A few prominent pyramids were also seen. These findings were indicative of transplant rejection. The patient had shaking and chills during ALG treatment, and the ALG was temporarily discontinued. ALG was restarted after skin testing, and the serum creatinine fell to 2.1 mg per dl after nine doses of ALG. The graft function continued to deteriorate slowly because of chronic rejection necessitating multiple courses of ALG, and a nephrectomy was performed at the time of a

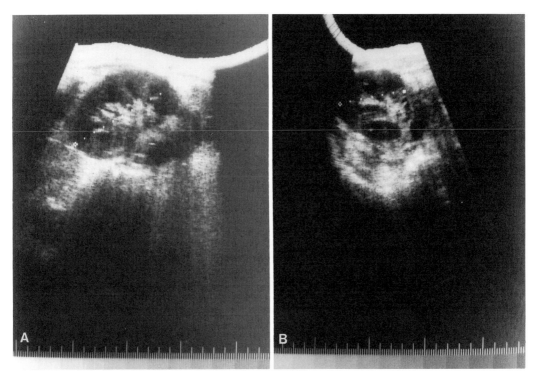

Figure 16–8.

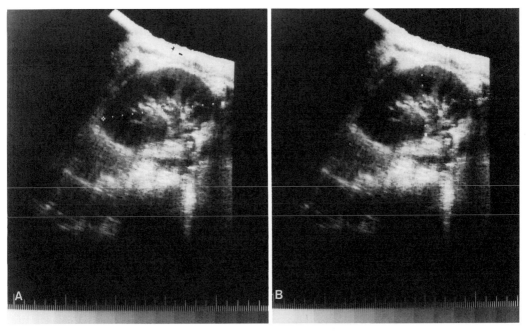

Figure 16–9.

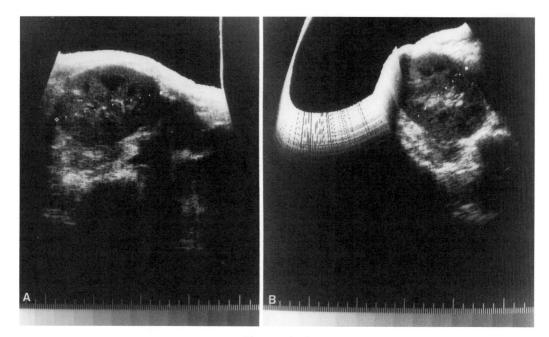

Figure 16–10.

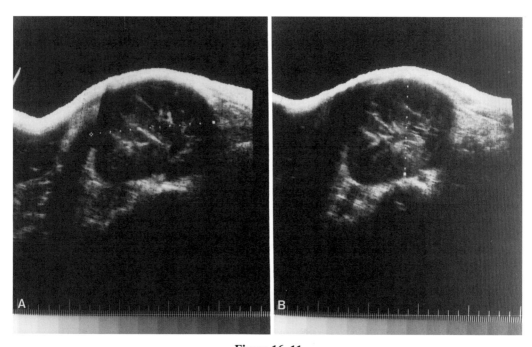

Figure 16–11.

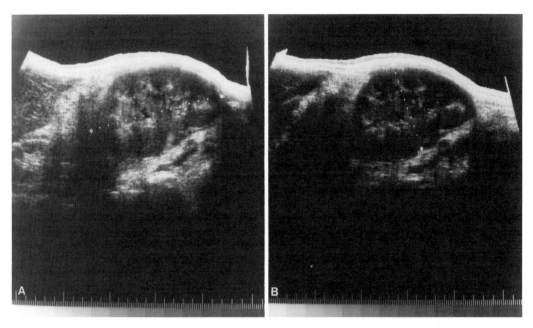

Figure 16–12.

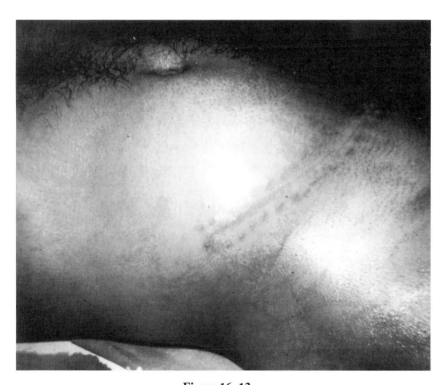

Figure 16–13.

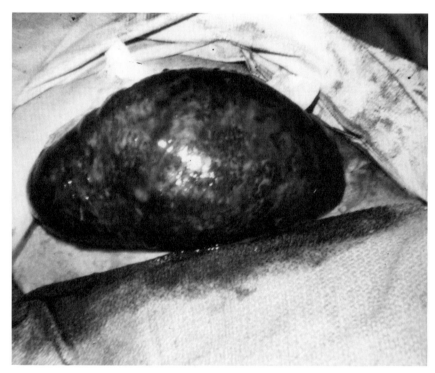

Figure 16–14.

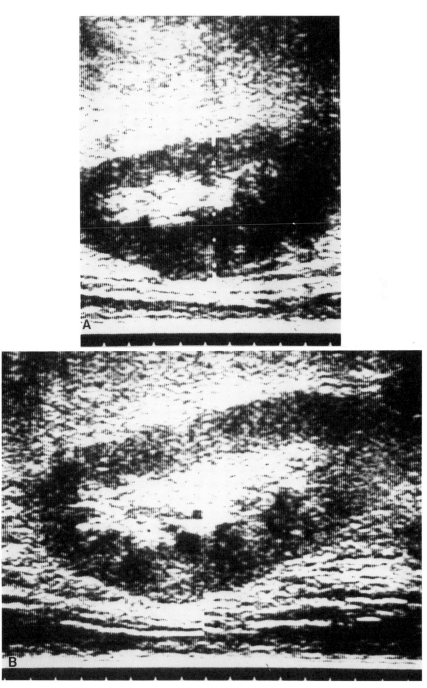

Figure 16–15.

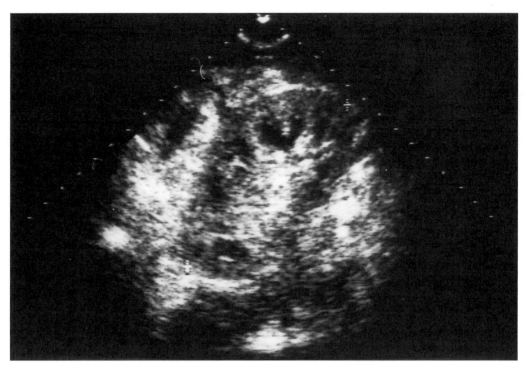

Figure 16–16.

second cadaver transplant almost 5 years after the first procedure.

Patient 3

This patient received a living related transplant, and oliguria set in on the third postoperative day. A renogram performed 3 days posttransplantation demonstrated decreased perfusion of the renal allograft and accumulation of dye. Findings of an echogram at that same time were consistent with accelerated rejection. Prominent renal pyramids, hypoechoic in nature, were seen. An obliteration of sinusoidal echoes was also observed (Fig. 16–16). (Figure 16–2 shows an arteriogram of this patient on the fourth postoperative day.) On the eighth postoperative day, renal vein thrombosis was discovered on exploration and a transplant nephrectomy was performed.

REFERENCES

1. Williams, GM, et al: "Hyperacute" renal-homograft rejection in man. N Engl J Med 279:611, 1968.

2. Beachley, MC, et al: The angiographic evaluation of human renal allotransplants. Arch Surg 111:134, 1976.

3. Busch, GJ, et al: Human renal allografts: The role of vascular injury in early graft failure. Medicine 50:29, 1971.

4. Williams, GM: Clinical course following renal transplantation. In Morris, PJ (ed): Kidney Transplantation, ed 2. Grune & Stratton, Orlando, 1984.

5. Jaffers, GJ and Cosimi, AB: Antilymphocyte globulin and monoclonal antibodies. In Morris, PJ (ed): Kidney Transplantation, ed 2. Grune & Stratton, Orlando, 1984.

6. Najarian, JS, et al: A single institution, randomized, prospective trial of cyclosporine versus azathioprine-antilymphocyte globulin for immunosuppression in renal allograft recipients. Ann Surg 201:142, 1985.

7. Howard, RJ: Definition, diagnosis and treatment of acute kidney rejection, the first 30 days. Transplant Proc 18:92, 1986.

8. Finkelstein, FO, et al: Kidney transplant biopsies in the diagnosis and management of acute rejection. Kidney Int 10:171, 1976.

9. Mozes, MF, et al: The prognostic value of the postrejection treatment biopsy in renal transplantation. Transplant Proc 19:1625, 1987.

10. Laasonen, L, Edgren, J, and Wattson, T: Magnification angiography in the evalua-

tion of transplanted kidneys. Acta Radiol 17:200, 1976.

11. Kreis, H: Transplanted kidney: Natural history. In Hamburger, J (ed): Renal Transplantation: Theory and Practice, ed 2. Williams & Wilkins, Baltimore, 1981.

12. Hricak, H, et al: Evaluation of acute posttransplant renal failure by ultrasound. Radiology 133:443, 1979.

13. Hricak, H, et al: The role of ultrasound in the diagnosis of kidney allograft rejection. Radiology 132:667, 1979.

14. Bergren, CT, et al: The role of ultrasound in the diagnosis of cyclosporine toxicity in renal transplantation. Bol Assoc Med PR 78:50, 1986.

15. Pasternack, A: Fine needle aspiration biopsy of human renal homografts. Lancet 2:82, 1968.

16. Hayry, P and Von Willebrand, E: Monitoring of human renal allograft rejection with fine needle aspiration cytology. Scand J Immunol 13:87, 1981.

17. Atkins, RC, et al: Cellular immune mechanisms in human glomerulonephritis: The role of mononuclear leukocytes. Springer Semin Immunopathol 5:269, 1982.

18. Egidi, F, et al: Patterns of inflammation in fine needle aspiration biopsies in renal transplant patients treated with different immunosuppressive regimens. Transplant Proc 17:209, 1985.

19. Wood, RFM: Immunological monitoring after renal transplantation. In Morris, PJ (ed.): Kidney Transplantation: Principles and Practice, ed 2. Grune & Stratton, Orlando, 1984, p 383.

20. Campos, H, et al: Fine needle aspiration biopsy in the follow-up of kidney transplant recipients. Transplant Proc 17:2077, 1985.

21. Salaman, JR and Griffin, PJA: Fine needle intrarenal manometry: A new test for rejection in cyclosporin-treated recipients of kidney transplants. Lancet 2:709, 1983.

22. Diethelm, AG, et al: Diagnosis of impaired renal function after kidney transplantation using renal scintigraphy, renal plasma flow, and urinary excretion of hippurate. Ann Surg 191:604, 1980.

23. Matas, AJ, et al: Factors mimicking rejection in renal allograft recipients. Ann Surg 186:51, 1977.

24. Kim, YC, Massari, PU, and Brown, ML: Clinical significance of 99m technetium sulfur colloid accumulation in renal transplant patients. Radiology 124:745, 1977.

25. Leonard, JC, et al: 99m technetium sulfur colloid scanning in diagnosis of renal transplant rejection. J Urol 123:815, 1980.

26. Smith, N, et al: Indium-labelled autologous platelets as diagnostic aid after renal transplantation. Lancet 2:1241, 1979.

27. Fenech, A, Nicholas, A, and Smith, FN: Indium (^{111}In)-labelled platelets in the diagnosis of renal transplant rejection: Preliminary. Br J Radiol 54:325, 1981.

28. Jurewicz, WA, et al: Indium-111 platelets as a diagnostic aid in posttransplant monitoring of renal allografts in humans. Transplant Proc 16:1481, 1984.

29. Desir, G, et al: Detection of acute rejection by indium-111 labelled platelet scintigraphy in renal transplant patients. Transplant Proc 19:1677, 1987.

30. Hau, T, et al: Nuclear magnetic resonance imaging of the transplanted kidney. Transplant Proc 17:122, 1985.

31. Jordan, ML, et al: Imaging of the transplanted kidney with nuclear magnetic resonance. Transplant Proc 17:32, 1985.

32. Barnes, RMR, Alexander, LC, and Sells, RA: Beta-2-microglobulin quantitation by rocket immunoelectrophoresis and renal graft function. Transplant Proc 15:1189, 1983.

33. Edwards, LC, et al: Noninvasive monitoring of renal transplant function by analysis of beta-2-microglobulin. Kidney Int 23:767, 1983.

34. Light, JA, et al: Serum beta-2-microglobulin: an adjunctive monitoring test in renal transplantation. Proc Dial Transplant Forum 10:67, 1980.

35. Vincent, C, et al: Beta-2-microglobulin in monitoring renal transplant function. Transplant Proc 11:438, 1979.

36. Vernon, WB, et al: Renal transplant monitoring with serum beta-2-microglobulin and creatinine. Transplant Proc 17:646, 1985.

37. Schaefer, AJ, et al: Assessment of plasma neopterin in clinical kidney transplantation. Transplantation 41:454, 1986.

38. Magalini, SC, et al: Possibility of recognizing immunologic and cyclosporine A damage by urinary neopterin excretion in kidney transplant recipients. Transplant Proc 19:1686, 1987.

39. Noel, C, et al: Neopterin excretion for kidney transplant monitoring: Relationship with antilymphocyte globulin treatment. Transplant Proc 19:1689, 1987.

40. Mortensen, RF, et al: Interaction of C-reactive protein with lymphocytes and monocytes: Complement-dependent adherence and phagocytosis. J Immunol 117:774, 1976.

41. Kushner, I and Feldman, G: Control of the acute phase response: Demonstration of C-reactive protein synthesis and secretion by hepatocytes during acute inflammation in the rabbit. J Exp Med 148:466, 1978.

42. Groth, J, et al: C-reactive protein and clinical kidney transplantation. Nephron 37:236, 1984.

43. White, J, Meyer, E, and Hardy, MA: Prediction of onset and termination of renal allograft rejection by serum levels of C-reactive protein. Transplant Proc 13:682, 1981.

44. Freed, B, et al: Early detection of renal allograft rejection by serial monitoring of serum C-reactive protein. Transplantation 37:315, 1984.

45. Lempert, N, et al: C-reactive protein: An indicator of rejection episode severity in renal allograft recipients pretreated with donor-specific transfusions. Transplant Proc 17:662, 1985.

46. Lempert, N, et al: Elevation of serum C-reactive protein levels during graft rejection. Transplant Proc 19:1683, 1987.

47. Pellet, H, et al: Urinary cytology after renal transplant: Early diagnosis of rejection. Arch Anat Cytol Pathol 29:39, 1981.

48. Madras, PN, et al: Correlation between urine sediment cytology analysis and clinical state in cyclosporine treated renal recipients. Transplant Proc 19:1664, 1987.

49. Simpson, MA, et al: Correlation of binding of human immunoglobulin, urinary cytology and needle biopsy in the early posttransplant period. Transplant Proc 19:1662, 1987.

50. Vangelista, A, et al: Flow cytometry analysis of urinary cytology in renal transplantation. Transplant Proc 19:1665, 1987.

51. Kano, T, et al: A new and sensitive method to detect acute rejection in renal transplantation. Transplant Proc 19:1691, 1987.

52. Flechner, SM, et al: The nephrotoxicity of cyclosporine in renal transplant recipients. Transplant Proc 15:2689, 1983.

53. Klintmalm, G, Ringden, O, and Groth, CG: Clinical and laboratory signs in nephrotoxicity and rejection in cyclosporine-treated renal allograft recipients. Transplant Proc 15:2815, 1983.

54. Cantarovich, F: Personal communication. May 1986.

55. Mihatsch, MJ, et al: Morphological findings in kidney transplants after treatment with cyclosporine. Transplant Proc 15:2821, 1983.

56. d'Apice, AFJ: Non-specific immunosuppression. In Morris, PJ (ed): Kidney Transplantation, ed 2. Grune & Stratton, Orlando, 1984.

57. Hardy, MA, et al: Use of ATG in treatment of steroid-resistant rejection. Transplantation 29:162, 1980.

58. Cosimi, AB: The clinical usefulness of antilymphocyte antibodies. Transplant Proc 15:583, 1983.

59. Monaco, AP: Antilymphocyte globulin: A clinical research opportunity. Am J Kid Dis 2:67, 1982.

60. Toledo-Pereyra, LH: New perspectives in antilymphocyte globulin therapy for renal transplantation. Dial Transplant 14:682, 1985.

61. Howard, RJ, et al: The use of antilymphoblast globulin in the treatment of renal allograft rejection. Transplant Proc 13:473, 1981.

62. Filo, RS, Smith, EJ, and Leapman, SB: Reversal of acute renal allograft rejection with adjunctive ATG therapy. Transplant Proc 13:482, 1981.

63. Nowygrod, R, Appel, G, and Hardy, MA: Use of ATG for reversal of acute allograft rejection with adjunctive ATG therapy. Transplant Proc 13:469, 1981.

64. Streem, SB, et al: Antilymphoblast globulin for treatment of acute allograft rejection. Transplant Proc 15:590, 1983.

65. Hardy, MA, et al: Use of ATG in treatment of steroid resistant rejection. Transplantation 29:162, 1980.

66. Novick, AC, et al: Prophylactic antilymphoblast globulin, low-dose prednisolone and antilymphoblast globulin for first rejection: A steroid-sparing approach to immunosuppressive therapy. Transplant Proc 15:599, 1983.

67. Shield, CF, et al: Use of antithymocyte globulin for reversal of acute allograft rejection. Transplantation 28:461, 1979.

68. Simonian, SJ, et al: Reversal of acute cadaveric renal allograft rejection with added ATG treatment. Transplant Proc 15:604, 1983.

69. Toledo-Pereyra, LH, et al: Nonsteroid treatment of rejection in kidney transplantation: A new approach including long term treatment of rejection with antilymphoblast globulin in a high risk population. Transplantation 33:325, 1982.

70. Howard, RJ, et al: The use of antilymphoblast globulin in the treatment of renal allograft rejection. Transplant Proc 13:473, 1981.

71. Hoitsma, AJ, et al: Treatment of acute rejection of cadaveric renal allografts with rabbit antithymocyte globulin. Transplantation 33:12, 1982.

72. Glass, NR, et al: A comparative study of steroids and heterologous antiserum in the treatment of renal allograft rejection. Transplant Proc 5:617, 1983.

73. Light, JA, et al: Sequential antilymphocyte globulin (ALG) therapy (Rx) improves graft and patient survival. Transplant Proc 15:622, 1983.

74. Light, JA, et al: Antilymphocyte globulin (ALG) reverses "irreversible" allograft rejection. Transplant Proc 13:475, 1981.

75. Hoitsma, JA, et al: Treatment of acute re-

jection of cadaveric renal allografts with rabbit antithymocyte globulin. Transplant Proc 17:72, 1985.

76. Cosimi, AB: Treatment of rejection: Antithymocyte globulin versus monoclonal antibodies. Transplant Proc 17:1526, 1985.
77. Kreis, H, et al: Prophylactic treatment of allograft recipients with a monoclonal anti-T3 cell antibody. Transplant Proc 17:1315, 1985.
78. Goldstein, G, et al: Orthoclone OKT3 treatment of acute renal allograft rejection. Transplant Proc 17:129, 1985.
79. Norman, DJ, et al: Reversal of acute allograft rejection with monoclonal antibody. Transplant Proc 17:39, 1985.
80. Takahaski, H, et al: Reversal of transplant rejection by monoclonal antiblast antibody. Lancet 2:1155, 1983.
81. Oei, J, et al: Treatment of kidney graft rejection with CHAL 1 and CBL1 monoclonal antibodies. Transplant Proc 17:2740, 1985.
82. Kirkman, RL, et al: Treatment of acute renal allograft rejection with monoclonal anti-T12 antibody. Transplantation 36:620, 1983.
83. Cardella, CJ, et al: Intensive plasma exchange and renal transplant rejection. Lancet 1:264, 1977.
84. Cardella, CJ, et al: Effect of intensive plasma exchange on renal transplant rejection and serum cytotoxic antibody. Transplant Proc 10:617, 1978.
85. Niak, RB, et al: The role of plasmapheresis in renal transplantation. Transfusion 20:337, 1980.
86. Kurland, J, Franklin S, and Goldfinger, D: Treatment of renal allograft rejection by exchange plasmalymphocytopheresis. Transfusion 20:337, 1980.
87. Darr, FW, et al: Treatment of steroid-resistant renal allograft rejection with lymphocytopheresis. Plasma Ther Transfus Technol 3:423, 1982.
88. Cardella, CJ, et al: Renal allograft rejection and intensive plasma exchange. Proceedings of the Aemonetics Research Institute Advanced Component Seminar, 1979.
89. Kirubakaran, MS, et al: A controlled trial of plasmapheresis in the treatment of renal allograft rejection. Transplantation 32:164, 1981.
90. Helderman, JH, Gailiunas, P, and Silva, F: Plasmapheresis and renal transplant rejection. In Therapeutic Apheresis and Plasma Perfusion. Alan R. Liss, New York, 1982.
91. Langley, J, et al: Treatment of renal allograft rejection by plasmapheresis. Transplant Proc 17:2773, 1985.
92. Cardella, C, et al: Factors influencing the effect of intensive plasma exchange on acute transplant rejection. Transplant Proc 17:2777, 1985.
93. Toledo-Pereyra, LH, et al: Treatment of chronic repetitive cadaver kidney rejection episodes with antilymphoblast globulin. Dial Transplant 11:380, 1982.
94. Kahan, BD, et al: Allograft rejection in renal allograft recipients under cyclosporine-prednisolone immunosuppressive therapy. In Williams, GM, Burdick, JF, and Solez, K (eds): Kidney Transplant Rejection. Marcel Dekker, New York, 1986.

Chapter 17

Transplantation Pathology

THEODORE A. REYMAN

The renal allograft is subjected to a variety of potentially hazardous environments before and after transplantation. In each, injury that may influence graft function and survival can occur. Accurate identification and classification of any tissue alterations in the graft not only help to delineate pathogenic mechanisms but also may dictate therapy or the need for procedural changes.

Kidneys, whether from living related or cadaveric donors, may contain pre-existing diseases.[1,2] Harvesting, perfusion, or storage of the potential allograft may result in significant tissue alterations.[3-18] The function of the recipient's immune system can produce additional changes that when severe and irreversible cause failure of the graft.[1,2,19,20] Uncommonly, graft failure may result from recurrence of the patient's original disease or development of de novo disease in the allograft.[1,2,21] Finally, alterations relating to drug toxicity, principally cyclosporine,[22,23] or infections[1,2,24] further complicate the picture.

This chapter utilizes the patient material at our center to present the topic of transplantation pathology. Three hundred seventy-six renal transplants have been performed at Mount Carmel Mercy Hospital. Thirty-three patients have received their second transplantation and seven, their third. Three patients were provided a kidney plus a segmental pancreatic transplant. Thirty patients obtained their renal allografts from living related donors.

THE IMMEDIATE BIOPSY

For the past 27 months needle biopsies have been taken regularly at the time of arterial anastomosis of the allograft into the recipient. These biopsies have enabled us to evaluate the kidney for pre-existing disease and for changes relating to harvesting and storage. They further serve as a histologic baseline against which to interpret subsequent biopsies during the patient's posttransplantation clinical course. Additionally, any changes in the handling of the allograft prior to transplantation can be monitored by comparing any tissue alterations associated with the old and new methods.

PRETRANSPLANTATION CHANGES

Pre-existing Disease

Although all of the immediate biopsies revealed some microscopic abnormality, a small percentage contain changes that could be interpreted with some assurance as pre-existing and not related to harvesting or storage of the kidney. These include glomerular, vascular, and interstitial abnormalities.

Thickening of the focal glomerular basement membrane was noted in three cases. The thickening, evaluated by silver stain, was segmental and not severe. In one biopsy an entire glomerular lobule demonstrated thickening and wrinkling of the basement membrane with capillary collapse. Adjacent glomeruli were normal. The most severe form was total hyalinization of the glomerulus (Fig. 17–1A). In one biopsy 2 sclerotic glomeruli were noted in the 13 present in the biopsy. No biopsy showed evidence of pre-existing glomerulitis.

Abnormalities in the endothelial and epithelial cells of the glomeruli were minor and when present were believed to be a result of harvesting and storage. Isolated focal thickening of Bowman's capsule and focal periglomerular sclerosis were occasionally noted.

Vascular changes included mild thickening of arteriolar walls with slight luminal narrowing. These changes were often but not invariably associated with some degree of glomerular change.

Interstitial fibrosis, with or without mononuclear cell infiltrates, was present in a few biopsies (Fig. 17–1B). Vascular sclerosis was more common in these areas. Periglomerular fibrosis, tubular atrophy, and focal or total glomerular sclerosis, when associated with this change, were considered to represent nephrosclerotic scars and occurred most commonly in the immediate subcapsular cortex. The age range for donors whose allografts exhibited this change was 27 to 52 years, and the group included both men and women.[25] A single small tubular adenoma was present in one biopsy.

The focal glomerular basement membrane thickening was again noted by electron microscopy. No splitting or duplication of basement membranes could be detected and no deposits were identified. Immunofluorescent studies were negative.

An occasional biopsy also revealed mild widening of mesangial areas. No deposits or amyloid was found. A variety of cytoplasmic abnormalities were present but were thought to be related to harvesting and storage of the allograft and will be described. None of the donors had any clinical or laboratory evidence of renal disease. The possibility of focal glomerular sclerosis as a disease entity cannot be absolutely excluded, but the lack of associated epithelial cell changes in cases with focal glomerular basement membrane changes makes it unlikely.

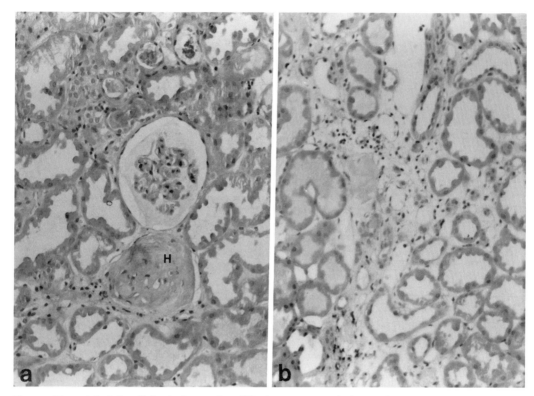

Figure 17–1. (*A*) A hyalinized glomerulus (H) abuts a normal glomerulus. Tubules exhibit minor degenerative changes in this preserved allograft. (*B*) A focus of interstitial fibrosis contains sparse mononuclear inflammatory cells from the same case (hematoxylin and eosin, 40×).

Harvesting and Storage

A variety of alterations can occur in the allograft prior to implantation into the recipient.[3,4,5] In vivo warm ischemia can result from poor renal perfusion during that agonal period preceding death. This may be related to cardiogenic shock, hypovolemia, hypoxia, or a combination of factors. Additional injury to the renal parenchyma may develop secondary to nephrotoxic drugs used therapeutically during life.[26] Ex vivo ischemia, both warm and cold, occurs during harvesting and subsequent perfusion and storage. Mechanical and osmotic damage can result from perfusion and storage of the graft.[10–16] Generally speaking, proper donor selection and efficient harvesting of renal allografts have kept the combined effects of these at a minimum. The degenerative changes, except in severe cases, appear to be reversible.[10]

Degenerative changes in the proximal tubular epithelial cells were always greater than in the distal tubules, Henle's loop, and the collecting tubules. Under light microscopy the proximal tubular cells in some cases appeared swollen and pale, containing large or small vacuoles, particularly in the apical portions of the cells. Often the apical portion was sloughed into the lumen, where it was seen as fragmented or granular debris. Hydropic apical blebs and occasionally entire cells became detached and entered the lumen. In more severe instances, many cells revealed a granular degeneration with loss of nuclear detail and staining, signaling tubular necrosis.[9,17,18] If cell necrosis was associated with red blood cells in the tubular lumens, this suggested antemortem injury. Hemosiderin pigment in tubular epithelial cells was quite uncommon and present only in small quantities. Interstitial edema was mild or absent. The tubules of the distal portions of the nephron unit revealed little abnormality, although occasional cells demonstrated small cytoplasmic vacuoles or pale staining cytoplasm.

The arterioles and venules generally had

normal appearing microarchitecture. The endothelial cells often had prominent nuclei and pale staining cytoplasm. Occasionally the cytoplasm was hydropic and appeared to have separated from the underlying basement membrane.[10]

Similar endothelial changes were present within the glomerular capillaries. Small amounts of granular debris could be seen within the capillary lumens, and rare inflammatory cells, both mononuclear and polymorphonuclear types, were noted.[10] In some cases with hematoxylin and eosin staining, the glomerular basement membrane appeared focally or diffusely thickened. However, with silver stains they had normal contours, although the lumens were somewhat elongated and collapsed due to loss of tissue turgor. Epithelial cells covering the capillary loops and lining Bowman's space generally appeared pale and mildly hydropic, with enlarged, or perhaps merely accentuated, nuclei.

Under electron microscopy the proximal tubular epithelial cells commonly revealed dilatation of the endoplasmic reticulum, which when severe became coalescent into cystlike spaces.[10] Occasional mitochondria appeared swollen, with rarefied matrices and loss of cristae centrally.[10] Focal loss of the microvillous brush border of the proximal tubular cells was common (Fig. 17–2). Occasionally the entire surface was lost with sloughing of cytoplasmic fragments into the tubular lumen. In some instances portions of the brush border were lost because of protrusions of cytoplasmic blebs from the cell surface.[10] More severe changes included fragmentation of cellular organelles and partial or total granular degeneration of cytoplasmic structures. When more than an occasional cell was involved, the pattern usually indicated acute tubular necrosis.

Interstitial edema was mild or absent. Vascular endothelial cells occasionally appeared hydropic, with cytoplasmic blebs extending from the cell surface.[10,13,16]

In the glomeruli, epithelial cell cytoplasm was commonly hydropic-appearing but occasionally revealed an increase in density and contained an increased amount of endoplasmic reticulum. The epithelial foot processes often appeared somewhat swollen and blunted, but not fused.[10] In a few biopsies the basement membrane was

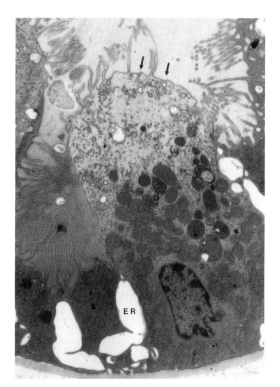

Figure 17–2. Minor ultrastructural changes in a preserved allograft include cystically dilated endoplasmic reticulum (ER) and focal loss of microvillous brush border (arrows) (uranyl acetate-lead citrate, 14,000×).

focally thickened and wrinkled but without other associated glomerular abnormalities. In many cases in which the allograft had been treated by pulsatile perfusion, focal or diffuse widening of the lamina rara interna was noted (Fig. 17–3). This portion of the basement membrane was irregularly pale staining with occasional aggregates of granular electron dense material, associated in some instances with detached endothelial cells. This basement membrane lucency has also been noted in transplantation rejection[1,2] and in cases of hemolytic-uremic syndrome.[1,11] A common pathogenic mechanism may be an alteration in endothelial integrity with deposition of proteinaceous material and imbibing of water into the lamina rara interna. When present in pretransplantation allografts, these vascular abnormalities have been labeled perfusion nephropathy and incriminated in the development of a nonimmunologic microangiopathic process mimicking hyperacute rejection.[27,28,29,30]

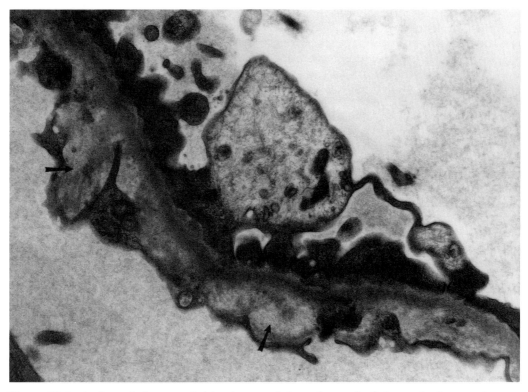

Figure 17-3. An irregularly expanded lamina rara interna (arrows) of glomerular basement membrane is noted in an allograft preserved by hypothermic pulsatile perfusion (uranyl acetate-lead citrate, 28,000×).

None of the allografts treated with hypothermic storage revealed these basement membrane changes. However, these non-perfused grafts did demonstrate an increase in the size of the fenestrations between adjacent endothelial cells[16,36] (Fig. 17-4). In both types of graft treatment, glomerular endothelial cells were often hydropic-appearing, with cytoplasmic blebs extending from the surface of the cells.[13,16] Occasional neutrophils, platelets, and red blood cells were noted in capillary loops in allografts treated both by hypothermic pulsatile perfusion and hypothermic storage.[10] None subsequently developed hyperacute rejections.

Our biopsy material suggested that graft preservation was better with colloid solutions than with crystalloid solutions,[32,33] regardless of whether hypothermic pulsatile perfusion or hypothermic storage was used. Grafts treated with crystalloid solutions had an average cold ischemic time of 21 hours, while those treated with colloid so-

lutions had an average cold ischemic time of 36.4 hours. Warm ischemic time varied from 1 to 10 min in these cases, generally less than 5 min.

IMMUNOLOGY OF REJECTION

Having survived harvesting and storage and the potential for injury in those procedures, the allograft is introduced to yet another hostile environment following implantation into the recipient. The immunologic surveillance system of the host has the ability to recognize and attack the graft as foreign.[1,2,19,20] This may be accomplished through the T lymphocyte cellular arm of the immune system, or by cytotoxic antibodies produced in B lymphocytes, or both. These actions may be aided and abetted by components of the complement[34] and the coagulation systems.[19] This attempt to destroy the graft is often violent but at

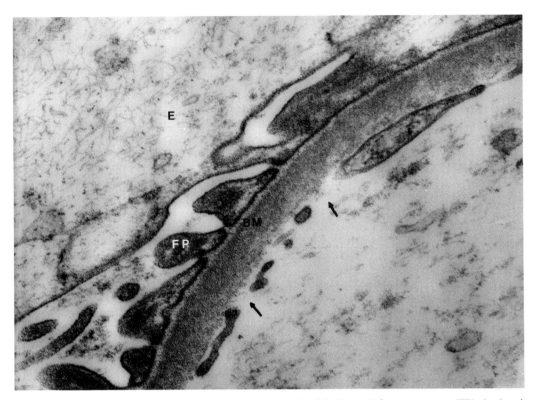

Figure 17–4. A normal basement membrane (BM) and epithelial cell foot processes (FP), hydropic epithelial cell cytoplasm (E), and widened endothelial cell fenestrations (arrows) are present in this allograft preserved by nonpulsatile hypothermic storage (uranyl acetate-lead citrate, 70,000×).

times may be indolent and inapparent.[35] In either case, rejection of the allograft is based on recognition that the tissue antigens of the graft are different from those of the host.

The antigens involved are the serologically defined HLA-A, -B, -C, and -DR as well as the cellularly defined D locus antigens.[36,37] The class I HLA-A, -B, and -C antigens are found on all nucleated cells in the body, including lymphocytes, platelets, and most cells of the kidney. Class II DR antigens have been identified on B lymphocytes, some activated T lymphocytes, monocytes, capillary and glomerular endothelial cells, and some tubular cells in the kidney (see Chapter 1).

T lymphocytes, specifically T helper (T4) cells, recognize the foreign class II antigens of the graft.[38,39,40] They secrete migration inhibition factor (MIF), which is chemotactic for macrophages. These phagocytic cells probably help process antigen and in turn secrete interleukin-1 (Il-1). This substance activates some T helper cells to produce another lymphokine, interleukin-2 (Il-2) and others to develop Il-2 receptors. Il-2 also stimulates another subset of T lymphocytes, the T cytotoxic cell (T8), to proliferate and mature as cytotoxic cells directed against class I antigens. The T helper cells, through other lymphokines,[41] stimulate B lymphocytes, which produce specific antibodies against both class I and II antigens. The T cytotoxic or killer cells, along with T helper cells and specific antibodies, attack the graft cells, causing cell lysis. This action is aided by macrophages stimulated by gamma interferon produced by T cytotoxic cells.[38,40]

Although this pattern of antigen recognition and immunologic reactivity has been clarified in recent years, a number of peculiarities within this complex system have been identified. Genetically identical twins have virtually 100 percent success in transplantation.[1] However, phenotypically identical but genetically nonidentical twins or siblings have a significant rejection rate despite no mismatches at the HLA-A, -B, -C, or -DR loci. This is probably due for the most part to antigenic differences at the D locus, which can be identified by the mixed lymphocyte culture.[36,37] Nonresponders in this test have a low rejection rate as a result of nearly identical antigen status.

In most cases achieving antigenic identity between donor and recipient is highly unlikely. Still, there are factors that may improve graft survival. The antigens at the DR locus appear to be the most antigenic, with those at the B locus less so, and A-locus antigens the least.[37] Cadaveric grafts fare the best if matched at the DR locus, and survival is enhanced if there is additional matching of antigens at the B and A loci as well.[36,37] For reasons not yet known, multiple blood transfusions prior to transplantation appear to augment graft survival over and above the enhancement due to HLA antigen matching.[42,44] This phenomenon may be related to the induction of unresponsiveness in the recipient.

DR-6-negative recipients, mismatched at the DR locus, have better graft survival than mismatched DR-6-positive recipients,[45] suggesting that patients with DR-6 react more strongly to antigenic differences.[36,37] Patients with DR-3 appear to react less strongly to mismatches at the locus than the average.[46] My own material seems to bear this out.

Patients who are Lewis-antigen-negative have poorer graft survival than those who are Lewis-positive (Le$_{a+}$ Le$_{b-}$, Le$_{a-}$ Le$_{b+}$), perhaps because a high percentage of the donor population is Lewis-antigen-positive.[36,47]

Statistically, older recipients tend to have poorer graft survival than their younger counterparts when correlated with other factors such as HLA antigen matching.[48] Certainly graft survival is enhanced by the use of immunosuppressive drugs, cyclosporine in particular. The combination of good antigenic matching with all its vagaries, pretransplantation blood transfusion, and the use of regulated immunosuppressive therapy has improved allograft survival.[49] Despite these innovations, however, few allografts entirely elude the ever-vigilant immune system of the host.

TRANSPLANTATION REJECTION PATTERNS

Based on the type of immunologic reaction and the time interval from grafting to rejection, several histologic patterns have been identified[1,2,11] (Table 17–1). These are hyperacute, accelerated acute, acute vascular, acute cellular and chronic vascular rejection, and finally transplant glomerulopathy.

Hyperacute Rejection

Hyperacute rejection occurs within minutes of the completed arterial anastomosis and is based on the presence of preformed cytotoxic antibodies.[1,2,11] The preformed antibodies may be the result of previous transplants, pregnancies, or blood transfusions.

The same pattern can be seen when ABO incompatibilities occur between donor and recipient and arises from the presence of naturally occurring isoagglutinins.[36] Although of a nonimmunologic type, the perfusion nephropathy secondary to injury

| Table 17–1 Types of Immunologic Rejection |||
Type	Immunologic Mechanism	Time of Occurrence
Hyperacute	Humoral	Immediate:minutes to hours
Accelerated acute	Humoral or cellular	Hours or days
Acute	Humoral or cellular (or mixed)	Usually in first few months, but may occur late
Chronic	Humoral	Months to years
Transplant glomerulopathy	Humoral	Months to years

during storage or perfusion may closely resemble hyperacute rejection, both clinically and microscopically.[28,29] Nonspecific cytotoxic antibodies or cold agglutinins present in perfusing fluids have been incriminated in hyperacutelike rejection episodes.[1,36] Improvements in antigen typing, the use of the cytotoxic antibody screen, and development of safer perfusion techniques and fluids have made this type of rejection uncommon.

Shortly after arterial anastomosis, the graft loses turgor and becomes pale or blue,[1,2] the time interval varying from a few minutes to several hours. The binding of cytotoxic antibodies results in damage to vascular endothelium. Fixation of complement protein aids cell lysis, and fragments of complement molecules are chemotactic for neutrophils and macrophages.[34] Exposure of the underlying basement membrane results in platelet adhesion and aggregation. Plasma coagulation contact factors enhance the agglutination of red blood cells so that capillaries are filled and occluded with

platelet-erythrocyte plugs. The kidney rapidly becomes ischemic and eventually undergoes infarction. The graft never functions and nephrectomy is indicated. In the mechanical endothelial injury of perfusion nephropathy, the reaction may be less severe and the graft may survive.[11]

Depending on the time interval from anastomosis to biopsy or nephrectomy, several microscopic patterns may be noted. Very early in the hyperacute rejection process, the glomerular and peritubular capillaries become dilated and neutrophils begin to accumulate (Fig. 17–5) and may be seen in an immediate postanastomosis biopsy.[1,2,11] However, small numbers of neutrophils within glomerular capillaries may represent residual cells not removed during perfusion or storage[10] and do not necessarily indicate rejection. The presence of more than six neutrophils in each of several glomeruli, or in peritubular capillaries, is usually indicative of endothelial injury of some type. Following this, the capillaries become packed with red blood cells and amorphous

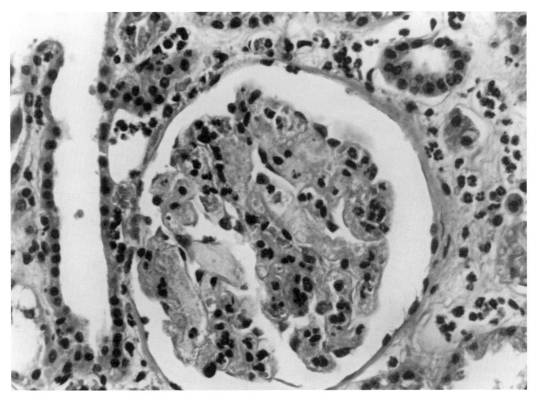

Figure 17–5. Glomerular and peritubular capillaries contain many neutrophils and amorphous platelet aggregates (hematoxylin and eosin, 200×).

platelet plugs may be noted. Within minutes or hours, the capillary occlusion results in cortical infarcts or extensive necrosis. In the later stages, fibrin thrombi may be seen as well. The entire graft may undergo hemorrhagic necrosis. Immunofluorescent studies reveal linear localization of IgG and C3 complement in the walls of the blood vessels.[1,2] Because of necrosis and leakage of serum proteins into the surrounding tissues, larger aggregates of various immunoglobulins may be found.

Ultrastructurally the electron microscopic pattern mimics the light microscopic studies. Early in the rejection episode, neutrophils and platelets accumulate within glomerular and peritubular capillaries (Fig. 17–6). Many platelets may be degranulated and undergo viscous metamorphosis. Small amounts of fibrin may be present. Later, endothelial and epithelial cells swell and their identity is lost as these cells become necrotic. Hemorrhage and interstitial edema may be conspicuous. Vascular basement membranes become disrupted as the inflammatory reaction continues toward frank infarction. Mononuclear cell infiltrates are either absent or not prominent. Larger vessels can exhibit a similar spectrum of changes, progressing to fibrinoid necrosis and thrombosis.

Accelerated Acute Rejection

An almost identical pattern may develop somewhat more slowly, occurring 24 hours to 48 hours later, and is termed accelerated acute rejection.[1] This phenomenon may be due to the presence of low titer or low avidity cytotoxic antibodies or alterations in other components of the cytolytic systems involved. A second form of accelerated acute rejection results from the presence of presensitized T lymphocytes[1,40] and otherwise has a microscopic pattern like that described under acute cellular rejection. This type of rejection is most often

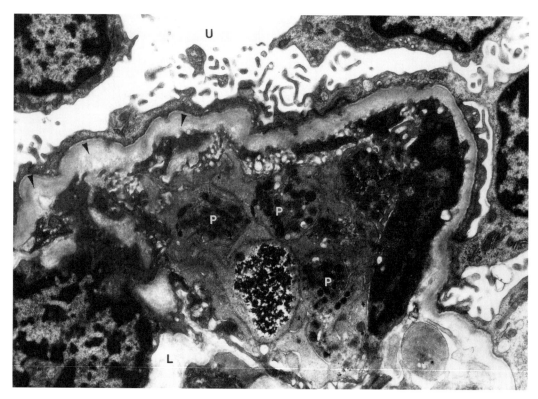

Figure 17–6. Several platelets (P) fill a capillary. The basement membrane has an irregularly lucent subendothelial zone (arrowheads) with adjacent vacuolated endothelial cells. U = urinary space; L = capillary lumen (uranyl acetate-lead citrate, 14,000×).

seen in second or third allografts in the same patient;[40] it develops within a few days of transplantation.

Acute Rejection

Acute rejection episodes generally occur within the first few weeks after transplantation but may develop many months later. This type of rejection is heralded by development of oliguria, rising creatinine, fever, and a swollen, painful allograft. Any of several different gross and histologic patterns may be seen, depending on the time interval and the major form of immunologic attack. In the first few days following transplantation, biopsy may be necessary to differentiate acute rejection from acute tubular necrosis, particularly if the graft has not produced good urinary output. In later stages, acute rejection and cyclosporine nephrotoxicity enter into the differential diagnosis along with rapidly failing allograft function.

The gross appearance of nephrectomy specimens in acute rejection is variable. If relatively soon after transplantation, the graft will be very heavy, swollen, and severely congested. Serosanguineous fluid oozes from the cut surface. Cortical petechial hemorrhages and areas of frank necrosis may be present. If unabated, the acute rejection episode results in a totally infarcted graft. If months after transplantation, when acute changes may be superimposed on chronic rejection, the graft will be less swollen and congested but with areas of hemorrhage and infarction (Fig. 17–7).

Acute cellular rejection has the appearance of an interstitial nephritis in the earliest form.[1,2,11] Interstitial edema and congestion of peritubular capillaries and venules are prominent features. Mononuclear cell infiltrates are relatively sparse and focal. As the rejection episode proceeds, the cellular infiltrates increase and become confluent, disrupting vessels and invading tubules (Fig. 17–8). Tubular epithelium un-

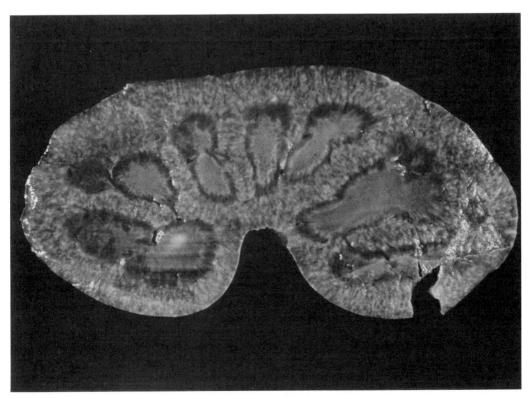

Figure 17–7. A soft, swollen allograft acutely rejected 16 days posttransplantation exhibits focal cortical hemorrhages that correlated with microscopic hemorrhagic infarcts.

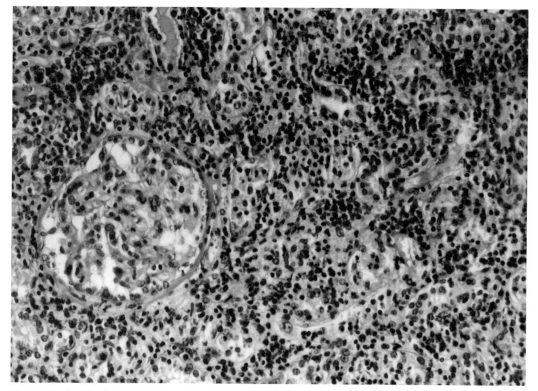

Figure 17–8. Confluent aggregates of mononuclear inflammatory cells disrupt and obliterate tubules and peritubular capillaries in an allograft undergoing acute cellular interstitial rejection. Note sparing of the glomerulus (hematoxylin and eosin, 100×).

dergoes necrosis and renal tubular epithelial antigens may appear in the serum.[50] If rejection is reversed by therapy, the antigens revert to prerejection levels. The inflammatory infiltrate changes from large immunoblastlike cells to an admixture of lymphocytes, macrophages, plasma cells, and occasional eosinophils and neutrophils.[11] Immunochemical studies indicate that a large percentage of the lymphocytes are cytotoxic T cells (T8).[19,20,51,52] The glomeruli are generally unaffected unless secondarily involved by ischemic changes. Immunofluorescent stains for immunoglobulin and C3 complement are usually negative.[1,2,11]

Acute vascular rejection has many of the features already described in hyperacute and acelerated acute rejection, being an antibody-mediated process. In this case, however, the larger arteries, arterioles, and veins appear to be primarily involved (Fig. 17–9). Endothelial cells swell and become necrotic. Platelet aggregates form in the vessels and may be accompanied by mononuclear cells and occasional neutrophils and fibrin. Medial smooth muscle cells may become vacuolated and degenerated, leading to vascular fibrinoid necrosis. If the rejection process is more indolent and prolonged, varying degrees of intimal proliferation can be seen. Vascular thrombosis is common. Infiltrating lymphocytes are mainly B cells. Immunoglobulins can be identified in these vessels and feature IgG and/or IgM as well as C3 complement and fibrin.[1,2,11] Occasional grafts reveal no immunoglobulin localization and have mononuclear cells infiltrating the vascular intima, suggesting a cell-mediated attack against vascular endothelial antigens. This process may be antibody-dependent.[1]

A characteristic feature is noted on electron microscopy. An irregular lucent zone can be seen in the glomerular basement membrane in the area of the lamina rara in-

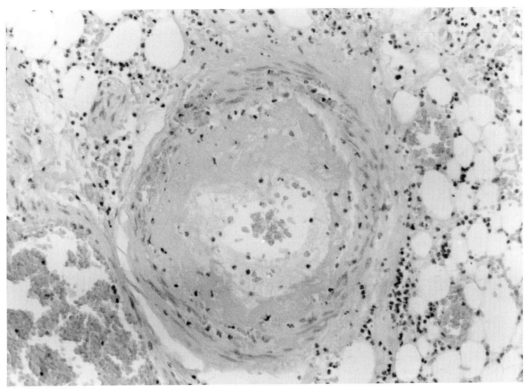

Figure 17–9. A pale staining small artery is virtually occluded by platelet-fibrin thrombus in an allograft undergoing acute vascular rejection. A few neutrophils are present in the vessel and the surrounding tissue (hematoxylin and eosin, 200×).

terna and is often associated with detached or necrotic endothelial cells[1,2,11] (Fig. 17–10). Inflammatory cells are usually sparse.

In many cases the pattern seems to be a mixture of the two types of immune rejection.[35] Labeling a specimen as one or the other is sometimes subjective, based on which one appears to be the predominant pattern.

Chronic Rejection

This type of rejection takes two forms.[1,11] Chronic vascular rejection is usually seen months or years after transplantation. Most patients have heavy proteinuria, hypertension, and progressively failing allograft function.[1,2] The major abnormality is marked and often occlusive intimal proliferative arterial disease, probably mediated by antibodies to vascular antigens[53] (Fig. 17–11). Grossly, the graft is only slightly enlarged and pale, although occasional punctate hemorrhages or infarcts may be present. The large interlobular and arcuate arteries of the graft reveal the most significant alteration, secondary to long-standing vascular injury. Platelet aggregates and deposited fibrin become incorporated into the vascular wall and the vessel forms a new endothelial layer. Fibroblasts and smooth muscle cells proliferate in an attempt to repair the damage. Repeated episodes result in marked concentric narrowing or virtually total occlusion of the artery. The internal elastic lamina frequently is fragmented, duplicated, or lost entirely in a segmental fashion. Lipid-laden foam cells can be seen, but inflammatory cells are sparse. Similar though generally less severe changes will be seen in smaller arteries and arterioles. These vascular changes may result in cortical infarcts. Glomerular changes are often present and consist of basement membrane thickening, expanded

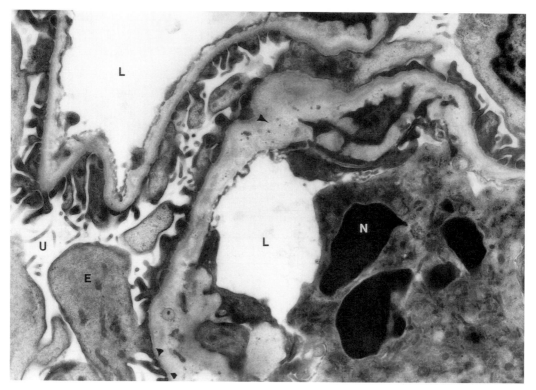

Figure 17–10. An irregular, lucent expansion of the lamina rara interna (arrowheads) of the glomerular basement membrane entraps endothelial cell cytoplasm. Note neutrophil (N) in capillary lumen (L). U = urinary space; E = epithelial cell (uranyl acetate-lead citrate, 28,000×).

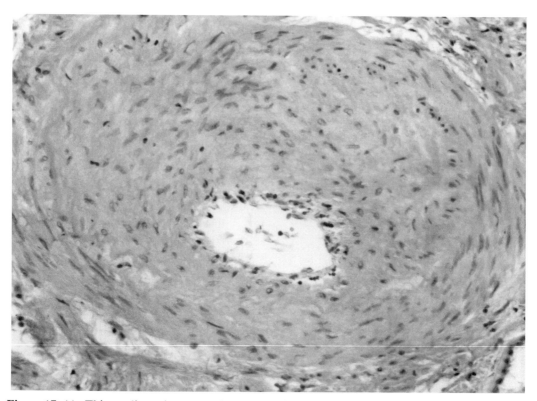

Figure 17–11. This medium-size artery shows extensive narrowing of the lumen because of intimal fibrous proliferation in a case of chronic vascular rejection. A meager mononuclear cell infiltrate is present (hematoxylin and eosin, 400×).

mesangial matrix, ischemic collapse of glomerular capillaries, and degenerative changes in the epithelial and endothelial cells.[1,2,11] Tubular epithelial atrophy with thickened basement membranes is characteristic. The interstitium is fibrotic and inflammatory cells are sparse. Immunoglobulins can be seen in the larger vessels and usually consist of IgM, C3 complement, and fibrin within the arterial wall. Similar deposits may be seen along the glomerular basement membrane in a granular or occasionally linear pattern.[1,2]

Transplantation glomerulopathy is the second form of chronic rejection.[11] There are many similarities between these two types of chronic patterns. However, in transplant glomerulopathy, the glomerular lesions are more pronounced, with only modest arterial thickening (Fig. 17–12). The tubular and interstitial changes are much the same. The glomerular abnormality may be global or segmental and may have a variety of expressions. Basement membrane thickening and capillary collapse with sclerosis is common. Ultrastructurally, the thickening of the basement membrane can be due to the presence of basement membrane duplication (Fig. 17–13), mesangial cell interposition, and/or the presence of an irregularly thickened electron lucent subendothelial zone.[2,11] Granular and sometimes filamentous inclusions in this area probably are the result of entrapment of cytoplasmic debris from necrotic endothelial or mesangial cells.

This peculiar pale expansion of the lamina rara interna can be seen in other forms of vascular rejection and in perfusion nephropathy. If dense deposits are found in the basement membrane, differentiation from de novo and recurrent glomerulonephritis in the allograft may be impossible.

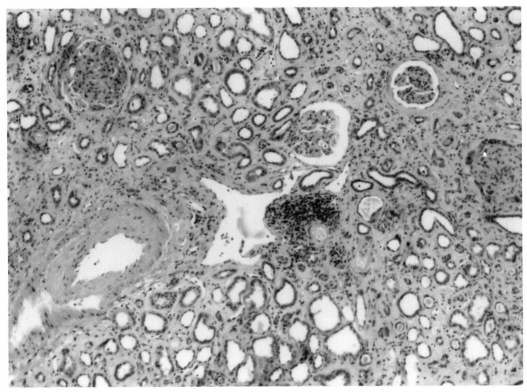

Figure 17–12. Extensive interstitial fibrous tubular atrophy and glomerular sclerosis but mild vascular narrowing feature in transplant glomerulopathy. A mononuclear aggregate is present around a dilated venule (hematoxylin and eosin, 40×).

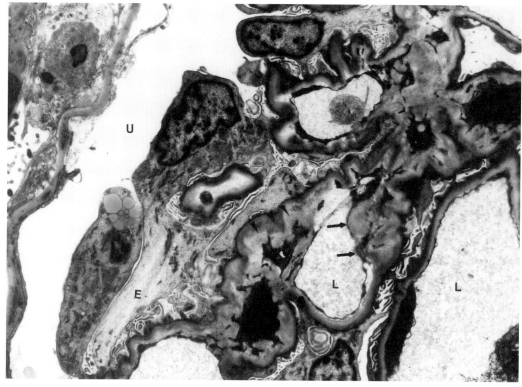

Figure 17–13. The thickened glomerular basement membrane is focally duplicated (arrows) and has an expanded lucent subendothelial zone (arrowheads). Epithelial foot processes are focally fused. U = urinary space; E = epithelial cell; L = capillary lumen (uranyl acetate-lead citrate, 6400×).

CYCLOSPORINE NEPHROPATHY

Cyclosporine has proven to be a very important drug in transplantation of organs. Having a direct toxic action against human T lymphocytes,[54] its immunosuppressive capability has benefited many patients. Unfortunately, it is also a nephrotoxic agent,[55-57] not only in renal allograft patients,[58-62] but also in the native kidneys of patients receiving bone marrow, hepatic, and cardiac transplants.[63-66] The primary site of action is proximal renal tubular epithelium,[57] although other mechanisms may contribute to the acute renal failure.[56] Attempts to isolate the mechanism of cellular injury have been hampered in renal transplantation patients by concomitant occurrence of acute tubular necrosis early in the course of the transplantation and by immunologic rejection later in the life of the graft. The nephrotoxic effects of cyclosporine can occur alone or in combination with ischemia or rejection and may enhance the renal dysfunction secondary to those processes.[55,56,67] Even studies involving nonrenal transplantation,[63-66] where the masking effect of these types of tubular damage is not present, do not reveal a specific diagnostic microscopic picture of cyclosporine toxicity.

The toxic actions of the drug can be roughly correlated with the serum trough levels, and general recommendations have been to keep the serum level as low as possible by combining cyclosporine with corticosteroids, azathioprine, and/or antilymphocyte globulin. When we used this type of combined therapy in our patients, serum trough levels have rarely exceeded 300 ng per ml, and clinical and microscopic evidence of cyclosporine toxicity has been uncommon.

When presented with a biopsy of the allograft from a patient with suspected cyclosporine toxicity, what are the parameters to be assessed? An excellent review of this subject is recommended to those dealing with these biopsies.[23]

Glomerular

Glomerular lesions may be present but are nonspecific and probably relate to changes in the arterial system within the graft. Early in the course of cyclosporine therapy, focal and mild thickening of the glomerular basement membrane has been noted.[58] Mild mesangial sclerosis has been present in some cases and consists of slight expansion of the mesangial matrix with an increase in argyrophilic fibrils. Thrombosis of glomerular capillaries has been described[68,69] but is unusual. None was seen in our material. Mild degenerative changes in the glomerular endothelial and epithelial cells may be found.

As the course of treatment is prolonged, the thickening of the basement membrane may progress to segmental collapse and may go on to partial or total glomerular sclerosis.[58]

Blood Vessels

Significant alterations occur only in the arterioles of the graft. Progressive hyaline degeneration or necrosis of the arteriolar wall (Fig. 17–14), similar to that seen in severe hypertension, has been identified in serial biopsies of cyclosporine-treated patients.[22,58] A second arteriolar lesion noted in these cases consists of a mucoid intimal thickening, rich in proteoglycan substances.[58] The hyaline change has been associated with electron microscopic deposits of lumpy protein masses.[58] Granular deposits of IgM and/or complement have been observed by immunofluorescence. These arteriolar lesions do not involve the glomerulus directly but may result in ischemic

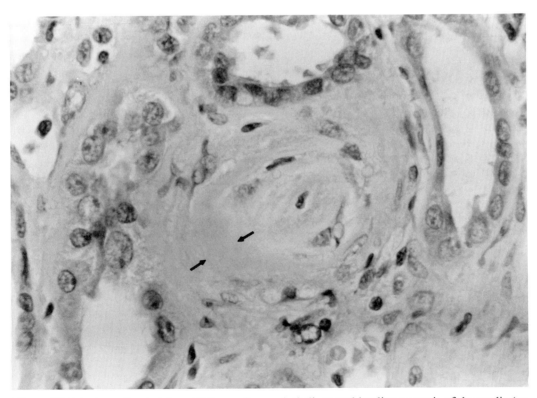

Figure 17–14. A small arteriole exhibits swollen endothelium and hyaline necrosis of the media (arrows) in this case of suspected cyclosporine toxicity (hematoxylin and eosin, 400×).

obsolescence. The presence of arteritis is probably related to immunologic rejection and not cyclosporine toxicity. Chronic vascular rejection often produces extensive intimal thickening but involves primarily larger arteries or both arteries and arterioles.

Interstitium

Interstitial fibrosis of a segmental or striped form has been noted, and when associated with tubular atrophy, is thought to be related to cyclosporine-induced damage.[58,59,60] In this lesion segmental fibrosis abuts normal-appearing tubules and interstitium. Peritubular capillary dilation[58] and congestion have also been related to this process. Interstitial inflammation generally is mild and consists of mononuclear cells. In contrast to immunologic rejection, wherein most of the mononuclear cells have been noted to be T8 cytotoxic cells,[51] the infiltrate in the cyclosporine toxicity appears to be primarily T4 helper lymphocytes.[58] In our material, eosinophils have been prominent in three cases and could be found singly in tubular lumens or in dilated peritubular capillaries in two other cases. Whether they herald drug-induced injury remains to be seen.[11] Diffuse fibrosis or heavy mononuclear inflammation suggests rejection rather than cyclosporine toxicity. Also, focal fibrosis with tubular atrophy and mononuclear cell aggregates has been seen in some of our biopsies from functioning grafts not treated with cyclosporine. Interstitial edema is minimal. If edema is present to a significant degree, acute tubular necrosis or rejection can be considered.

Tubules

Tubular changes may be mild or absent under light microscopy. Tubular cell degeneration consisting of apical blebs or focal irregular vacuolation is common but nonspecific (Fig. 17–15). More advanced lesions

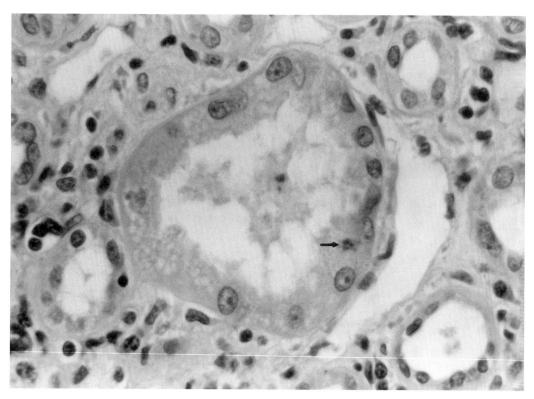

Figure 17–15. A proximal tubule exhibits fine cytoplasmic vacuolization and a mitotic figure (arrow) in a case of suspected cyclosporine toxicity (hematoxylin and eosin, 400×).

are isometric vacuolization,[22,58] punctate or aggregated tubular calcifications,[58] and the presence of large inclusions in the epithelial cells.[58] Isometric vacuolation can also be seen in osmotic nephrosis, and the use of mannitol and similar compounds should be excluded. Tubular calcification is probably secondary to cell death. The cellular inclusions correlated with giant mitochondria and clusters of lysosomes seen with electron microscopy.[58,59] Coils of hyperplastic, rough endoplasmic reticulum within tubular epithelial cells unassociated with mitochondria have been seen in one of our biopsies. Pleomorphism of tubular cell nuclei and the presence of mitotic figures in tubular and interstitial cells have been described[57] and were common in our material. Occasional multinucleated tubular cells also occurred in our cases. These changes appear to signal cellular injury with regenerative efforts but unfortunately are not specific for cyclosporine toxicity. Circulating serum renal tubular epithelial antigens have been identified in cyclosporine toxicity cases but may also be seen in immunologic rejection.[50]

Infiltration of mononuclear inflammatory cells into the tubules and within tubular epithelium probably represents rejection. Extensive tubular degeneration or necrosis is not commonly seen in cyclosporine toxicity and would be more typical of ischemic injury or immunologic rejection.

Renal failure in an allograft may result from several etiologies. Acute tubular necrosis, immunological rejection, and cyclosporine toxicity are the most common. Rarely, glomerulonephritis may recur or develop de novo in the graft and produce progressive impairment of function. Infections with cytomegalovirus and pyogenic organisms, as either an ascending pyelonephritis or emboli, must be considered as well. However, these usually can be identified, and we are left with the difficult problem of differentiating ischemic or rejection-

Table 17–2 Histologic Changes in Acute Tubular Necrosis, Immunologic Rejection, and Cyclosporine Toxicity

Microscopic Change	Acute Tubular Necrosis	Acute* Rejection	Chronic† Rejection	Cyclosporine Toxicity
Glomeruli				
Basement membrane thickening	0	±	++	±
Capillary thrombosis	0	+++	+	±
Tubules				
Isometric vacuoles	0	±	0	++
Cell necrosis	+++	+++	+	+
Tubular inflammatory cells	0	+++	+	+
Blood Vessels				
Arteriolonecrosis	0	++	0	++
Arterial sclerosis	0	+	+++	0
Arteritis	0	+++	+	0
Thrombosis	0	+++	+	±
Interstitium				
Edema	++	+++	+	+
Fibrosis	0	+	+++ diffuse	++ focal
Heavy cell infiltrate	0	+++	+	+
T4 lymphocytes	0	+	+	++
T8 lymphocytes	0	+++	+	±

0 = absent; ± = rarely present; + = uncommonly present; ++ = commonly present; +++ = usually present and extensive
*Humoral and cellular types
†Chronic vascular and transplant glomerulopathy

related injury, in its various forms, from cyclosporine toxicity (Table 17–2). Historical data or clinical parameters may be helpful when correlated with equivocal microscopic changes. Withdrawal or reduction of the dose of cyclosporine with substitute immunosuppression may be necessary in suspected cases.[62,68,70] An improvement in renal function following such a therapeutic change would imply cyclosporine toxicity.

INFECTIONS IN THE ALLOGRAFT

Infections in transplantation patients are not uncommon.[24,71,72] Improvements in technical transplantation and immunosuppression as well as early antibiotic therapy, however, have reduced the incidence of sepsis. Infections directly involving the allograft are unusual. In our series nine cases (2.4 percent) with infection could be identified from allograft nephrectomy specimens, and in patients dying with their grafts in place, at the time of autopsy. All had failing grafts that revealed evidence of acute vascular or acute cellular rejection. There probably were more cases that went undiscovered, being masked by intensive antibiotic therapy.

Eight cases were due to bacteria and one had cytomegalovirus infection in the graft (Table 17–3). Five of the nine patients had wound infections with perinephric allograft abscesses.[72] Four were due to *Pseudomonas aeruginosa* and/or *Staphylococcus aureus.*

The fifth patient's wound culture grew *Klebsiella pneumoniae* from the abscesses. Two patients had septicemia with septic emboli involving the graft.[71,72,73] *Enterobacter cloacae* and *Pseudomonas aeruginosa* were cultured from the grafts, the blood, and the primary infected sites (lungs and peritoneal cavity) in these two cases, respectively. One patient developed acute pyelonephritis (Fig. 17–16) with parenchymal abscesses.[71–73] The urine and allograft both grew *Escherichia coli* on culture. Finally, one patient had extensive pneumonia and died with cytomegalovirus present in both lungs and allograft.[24,71] All of these patients had their immunosuppressive drug dosage increased in the face of rejection, and this may in part be responsible for dissemination of the sepsis. Because most of these infections were due to gram-negative bacteria, the use of aminoglycosides may have also had a nephrotoxic effect[26] superimposed on the effects of immunologic rejection and the septic process.

A variety of other unusual infections developed in our patients during the post-transplantation period. One patient developed gas gangrene secondary to extensive enterocolitis and died. *Clostridium perfringens* was cultured from multiple sites but not the graft. The allograft was functioning until the time of death with no evidence of rejection. Two patients developed reactivation tuberculosis without involvement of the allografts. Other organisms that were isolated from transplant patients included *Listeria monocytogenes, Pneumocystis carinii,* cytomegalovirus and a variety of

Table 17–3 Infections in Renal Allografts (Nine Cases)		
Type	**Number**	**Organism(s)**
Perinephric (allograft) abscess	5	*Staphylococcus aureus* *Pseudomonas aeruginosa* *Klebsiella pneumoniae*
Septic emboli	2	*Pseudomonas aeruginosa* *Enterobacter cloacae*
Acute pyelonephritis	1	*Escherichia coli*
Viral nephritis	1	Cytomegalovirus

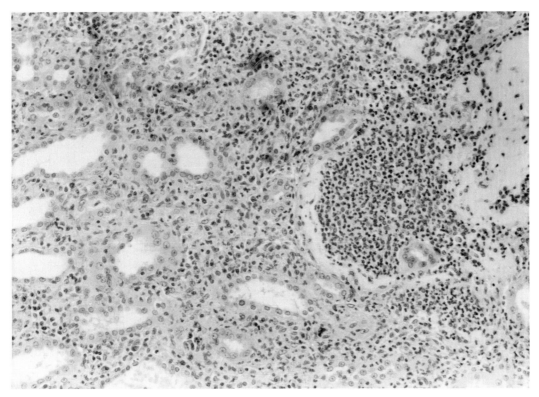

Figure 17–16. A pyelonephritic microabscess is present in the right of the photograph. Extensive interstitial mononuclear cell infiltrate is the result of acute cellular rejection (hematoxylin and eosin, 40×).

gram-negative bacilli.[71] Many patients had bouts of pneumonia and some had septicemia, but none of this latter group had any involvement of the allograft. One interesting case resulted from transplanting an allograft from a patient who was subsequently found to be a carrier of hepatitis B virus. The kidney was rejected within hours with a pattern suggesting hyperacute rejection. The recipient immediately exhibited a viremia and several weeks later developed stigmata of hepatitis.[27] Immunoperoxidase stains for hepatitis B virus in this allograft were negative.

The infections that transplantation patients develop are serious and often difficult to identify. Few, however, directly affect the allograft. They seem to occur in cases with disseminated infections, perhaps augmented by increased immunosuppression as therapy for a rejecting graft. What functional effect these superimposed infections may have had on the failing allograft is difficult if not impossible to determine.

GLOMERULONEPHRITIS IN THE ALLOGRAFT

Pre-existing Disease

Yet another problem that can beset the renal transplant patient is glomerulonephritis in the allograft.[1,2,74] This rarely occurs as a result of disease existing in the donor kidney before transplantation. Careful screening of donors usually eliminates those with questionable renal status. Our routine use of the immediate or 1-hour biopsy has not identified any cases. Potentially much more serious is the development of de novo glomerulonephritis or the recurrence of the recipient's original disease in the allograft. As we have seen, a major difficulty in determining the incidence of these post-transplantation nephropathies is the masking effect of perfusion-related changes, immunologic rejection, toxic changes, and infections.

One of the commonest pre-existing diseases found in the donor allograft appears to be IgA nephropathy.[75,77] Because these donors often have no overt symptoms of renal disease and have microscopic or no hematuria at all, sporadic cases may continue to occur. Fortunately, the presence of this form of nephropathy has not caused serious functional alterations in the allograft[75-77] in reported cases. Other focal lesions may likewise avoid detection. Minimal change glomerulitis, or nil disease, may be impossible to differentiate from perfusion-related changes in the 1-hour or immediate biopsy. Because most cases respond to immunosuppression, the undetected presence of this disease in the allograft appears unlikely to cause problems.

De Novo Disease

De novo glomerulonephritis or new disease arising primarily in the allograft is equally uncommon,[11,21] perhaps a byproduct of the intense immunosuppression in transplantation patients. However, because of the many bacterial and viral infections that afflict these patients, occasional reports of typical postinfectious glomerulonephritis are not suprising.[21,74] Other types of de novo glomerulonephritis identified in allografts include membranous glomerulonephritis,[78-80] mesangiocapillary (membranoproliferative) glomerulonephritis,[11,74] hemolytic uremic syndrome,[11] and antiglomerular basement membrane disease.[11] In our series one case appeared to represent de novo disease. The patient's original disease was diabetic nephropathy. Following transplantation, he developed nephrotic syndrome. The allograft biopsy revealed by both immunofluorescence and electron microscopy a diffuse membranous glomerulonephritis with immune complexes present in the subepithelial portion of the thickened glomerular basement membrane and in the mesangial areas (Fig. 17-17). The allograft eventually failed, requiring graft nephrectomy.

Recurrent Disease

Recurrence of the patient's original disease in the transplanted kidney is more common than pre-existing disease or de novo glomerulonephritis. The disorders reported to have a high recurrence rate in the allograft include not only those with immune deposits[11,82] but also focal glomerular sclerosis[83] and the metabolic diseases oxalosis[84] and cystinosis.[84] IgA glomerulitis commonly recurs in the allograft with a pattern like that in native kidneys.[11,77] However, the clinical course appears to be less severe in the allograft than in the native kidneys. Mesangiocapillary glomerulonephritis, type II, or dense deposit disease, also has a high recurrence rate, but the disease in the allograft may be milder than in the original kidneys.[1,21] Focal segmental glomerular disease may be difficult to categorize because of the nonspecific injury that may result from toxic damage, infections, embolic phenomena, and reversible immunologic rejection episodes, which persist as focal proliferative or sclerotic lesions. Crystal deposition in the allografts of patients with oxalosis and cystinosis has often been noted, with altered function and loss of allograft usual in the former and unusual in the latter.[84-86]

Diseases that infrequently recur or have indeterminate recurrence rate in the allograft include membranous glomerulonephritis,[87,88] diabetic glomerulosclerosis,[89] amyloidosis,[11,80] and antiglomerular basement membrane (anti-GBM) disease.[2,11] In the last disorder, the change of recurrence may be lessened if the serum level of anti-GBM antibodies is allowed to fall to minimal levels prior to transplantation.[1] The rate of recurrence for type I mesangiocapillary glomerulonephritis is reported to be high, with significant graft failure[21,74,82] as a consequence. Its true incidence is clouded by the similarity of microscopic changes to those noted in transplant glomerulopathy.

The diagnosis of glomerulonephritis in the allograft is problematic. Clinical parameters, light and electron microscopic findings, and immunofluorescent studies must be used to assess the changes noted in a malfunctioning allograft. Nonetheless, there are a few alterations that can enable us to say with some degree of certainty that glomerulonephritis or other disease has developed in the graft. Certainly the deposition of oxalate or cystine crystals or amyloid within the graft is not difficult to interpret. Because de novo or recurrent glomerulonephritis in the allograft has the same appearance as in native kidneys, specific patterns of immune complex deposi-

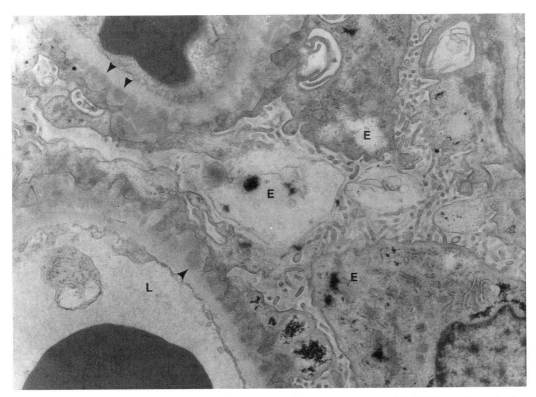

Figure 17–17. Thickened basement membranes contain numerous subepithelial dense deposits (arrowheads) in this case of de novo membranous glomerulonephritis. The urinary space is virtually obliterated by swollen epithelial cells with microvillus formation. L = capillary lumen; E = epithelial cell (uranyl acetate-lead citrate, 20,000×).

tion unequivocally demonstrated in the allograft by immunofluorescent and electron microscopy probably represent glomerulonephritis. However, differentiation from transplantation glomerulopathy may not be possible in some cases. The presence of many epithelial crescents and linear deposits of IgG appear to be specific findings for anti-GBM disease. Focal sclerotic or proliferative lesions or other nonspecific irregularities noted by light or immunofluorescent microscopy alone should be viewed skeptically. This is particularly true if these histologic changes appear to be commingled with one of the known patterns of transplantation rejection.

MALIGNANCIES IN TRANSPLANTATION PATIENTS

The alterations of cellular immunity in transplantation patients following immunosuppressive therapy have resulted in an-other undesirable side effect. Collectively, these patients have developed a variety of malignancies. In a recent study,[91] a comparison was made between the types of tumors that occurred and their rate of occurrence in patients receiving cyclosporine versus patients receiving noncyclosporine therapy. The cyclosporine-treated patients developed malignancies sooner (average 14 months) than did the noncyclosporine group (average 59 months). Other differences were also noted. The cyclosporine group had higher rates for non-Hodgkin's lymphoma and Kaposi's sarcoma and lower rates for cutaneous malignancies than did the noncyclosporine group. No malignant melanomas[92] were identified in the cyclosporine-treated group. The age at occurrence of tumor and the male to female ratio was the same for both groups.

In the non–cyclosporine-treated patients, the lymphomas tended to be extranodal and to affect the central nervous system. In the cyclosporine-treated cohort, the lymphomas had nodal involvement in a pattern more like that seen in lymphomas that develop in the nontransplant population, with central nervous system involvement particularly uncommon. When extranodal, lymphomas in the cyclosporine group appeared to have a predilection for the gastrointestinal tract and lungs.[91] Also, tumors in the cyclosporine group, particularly the lymphomas and skin cancers, appeared to be more localized and less prone to metastasize, and they responded more favorably to a variety of therapeutic modalities than the non–cyclosporine-treated group.[91] The lymphomas in both groups commonly were B cell types and were associated with Epstein-Barr virus markers in many cases.

Cyclosporine-treated nonrenal transplant recipients had a very high incidence of malignancy compared with the renal transplant group.[91] A relatively small number of other types of malignancies (kidney, lung, testis, ovary, breast) also were noted in cyclosporine-treated transplantation recipients. However, because of the short period during which cyclosporine has been used as an immunosuppressive agent, this pattern may change.

A disquieting similarity emerges between these immunosuppressed transplant patients and those with acquired immunodeficiency syndrome (AIDS).[93,94] A plethora of opportunistic infections occur in both groups. In AIDS the patients have a high incidence of squamous cell carcinomas of the tongue and cloacogenic carcinomas of the anal canal.[93,95] Both groups have EB virus infections involving B lymphocytes and a common deficit in T cell immunity.[91,94] A major difference appears to be the generally poor prognosis with tumors presenting in AIDS patients compared with the more favorable outlook in transplantation patients treated with cyclosporine.[91] Only time will further delineate these and other disorders with defective T lymphocyte immunologic surveillance.

REFERENCES

1. Porter, KA: Renal transplantation. In Heptinstall, RH (ed): Pathology of the Kidney, Vol 3, ed 3. Little, Brown, Boston, 1983, p 1455.
2. Dunnill, MS: Histopathology of rejection in renal transplantation. In Morris, PJ (ed): Kidney Transplantation, Principles and Practice, ed 2. Grune & Stratton, London, 1984, p 355.
3. Santiago-Delpin, EA: Pharmacological principles during organ harvesting. In Toledo-Pereyra, LH (ed): Basic Concepts in Organ Procurement, Perfusion and Preservation for Transplantation. Academic Press, New York, 1982, p 73.
4. Grundmann, R: Fundamentals of preservation methods. In Toledo-Pereyra, LH (ed): Basic Concepts in Organ Procurement, Perfusion and Preservation for Transplantation. Academic Press, New York, 1982, p 93.
5. Fahy, GM: Viability concepts in organ preservation. In Toledo-Pereyra, LH (ed): Basic Concepts in Organ Procurement, Perfusion and Preservation for Transplantation. Academic Press, New York, 1982, p 121.
6. Toledo-Pereyra, LH: Kidney perfusion. In Toledo-Pereyra, LH (ed): Basic Concepts in Organ Procurement, Perfusion and Preservation for Transplantation. Academic Press, New York, 1982, p 183.
7. Collins, GM: Kidney hypothermic storage. In Toledo-Pereyra, LH (ed): Basic Concepts in Organ Procurement, Perfusion and Preservation for Transplantation. Academic Press, New York, 1982, p 203.
8. Reidy, MA: A reassessment of endothelial injury and arterial lesion formation. Lab Invest 53:513, 1985.
9. Brophy, D, Najarian, JS, and Kjellstrand, CM: Acute tubular necrosis after renal transplantation. Transplantation 29:245, 1980.
10. Hall-Craggs, M, et al: Structural changes following hypothermic preservation of human cadaveric kidneys. Hum Pathol 11:23, 1980.
11. Spargo, BH, Seymour, AF, and Ordonez, NG: Renal Biopsy Pathology with Diagnostic and Therapeutic Implications. Wiley Medical Publishers, New York, 1980, p 431.
12. Spees, EK, et al: Why some preserved kidneys do not function: A review of preservation-related injuries. Transplant Proc 14:80, 1982.
13. Evan, AP, et al: Glomerular endothelial injury related to renal perfusion: A scanning electron microscopy study. Transplantation 35:436, 1983.
14. Marshall, VC: Renal Preservation. In Morris, PJ (ed): Kidney Transplantation, Principles and Practice, ed 2. Grune & Stratton, London, 1984, p 129.
15. Belzer, FO, et al: Combination perfusion-cold storage for optimum cadaver kidney function and utilization. Transplantation 39:118, 1985.
16. Gattone, VH II, et al: Time course of glomerular endothelial injury related to pulsa-

tile perfusion preservation. Transplantation 39:396, 1985.

17. Schurek, H-J and Wilhelm, K: Morphologic and functional evidence for oxygen deficiency in the isolated perfused rat kidney. Lab Invest 53:145, 1985.

18. Tiggeler, RGWL, et al: Prevention of acute tubular necrosis in cadaveric kidney transplantation by the combined use of mannitol and moderate hydration. Ann Surg 201:246, 1985.

19. Hayry, P: Intragraft events in allograft destruction. Transplantation 38:1, 1984.

20. Sanfilippo, F, et al: Renal allograft infiltrates associated with irreversible rejection. Transplantation 40:679, 1985.

21. Cameron, JS and Turner, DR: Recurrent glomerulonephritis in allografted kidneys. Clin Nephrol 7:47, 1977.

22. Mihatsch, MJ, et al: Morphological findings in kidney transplants after treatment with cyclosporine. Transplant Proc (Suppl) 15:2821, 1983.

23. Kahan, BD (ed): Proceedings of an international symposium on cyclosporine-associated renal injury. Transplant Proc (Suppl) 17:1, 1985.

24. Fryd, DS, et al: Cytomegalovirus as a risk factor in renal transplantation. Transplantation 30:436, 1980.

25. Tracy, RE, et al: Quantitation of hypertensive nephrosclerosis on an objective rational scale of measurement in adults and children. Am J Clin Pathol 85:312, 1986.

26. Hook, JB and Smith, JH: Biochemical mechanisms of nephrotoxicity. Transplant Proc (Suppl)17:41, 1985.

27. Hill, GS, Light, GA, and Perlott, LJ: Perfusion-related injury in renal transplantation. Surgery 79:440, 1976.

28. Spector, D, et al: Perfusion nephropathy in human transplants. N Engl J Med 295:1217, 1976.

29. Curtis, JJ, et al: Hyperacute rejection due to perfusion injury. Clin Nephrol 7:120, 1977.

30. Cerra, FB, et al: The endothelial damage of pulsatile renal preservation and its relationship to perfusion pressure and colloid osmotic pressure. Surgery 81:534, 1977.

31. Ghadially, FN: Ultrastructural Pathology of the Cell and Matrix, ed 2. Butterworth, London, 1982, p 768.

32. Besarab, A, et al: Effect of plasma proteins and buffer in flushing solutions on rat kidney preservation by cold storage. Transplantation 37:239, 1984.

33. Toledo-Pereyra, LH: A new generation of colloid solutions for preservation. Dial Transplant 14:143, 1985.

34. Bisecker, G: Membrane attack complex of complement as a pathologic mediator. Lab Invest 49:237, 1983.

35. Rao, KV and Rose, JK: Incidence, histological pattern, and clinical outcome and rejection episodes occurring in the late posttransplant period. Transplant 40:631, 1985.

36. Braun, WE: Histocompatibility testing in clinical renal transplantation. Urol Clin North Am 10:231, 1983.

37. Zmijewski, CM: Human leukocyte antigen matching in renal transplantation: Review and current status. J Surg Res 38:66, 1985.

38. Strom, TB, et al: The cellular and molecular basis of allograft rejection: Fact and fancy. Transplant Proc 17:801, 1985.

39. Boral, LI and Cheung, K W-K: The HLA antigens in organ grafting. I: Pretransplantation tests. Lab Manage 24:45, 1986.

40. Cheung, K W-K and Boral, LI: The HLA antigens in organ grafting. II: Rejection and posttransplantation monitoring. Lab Manage 24:61, 1986.

41. Maizel, AL, Lawrence, BL: Biology of disease: Control of human lymphocyte proliferation by soluble factors. Lab Invest 50:369, 1984.

42. Opelz, G and Terasaki, PI: Dominant effect of transfusions on kidney graft survival. Transplantation 29:153, 1980.

43. Burlingham, WJ, et al: Improved renal allograft survival following donor specific transfusions. Transplantation 39:12, 1985.

44. Norman, DJ, Babby, JM, and Wetzsteon, PJ: Successful cadaver kidney transplantation in patients highly sensitized by blood transfusions. Transplantation 39:293, 1985.

45. Soulillow, JP and Brignon, JD: Poor kidney graft survival in recipients with DRw6. N Engl J Med 308:969, 1983.

46. Cicciarelli, JC, Perome, S, and Terasaki, PI: HLA-DR3 associated with improved kidney transplant survival. Transplant Proc 14:308, 1982.

47. Oriol, R, et al: The Lewis system and kidney transplantation. Transplantation 29:397, 1980.

48. Oriol, R, et al: Combined effects of HLA matching and age in renal transplantation. Transplantation 29:125, 1980.

49. Opelz, G: Correlation of HLA matching with kidney graft survival in patients with or without cyclosporine treatment. Transplantation 40:240, 1985.

50. Shen, SY, et al: Enzyme-linked immunosorbent assay for serum renal tubular antigen in kidney transplant patients. Transplantation 40:642, 1985.

51. Hancock, WW, et al: Immunohistological analysis of serial biopsies taken during human renal allograft rejection. Transplantation 39:430, 1985.

52. Kolbeck, PC, Sheinman, JI, and Sanfilippo, F: Acute cellular rejection and cyclosporine nephrotoxicity monitored by biopsy in a

renal allograft recipient. Arch Pathol Lab Med 110:389, 1986.

53. Paul, LC, Baldwin, WM, and van Es, LA: Vascular endothelial alloantigens in renal transplantation. Transplantation 40:117, 1985.

54. Kahan, BD: Cyclosporine: The agent and its actions. Transplant Proc (Suppl)17:5, 1985.

55. Flechner, SM, et al: The nephrotoxicity of cyclosporine in renal transplant recipients. Transplant Proc (Suppl)15:2689, 1983.

56. Humes, HD, et al: Pathogenetic mechanisms of nephrotoxicity: Insights into cyclosporine nephrotoxicity. Transplant Proc (Suppl)17:51, 1985.

57. Weinburg, JM: Issues in the pathophysiology of nephrotoxic renal tubular cell injury pertinent to understanding cyclosporine nephrotoxicity. Transplant Proc (Suppl) 17:51, 1985.

58. Mihatsch, MJ, et al: Morphological patterns in cyclosporine-treated renal transplant recipients. Transplant Proc (Suppl)17:101, 1985.

59. Wallace, AC: Histopathology of cyclosporine. Transplant Proc (Suppl)17:117, 1985.

60. Solez, K, et al: Reflections on the use of the renal biopsy as the "gold standard" in distinguishing transplant rejection from cyclosporine nephrotoxicity. Transplant Proc (Suppl)17:123, 1985.

61. Taube, D, et al: A comparison of the clinical, histopathologic, cytologic and biochemical features of renal transplant rejection, cyclosporine A nephrotoxicity and stable renal function. Transplant Proc (Suppl) 17:179, 1985.

62. Myers, BD, et al: Cyclosporine-associated chronic nephropathy. N Engl J Med 311:699, 1984.

63. Hows, JM, et al: Nephrotoxicity in marrow graft recipients treated with cyclosporine. Transplant Proc (Suppl)15:2708, 1983.

64. Moran, M, Tomlanovich, S, and Myers, BD: Cyclosporine induced chronic nephropathy in human recipients of cardiac allografts. Transplant Proc (Suppl)17:185, 1985.

65. Iwatsuki, S, et al: Nephrotoxicity of cyclosporine in liver transplantation. Transplant Proc (Suppl)17:191, 1985.

66. Yee, GC, et al: Cyclosporine associated renal dysfuncton in marrow transplant recipients. Transplant Proc (Suppl)17:196, 1985.

67. Gonwa, TA, et al: Cyclosporine use in early graft dysfunction. Transplant Proc (Suppl)18:104, 1986.

68. Shulman, H, et al: Nephrotoxicity of cyclosporin A after allogeneic marrow transplantation: Glomerular thromboses and tubular injury. N Engl J Med 305:1392, 1981.

69. Wolfe, JA, McCann, RL, and Sanfilippo, F: Cyclosporine-associated microangiopathy in renal transplantation: A severe but potentially reversible form of early graft injury. Transplantation 41:541, 1986.

70. Diethelm, AG: Clinical diagnosis and management of the renal transplant recipient with cyclosporine nephrotoxicity. Transplant Proc (Suppl)18:82, 1986.

71. Winearls, GG, Lane, DJ, and Kurtz, J: Infectious complications after renal transplantation. In Morris, PJ (ed): Kidney Transplantation, Principles and Practice, ed 2. Grune & Stratton, London, 1984, p 427.

72. Feduska, NJ, et al: Clinical management of immunosuppressive therapy for cyclosporine-treated recipients of cadaver kidney transplants at one to six months. Transplant Proc (Suppl)18:136, 1986.

73. Calne, RY, et al: Cyclosporin A in patients receiving renal allografts from cadaver donors. Lancet 2:1323, 1978.

74. Mathew, TH, et al: Glomerular lesions after renal transplantation. Am J Med 59:177, 1975.

75. De La Riviere, GB and van de Putte, LBA: Preexisting glomerulonephritis in allografted kidneys. Arch Pathol Lab Med 100:196, 1976.

76. Silva, FG, Chandler, P, and Pirani, CL: Disappearance of glomerular IgA deposits after renal allograft transplantation. Transplantation 33:214, 1982.

77. Sanfilippo, F, Croker, BP, and Bollinger, RR: Fate of four cadaveric donor renal allografts with mesangial IgA deposits. Transplantation 33:370, 1982.

78. Peterson, VP, et al: Late failure of human renal transplants: An analysis of transplant disease and graft failure among 125 recipients surviving for one to eight years. Medicine (Baltimore) 54:45, 1975.

79. Smith, WE and McMorrow, RC: Membranous glomerulonephritis in renal allografts. N Engl J Med 302:1207, 1980.

80. Grizzle, WE and Johnson, KH: Membranous nephropathy in renal allograft. Arch Pathol Lab Med 105:71, 1981.

81. Milliner, DS, Pierides, AM, and Holley, KE: Renal transplantation in Alport's syndrome: Antiglomerular basement membrane glomerulonephritis in the allograft. Mayo Clin Proc 57:35, 1982.

82. McLean, RH, et al: Recurrence of membranoproliferative glomerulonephritis following kidney transplantation. Am J Med 60:60, 1976.

83. Pinto, J, et al: Recurrence of focal segmental glomerulosclerosis in renal allografts. Transplantation 32:83, 1981.

84. Barnes, BA, et al: Renal transplantation in congenital and metabolic diseases: A report

from the ASC/NIH Renal Transplant Registry. JAMA 232:148, 1975.

85. Lenmann, EP, Wegmann, W, and Larglader, F: Prolonged survival after renal transplantation in primary hyperoxaluria of childhood. Clin Nephrol 9:29, 1978.

86. Malekzadeh, MH, et al: Cadaver renal transplantation in children with cystinosis. Am J Med 63:525, 1975.

87. Berger, BE, et al: De novo and recurrent membranous glomerulonephropathy following kidney transplantation. Transplantation 35:315, 1983.

88. Obermiller, LE, et al: Recurrent membranous glomerulonephritis in two renal transplants. Transplantation 40:100, 1985.

89. Maryniak, RK, et al: Recurrence of diabetic nodular glomerulosclerosis in a renal transplant. Transplantation 39:35, 1985.

90. Light, PD and Hall-Craggs, M: Amyloid deposition in a renal allograft in a case of amyloidosis secondary to rheumatoid arthritis. Am J Med 66:532, 1979.

91. Penn, I and First, MR: Development and incidence of cancer following cyclosporine therapy. Transplant Proc (Suppl)18:210, 1986.

92. Sheil, AGR, et al: Cancer development in patients progressing to dialysis and renal transplantation. Transplant Proc 17:1685, 1985.

93. Redfield, RR, Wright, DG, and Tramong, EC: The Walter Reed staging classification for HTLV III/LAV infection. N Engl J Med 314:131, 1986.

94. Birx, DL, Redfield, RR, and Tosato, G: Defective regulation of Epstein-Barr virus infection in patients with acquired immunodeficiency syndrome (AIDS) or AIDS-related disorders. N Engl J Med 314:874, 1986.

95. Longo, DL, et al: Malignancies in the AIDS patient: Natural history, treatment strategies and preliminary results. Ann NY Acad Sci 437:420, 1984.

Chapter 18

Transplantation Complications

LUIS H. TOLEDO-PEREYRA
ELEANOR D. LEDERER
WADI N. SUKI

Oncologic Complications
Endocrine Abnormalities
Hematologic Complications
Neurologic Complications
Ophthalmologic Complications

Complications occurring after renal transplantation may be of technical origin and affect the graft directly or may affect other organs and systems. Most technical complications are uncommon; however, when they occur, they may lead to graft loss or even patient mortality. It is important, therefore, that these complications be diagnosed early so that appropriate treatment may be instituted. Other complications not surgically related are caused by pre-existing disease and postoperative factors such as immunosuppression. This chapter discusses the complications occurring mainly in the outpatient period, including early and late vascular complications, urologic and renal complications, perirenal fluid collections, and treatment of acute renal failure. Also presented are the spectrum of infectious and cardiovascular as well as metabolic, gastrointestinal, immunosuppressive, and other complications. The immediate postoperative course and care of the renal transplant recipient were discussed in detail in Chapter 7.

VASCULAR COMPLICATIONS

In the renal transplantation experience of more than 379 cases at our center (Mount Carmel Mercy Hospital, Detroit, Michigan), vascular complications have been uncommon (7 of 379, or 1.8 percent). Early vascular complications include hemorrhage from the wound, the transplanted kidney, or the arterial or venous anastomosis; thrombosis of the renal artery; and spontaneous rupture of the kidney. The development of renal artery aneurysms, anastomotic or mycotic, and renal artery stenosis occur as late vascular complications (Table 18–1).

Early Vascular Complications

Hemorrhage

Nonanastomotic intraoperative bleeding may occur from untied or torn hilar vessels or accidentally cut vessels of the donor kidney and will be evident after vascular anastomosis. This type of bleeding may be controlled by clamping and tying or by suture. Bleeding from the arterial or venous anastomosis is a serious complication and can occur because of imperfect operative hemostasis, which may be related to uremic coagulopathy or anticoagulation given for preoperative hemodialysis. It may be observed either intraoperatively or postoperatively.[1,2,3,4] Often this bleeding can be controlled by simple packing with dry gauze sponges around the anastomosis. This may be followed by thrombin-soaked gelfoam pledgets. Brisk bleeding will require additional suture for hemostasis. Perivascular and perinephric hemorrhage may develop after renal transplantation, especially if the patient has been recently dialyzed. Regional heparinization may reduce the incidence; however, platelet abnormalities may still contribute to bleed-

Table 18–1 Vascular Complications After Renal Transplantation
Early Vascular Complications
Hemorrhage
Spontaneous rupture
Renal artery thrombosis
Renal vein thrombosis
Late Vascular Complications
Massive hemorrhage
Renal artery stenosis
Aneurysm

ing. Meticulous care with securing hemostasis will help to avert this complication. Early exploration may be indicated for evacuation of large and enlarging hematomas.

Spontaneous Rupture

This complication is extremely rare in our experience (1 of 370, or 0.2 percent) and in the experience of other transplant centers.[5,6,7] Rupture is characterized by pain, swelling over the graft, oliguria, and vascular collapse. It occurs usually within the first two weeks after surgery and is always preceded by the classic signs of allograft rejection. Causes of spontaneous renal allograft rupture include renal biopsy, ischemic damage during organ procurement or implantation, urinary obstruction, emboli secondary to perfusion, and trauma. The convex surface along the longitudinal axis of the kidney is the usual site of spontaneous rupture. Routine capsulotomy to prevent this complication has been applied at many centers but remains controversial.[8] We recommend early diagnosis and aggressive treatment of acute rejection episodes as the best prophylaxis. When spontaneous rupture is detected too late, transplant nephrectomy is the most common treatment. Sometimes repair is attempted in select cases. Overall mortality from renal rupture is 10 percent.[8,9] In our experience of 379 cases, only one spontaneous rupture has occurred in a patient with a posttransplantation biopsy on the longitudinal convex border of the kidney. We could not save the graft, and nephrectomy was necessary.

Renal Artery Thrombosis

This is also a relatively rare complication, occurring in slightly more than 1 percent of renal transplant recipients.[2] In our experience renal artery thrombosis has occurred in only 1 of 379 patients (0.2 percent). Thrombosis may be due to an unidentified flap that has not been tacked down. It is more commonly seen when end-to-side anastomosis to the external iliac artery is used. There may also be a predisposition to stenosis and thrombosis with an end-to-end anastomosis to the internal iliac artery if there is a large disparity in size between the recipient and donor arter-

ies. Other factors that can contribute to the development of renal artery thrombosis are multiple anastomosis with multiple renal arteries, internal damage due to preservation or trauma from rough handling, rejection, and stenosis.[1] A sudden cessation of urine output in a functioning kidney should lead to suspicion of renal artery thrombosis. The Foley catheter should be irrigated to rule out plugging by a clot. If the central venous pressure is low, a fluid challenge should be given. If it is still low, a furosemide challenge is indicated. If there is no resulting increase in urine output, an arteriogram is performed to rule out thrombosis or renal artery stenosis.

Renal Vein Thrombosis

In 1 to 4 percent of transplants (1 of 379 patients in our series) renal vein thrombosis occurs as a complication.[3,10] It is thought to occur as a result of intimal injury during organ retrieval; because of kinking of the anastomosis or the iliac vein; as an extension of thrombosis from the iliac-venous system; because of pressure on the iliac due to a lymphocele, urinoma, hematoma, or silent left iliac vein compression syndrome; or occasionally because of severe rejection. The presence of renal vein thrombosis should be suspected if there is oliguria or anuria, reduction of renal function, graft swelling, or massive proteinuria or hematuria. A deep vein thrombosis may be associated with ipsilateral leg swelling. Venography is the confirmatory test for renal vein thrombosis. When thrombosis is incomplete, either heparin treatment or thrombectomy or both should be done. Nephrectomy will be necessary if thrombosis is complete. Heparinization is indicated in either event because of the risk of pulmonary embolism.

Late Vascular Complications

Massive Hemorrhage

This complication may be due to infection, mycotic aneurysms from perinephric abscess or hematoma infection, and rarely, from infected urinary leakage. Symptoms may include intense graft site pain or back pain radiating to the flank and rectum, a decrease in hematocrit, and vascular collapse. Expeditious exploration to control the hemorrhage is necessary to save the patient; mortality may be as high as 50 percent.[1,2,3,4] If bleeding is from the arterial suture line, nephrectomy is usually necessary. Ligation of the iliac artery on the side of the transplant may be indicated if the anastomosis is end-to-side with the common or external iliac. A femorofemoral or axillofemoral bypass may be used to provide blood supply to the leg on the side of the transplant. This complication has not occurred in our renal transplantation experience of 379 cases.

Renal Artery Stenosis

This complication is usually investigated only in patients with postoperative hyper-

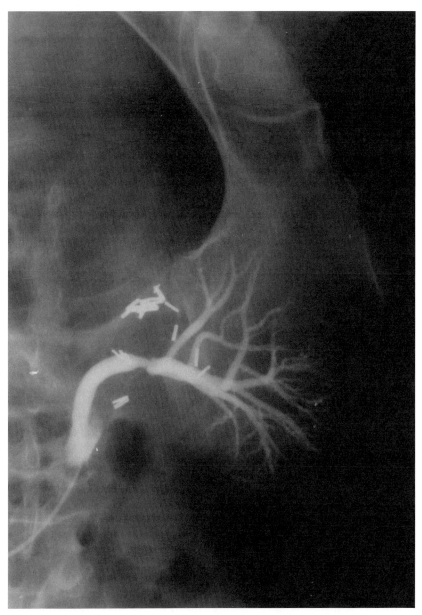

Figure 18–1. Severe renal artery stenosis developed in this recipient of a living related allograft after 4½ years of good renal function. This angiogram shows the renal artery stenosis before dilation using balloon angioplasty. (From Whitten and Toledo-Pereyra,[14] with permission.)

tension; it occurs in 0.6 to 13.5 percent of total renal transplant cases.[11] It can be seen early or late in the posttransplantation course. In our experience, 4 of 379 cases (1.05 percent) have developed renal artery stenosis. The actual occurrence may be higher because of the potential for stenosis in patients without postoperative hypertension. New onset of difficult-to-control hypertension, an unexplained decline in renal function, or the presence of a bruit over the iliac artery should arouse suspicion of renal artery stenosis. Arteriograms are necessary to confirm diagnosis and to assist in classification of the type and degree of stenosis present. Stenosis > 50 percent is considered hemodynamically significant. The various types of renal artery stenosis are classified

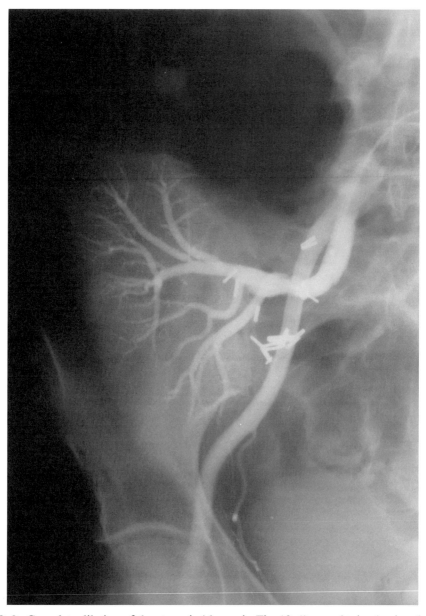

Figure 18–2. Complete dilation of the stenosis (shown in Fig. 18–1) was obtained using the balloon angioplasty procedure. The patient was discharged with satisfactory renal transplant function. (From Whitten and Toledo-Pereyra,[14] with permission.)

as follows, according to their location and etiology;[1,12-14]

1. A short stenotic segment localized to the area of anastomosis
2. A lesion in the donor artery
3. Stenosis secondary to renal allograft rejection.

Depending on the characteristics of the stenosis, resection and reanastomosis or percutaneous transluminal angioplasty may be used to correct the problem[15,16] (Figs. 18-1 and 18-2).

Aneurysm

This late vascular complication may be anastomotic (pseudoaneurysm) or infected (mycotic). An aneurysm may present with rupture, bleeding, and shock. Distal embolization to the lower extremity may also occur if the anastomosis is to the external iliac artery. Thrombosis of the aneurysm can occur with sudden cessation of the renal function.

In the absence of rejection, anastomotic aneurysms are rare.[17] Etiologic mechanisms may include suture breakage or the use of biodegradable suture such as chromic or catgut. Anastomotic leakage with surrounding hematoma that is eventually resolved may leave a pseudoaneurysm. Vessel wall ischemia resulting from suture bites that are too small or tied too tightly may eventually lead to the development of a pseudoaneurysm. Good technique and choice of appropriate suture material, such as 6-0 or 5-0 Tevdek or silk cardiovascular suture, will generally prevent pseudoaneurysms. Diagnosis may be confirmed by arteriogram, and repair should include resection and reanastomosis.

In mycotic aneurysms, the source of the infection is usually thought to be the kidney itself. A positive culture from the perfusate or donor vein or artery should alert the surgeon to the possibility of subsequent infection. A rapidly expanding, warm, tender pulsatile mass in the iliac fossa should be suspect as possible mycotic aneurysm. Usually fever and leukocytosis are also present. Diagnosis can be made by ultrasound. Treatment must include removal of all infected tissue. If limb ischemia is present, an extra-anatomic bypass such as axillofemoral or femorofemoral crossover

graft will be necessary. Open wound drainage is established and appropriate antibiotic therapy is instituted.

PERIRENAL FLUID COLLECTIONS

Lymphocele

A collection of lymph surrounding the kidney or lymphocele may occur weeks or months postoperatively in 0.6 to 22 percent of transplant recipients.[18-20] They are frequently asymptomatic, discovered only on routine ultrasound. In our experience, 7 of 370 patients (1.8 percent) have developed lymphoceles posttransplant. The divided lymphatics of the graft may be a source of lymph; however, most believe the lymph comes from the divided lymphatics of the recipient. With end-to-end anastomosis the incidence is near zero if the peri-iliac lymphatics are not disturbed. Most lymphoceles have been noted after end-to-side anastomosis to the iliac artery. The use of electrocautery to control lymphatics is associated with a higher incidence of lymphoceles than when ligation is used. A large lymphocele may present with swelling of the wound, edema of the scrotum or labia, or as an iliac or abdominal mass. If the ureter is compressed, deterioration of renal function may be observed. Edema of the ipsilateral leg may also be present. Ultrasound is the most useful diagnostic study, and initial conservative management includes needle aspiration. Persistent lymphocele formation after repeated needle aspiration may indicate surgery. Preferably the lymphocele should be surgically drained internally with a window into the peritoneal cavity with or without omental patch, or it can be marsupialized externally. Asymptomatic lymphoceles do not require therapy.

Seroma

In a small number of cases, a perirenal collection of serous fluid may develop after renal transplantation.[21] We have encountered this complication in 4 of 370 transplant cases (1.0 percent) reviewed in our series. Detection and drainage of this accumulation is important because it may foster bacterial infection. A small seroma may go undetected and may cause no observable problems; however, a large seroma may cause pressure on the ureter, resulting in decreased urinary output and increased serum creatinine levels. Initial conservative management includes aspiration. If multiple aspirations are necessary, a catheter may be placed for external drainage with negative suction.

Urinoma

The development of urinomas after transplantation surgery should be considered significant, since they are associated with a mortality between 14 and 60 percent.[22-25] The most frequent manifestations are pain, mass, and infection requiring drainage. Diagnosis is made by aspiration of the fluid and determination of urea nitrogen and creatinine, or by retrograde ureterography, which will show leakage of dye into a fluid-filled cavity.[23-25] Leakage of urine at the site of the ureteral anastomosis most often follows pyeloureterostomy and least often ureteroneocystostomy. Necrosis and sloughing of the transplant ureter is the major cause of urinoma. The cause of ureteral necrosis is thought to be vascular damage occurring during handling of the donor ureter. Some investigators have postulated a role for rejection in this process. Urinomas are not surgically correctable and may require extended time to heal. Often percutaneous nephrostomy and the placement of a ureteral stent are used to divert the urinary stream and prevent obstructive nephropathy while awaiting healing.

UROLOGIC AND RENAL COMPLICATIONS

Although there has been significant improvement in graft and patient survival in the last decade, urologic and renal complications continue to be a major source of morbidity and mortality after renal transplantation. Devascularization of the ureter may lead to ureteral necrosis and fistula formation within the first few days or weeks after transplantation. Less severe ureteral ischemia may result in occasional late distal ureteral stenosis followed by partial or total occlusion. Fluid from wound drains or needle aspiration may be identified as urine by its increased urea content as compared to serum or lymph.

Prevention of these complications begins with meticulous surgical technique and gentle handling of the kidney, vessels, ureter, and bladder at the time of donor nephrectomy and subsequent recipient transplantation. This includes proper identification and handling of multiple renal vessels, preparation of the iliac fossa, proper techniques for ureteroneocystostomy or cystotomy, and recognition of pretransplant urologic problems in the recipient.

Immediate postoperative care also plays a role in preventing urologic and renal complications. Most centers advocate early removal of the urinary catheter (after 3 days) to prevent infection.[26] Posttransplantation urologic complications, which are most frequently encountered, are reviewed in Table 18–2. These include ureteral obstruction,[26,27,28] ureteral fistulas,[29,30,31,32] vesical fistulas,[26,33,34,35] and calyceal fistulas.[33,34] Other renal complications include hematuria, tubular dysfunctions, hypomagnesemia, proteinuria, glomerulonephritis, and urinomas, which are discussed in other sections. Acute posttransplantation renal failure and scrotal complications after renal transplantation are also discussed. At our center, urologic complications have been identified in 31 of 379 patients (8.2 percent). The incidence in diabetics is somewhat higher (12 to 15 percent).

The most common cause of sudden cessation of urinary output in the immediate postoperative period is a clot in the bladder or in the urethral catheter. This may be corrected by irrigation. Other causes of obstruction are vascular occlusion, acute tubular necrosis, and rejection. The ureteroneocystostomy may be occluded by hematoma at the site of the mucosal tunnel in the bladder or by a technically unsatisfactory anastomosis. Partial obstruction may also be caused by an adynamic ureter or edema at the orifice in the bladder.

Diagnosis of these complications is usu-

Table 18–2 Potential Posttransplantation Urologic Complications

Complication	Symptoms/Diagnosis	Treatment
Ureteral obstruction	May mimic acute or chronic rejection. Patient may present with oliguria, anuria, sepsis, local pain, and/or a gradual rise in serum creatinine. Diagnosis confirmed by ultrasonography. If renal function is sufficient, an intravenous pyelogram may reveal degree and site of obstruction. Renal scan may demonstrate hydronephrosis. CT or MRI scan may be used if ultrasound is nondiagnostic.	Surgical re-establishment of patency. Mortality rate = 9–19%. Graft salvage rate = 78–90%
Ureteral fistula	Clinical symptoms usually present early (before 5th post-transplantation week). Patient presents with pain and swelling over the graft area, fever, progressive creatinine elevation, oliguria, cutaneous urinary drainage, or sepsis. May mimic acute rejection or a vascular problem. Ultrasound will reveal periuteral collection and/or hydronephrosis. Renal scan may show extravasation out of ureter. Intravenous pyelogram (if serum creatinine less than 2.0 mg/dl). Cystogram to rule out vesical fistula. CT or MRI scan if others are nondiagnostic.	Early definitive operative treatment suggested because of high morbidity and mortality. Surgical reconstruction depends on the extent and location of the ureteral slough, the conditions of the ureter, and the presence of a native ureter. Significant morbidity and morality. Graft survival around 60–65%.
Vesical fistula	Usually manifested in the first 2 postoperative weeks. If drain is present, extravasation of the urine may be seen. If there is no drain, serum creatinine may be elevated and there may be a palpable mass above the pubis. May be fever or pain in the suprapubic area or around the graft. Diagnosis by ultrasound will demonstrate perivesical fluid collection.	Conservative treatment with continuing vesical drainage, with sump drainage apparatus, if preferred. Some advocate immediate repair.
Calyceal fistula	At the time of transplantation an area of ischemia may indicate ligation of an accessory artery. Urinary extravasation may be present through the wound. A mass, fever, and/or sepsis will manifest. Diagnosis defined by an excretory urogram. CT scan and/or angiography may be helpful in some cases.	Nephrostomy drainage or resection with closure with or without the aid of omentum.

(continued)

Table 18–2 Potential Posttransplantation Urologic Complications *(Continued)*		
Complication	Symptoms/Diagnosis	Treatment
Renal rupture	Presents with dramatic symptomatology at the graft site and signs of acute blood loss. Usually occurs within the first 3 weeks posttransplantation. Graft site pain and swelling, oliguria, and/or hematuria. Hypovolemia or shock may present. Diagnosis confirmed by ultrasonography or CT scan. Intravenous pyelography or retrograde pyelography or more rarely angiography may help confirm diagnosis.	Surgical exploration of the graft after suspected diagnosis. High incidence of graft removal (up to 74%). Nephrectomy performed in most cases. Routine capsulotomy not recommended.

ally determined by intravenous pyelogram, cystogram, or retrograde pyelogram or at the time of surgical exploration. Recent advances in diagnostic testing also include ultrasonography,[36] renal isotope scanning,[37] CT scanning,[38] MRI scanning,[39] and endourologic percutaneous techniques.[37,40]

Ureteral Obstruction

This complication has been reported to occur in 1 to 9.7 percent of transplant recipients.[26–28] Extrinsic causes include periureteral fibrosis, periureteral collection, periureteral inflammation, ureteral compression by kidney, and spermatic cord obstruction. Intrinsic causes include strictures, kinking, torsion, stones, infection, tumor, and blood clots. Diagnosis may be confirmed by ultrasonography, which demonstrates hydronephrosis with ureterectasis. An intravenous pyelogram will give information as to the degree and site of the ureteral obstruction. If renal function is impaired, however, the renal scan can be used to show hydronephrosis. CT or MRI scan should be used only when ultrasound studies are nondiagnostic or when further detail is necessary to investigate a suspect extrinsic periureteral process. Retrograde pyelography will give accurate information when the procedure is feasible.

After diagnosis of ureteral obstruction, the strategy is to re-establish patency of the ureter. This has traditionally been done by reimplantation of the ureter, ureteroureter-ostomy or a ureteropyelostomy with the use of the native ureter. Ureteroureterostomy or pyelostomy has been associated with significant graft loss and mortality (9 to 19 percent).[40,41] A more conservative approach used in recent years has been the placement of a percutaneous nephrostomy tube to allow for stabilization of the patient.[23] An internal double J stent may be passed in an antegrade fashion to avoid external tubes.[37,40,42] Balloon dilation of the stricture has also been reported by some investigators.[43,44] When the obstruction is at the ureteropelvic junction, a pyeloplasty or pyeloureterostomy is the procedure of choice.[45]

Ureteral stenosis may also cause obstruction and is generally seen early in the posttransplantation period. However, ureteral stenosis can occur even years after the transplant.[46] As a consequence, chronic partial obstruction may produce progressive renal insufficiency and, if unrecognized, renal failure.[47] Generally, renal ultrasound will show hydronephrosis. However, more precise determination of the site of obstruction will require cystoscopy and retrograde pyelography. Increasingly, percutaneous techniques are being successfully employed to treat these conditions, thus sparing the patient a major surgical procedure. As a general rule, however, late urologic complications require an open procedure for complete resolution.[23,48–52]

Other causes of obstruction occur less frequently than stenosis. Calculi may present as pain, hematuria, infection, or obstruction. The major metabolic abnormality present is severe hyperparathyroidism with or without hypercalcemia. Urodynamic abnormalities, recurrent urinary tract infections, hyperoxaluria, renal tubular acidosis, and the presence of surgical material such as staples have also been implicated as contributory factors. Stasis is thought to play a crucial role in stone formation associated with transplants emptying into ileal conduits. Rarely, a calculus may accompany the donor kidney or originate from the recipient's native kidney. Fungus balls are an even rarer cause of obstruction. Declining renal function associated with funguria may alert one to this unusual complication.[53-57]

Ureteral Fistula

Devascularization of the ureter or ureteral ischemia may lead to the development of ureteral fistulas in the first few days or weeks after transplantation.[29-31,35] The high morbidity and mortality associated with the development of ureteral fistulas after transplantation make them a very serious complication. Signs and symptoms include pain, swelling over the graft area, fever, progressive creatinine elevation, oliguria, cutaneous urinary drainage, and sepsis. Signs of ureteral fistulas may mimic acute rejection or a vascular problem. Ultrasonography, renal scan, cystogram, CAT or MRI scan, retrograde pyelogram or antegrade pyelogram may be used to confirm diagnosis. Early operative treatment is indicated due to high mortality and morbidity. The extent of surgical reconstruction depends on the individual situation. Graft survival has been reported to be 63 percent in these patients.[26,34]

Vesical Fistula

This type of fistula develops at the site of anterior cystostomy closure or at the ureteral hiatus. Usually the fistula forms from the anterior cystostomy suture line. Vesical fistulas after renal transplantation have been reported in 0.6 to 4.4 percent of the recipients in the first 2 weeks after transplantation.[26,33-35] Extravasation of urine may occur in the first 2 weeks with a drain.

Without a drain indications are decreased urinary output, elevated serum creatinine, a palpable mass over the pubis, and fever or pain or both in the suprapubic area or around the graft. Ultrasonography will demonstrate perivesical fluid collection. Radioisotope scan may be used to show urinary extravasation but is not useful for determining the source. Vesical fistulas are treated by continuing vesical catheter drainage[45] or immediate repair.[31]

Calyceal Fistula

This complication may develop if ligation of an accessory renal artery leads to segmental renal ischemia. The incidence of this complication has been reported to be between 1.3 and 2.2 percent in renal transplant recipients.[33,34] Calyceal fistula may present with urinary extravasation through the wound, a mass, fever, and/or sepsis. Excretory urogram may be used; however, retrograde studies are preferred. CT scans and/or angiography may also be used for diagnosis. In some cases treatment consists of nephrostomy drainage[58] or segmental resection with or without omentum.[59]

Acute Posttransplant Renal Failure

Although, ideally, the renal graft functions immediately after transplantation, normal function is delayed in about 10 to 60 percent of the cadaver donor transplants.[60] Our experience with this complication is summarized in Table 18–3. Acute posttransplant renal failure is generally defined in the literature as requirement for hemodialysis within one week after transplantation. Acute posttransplant renal failure ·is dependent on many factors. Donor age, oliguria, shock, the use of vasopressors, and prolonged warm ischemia can affect immediate function of the renal graft.[60-62] During surgery it is important for the surgeon to handle the kidney carefully, to avoid prolonged periods of rewarming during anastomosis, and to handle multiple vessels properly. Vascular technical complications, including arterial or venous thrombosis and compression of the kidney

Table 18–3 Incidence of ATN in Cadaver Kidney Transplantations at Mount Carmel Mercy Hospital			
Method of Preservation	Hours	N	Incidence of ATN (%)
HS	0–12	2	0
HS	>12–24	19	16
HS	>24–36	7	78
HS	>36–48	19	39
HPP	0–12	10	40
HPP	>12–24	80	29
HPP	>24–36	53	36
HPP	>36–48	38	53
HPP	>48	9	55

HS: Hypothermic storage; HPP: Hypothermic pulsatile perfusion.

fluid challenge. The patency of the vascular supply of the graft may first be demonstrated by radionuclide scanning and then confirmed with angiography if needed.

The greatest difficulty in acute renal failure with oliguria is differentiating between acute tubular necrosis and acute rejection superimposed on acute tubular necrosis. This has become an even greater problem since the advent of cyclosporine for immunosuppression.[64] We have found, however, that close attention to systemic cyclosporine levels, as well as a better understanding of the pathology of cyclosporine nephrotoxicity, may improve this situation, as the incidence of ATN has not increased overall with administration of cyclosporine to transplant patients in Michigan (Table 18–4). The effect of acute renal failure on long-term graft and patient survival has been somewhat controversial. Several centers have reported that acute renal failure has no effect on ultimate graft and patient survival.[65,66] However, recent reports indicate that long-term graft survival is compromised in kidneys with delayed function after transplantation.[67,68] Patient survival appears to be unaffected by acute renal failure, even in recent reports.

or ureter by lymphatic accumulation or hematoma may also result in acute renal failure. The possibility of a clot in the Foley catheter should be ruled out by gentle irrigation. If the urine output is <30 ml per hour, it is important to determine if the patient is well hydrated. Dehydration may occur posttransplantation, especially if the patient was dialyzed prior to transplantation surgery. If the central venous pressure is low (5 to 10 cm H_2O), fluid should be administered. As the central venous pressure reaches 4 to 5 cm H_2O, intravenous furosemide may be given to encourage urinary output. Ultrasonography is used to rule out perirenal collections as the cause of the oliguria if the patient fails to respond to the

Hematuria

In the transplantation patient, hematuria carries the same significance as in nontransplanted patients and necessitates a similar approach. Identifying the source of bleeding is complicated by the fact that the patient now has both native and implanted

Table 18–4 Comparison of Incidence of ATN in Pre-Cyclosporine and Cyclosporine Eras—Michigan Experience			
Group	N	Mean Preservation Time (hrs)	ATN (%)
Pre-Cy A era-HS	100	25.2	62
Pre-Cy A era-HPP	106	25.2	57
Cy A era-HS	136	22.3	45
Cy A era-HPP	169	26.1	35

Cy A: Cyclosporine; HS: Hypothermic storage; HPP: Hypothermic pulsatile perfusion.

kidneys. Special diagnoses to be aware of in this population are acquired cystic disease of the native kidneys, arteriovenous malformation secondary to a prior biopsy, flare of the original disease (such as glomerulonephritis or polycystic kidney disease) in the native kidney, development of the original disease (such as glomerulonephritis) in the transplanted kidney, and the presentation of a neoplasm in the native or transplanted urinary tract. Additionally, hypercalciuria has been associated with hematuria in this population.[69]

Proteinuria

The finding of clinical proteinuria, especially of nephrotic range, signifies the development of one of three conditions: transplant glomerulopathy (chronic rejection), recurrent glomerulonephritis, or de novo glomerulonephritis. The histologic features of chronic allograft rejection include obliteration of small renal vessels secondary to progressive intimal thickening and widening of the glomerular basement membrane. Transplant glomerulopathy may or may not be an entity distinct from chronic rejection, depending on the reviewing pathologists. In many reported series, however, the distinction between the two is not made. The characteristic findings of transplant glomerulopathy on biopsy are enlarged glomeruli with increased mesangial matrix. These one or two processes account for about two thirds of the cases of posttransplantation nephrotic range proteinuria. Recurrent and de novo glomerulonephritis comprise almost all of the remaining cases. The exact percentage contribution of one versus the other cannot be determined, since in many cases the original disease-producing renal failure is unknown. Furthermore, the incidence of recurrent disease as defined histologically may far exceed clinical illness.

Glomerulonephritides

Focal glomerulosclerosis and type II membranoproliferative glomerulonephritis may recur after transplantation, commonly producing significant clinical manifestations. Focal glomerulosclerosis may recur within days of the transplantation. Factors predicting early aggressive recurrence include significant mesangial proliferation and less than 36 months between the onset and the end stage of renal disease. Reflux involving the transplanted kidney may also play a role. Interestingly, the extent of HLA matching and the donor source do not seem to be important. Few patients with membranoproliferative glomerulonephritis type II have undergone transplantation. Histologically the rate of recurrence is quite high, nearly 90 percent. However, only 25 percent have clinically significant disease.

Other glomerulonephritides may frequently recur histologically but rarely lead to clinical problems. These include membranous nephropathy, IgA nephropathy, and Henoch-Schonlein purpura. On the other hand, antiglomerular basement membrane disease, nonantiglomerular basement membrane extracapillary glomerulonephritis, systemic lupus erythematosus, and Alport's syndrome rarely recur.

Virtually every form of glomerulonephritis has been reported to occur de novo in transplanted kidneys. The two most common entities are membranous glomerulonephritis and focal glomerulosclerosis. In fact, membranous glomerulonephritis occurs more commonly de novo than as a recurrent illness and is frequently seen when the original disease was not glomerular. Focal glomerulosclerosis may be seen in grafts exposed to chronic reflux or multiple ischemic insults. As in other instances of glomerulosclerosis, hemodynamic factors may play a vital role in the pathogenesis of this disorder.

Although clinical circumstances may suggest one or another type of glomerular involvement, it is virtually impossible on clinical grounds alone to be certain of the underlying pathology. Renal biopsy is indicated for diagnostic and prognostic purposes. However, it is unlikely that the findings would alter therapy.[70-87]

Scrotal Complications

Posttransplantation scrotal complications may include hydrocele, testicular atrophy, testicular necrosis, and recurrent pain.[88] With these scrotal complications, the patient may also risk infertility. Preservation of the spermatic cord appears to be important for avoiding these problems.[88] The ureter should pass below the cord toward the bladder.[5] Hydrocele should be treated by hydrocelectomy. Epididymitis is treated with appropriate broad-spectrum antibiotics. In severe cases orchiectomy should be performed to avoid sepsis.

INFECTIOUS COMPLICATIONS

Infectious complications are a major problem in renal transplant patients for a number of reasons. Kidney transplantation is a major surgical operation involving both vascular and urologic procedures. Surface defenses are breached by urinary catheters, intravenous cannulae, and peritoneal dialysis catheters. The patient is uremic and therefore already immunosuppressed. In addition, patients are usually anemic and may have coagulation defects. The immunosuppressive drugs administered postoperatively reduce immunological defenses against infection. If prednisolone is given, its anti-inflammatory effects may delay wound healing.

Pretransplantation Period

It is important to screen the transplantation candidate for latent infections as part of the pretransplantation work-up to detect respiratory tract infection, urinary tract infection, and other sources of infection. Patients undergoing continuous ambulatory peritoneal dialysis (CAPD) should have the peritoneal fluid examined on a regular basis. Previous infections with hepatitis B, cytomegalovirus (CMV), and varicella zoster should be noted in the patient's history. Potential transplant recipients should also be screened for AIDS and intravenous drug abuse. In our program transplantation candidates who have abused intravenous drugs must successfully complete a drug rehabilitation program before they are eligible to receive a kidney allograft.[89]

Perioperative Period

Proper evaluation of prospective cadaver donors should be performed prior to kidney harvesting to rule out sepsis, AIDS, syphilis, and tuberculosis. Bacterial cultures of blood and urine should be done at the time of harvest, with communication of positive results to the recipient transplantation center. The organ preservation procedure is another source of infectious contamination. It is important for all technical personnel to observe strict aseptic technique during preparation of the preservation solutions, flushing of the organ, and hypothermic perfusion or storage. During the transplant operation meticulous surgical technique is important to prevent the development of hematomas, urine leaks, and lymphoceles, which may serve as potential foci of infection. The routine use of wound drains remains controversial, but we always use a Jackson-Pratt drain postoperatively. Prophylactic antibiotic therapy is recommended to prevent infection in the immediate postoperative period.[90]

Postoperative Period

After renal transplantation the leukocyte count should be monitored on a regular basis so that extremely low levels can be avoided. At some centers immunologic monitoring of T cell subsets is also performed if antithymocyte preparations such as ALG, ATG, and monoclonal antibodies are administered. With severe infections a reduction or withdrawal of immunosuppression is recommended. A fever in the postoperative period is never insignificant. Table 18–5 shows potential sites of origin for unexplained fever in the post-transplantation period.[91] Table 18–6 diagrams a decision tree for diagnosis of unexplained fever in transplant recipients.

After the possible sources of fever are considered, several diagnostic tests may be used to assist diagnosis;[92] a chest roentgenogram should be performed to compare previous and current films if pulmonary infection is suspected; ultrasound of the transplant wound and bed, if infection is

Table 18–5 Diagnosis of Unexplained Fever in Renal Transplant Recipients: Potential Sites of Origin*

Central nervous system
  Listeria
  Cryptococcus
  Asperigillus
  M. tuberculosis
Chest
  Pulmonary infection
  Pericarditis
  Endocarditis
Lower limb
  Deep vein thrombosis
Mouth
  Candida
Peritoneum
  Dialysis catheter sites
  Peritoneal fluid
  Pancreas
  Colon
Soft tissues
  Skin (fungi, *Nocardia,* atypical
    mycobacteria)
  Joints
  Wound
Systemic
  Viral
  M. tuberculosis
  Malignancy
Transplant site
  Rejection
  Abscess
  Hematoma
  Urine leakage
Urinary tract
  Bladder
  Prostate
  Native Kidneys
Vascular access site and cannula

*Modified from Winearls et al,[47] with permission.

onella, and *Pneumocystis.* Fever in the early posttransplantation period may arise from rejection, hematoma, or deep venous thrombosis. Of these complications, rejection is the most common; however, it may be difficult to distinguish it from infection. Table 18–7 shows the most common infections in renal transplant recipients during the first 6 months after surgery and their usual time of occurrence after transplantation.

Wound Infections

Early transplant experience reported a high incidence of wound complications (14 to 34 percent);[93] however, these have decreased in the more recent years (1 to 3 percent).[90,94] In our transplantation experience, a similar decrease was noted between the pre-ALG, ALG, and cyclosporine eras (21 percent, 1.2 percent, and none, respectively).[90] Many factors contribute to the incidence of wound infection after renal transplantation. However, surgical technique is one of the most important factors in posttransplantation wound infections, since complications of the operation itself may contribute to many early wound and urinary tract infections. Because of the uremic and malnourished state of the average renal transplant recipient and the posttransplant immunosuppression, a high risk for infection exists. This is especially increased if the primary transplant wound is reopened for reoperation or transplant nephrectomy. Wound infection should always be considered a serious complication; it may lead to subsequent infection of the arterial anastomosis and massive bleeding or sepsis in wounds that are slow to heal.

Prevention of wound infections is accomplished by attention to several factors. Adequate surgical technique is extremely important for preventing wound infection; this includes minimizing tissue damage and control of hemostasis. Prophylactic antibiotics such as cefotaxime sodium and cefotoxin sodium should be considered. Choice of suture material may affect the potentiation of infection. Choice of techniques for wound closure and dressing may also be important. Decisions regarding the

suspected at the transplant site; cultures of blood, urine, sputum, stool, access sites, and gastric washings, when appropriate; serologic evaluation for CMV IgM appearance or rise in CMV IgG; and lumbar puncture to detect Epstein-Barr virus. Among the pathogens that are difficult to exclude are cytomegalovirus, *Listeria, Nocardia asteroides, Mycobacterium tuberculosis* and atypical mycobacteria, *Cryptococcus, Legi-*

Table 18–6 Diagnosis of Unexplained Fever*

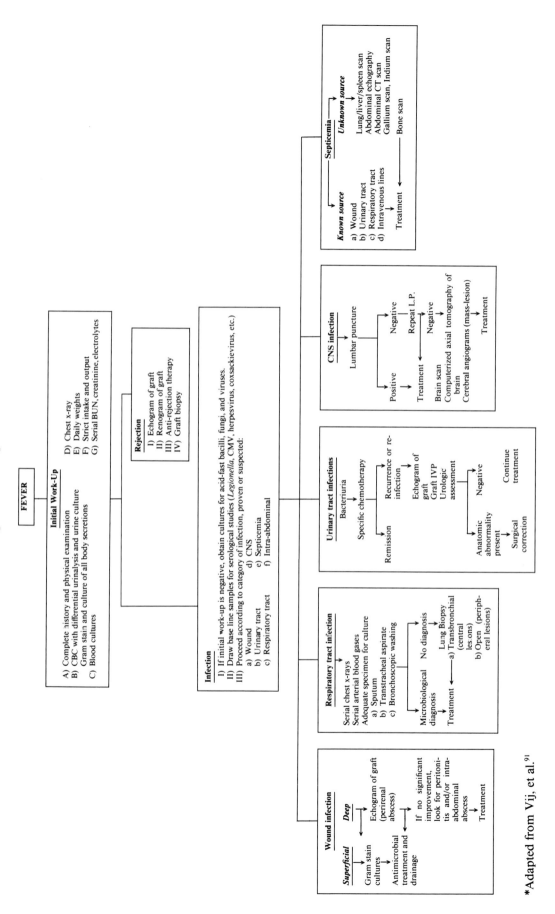

FEVER

Initial Work-Up

A) Complete history and physical examination
B) CBC with differential urinalysis and urine culture
   Gram stain and culture of all body secretions
C) Blood cultures
D) Chest x-ray
E) Daily weights
F) Strict intake and output
G) Serial BUN, creatinine, electrolytes

Rejection

I) Echogram of graft
II) Renogram of graft
III) Anti-rejection therapy
IV) Graft biopsy

Infection

I) If initial work-up is negative, obtain cultures for acid-fast bacilli, fungi, and viruses.
II) Draw base line samples for serological studies (*Legionella*, CMV, herpesvirus, coxsackievirus, etc.).
III) Proceed according to category of infection, proven or suspected:
   a) Wound   d) CNS
   b) Urinary tract   e) Septicemia
   c) Respiratory tract   f) Intra-abdominal

Septicemia

Known source
a) Wound
b) Urinary tract
c) Respiratory tract
d) Intravenous lines
   Treatment

Unknown source
Lung/liver/spleen scan
Abdominal echography
Abdominal CT scan
Gallium scan, Indium scan
Bone scan

CNS infection

Lumbar puncture
Positive → Treatment
Brain scan
Computerized axial tomography of brain
Cerebral angiograms (mass-lesion)
Negative → Repeat L.P.
Negative → Treatment

Urinary tract infections

Bacteriuria
Specific chemotherapy
Remission
Recurrence or re-infection
Echogram of graft
Graft IVP
Urologic assessment
Anatomic abnormality present → Surgical correction
Negative → Continue treatment

Respiratory tract infection

Serial chest x-rays
Serial arterial blood gases
Adequate specimen for culture
a) Sputum
b) Transtracheal aspirate
c) Bronchoscopic washing
Microbiological diagnosis
No diagnosis
Treatment
Lung Biopsy
a) Transbronchial (central lesions)
b) Open (peripheral lesions)

Wound infection

Superficial
Gram stain cultures
Antimicrobial treatment and drainage

Deep
Echogram of graft (perirenal abscess)
If no significant improvement, look for peritonitis and/or intra-abdominal abscess
Treatment

*Adapted from Vij, et al.[91]

Table 18–7 Timetable of Infection in the Renal Transplantation Patient*	
Pathogen	**Occurrence Post Transplantation**
Viral	
Herpes simplex virus	0–12 weeks
Cytomegalovirus (onset)	4–12 weeks
Epstein-Barr virus	>7 weeks
Varicella/zoster virus	>7 weeks
Papovavirus	>7 weeks
Adenovirus	>7 weeks
Bacterial	
Wound	0–4 weeks
Line associated	0–4 weeks
Pneumonia (nosocomial)	0–4 weeks
Pneumonia (non-nosocomial)	>11 weeks
Urinary tract infections (relapsing)	0–16 weeks
Benign urinary tract infections	>24 weeks
Listeria septicemia and central nervous system infection	>4 weeks
Mycobacterial	>4 weeks
Fungal	
Candida	0–24 weeks
Cryptococcus	>16 weeks
Aspergillus	>4 weeks
Others	
Pneumocystis	>4 weeks
Nocardia toxoplasma	>4 weeks

*During first 6 months posttransplantation.
(Modified from Rubin et al: Infection in the renal transplant patient. Am J Med 70:405, 1981, with permission.)

use of drains may contribute to subsequent outcome, since they may serve as conduits for bacteria and may affect resistance to infection. A very high infection rate has been associated with transplant nephrectomy (17 to 50 percent).[95]

CARDIOVASCULAR COMPLICATIONS

Similar to what is seen in dialysis patients, cardiovascular complications are a major cause of morbidity and mortality in the renal transplantation population. Myocardial infarction, cerebrovascular accident, and other forms of peripheral vascular disease occur many times more frequently than in the general population. As a subgroup, diabetics are particularly prone to cardiovascular complications, with as many as 25 percent undergoing amputation of an extremity after transplantation.[96,97] The major predisposing factors are underlying atherosclerosis, hypertension, and hyperlipidemia.

Hypertension occurs in a significant percentage of the population, with most centers reporting between 50 and 60 percent prevalence. Risk factors include dysfunction and a cadaveric renal transplantation. On the other hand, other factors such as age, race, sex, and family history are not important in this entity. The causes of hypertension in this population are probably multifactorial, even for the individual patient. They include chronic rejection and other renal pathology, renal artery stenosis, abnormalities of the renin-angiotensin system, elevation of aldosterone levels, decrease in kinin production, steroid effect, native kidney effect, and hypercalcemia.[98-106] Recently cyclosporine has been associated with a markedly increased incidence of hypertension when used for non-renal transplantation patients and may be associated with the development of hypomagnesmia.[49]

As well, most patients with transplants are hyperlipidemic, presumably exacerbated by the chronic steroid therapy. The most frequent patterns are type II and type IV. In general, hyperlipidemia occurs immediately posttransplantation and may diminish in severity over time, especially if steroids are discontinued or switched to an alternate-day regimen. The protective effect of alternate-day steroid therapy has not been a universal finding; however, in view of the equivalent immunosuppressive efficacy of high- and low-dose regimens and the documented cardiovascular risk in this group of patients, it would seem prudent to opt for lower-dose regimens.[106-110]

It has recently been estimated that between 20 and 40 percent of all deaths in renal transplant patients in the United States are related to cardiovascular problems.[111] Individuals dying of cardiovascular complications generally have a higher mean age at the time of transplantation. In addition, the reduced survival of renal transplant recipients, with ESRD secondary to hypertension or diabetes mellitus, is probably related to the greater prevalence of cardiovascular disease associated with these disorders.[112] The cardiovascular complications that contribute to increased mortality in the renal transplant recipient population include cerebrovascular accident, cardiac arrest, pulmonary embolism, myocardial infarction, stroke, and venous thromboembolism. More detail on this subject may be found in Chapter 8.

MINERAL METABOLISM COMPLICATIONS

Although successful renal transplantation improves abnormalities in mineral metabolism, it does not completely correct them[113] (Table 18–8). The derangements in intestinal calcium absorption and vitamin D metabolism that were seen after transplantation in the precyclosporine era have become less prevalent with reduced steroid administration in the cyclosporine era.

Table 18–8 Potential Complications of Mineral Metabolism
Decreased calcium absorption
Altered vitamin D metabolism
Hyperchloremia
Hypobicarbonatemia
Impaired urine acidification
Hyperkalemia
Hypoaldosteronism
Renal tubular acidosis
Phosphate wasting
Hypomagnesemia

Newer approaches include attention to antacid therapy, magnesium depletion, and vigorous treatment of hypophosphatemia. At some centers pretransplantation determinations of parathyroid mass have helped to identify patients at increased risk for mineral metabolic problems in the posttransplantation period.[114] In patients with abnormal mineral metabolism it is important to determine the optimal level of serum calcium that will permit healing of osteodystrophy without stimulating the parathyroid.[114,115] Intrinsic leaks of phosphorus and/or calcium, which may cause persistently altered mineral metabolism, can be treated by phosphorus or hydrychlorothiazide replacement therapy.[116-118] Rarely, optimum serum calcium levels cannot be maintained and surgery is pursued.[115]

A number of tubular dysfunctions have been observed and studied in these patients. Hyperkalemia, renal tubular acidosis (RTA), and phosphate wasting may all occur, particularly within the first 3 months. They may also presage the onset of either acute or chronic rejection any time during the posttransplantation course. Both proximal and distal renal tubular acidosis have been described, though on the whole, distal defects are more common. The patients may manifest frank distal RTA with hyperchloremia, hypobicarbonatemia, and impaired urine acidification, as demonstrated by depressed U-BpCO$_2$ levels. Another common abnormality is hyperkalemia-distal RTA, particularly in cyclosporine-treated patients. In some individuals, hypoaldosteronism has been documented; in others, however, aldosterone levels have been normal, suggesting a tubular unresponsiveness to aldosterone as the mechanism.[119-123] Where they have been searched for, other manifestations of distal tubular defects such as inability to concentrate or dilute the urine maximally have been demonstrated. Both distal forms of RTA are more common than proximal RTA, and full-blown Fanconi's syndrome is rarer still. Proximal RTA in some cases may be related to severe hyperparathyroidism. Phosphaturia has also been seen in a sizable percentage of patients. Several factors may play a role in this phenomenon, including a direct steroid effect, hyperparathyroidism, and immunologic injury to the renal tubule. Generally, phosphate wasting is a transient phenomenon but may produce significant clinical symptoms, including muscle weakness and twitching. The problem frequently is self-limited and can be controlled with oral phosphate supplementation. Renal glycosuria, uric acid wasting, and generalized aminoaciduria are quite rare.

Hypomagnesemia has become increasingly frequent with the widespread use of cyclosporine. Inappropriate renal magnesium wasting has been observed in a significant percentage of renal transplantation patients treated with cyclosporine and of patients on cyclosporine for other indications. The mechanism of this disorder is unknown. Neither hypocalcemia nor hypokalemia accompanies this defect, and it may occur independent of treatment with other magnesuric agents, such as diuretics and aminoglycosides. It has also been implicated in some cases of cyclosporine toxicity.[124]

GASTROINTESTINAL COMPLICATIONS

Although septic and cardiovascular complications are generally cited as the most significant causes of mortality, at least one center has reported hepatic failure as the leading cause of death in patients with functional transplants greater than 5 years.[125] Compared with patients who do not have abnormalities of hepatic function, those with chronic liver disease have an increased mortality, reaching 30 percent in 5 years. The most common cause in the above-cited series was hepatitis B, with ethanol use being the next most frequently implicated agent. Interestingly, in patients dying of hepatic failure, 80 percent underwent an immediately premorbid septic episode. This finding reflects the additional immunosuppressive effect of hepatic dysfunction, an effect that has been previously attributed to enhancement of T cell suppressor/cytotoxic activity relative to helper activity.

Additional potentially hepatotoxic elements also need to be considered (Table 18-9). CMV, EBV, and non-A, non-B hepatitis viruses afflict transplant patients, and are all capable of producing chronic hepatic damage. However, the percentage of patients exposed to these agents who subsequently develop chronic liver disease is unknown. Equally unclear is the role of drug toxicity in producing chronic liver disease, although both azathioprine and cyclosporine are known hepatotoxins. Other less common causes of hepatic damage reported in renal transplant recipients include hepatic veno-occlusive disease,[126,127] idiopathic portal fibrosis,[128] and hemochromatosis.[129] Interestingly, in one series, the etiology of most of the patients (27 of 38) who developed chronic liver disease could not be determined.[130,131]

On the other hand, acute hepatic damage occurred in 24 of 162 patients who were followed an average of 36 months posttransplantation. CMV was identified as the most frequent etiologic agent in this group, fol-

Table 18-9 Potential Causes of Hepatic Failure or Hepatic Toxicity in the Patient with a Transplant
Hepatitis B*
Ethanol
Cytomegalovirus
Epstein-Barr virus
Non-A, Non-B hepatitis viruses
Azathioprine
Cyclosporine
Hepatic veno-occlusive disease
Idiopathic portal fibrosis
Hemochromatosis
*Most common cause of hepatic failure

lowed by azathioprine. A large percentage, 9 of 34, had no identifiable cause of acute liver disease. Hepatitis B and EBV and other drugs played a far lesser role. No patients had hepatitis A.[130]

It is apparent, therefore, that liver disease, acute or chronic, is a common complication of renal transplantation. The effect of transplantation on established chronic liver disease remains controversial. In addition, whether patients who have positive hepatitis serology should be transplanted has not been determined. Studies examining the progression of liver disease have yielded conflicting results. Parfrey and coworkers[132] witnessed an increased mortality and a significant incidence of progression of liver disease as documented by liver biopsy. Progression generally occurred in HBsAg-positive patients and was unrelated to the pretransplantation histologic picture on liver biopsy. A follow-up study comparing HBsAg-positive and -negative transplantation and dialysis patients indicated that chronic hepatitis was both more common and more lethal in transplant patients, and it reconfirmed the significance of ABsAg positivity.[133] Whether HBsAg positivity should influence the choice of uremic therapy is a hotly debated issue. Clearly there are reports of individuals with HBsAg-positive chronic persistent hepatitis progressing to frank chronic active hepatitis after transplantation, thus transforming a generally benign illness into a more malignant disease. Additionally, cirrhosis, portal hypertension with its sequelae, and hepatoma have also been reported.[134–140] Attribution of these outcomes to transplantation alone has been challenged by other investigators, who have failed to reproduce an increased mortality or an increased incidence of hepatic failure in hepatitis-B-positive patients or who have discovered other causes of hepatic disease such as azathioprine toxicity or hemochromatosis.[141–148] In fact, some investigators have suggested that HBsAg positive patients may in fact accept transplants more readily and that liver function deterioration may be beneficially affected by a reduction in azathioprine dose. Thus HBsAg positive patients should not be denied a transplant on the basis of seropositivity alone. The resolution of this controversy will come only with more complete

comparative histologic and serologic studies between dialysis and transplantation patients. In our opinion, all HBsAg positive patients should be considered for liver biopsy prior to transplantation and be apprised of the potential increased mortality. However, at this time seropositivity alone should not preclude transplantation.

Another major gastrointestinal complication, upper tract bleeding, is discussed in Chapter 7. Further complications that warrant mention include pancreatitis, acalculous perforation of the gallbladder, and infectious diseases of the gut. Necrotizing pancreatitis is a rare but highly lethal complication, carrying a mortality in excess of 70 percent.[149] The major predisposing factors are immunosuppression, surgery, hypercalcemia, and infection, especially CMV. These patients generally require early surgical intervention. Less severe pancreatitis is also seen, and in these cases alcohol and cholelithiasis may be important factors. Perforation of an acalculous gallbladder is an equally rare complication.[150] Clinicians have considered predisposing factors to be recent surgery, the immunosuppressed state, and possible CMV infection.

If one considers infections of the oropharynx and esophagus, then infectious gastroenteritis is a fairly common complication.[151] Herpes virus and *Candida* infections frequently affect the upper tract, though they can be quite easily and effectively prevented by appropriate prophylactic therapy. On the other hand, infectious complications of the lower gastrointestinal tract are less common. Pseudomembranous colitis generally results from prolonged antibiotic therapy. Disseminated CMV infection may involve any portion of the gastrointestinal tract and produce ulceration, bleeding, and possibly perforation. In one series this complication was universally fatal, even with colon resection.

Intrinsic defense mechanisms of the gastrointestinal tract are affected in a variety of ways by transplantation (Table 18–10). Surgical trauma directly disrupts barriers to infection. Ileus associated with surgical procedures and the frequent use of nasogastric tubes disrupts normal flora, traumatizes the mucosa and allows unusual pathogens to attach, replicate, or cause direct injury to mucosal surfaces that would oth-

---

Table 18–10 Potential Effects of Transplantation on Defense Mechanisms of Gastrointestinal Tract

Disruption of barriers to infection by surgical trauma.

Ileus associated with surgical procedures disrupts normal flora and traumatizes mucosa, allowing unusual pathogens to invade and cause injury.

Use of antibiotics and immunosuppressive drugs may alter rate and type of secretions of gastrointestinal tract.

Balance of endogenous flora changed.

Drugs administered may be toxic to gastrointestinal tract.

Immunosuppression may disturb phagocytic activity of polymorphonuclear and mononuclear cells.

---

erwise not be susceptible to this type of injury.[152] In addition, the use of antibiotics and immunosuppressive drugs greatly impairs the natural defense mechanisms of the gastrointestinal tract by altering the rate and type of secretions. The fine balance of the various types of endogenous flora is also changed, allowing one or another organism to predominate or new organisms to take hold. Administration of these drugs also can be toxic to the gastrointestinal tract and its appendages.[152] Secondary defenses such as phagocytic activity of the polymorphonuclear and mononuclear cells of the lamina propria are also disturbed by drugs used for antirejection therapy.

The most common fungal infection posttransplantation is caused by *Candida albicans.* It affects the upper gastrointestinal tract, including the mouth, pharynx, esophagus, and stomach. The second most common fungal pathogens are *Aspergillus* organisms, which may cause lesions at any part of the gastrointestinal tract; however, the esophagus and stomach are frequent sites.

The most common viral infections of the gastrointestinal tract are due to herpes, cytomegalovirus (CMV), Epstein-Barr virus (EBV), adenovirus, and the various hepatitis viruses.

In transplant patients bacterial infections of the gastrointestinal tract are usually associated with local trauma or tissue injury. Since many bacterial gastrointestinal infections present with diarrhea with overt or more often occult bleeding, biopsy or culture is often necessary to identify the particular organism. Besides encouraging opportunistic infections, administration of antirejection drugs can also produce atro-

phy of intestinal villi. It is important to monitor cyclosporine doses, since this drug can be hepatotoxic in high doses.

ONCOLOGIC COMPLICATIONS

Neoplasm is another significant complication of the long-term transplant patient, occurring with a frequency ranging from 2 to 25 percent depending on the series and the types of malignancies reported.[153] Tumors presenting in these individuals may be of three origins: inadvertent transplantation of a tumor from a donor, recurrence of a tumor previously present in the recipient, or de novo development of a malignancy. Tumors originating from the donor occur rarely and may be primary renal cell carcinoma, metastatic carcinoma, or lymphoma. Transplantation has been used as a modality of treatment for certain tumors such as renal cell carcinoma. Up to 41 percent of patients have suffered a recurrence of the tumor under these circumstances.[154] De novo malignancies tend to be of certain types most frequently seen in skin cancer, particularly in certain areas of the world such as New Zealand and Australia. Interestingly, some areas of skin are highly overrepresented in the statistics, in particular, the anus, vulva, and lip.[152] Another commonly seen tumor is non-Hodgkins lymphoma. The very high incidence of this tumor initially seen after cardiac and renal transplantation may have been related to the significantly higher doses of immunosuppression used in the early days of cyclosporine use. Although further follow-up on the incidence of lymphoma with cyclosporine has failed to confirm the initial statistics, the incidence of lymphoma is still significantly elevated over the general population and represents one of the most common tumors seen. There may be some predilection for the central nervous system. For the most part, these tumors have been described as quite aggressive and resistant to therapy. However, several case reports now suggest that withdrawal or reduction of immunosuppression as well as early and aggressive therapy may be warranted. Other tumors seen with increased frequency in the transplant population include carcinoma in situ of the uterine cervix, Kaposi's sarcoma, and in one series, carcinoma of the colon. Interestingly, tumors common in the general population such as cancer of the lung and breast are not seen with increased frequency.[155-167]

The risk factors for the development of tumors are not fully delineated. It would appear that the incidence of malignancy is approximately the same in individuals receiving azathioprine as in those receiving cyclosporine. The vast majority of people developing tumors have received more than one immunosuppressive agent such as prednisone, antithymocyte globulin, cyclophosphamide, azathioprine, and irradiation.[168-174] In addition, there is increasing evidence for oncogenic viral involvement, particularly EBV and lymphoma, hepatitis B virus and hepatoma, polyoma virus and skin cancer, and herpes virus and carcinoma of the cervix. Whether the presence of prior infection with these or other viral agents will prove to be independent risk factors in posttransplantation patients is not known.[175-185] Individuals who develop tumors tend to have the best renal function, suggesting that diminished immune surveillance allows the persistence of good graft function but exposes patients to a higher risk of developing an unchecked tumor. In view of the high incidence of skin cancer, it seems prudent to recommend avoidance of heavy sun exposure as well as the use of a sun-blocking agent. Lesions in transplant patients frequently mimic cancer, so any suspicious areas should be biopsied. Follow-up of female patients should include routine pelvic examinations and cervical smears for early detection of lesions. Reduction in immunosuppressive drugs where possible and conservative cancer treatment are the usual approaches for the rare occurrences of cancer after transplantation. New neurological signs should prompt a search for a central nervous system tumor.

ENDOCRINE ABNORMALITIES

Endocrine abnormalities of uremia have been well characterized and studied. Successful renal transplantation may completely reverse or at least ameliorate many of these disturbances. Bonomoni[186] has documented normalization of hormonal status in 57 percent of patients with normally functioning grafts, more frequently in living related than in cadaveric transplants. Specifically, increase in erythropoietin leads to improvement in uremic anemia. Vitamin D metabolism normalizes. Most young men and women regain normal sexual and reproductive function within 6 months. Recognition of this phenomenon and contraceptive counseling are important aspects of outpatient care. It is advisable for the transplant patient to defer pregnancy until the stability of the transplant can be ascertained. Thyroid, parathyroid, gastrointestinal, and pituitary hormones also tend to normalize. It stands to reason that graft dysfunction interferes with correction of these abnormalities. The importance of the kidneys in hormonal metabolism is underscored by the fact that during acute rejection there is rapid recurrence of biochemic evidence of uremic hormonal dysfunction, which is reversible with resolution of the rejection. On the other hand, progressive endocrinologic abnormalities accompany chronic allograft rejection, as with the initial uremic state.

Approximately two thirds of transplant recipients experience reversal of uremic endocrinopathies and one third suffers from persistent abnormalities after transplantation. It is thought by some investigators that the extent of pretransplantation damage is a vital factor in predicting persistence of these abnormalities. In Bonomoni's series the most common problems were hyperparathyroidism, sexual dysfunction, and growth retardation. Biochemical hyperparathyroidism is common in the immediate posttransplantation period.[187-194]

In most cases early severe hypercalcemia is related to the large size of parathyroid glands secondary to poor control of hyperparathyroidism before transplantation. Contributory factors often include phosphate depletion, mobilization of soft tissue calcium deposits, steroid withdrawal, and vitamin D intoxication. This early state tends to subside within a few weeks. In only a small percentage of patients, probably less than 10 percent, one will have to address the problem of clinical hyperparathyroidism. These patients may present with hypercalcemia, hypophosphatemia, and elevated PTH levels. Fatigue is a common complaint, but any of the features of this disorder may be present, including bone and abdominal pain, depression, and renal stones. Rarely, severe hyperparathyroidism may result in ischemic necrosis of the digits. Early severe disease appears to correlate with the degree of hyperparathyroidism. In most cases persistent delayed hypercalcemia is also related to residual hyperparathyroidism and responds to usual surgical treatment.

The long-term complications of uncontrolled hypercalcemia include peptic ulcer disease, dystrophic metastatic calcifications, and renal functional abnormalities such as tubular acidosis, inability to concentrate the urine, and insufficiency. Since hyperparathyroidism has been implicated in aseptic necrosis, hypertension, and arterial disease, it is advisable to treat this entity aggressively. The choice of surgical procedure depends on the underlying anatomy and the expertise of the surgeon. Removal of a single hyperfunctioning adenoma, subtotal parathyroidectomy, or total parathyroidectomy with forearm implant are all viable options. Other causes of hypercalcemia, neoplasm in particular, must be considered and excluded.

Osteoporosis and aseptic necrosis may occur with or without hyperparathyroidism. A number of variables have been investigated and may help to predict which patients will develop aseptic necrosis. These include underlying renal disease, the length of time on dialysis, the severity of bone disease prior to transplantation, calcium and phosphate levels, and the total dose of steroids received. Thus far none of these factors have proved to be significant discriminating variables.[195-201] The most frequent presenting symptom of aseptic necrosis is bone pain, particularly while bearing weight. The plain radiograph may not be revealing. However, CT scan and more recently MRI technique have been shown to be very effective in early diagnosis. Yearly bone scans may show increased focal activity even before clinical symptoms are apparent. After early diagnosis surgical intervention such as the Hungerford decompression procedure may abort frank aseptic necrosis and obviate the need for a more extensive surgical procedure. While the hip is the most common site of involvement, virtually any other bone may suffer the same degenerative process. Minimizing steroid dose, for example, to an alternate-day regimen, may also help to slow the progression of this process.[202]

The risk of osteoporosis after transplantation has been well documented. Steroid dose is a well-established risk factor for it; other endocrinopathies such as diabetes and estrogen deficiency may also accompany the uremic state. Correctable risk factors for the development of osteoporosis must be identified and treated. Alternate-day steroid regimens may also be beneficial in the treatment of this disorder. As well, it is imperative to determine that osteoporosis rather than hyperparathyroidism or osteomalacia is the underlying process. Patients with steroid-induced osteoporosis have normal levels of serum calcium, phosphorus, and alkaline phosphatase.

Persistent sexual and reproductive dysfunction occurs more commonly in men than women, probably because of pre-existing uremic damage. Testosterone levels, basal and stimulated, may be lower than normal, and testicular biopsies show marked interstitial fibrosis. Persistently elevated FSH levels may be a clue to this unfortunate outcome.[203-207] Details of female reproductive function are found in Chapter 13.

Finally, persistent growth retardation has been a disappointing result in the majority of children. Virtually all children with renal failure suffer significant growth retardation. Transplantation has been associated with normalization of basal and stimulated growth hormone levels. Therefore, the impairment in growth has been postulated to be related to other factors. Steroids may play a crucial role in this because they are known to impair bone metabolism and cause phosphaturia, and they may cause peripheral resistance to somatomedins, thus inhibiting growth hormone action.[208,209]

Acquired endocrinopathies have also been observed in transplant patients. Diabetes mellitus occurs within the first 3 weeks in as many as 1 percent of transplant recipients. In one long-term series, diabetes mellitus affected transplant patients at a rate of about 15 percent per year. Hyperinsulinism related to high-dose steroids generally occurs early in the posttransplant course and resolves with decrease in the steroid dose, yielding no significant sequelae. However, when persistent hyperinsulinism is associated with glucose intolerance, it may contribute to hyperlipidemia and consequent cardiovascular risk. About 50 percent of these patients will respond to diet alone. Significantly, when compared with nondiabetic recipients, survival was decreased: 67 percent as opposed to 83 percent at 2 years. The factors related to the development of this complication include the black race, older age, family history, and the development of obesity.[210–213] Other recently implicated factors include cyclosporine A and CMV infection.[214,215]

HEMATOLOGIC COMPLICATIONS

Correction of uremia-induced anemia is the expected result with resumption of normal renal function posttransplantation. In one series 18 percent of patients with transplant not only corrected this anemia but developed erythrocytosis.[216] Some investigators have found that erythropoietin levels are higher in erythrocytotic than in non-erythrocytotic patients, implicating increased erythropoietin production as the etiology. However, others have not reproduced this finding, instead suggesting an increased sensitivity to erythropoietin. This generally occurs within the first year and abates spontaneously, though it may take 3 to 5 years. Phlebotomy is indicated only for symptoms related to polycythemia or when the hematocrit exceeds 60. More rarely, erythrocytosis may signal the development of renal artery stenosis or a neoplasm.[217]

Anemia, leukopenia, and thrombocytopenia are well-known complications of cytotoxic drug therapy. Marrow suppression secondary to azathioprine occurs rarely if hematologic status is checked with reasonable frequency. The white blood cell count is generally the first to decrease, and if recognized early enough, it responds to simple dose reduction or withdrawal. More rarely persistent marrow depression may necessitate discontinuance of the drug for an extended period. Generally, if the white cell count drops below 5000, it is advisable to decrease the dose of azathioprine by half. Holding the drug is advisable for white cell counts less than 3500. Significant marrow toxicity may occur, particularly as steroid doses are being lowered, with concomitant allopurinol therapy, and with long-term trimethoprim sulfamethoxazole therapy.[218] In some patients bone marrow suppression may prevent administration of adequate immunosuppression. If the patient is leukopenic prior to transplantation, a steroid challenge to assess white cell response can help predict azathioprine intolerance. An inadequate rise in the white cell count suggests future intolerance to the drug.[219] In those cases there are two options. Splenectomy, whether complete or subtotal, may restore white blood cell counts closer to normal levels. However, splenectomy is associated with both significant immediate morbidity and long-term mortality. The preferable option is simply to use cyclosporine instead of azathioprine.

Long-term azathioprine use is associated with two significant hematologic effects: macrocytic anemia and myelodysplasia.[220–223] Evaluation of the bone marrow of 25 patients revealed a greater percentage of young red blood cells and a greater frequency of megaloblasts and sideroblasts. The significance of development of this maturation arrest is not known at this time but may represent a preleukemic state. Myelodysplasia has rarely been reported and is most frequently associated with prolonged antimetabolitic therapy. In general the onset is insidious, is associated with cytogenetic abnormalities, and culminates in death within months. Besides long-standing immunosuppressive therapy, no other predisposing conditions have been found.

Cyclosporine does not share the marrow-suppressive properties of the cytotoxic agents, so cytopenias are generally not a limiting toxicity in using this agent. However, cyclosporine has been associated with the development of the hemolytic uremic syndromes in which thrombocytopenia is a nearly universal finding.[224-225] As well, cyclosporine toxicity has been associated with elevated levels of factor-VIII-related antigen, presumably as an index of its endothelial toxicity.[226]

NEUROLOGIC COMPLICATIONS

The most common neurologic complications, cerebrovascular accident, infection and seizures, have been discussed in Chapter 7. *Listeria,* fungi (particularly *Cryptococcus* and *Aspergillosis*), and herpes virus are the major infectious agents.[227]

Uremic neuropathy as measured by nerve conduction velocity and electromyelogram studies generally improves after transplant, with the greatest improvement seen in patients most severely afflicted prior to transplantation.[228,229] Autonomic dysfunction, however, may not improve after transplant; this was demonstrated in one series of 15 nondiabetic patients 12 months posttransplantation.[230] The long-term significance of this finding is unknown at this time.

The other major source of neurologic morbidity is drug-induced neurotoxicity. Prednisone has been associated with proximal myopathy and a multitude of psychiatric symptoms including euphoria, depression, sleep disturbances and even psychosis. Cyclosporine can also produce a variety of neurologic complaints. Seizures, tremor, paresis, blurred vision, and myoclonus may all occur.[231] With both drugs the symptoms are generally reversible on reduction or discontinuation. Other less common complications include lymphomatoid granulomatosis[232] and progressive multifocal leukoencephalopathy.[233]

OPHTHALMOLOGIC COMPLICATIONS

The three major ophthalmologic complications in renal transplant patients are infections, tumors, and cataracts.[234-238] The most common infections are caused by herpes virus. Herpetic keratitis and cyto-megalovirus (CMV) retinitis are chronic conditions that may result in blindness. CMV retinitis generally presents as the insidious development of visual impairment and may occur in the absence of disseminated illness. The treatment of choice is immunosuppressive withdrawal, although the experimental agent DHPG has show efficacy in other populations.[239] Keratoacanthoma and squamous cell carcinoma of the eyelid have been observed, an expected finding in view of the generally increased incidence of skin tumors.[240]

Posterior subcapsular cataracts have been associated with steroid use since 1960.[241,242] Factors other than steroid use that predispose to this complication have not been determined. In particular the total steroid dose, intensity, duration of therapy, and the age of the patient have demonstrated no predictive value. Instead, it appears that there is significant individual variability in susceptibility to this complication. An association with HLA-A1 has been demonstrated in one series.[243]

SUMMARY

A variety of complications, both surgical and nonsurgical in nature, can result after renal transplantation. Although some complications are rarely seen, others are more common and may be anticipated in a large number of cases. Close attention to early diagnosis and management is important to obtain acceptable transplantation results and to reduce patient morbidity and mortality.

REFERENCES

1. Lee, HM and Mendez-Picon, G: Complications of renal transplantation. In Greenfield, LJ (ed): Complications in Surgery and Trauma. JB Lippincott, Philadelphia, 1984, p 773.
2. Goldman, MH, et al: A twenty-year survey of arterial complications of renal transplantation. Surg Gynecol Obstet 141:758, 1975.
3. Palleschi, J, et al: Vascular complications of renal transplantation. Urology 16:61, 1980.
4. Robson, AJ, et al: Secondary hemorrhage

from the arterial anastomosis of renal allografts. Br J Surg 59:890, 1972.

5. Dostal, G, Medrano, J, and Eigler, FW: Die spontane nierentransplantruptur. Langenbecks Arch Chir 341:87, 1976.

6. Dryburgh, R, et al: Should the ruptured renal allograft be removed? Arch Surg 114:850, 1979.

7. Susan, LP, et al: Ruptured human renal allograft. Urology 11:53, 1978.

8. Lord, RSA, et al: Renal allograft rupture: Cause, clinical features and management. Ann Surg 177:268, 1973.

9. Kootstra, G, Meijer, S, and Elema, JD: Spontaneous rupture of homografted kidneys. Arch Surg 108:107, 1974.

10. Arruda, JAL, et al: Renal vein thrombosis in kidney allografts. Lancet 2:285, 1973.

11. Clunie, G: Renal transplantation: Selection and preparation of donors, immunosuppression, and surgical complications. In Chatterjee, S (ed): Organ Transplantation. John Wright PSG, Littleton, MA, p 151.

12. Kauffman, HM, et al: Prevention of transplant renal artery stenosis. Surgery 81:161, 1977.

13. Klarskov, P, et al: Renovascular hypertension after renal transplantation. Scand J Urol Nephrol 13:291, 1979.

14. Whitten, JI and Toledo-Pereyra, LH: Kidney transplantation: Vascular complications and perirenal fluid collections. In Toledo-Pereyra, LH (ed): Complications of Organ Transplantation. Marcel Dekker, New York, 1987, p 37.

15. Diamond, HG, et al: Dilatation of critical transplant renal artery stenosis by percutaneous transluminal angioplasty. AJR 133:1167, 1979.

16. Sniderman, KW, et al: Percutaneous transluminal angioplasty in renal transplant arterial stenosis for relief of hypertension. Radiology 135:23, 1980.

17. Banowsky, LHW: Surgical complications of renal transplantation. In Glenn, JF (ed): Urologic Surgery. JB Lippincott, Philadelphia, p 375.

18. Griffiths, AB, Fletcher, EW, and Morris, PJ: Lymphocele after renal transplantation. Aust NZ J Surg 49:626, 1979.

19. Howard, RJ, Simmons, RL, and Najarian, JS: Prevention of lymphoceles following renal transplantation. Ann Surg 186:700, 1977.

20. Lindstrom, BL, et al: Surgical complications in 500 kidney transplantations. Proc Eur Dial Transplant Assoc 14:353, 1977.

21. Fain, WR and Hardy, JD: Abdominal wounds and their complications. In Hardy, JD (ed): Rhoads Textbook of Surgery, Principles and Practice. JB Lippincott, Philadelphia, 1977, p 204.

22. Salvatierra, O, et al: 1,500 Renal transplants at one center: Evolution of a strategy for optimal success. Am. J Surg. 142:14, 1981.

23. Eklund, B, et al: Percutaneous nephrostomy: A therapeutic procedure for the management of urinary leakage and obstruction in renal transplantation. Transplant Proc 16:1304, 1984.

24. Pasternak, A: Lancet 2:82, 1968.

25. Hayry, P, et al: Monitoring of allograft by transplant aspiration cytology. Ann Clin Res 13:265, 1981.

26. Sagalowsky, AI, et al: Urologic complications in 505 renal transplants with early catheter removal. J Urol 129:929, 1983.

27. Goldstein, I, Cho, SI, and Olsson, CA: Nephrostomy drainage for renal transplant complications. J Urol 126:159, 1981.

28. Kinnaert, P, et al: Ureteral stenosis after kidney transplantation: True incidence and long term follow up after surgical correction. J Urol 133:17, 1985.

29. Hriko, GM, et al: Factors responsible for urinary fistula in the renal transplant recipient. Ann Surg 178:609, 1973.

30. Khauli, RB, et al: Preservation of the ureteral blood supply in rat renal transplantation. Microsurgery 4:225, 1983.

31. Smith, RB and Ehrlich, RM: The surgical complications of renal transplantation. Urol Clin North Am 3:621, 1976.

32. Starzl, RE, et al: Urological complications of 216 human recipients of renal transplants. Ann Surg 172:1, 1970.

33. Loughlin, KR, Tilney, NL, and Richie, JP: Urologic complications in 718 renal transplant patients. Surgery 95:297, 1984.

34. Schiff, M Jr., et al: Management of urinary fistulas after renal transplantation. J Urol 115:251, 1976.

35. Salvatierra, O Jr., Kountz, SL, and Belzer, FO: Prevention of ureteral fistula after renal transplantation. J Urol 112:445, 1974.

36. Koehler, PR, Kanemoto, HH, and Maxwell, JC: Ultrasonic "B" scanning in the diagnosis of complications in renal transplant patients. Radiology 119:661, 1976.

37. Lieberman, RP, et al: Non-operative percutaneous management of urinary fistulas and strictures in renal transplantation. Surg Gynecol Obstet 155:667, 1982.

38. Kartheuser, AH, et al: Anterior extravesical ureteroneocystostomy: The procedure of choice in kidney transplantation. Transplant Proc 17:176, 1985.

39. Jordan, ML, et al: Imaging of the trans-

planted kidney with nuclear magnetic resonance. Transplant Proc 17:32, 1985.

40. Lieberman, RP, et al: Fine needle antegrade pyelography in the renal transplant. J Urol 126:155, 1981.

41. Helling, TS, et al: The surgical approach to obstructive problems of the transplant ureter. Transplant Proc 14:751, 1982.

42. Berger, RE, et al: The use of self-retained ureteral stents in the management of urologic complications in renal transplant recipients. J Urol 124:781, 1980.

43. Lieberman, SF, et al: Percutaneous antegrade transluminal ureteroplasty for renal allograft ureteral stenosis. J Urol 128:122, 1982.

44. List, AR, et al: Balloon dilatations for ureteral strictures in graft kidneys: A viable alternative to further surgery. Transplantation 35:105, 1983.

45. Mendes, R and Vargas, AD: Kidney transplantation: Urological complications. In Toledo-Pereyra, LH (ed): Complications of Organ Transplantation. Marcel Dekker, New York, 1987, p 49.

46. Kinnaert, P, et al: Ureteral stenosis after kidney transplantation: True incidence and long-term follow-up after surgical correction. J Urol 133:117, 1985.

47. Feinstein, EI, et al: Fever and renal dysfunction in a renal transplant patient. Am J Nephrol 6:232, 1986.

48. Ehrlichman, RJ, et al: The use of percutaneous nephrostomy in patients with ureteric obstruction undergoing renal transplantation. Surg Gynecol Obstet 162:121, 1986.

49. Lamballe, AK, et al: Percutaneous nephrostomy in renal transplant patients. Transplant Proc 17:2143, 1985.

50. Burleson, RL and Marvarger, PD: Prevention of lymphocoele formation following renal allotransplantation. J Urol 127:18, 1982.

51. Gianello, P, et al: Ischemic necrosis of the allograft ureter. Transplant Proc 16:1301, 1984.

52. Thomalla, JV, et al: The manifestation and management of late urological complications in renal transplant recipients: Use of the urological armamentarium. J Urol 134:944, 1985.

53. Boyce, NW, et al: Acute renal transplant failure resulting from obstruction with a calculus. Transplant Proc 16:1364, 1984.

54. Brun, G, et al: Urolithiasis after kidney transplantation: Clinical and mineralogical aspects. Urol Res 8:211, 1980.

55. Motayne, GG, et al: Calculus formation in renal transplant patients. J Urol 132:448, 1984.

56. Narayana, AS, Loening, S, and Culp, DS: Kidney stones and renal transplantation. Urology 12:61, 1978.

57. Hulbert, JC, et al: The percutaneous removal of calculi from transplanted kidneys. J Urol 134:324, 1985.

58. Williams, G, et al: Urologic complications of renal transplantation. Br J Urol 42:21, 1970.

59. Fox, M and Tottenham, RC: Urinary fistula from segmental infarction in a transplanted kidney: Recovery following surgical repair. Br J Urol 44:336, 1972.

60. McDonald, JC, et al: Cadaver donor renal transplantation by centers of the Southeastern Organ Procurement Foundation. Ann Surg 193:1, 1981.

61. Toledo-Pereyra, LH: Organ harvesting. In Toledo-Pereyra, LH (ed): Basic Concepts of Organ Procurement, Perfusion, and Preservation for Transplantation. Academic Press, New York, 1982, p 57.

62. Toledo-Pereyra, LH: Risks of long-term preservation (cold ischemia) in renal preservation. Proc 18th International Course on Transplantation and Clinical Immunology, Lyon, France, May, 1986.

63. Lee, HM and Mendez-Picon, G: Complications of renal transplantation. In Greenfield, LJ (ed): Complications in Surgery and Trauma. JB Lippincott, Philadelphia, 1984, p 773.

64. Taube, D, et al: A comparison of the clinical, histopathologic, cytologic, and biochemical features of renal transplant rejection, cyclosporine A nephrotoxicity, and stable renal function. Transplant Proc 17:179, 1985.

65. Kjellstrand, CM, et al: Etiology and prognosis in acute posttransplant renal failure. Am J Med 61:190, 1976.

66. Brophy, D, Najarian, JS, and Kjellstrand, CM: Acute tubular necrosis after renal transplantation. Transplantation 29:245, 1980.

67. Heil, J, et al: Acute tubular necrosis of cadaver renal allografts does not correlate with organ sharing or preservation time but portends a poorer prognosis for long-term graft survival. Transplant Proc 16:270, 1984.

68. Cho, SI, et al: The influence of acute tubular necrosis on kidney transplant survival. Transplant Proc 17:16, 1985.

69. Springate, JE, et al: Hematuria and hypercalciuria following renal transplantation. Transplantation 41:664, 1986.

70. Case records of the Massachusetts General Hospital. New Engl J Med 301:1052, 1979.

71. Cameron, JS: Effect of the recipient's disease on the results of transplantation

(other than diabetes mellitus). Kidney Int (Suppl 14)23:S–24, 1983.

72. Cameron, JS: Glomerulonephritis in renal transplants. Transplantation 34:237, 1982.

73. Fische, FE, et al: Membranous glomerulopathy in transplant kidneys: Recurrent or de novo disease in four patients. Clin Nephrol 15:154, 1981.

74. First, MR, et al: Membranous glomerulopathy following kidney transplantation. Transplantation 38:603, 1974.

75. Ihle, BU, et al: Glomerulonephritis in a renal transplant. Transplant Proc 15:2147, 1983.

76. Leibowitch, J, et al: Recurrence of dense deposits in transplanted kidney: II, Serum complement and nephritic factor profiles. Kidney Int 5:396, 1979.

77. Lewis, EJ: Recurrent focal sclerosis after renal transplantation. Kidney Int 522:325, 1982.

78. Maizel, SE, et al: Incidence and significance of recurrent focal segmental glomerulosclerosis in renal allograft recipients. Transplantation 32:512, 1981.

79. Milliner, DS, Pierides, AM, and Holley, RE: Renal transplantation in Alport's syndrome: Anti-glomerular basement membrane glomerulonephritis in the allograft. Mayo Clin Proc 57:35, 1982.

80. Morzycka, M, et al: Evaluation of recurrent glomerulonephritis in kidney allograft. Am J Med 72:588, 1982.

81. Obermiller, LE, et al: Recurrent membranous glomerulonephritis in two renal transplants. Transplantation 40:100, 1985.

82. Parfrey, PS, et al: Glomerular sclerosis in a renal isograft and identical twin donor. Transplantation 38:343, 1984.

83. Petterson, E, Honkanen, E, and Tornroth, T: Recurrence of IgA nephropathy with nephrotic syndrome in renal allograft. Nephron 41:114, 1985.

84. Pommer, W, et al: De novo membranoproliferative glomerulonephritis in a renal allograft. Int Urol Nephrol 54:359, 1983.

85. Rivolta, E, et al: De novo focal glomerular sclerosis in an identical twin renal transplant recipient. Transplantation 35:328, 1983.

86. Turner, DR, et al: Transplantation in mesangiocapillary glomerulonephritis with intramembranous dense "deposits": Recurrence of disease. Kidney Int 9:439, 1976.

87. Walter, WC, et al: Allograft rejection and the nephrotic syndrome. Transplant Proc 17:1763, 1985.

88. Penn, I, et al: Testicular complications following renal transplantation. Ann Surg 176:697, 1972.

89. Cho, S, et al: Kidney transplantation in drug-addicts. Bol Asoc Med PR 77:136, 1985.

90. Cho, S, et al: Perioperative antibiotics in renal transplant wound infections. Infections in Surgery 4:591, 1985.

91. Vij, D, Dumler, F, and Toledo-Pereyra, LH: Infectious complications in renal transplantation: Approach to the problem of fever, urinary wound and pulmonary infections. Dialysis and Transpl 9:129, 1980.

92. Winearls, CG, Lane, DJ, and Kurtz, J: Infectious complications after renal transplantation. In Morris, PJ (ed): Kidney Transplantation, ed 2. Grune & Stratton, New York, 1984, p 427.

93. Walter, S, Pedersen, FB, and Vejlsgaard, R: Urinary tract infection and wound infection in kidney transplant patients. Br J Urol 47:513–516, 1975.

94. Ahonen, J: Wound complications in renal transplantation. In Toledo-Pereyra, LH (ed): Complications of Organ Transplantation. Marcel Dekker, New York, 1987, p 71.

95. Kyriakides, GR, Simmons, RL, and Najarian, JS: Wound infections in renal transplant wounds: Pathogenic and prognostic factors. Ann Surg 182:770, 1975.

96. Avram, MM: Treating diabetic nephropathy then and now. In Friedman, EA and L'Esperance, FA (eds): Diabetic Renal Retinal Syndrome. Grune & Stratton, New York, 1982.

97. Rimmer, JM, et al: Renal transplantation in diabetes mellitus. Nephron 42:304, 1986.

98. Cheigh, JS, et al: Hypertension and decreased graft survival in long-term kidney transplant recipients. Transplant Proc 17:174, 1985.

99. Colonna, JO, et al: Non-renin dependent hypertension in renal allograft rejections. Arch Pathol Lab Med 108:117, 1984.

100. Curtis, JJ: Hypertension and kidney transplantation. Am J Kidney Dis 7:181, 1986.

101. Curtis, JJ, et al: Surgical therapy for persistent hypertension after renal transplantation. Transplantation 31:125, 1981.

102. Curtis, JJ, et al: Remission of essential hypertension after renal transplantation. N Engl J Med 309:1009, 1983.

103. Kalbfleisch, JH, et al: Habitual excessive dietary salt intake and blood pressure levels in renal transplant recipients. Am J Med 73:205, 1982.

104. O'Connor, DT, et al: Urinary kallicrein excretion after renal transplantation. Am J Med 73:475, 1982.

105. Walter, WE, et al: Etiology and pathogenesis of hypertension following renal transplantation. Nephron 42:102, 1986.

106. June, CH, et al: Correlation of hypomagnesemia with the onset of cyclosporine-associated hypertension in marrow transplant patients. Transplantation 41:47, 1986.

107. Cattran, DC, et al: Hyperlipidemia after renal transplantation: Natural history and pathophysiology. Ann Intern Med 91:554, 1979.

108. Somer, J, et al: Lipoprotein lipids in renal transplant recipients of different pretransplant etiology of renal disease. Atherosclerosis 39:177, 1981.

109. Tsakiris, D, et al: Low density lipoprotein metabolism following renal transplantation. Transplantation 39:458, 1985.

110. Turgan, C, et al: The effect of renal transplantation with a minimal steroid regime on uraemic hypertriglyceridemia. Quarterly Journal of Medicine New Series 53:271, 1984.

111. Hiner, HH and Suki, WN: Cardiovascular complications of renal transplantation. In Toledo-Pereyra, LH (ed): Complications of Organ Transplantation. Marcel Dekker, New York, 1987, p 125.

112. Raine, AE, Ledingham, JGG: Cardiovascular complications after renal transplantation. In Morris, PJ (ed): Kidney Transplantation, ed 2. Grune & Stratton, 1984, p 470.

113. Sakhaee, K and Helderman, JH: Kidney transplantation: Mineral metabolism complications. In Toledo-Pereyra, LH (ed): Complications of Organ Transplantation. Marcel Dekker, New York, 1987, p 147.

114. McCarron, DA, et al: Post-transplantation hyperparathyroidism. Demonstration of retained control of parathyroid function by ionized calcium. Am J Clin Nutr 33:1536, 1980.

115. Parfitt, AM: Hypercalcemic hyperparathyroidism following transplantation: Differential diagnosis, management, and implications for cell population control in the parathyroid gland. Min Electrolyte Metab 8:91, 1982.

116. Sakhaee, K, et al: Disturbances in mineral metabolism after successful renal transplantation. Min Electrolyte Metab 11:167, 1985.

117. Rosenbaum, RW, et al: Decreased phosphate reabsorption after renal transplantation: Evidence for a mechanism independent of calcium and parathyroid hormone. Kidney Int 19:568, 1981.

118. Sakhaee, K, et al: Postmenopausal osteoporosis as a manifestation of renal hypercalciuria with secondary hyperparathyroidism. J Clin Endocrinol Metab 61:368, 1985.

119. Batlle, DC, et al: The pathogenesis of hyperchloremic metabolic acidosis associated with kidney transplantation. Am J Med 70:786, 1981.

120. Better, OS, et al: Syndrome of incomplete renal tubular acidosis after cadaver kidney transplantation. Ann Intern Med 71:39, 1969.

121. DeGronzo, RA, et al: Investigations into the mechanisms of hyperkalemia following renal transplantation. Kidney Int 11:357, 1977.

122. Foley, RJ, Hamner, RW, and Weinman, EJ: Serum potassium concentrations in cyclosporine and azathioprine-treated renal transplant patients. Nephron 40:280, 1985.

123. Mookerjee, B, Gault, UH, Dossetor, JB: Hyperchloremic acidosis in early diagnosis of renal allograft rejection. Ann Intern Med 71:47, 1969.

124. June, CH, et al: Profound hypomagnesemia and renal magnesium wasting associated with the use of cyclosporine for marrow transplantation. Transplantation 89:620, 1985.

125. Weir, MR, et al: Liver disease in recipients of long-functioning renal allografts. Kidney Int 28:839, 1985.

126. Katzka, DA, et al: Azathioprine and hepatic veno-occlusive disease in renal transplant patients. Gastroenterology 90:446, 1986.

127. Read, AE, et al: Hepatic veno-occlusive disease associated with renal transplantation and azathioprine therapy. Ann Intern Med 104:651, 1986.

128. Bredfeldt, JE, Enriquez, RE, and Groszmann, RJ: Idiopathic portal hypertension in a renal transplant recipient. J Clin Gastroenterol 4:157, 1982.

129. Rao, KV and Anderson, WR: Hemosiderosis and hemochromatosis in renal transplant recipients. Am J Nephrol 5:419, 1985.

130. Ware, AJ, et al: Etiology of liver disease in renal-transplant patients. Ann Intern Med 91:364, 1979.

131. LaQuaglia, MP, et al: Impact of hepatitis on renal transplantation. Transplantation 32:504, 1981.

132. Parfrey, PS, et al: The prevalence and progression of liver disease in renal transplant recipients: A histologic study. Transplant Proc 16:1103, 1984.

133. Parfrey, PS, et al: The impact of renal transplantation on the course of hepatitis B liver disease. Transplantation 39:610, 1985.

134. Pirson, Y, et al: Long-term effect of HB$_s$ antigenemia on patient survival after renal

transplantation. N Engl J Med 296:194, 1977.

135. Hillis, WD, Hillis, A, and Walker, WG: Hepatitis B surface antigenemia in renal transplant recipient. JAMA 242:329, 1979.

136. Degos, F, et al: Is renal transplantation involved in post-transplantation liver disease? Transplantation 29:100, 1980.

137. Disler, PB, et al: Hepatitis B virus-associated liver disease after renal transplantation. S Afr Med J 59:97, 1981.

138. White, AG, et al: Renal transplantation in hepatitis B surface antigen positive patients. Transplant Proc 19:2150, 1987.

139. London, WT, et al: Association of graft survival with host response to hepatitis B infection in patients with kidney transplants. New Engl J Med 296:241, 1977.

140. Rao, KV and Anderson, WR: The morphology and natural history of chronic liver disease in renal transplant recipients. Transplant Proc 17:165, 1985.

141. Shons, AR, et al: Renal transplantation in patients with Australia antigenemia. Am J Surg 128:699, 1974.

142. Chatterjee, SN, et al: Successful renal transplantation in patients positive for hepatitis B antigen. New Engl J Med 291:62, 1974.

143. Fine, RN, et al: HBs antigenemia in renal allograft recipients. Ann Surg 185:411, 1977.

144. Toussaint, C, et al: Prognostic significance of hepatitis B antigenemia in kidney transplantation. Nephron 17:335, 1976.

145. Berne, TV, Fitzgivvons, TJ, and Silberman, H: The effect of hepatitis B antigenemia on long-term success and hepatic disease in renal transplant patients. Transplantation 24:412, 1977.

146. Singar, DPS, Couture, RA, and Jindal, SL: Renal allograft outcome, patient survival and liver function in patients with HBsAg infections. Transplant Proc 16:1106, 1984.

147. Rivolta, E, et al: Prognostic significance of hepatitis B surface antigenemia in cadaveric renal transplant patients. Transplant Proc 19:2153, 1987.

148. Flagg, GL, et al: The influence of hepatitis B infection on the outcome of renal allotransplantation. Transplant Proc 19:2155, 1987.

149. Burnstein, M, et al: Necrotizing pancreatitis in renal transplant patients. Can J Surg 25:547, 1982.

150. Hopkinson, GB, Crowson, MC, and Barnes, AD: Perforation of the acalculous gallbladder following renal transplantation. Transplant Proc 17:2014, 1985.

151. Komorowski, RA, et al: Gastrointestinal complications in renal transplant recipients. Am J Clin Pathol 86:161, 1986.

152. Van Thiel, DH: Gastrointestinal and liver complications. In Toledo-Pereyra, LH (ed): Complications of Organ Transplantation. Marcel Dekker, New York, 1987, p 169.

153. Penn, I: Cancer and transplantation. In Toledo-Pereyra, LH (ed): Complications of Organ Transplantation. Marcel Dekker, New York, p 237.

154. Penn, I: Chemical immunosuppression and human cancer. Cancer 34:1474, 1974.

155. Penn, I: Some contributions of transplantation to our knowledge of cancer. Transplant Proc 12:676, 1980.

156. Penn, I: Malignancies following the use of cyclosporin A in man. Cancer Surveys 1:621, 1982.

157. Penn, I: Malignant lymphomas in organ transplant recipients. Transplant Proc 13:736, 1981.

158. Doyle, TJ, et al: Hodgkins disease in renal transplant recipients. Cancer 51:245, 1983.

159. Blohme, I and Brynger, H: Malignant disease in renal transplant patients. Transplantation 39:23, 1985.

160. Blohme, I and Larko, O: Premalignant and malignant skin lesions in renal transplant patients. Transplantation 37:165, 1984.

161. Shiel, AGR, et al: Cancer and survival after cadaveric donor renal transplantation. Transplant Proc 11:1052, 1979.

162. Penn, I: Development of cancer as a complication of clinical transplantation. Transplant Proc 9:1121, 1977.

163. Shiel, AGR: Cancer in renal allograft recipients in Australia and New Zealand. Transplant Proc 9:1133, 1977.

164. Akhtar, M, et al: Kaposi's sarcoma in renal transplant recipients. Cancer 53:258, 1984.

165. Bia, MJ and Flye, MW: Immunoblastic lymphoma in a cyclosporine-treated renal transplant recipient. Transplantation 39:673, 1985.

166. Eklund, B, et al: Lymphoproliferative disease after renal transplantation. Transplant Proc 18:95, 1986.

167. Harris, JP and Penn, I: Immunosuppression and the development of malignancies of the upper airway and related structures. Laryngoscope 91:520, 1981.

168. Matas, AJ, et al: Increased incidence of malignancy in uremic patients and its significance to transplantation. Transplant Proc 9:1137, 1977.

169. Sloan, GM, Cole P, and Wilson, RE: Risk indicators of de novo malignancy in renal transplant recipients. Transplant Proc 9:1129, 1977.

170. Kinlen, L, Doll, R, and Peto, J: The incidence of tumors in human transplant recipients. Transplant Proc 15:1039, 1983.

171. Kelly, GE and Sheil, AGR: Immuno-

depression as a contributing factor to a high incidence of skin cancer in kidney transplant recipients. Transplant Proc 16:1002, 1984.

172. Penn, I: Depressed immunity and the development of cancer. J Exp Immunol 46:459, 1981.

173. Penn, I: Cancer is a complication of severe immunosuppression. Surg Gynecol Obstet 162:603, 1986.

174. Kinlen, LJ: Immunosuppressive therapy and cancer. Cancer Surveys 1:565, 1982.

175. Halpert, R, et al: Human papillomavirus infection and lower genital neoplasia in female renal allograft recipients. Transplant Proc 17:93, 1985.

176. Hanto, DW, et al: Epstein-Barr virus-induced B-cell lymphoma after renal transplantation. N Engl J Med 306:913, 1982.

177. Hanto, DW, et al: Acyclovir therapy of Epstein-Barr virus-induced post-transplant lymphoproliferative diseases. Transplant Proc 17:89, 1985.

178. Penn, I: Kaposi's sarcoma in organ transplant recipients. Transplantation 27:8, 1979.

179. Sullivan, JL, et al: Epstein-Barr virus induced lymphoproliferation. N Engl J Med 305:1067, 1981.

180. Shafritz, DA, et al: Integration of hepatitis B virus DNA into the genome of liver cells in chronic liver disease and hepatocellular carcinoma. N Engl J Med 305:1067, 1981.

181. Matas, AJ, Simmons, RL, and Najarian, JS: Chronic antigenic stimulation, herpesvirus infection, and cancer in transplant recipients. Lancet 1:1277, 1975.

182. Hochberg, FH, et al: Central nervous system lymphoma related to Epstein-Barr virus. N Engl J Med 309:745, 1983.

183. Cleary, ML, Warnke, R, and Sklar, J: Monoclonality of lymphoproliferative lesions in cardiac transplant recipients. N Engl J Med 310:477, 1984.

184. Dummer, JS, et al: Epstein-Barr virus-induced lymphoma in cardiac transplant recipient. Am J Med 77:179, 1984.

185. Groopman, JE: Viruses and human neoplasia: Approaching etiology. Am J Med 75:377, 1983.

186. Bonomoni, V, et al: Hormonal abnormalities in renal transplantation. Contributions in Nephrology 48:56, 1985.

187. Conceicao, SC, et al: Hypercalcemia following renal transplantation: Causes and consequences. Clin Nephrol 16:235, 1981.

188. Cundy, T, et al: Calcium metabolism and hyperparathyroidism after renal transplantation. Quarterly Journal of Medicine New Series, 7:67, 1983.

189. Diethelm, AG, Edwards, RP, and Welchel, JP: The natural history and surgical treatment of hypercalcemia before and after renal transplantation. Surg Gynecol Obstet 154:481, 1982.

190. Friedlander, MA, Horst, RL, and Hawker, CD: Absence of effect of 24, 25-dihydroxycholecalciferol on serum immunoreactive PTH in patients with persistent hyperparathyroidism after renal transplantation. Clin Nephrol 22:206, 1984.

191. Garvin, PJ, et al: Management of hypercalcemic hyperparathyroidism after renal transplantation. Arch Surg 120:578, 1985.

192. McCarron, DA, et al: Total parathyrodectomy for posttransplantation hyperparathyroidism. Transplantation 40:266, 1985.

193. Memmos, DE, et al: The role of parathyroidectomy in the management of hyperparathyroidism in patients on maintenance hemodialysis and after renal transplantation. Nephron 30:143, 1982.

194. Vezzoli, G, et al: High plasma ionized calcium with normal PTH and total calcium levels in normal-function kidney transplant recipients. Nephron 42:290, 1986.

195. Adinoff, AD and Hollister, JR: Steroid-induced fractures and bone loss in patients with asthma. N Engl J Med 309:265, 1983.

196. Baylink, DJ: Glucocorticoid-induced osteosporosis. N Engl J Med 309:306, 1983.

197. Chesney, RW, Rose, PG, and Mazess, RB: Persistence of diminished bone mineral content following renal transplantation in childhood. Pediatrics 73:459, 1984.

198. Neubauer, E, et al: Bone mineral content after renal transplantation. Klin Wochenschr 62:93, 1984.

199. Parfrey, PS, et al: The decreased incidence of aseptic necrosis in renal transplant recipients: A case control study. Transplantation 41:182, 1986.

200. Scholz, D, et al: Prevention of osteonecrosis following renal transplantation by using vitamin D_2 (ergocalciferol). Proc Eur Dial Transplant Assoc 20:331, 1983.

201. Thompson, RC, Hauel, R, and Goetz, F: Presumed neurotrophic skeletal disease in diabetic kidney transplant recipients. JAMA 249:1317, 1980.

202. Dumler, F, et al: Advantage of long-term alternate day steroid therapy in renal transplantation: A controlled study. Proc Dialysis Transplant Forum 10:215, 1980.

203. Penn, I, Makowski, EL, and Harris, P: Parenthood following renal transplantation. Kidney Int 18:221, 1980.

204. Mies, R, et al: Investigation on Leydig cell function and regulation post renal transplantation. Clin Nephrol 4:86, 1975.

205. Lim, VS and Fang, VS: Gonadal dysfunction in uremic men: A study of the hypothalamo-pituitary testicular axis before

and after renal transplantation. Am J Med 58:655, 1975.

206. Holdsworth, SR, deKretser, DM, and Atkins, RC: A comparison of hemodialysis and transplantation in reversing the uremic disturbance of male reproductive function. Clin Nephrol 10:146, 1978.

207. Peces, R, et al: Prolactin in chronic renal failure, haemodialysis, and transplant patients. Proc Eur Dial Transplant Assoc 16:700, 1979.

208. Saenger, P, et al: Somatomedin and growth retardation after renal transplantation. Pediat Res 8:163, 1974.

209. Spencer, EM, Uthne, KO, and Arnold, WC: Growth impairment with elevated somatomedin levels in children with chronic renal insufficiency. Acta Endocrinol 19:36, 1979.

210. Friedman, EA, et al: Posttransplant diabetes in kidney transplant recipients. Am J Nephrol 5:196, 1985.

211. Ruiz, JO, et al: Steroid diabetes in renal transplant recipients: Pathogenetic factors and prognosis. Surgery 73:759, 1977.

212. Arner, P, et al: Some characteristics of steroid diabetes: A study in renal transplant recipients receiving high dose corticosteroid therapy. Diabetes Care 6:23, 1983.

213. Zawada, ET, et al: Hemoglobin A1 in renal transplant recipients. Arch Intern Med 145:82, 1985.

214. Engfeldt, P, et al: Impaired glucose tolerance with cyclosporine. Transplant Proc 18:65, 1986.

215. Lehr, H, et al: Cytomegalovirus-induced diabetes mellitus in a renal allograft recipient. Transplant Proc 17:2152, 1985.

216. Wickre, CG, et al: Posttransplant erythrocytosis: A review of 53 cases. Kidney Int 23:731, 1983.

217. Lamperi, S, et al: Erythropoietin-independent erythropoiesis in polycythemic transplanted patients. Transplant Proc 17:86, 1985.

218. Bradley, PP, et al: Neutropenia and thrombocytopenia in renal allograft recipients treated with trimethoprim sulfamethoxazole. Ann Intern Med 93:560, 1980.

219. Fisher, KA, et al: Prediction of azathioprine intolerance in transplant patients. Lancet 1:828, 1976.

220. Sjogren, U, Thysell, H, and Lindholm, T: Bone marrow morphology in patients in long-term treatment with azathioprine. Scand J Haematol 26:182, 1981.

221. Ihle, BU, et al: Myelodysplasia in cadaver renal allografts: A report of four cases. Am J Kidney Dis 5:251, 1985.

222. Kirchner, KA, et al: Chronic granulocytic leukemia after renal transplantation. Arch Intern Med. 143:1984, 1983.

223. Case Records Massachusetts General Hospital: Case 18-1983. N Engl J Med 308:1081, 1983.

224. Hows, JN, et al: Nephrotoxicity in bone marrow transplant recipients treated with cyclosporine A. Br J Haematol 54:69, 1983.

225. Atkinson, K, et al: Cyclosporin A associated nephrotoxicity in the first 100 days after allogeneic bone marrow transplantation: Three distinct syndromes. Br J Haematol 54:59, 1983.

226. Brown, Z, et al: Increased Factor VIII as an index of vascular injury in cyclosporine nephrotoxicity. Transplantation 42:150, 1986.

227. Beal, MR, et al: Aspergillosis of the central nervous system. Neurology 32:473, 1982.

228. Albertazzi, A, et al: Uremic polyneuropathy: Electrophysiologic findings after renal transplantation. Transplant Proc 17:127, 1985.

229. Yasbeck, S, Larbrisseau, A, and O'Regan, S: Femoral neuropathy after renal transplantation. J Urol 134:720, 1985.

230. Solders, G, Persson, A, and Wilczek, H: Autonomic system dysfunction and polyneuropathy in nondiabetic uremia. Transplantation 41:616, 1986.

231. Atkinson, K, et al: Cyclosporine-associated central nervous system toxicity after allogeneic bone marrow transplantation. Transplantation 38:34, 1984.

232. Michaud, J, Manerjee, D, and Kaufmann, JCE: Lymphomatoid granulomatosis involving the central nervous system complication of a renal transplant with terminal monoclonal B-cell proliferation. Acta Neuropathol 61:141, 1983.

233. Saxton, CR, et al: Progressive multifocal leukoencephalopathy in a renal transplant recipient. Am J Med 77:333, 1984.

234. Pfefferman, R, Gombos, GM, and Kountz, SL: Ocular complications after renal transplantation. Ann Ophthalmol 9:467, 1977.

235. Berkowitz, JS, David, DS, and Sakai, S: Ocular complications in renal transplant recipients. Am J Med 55:492, 1973.

236. Porter, R, Crombie, AL, and Gardner, PS: Incidence of ocular complications in patients undergoing renal transplantation. Br Med J 3:135, 1972.

237. Kern, R, Zaruba, A, and Scheitlin, W: Ocular side effects of long term immunosuppressive therapy in recipients of cadaver kidney transplants. Ophthalmic Research 1:21, 1970.

238. Hovland, KR and Ellis, PP: Ocular changes in renal transplant patients. Am J Ophthalmol 63:283, 1967.

239. Collaborative DHPG Treatment Study Group: Treatment of serious cytomegalo-

virus infections with 9-(1,3-dihydroxy-2-propoxymethyl) guanine in patients with AIDS and other immunodeficiencies. N Engl J Med 314:801, 1986.

240. Steward, WB, et al: Eyelid tumors and renal transplantation. Arch Ophthalmol 98:1771, 1980.

241. Manabe, S, Bucala, R, and Cerami, A: Nonenzymatic addition of glucocorticoids to lens proteins in steroid-induced cataracts. J Clin Invest 74:1803, 1984.

242. Shalka, HW, and Prchal, JT: Effect of corticosteroids on cataract formation. Arch Ophthalmol 98:1773, 1980.

243. Kollaritis, CR, et al: HLA-A1 and steroid-induced cataracts in renal transplant patients. Ann Ophthalmol 14:1116, 1982.

SECTION IV

LIVING RELATED
TRANSPLANTATION

Chapter 19

Living Donors: Selection, Availability, and Long-Term Follow-Up

DAVID A. OGDEN

SELECTION AND AVAILABILITY OF A LIVING DONOR

Introduction of the Patient to Renal Replacement Therapy

The patient with chronic, irreversible renal disease approaching the need for renal replacement therapy must make a choice among dialysis, transplantation, and progressive debilitation and death. These options, including the results and problems to be expected with each, should be thoroughly explained to the patient.

Since the patient with uremia is invari-

ably referred to a nephrologist as soon as the problem is appreciated, it is the nephrologist's role to introduce these options to the patient so that he or she can make an informed decision regarding subsequent care. In this process the renal social worker, dialysis nurse, transplantation nurse, transplantation coordinator, transplantation surgeon, a dialysis patient, and a transplantation patient serve as important resources. A visit to a dialysis or transplantation facility or both may be appropriate. Educational materials available from the National Kidney Foundation, its affiliates, and other sources are useful.

Few if any patients choose death, at least

initially, if they are offered options for living. Many, however, are emotionally incapacitated by learning of the severity and irreversibility of their renal failure. Depression and denial are frequent, and they interfere with the patient's ability to make an informed, positive decision. Many patients start dialysis as a sort of nondecision. For this reason patients must be presented with the options of renal replacement therapy not just before therapy has begun, but periodically thereafter as well. It is easy for the patient to become accustomed to the routine of center hemodialysis, which requires no new decisions, and difficult to make a decision for another form of therapy.

Potential transplant recipients, then, are identified both before and after initiation of dialysis. A few patients, probably fewer than 2 percent (Fig. 19–1), receive a transplant, usually from a living related donor, without prior dialysis. The remaining 98 percent start with dialysis. Of the total dialysis population, each year about 8 percent receive a transplant, 24 percent from a living donor and 76 percent from a cadaver donor. Most transplants are performed within the first year of starting dialysis (Fig. 19–2).

The number of patients receiving a transplant from either a living donor or a cadaver donor depends on a number of factors related to recipient suitability and organ availability as detailed in Table 19–1. Identification of a suitable recipient must precede selection of a donor.

Recipient Suitability

A number of studies show that patient survival with chronic dialysis, center or home, and living donor transplantation is no different when corrected for age and comorbid factors of diabetes, cardiovascular disease, chronic obstructive pulmonary disease, and nonskin malignancy.[1-4] The most recent data indicate that since 1982 cadaver donor patient survival is also equal to dialysis patient survival when both are corrected for comorbid factors, although graft loss with return to dialysis is more common than with living donor transplantation.[5,6] Patient morbidity is more difficult to assess. Measures of patient rehabilitation demonstrate better rehabilitation with successful renal transplantation than with chronic dialysis.[6,7] It is generally accepted that the patient with a successful living donor transplant has the least morbidity; the patient with successful cadaver transplantation suffers the next lowest morbidity; while the chronic dialysis patient, in

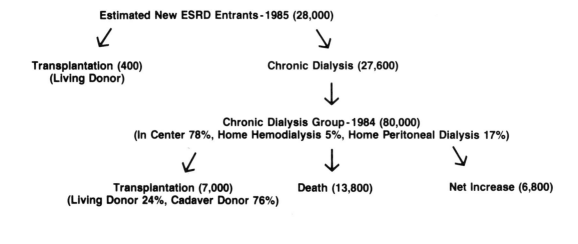

Estimated New ESRD Entrants - 1985 (28,000)

Transplantation (400) (Living Donor)　　　　**Chronic Dialysis (27,600)**

Chronic Dialysis Group - 1984 (80,000)
(In Center 78%, Home Hemodialysis 5%, Home Peritoneal Dialysis 17%)

Transplantation (7,000) (Living Donor 24%, Cadaver Donor 76%)　　　**Death (13,800)**　　　**Net Increase (6,800)**

(　　) = Number of Patients

Figure 19–1. Estimated treatment scheme for new ESRD entrants in 1985 reveals that fewer than 2 percent of new entrants receive a primary renal transplant, almost exclusively from a living donor. An additional 7000 transplants will be performed from the new entrants and existing group of dialysis patients, representing a transplantation rate of about 8 percent of the patients on dialysis.

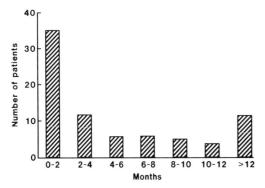

Figure 19–2. The duration of dialysis therapy before initial transplantation in a single transplant program shows that most patients who select and are suitable for transplantation are transplanted early in their plan of renal replacement therapy.

part simply by the time demands of any form of dialysis, has the greatest morbidity. There are, therefore, compelling reasons to identify all suitable potential transplant recipients and to transplant all identified as suitable.

Criteria for transplantation have evolved since the inception of transplantation, largely as a result of economic factors and organ availability. Initially only patients aged about 10 to 40 years without comor-

bid disease were considered suitable candidates, and then only if they could fund their care directly or indirectly, or if the transplantation center received federal or state research or feasibility grant funds or Veterans Administration support to perform renal transplantation. Most transplants were living donor transplants from immediate family, more distant family, prisoner "volunteers," and even nonhuman primates,[8] since the Uniform Anatomical Gift Act had not yet been enacted and cadaver organs were rarely available. With the advent of Medicare coverage of end-stage renal disease (ESRD), the adoption of the Uniform Anatomical Gift Act by more and more states, and general acceptance of brain death criteria, cadaver transplantation become dominant. In the last 5 years cadaver transplants have represented 70 to 75 percent of all transplants (Tables 19–2, 19–3). In 1984, the absolute number of living donor transplants actually decreased, and the percentage of living donor transplants fell sharply, since the number of cadaver transplants increased sharply at the same time.

Medical criteria for transplant suitability now include patients with diabetes but still exclude most patients with significant cardiovascular disease and older patients. All centers screen potential recipients with

Table 19–1 Factors Influencing the Role of Renal Transplantation in Renal Replacement Therapy		
	Living Donor	**Cadaver Donor**
Organ Availability		
Donor health	+ + + +	+ + +
Legal aspects (including brain death)		+ +
Request procedures	+	+ + + +
Ethical aspects	+	+
Patient Health		
Age	+ + +	+ + +
Comorbid disease	+ +	+ +
Transplant Results		
Patient's perception	+ + +	+ + +
Nephrologist's perception	+ +	+ +
Public's reception	+	+
Other		
Nephrologist-surgeon relationship	+ +	+ +
Financing of care (drugs)	+	+ +
Nephrologists' self-interest	+	+

Table 19–2 Trends: United States Kidney Transplants*					
Year	**1980**	**1981**	**1982**	**1983**	**1984**
Number and Source					
Living donor	1275 (27.4)	1458 (29.8)	1677 (31.3)	1796 (29.3)	1704 (24.5)
Cadaver donor	3422 (73.6)	3427 (70.2)	3681 (68.7)	4333 (70.7)	5264 (75.5)
Total	4647	4885	5358	6129	6968

( ) : % of total.
*From ESRD Systems Branch, Health Care Financing Administration, U.S. Department of Health & Human Services.

electrocardiograms, and some require stress tests of those over a certain age or with diabetes. Patients over the age of 40 have a significantly decreased survival, and transplant failure increases markedly over the age of 50.[5,9] Of course, age is also a significant determinant of survival with chronic dialysis. Since age is such an important factor in both dialysis and transplant survival, there is no demonstrated medical reason to limit renal transplantation on the basis of age. Patients aged a few days to over 70 have undergone successful transplantation, so extreme youth and older age are clearly only relative contraindications to transplantation. Those aged 6 to 30 show the best results, those 31 to 45 just slightly less patient survival and no less graft survival, while those 45 to 60 demonstrate significantly less patient and graft survival.[5] It is probable that absence of parents of suitable age, the relative unavail-ability of siblings free of medical problems, a reluctance to perform child-to-parent transplantation, and the absolute shortage of cadaver organs result in nonmedical rationing of transplantation to those most likely to survive and benefit. Artificial kidneys are made by humans, and their supply is limited only by the availability of funds, provided in abundance by Medicare from 1973 to date.

Recently, public awareness of organ transplantation has been greatly enhanced, due in part to the dramatic advances in immunosuppression and in liver and cardiac transplantation as well as the immediacy of the need of those requiring transplantation. If this awareness, exemplified by the National Organ Procurement and Transplantation Act of 1984, results in increased availability of cadaver organs, more elderly patients and more patients with comorbid disease factors may receive transplants in the future.

Functionally significant cardiovascular disease is at present an absolute contraindication to renal transplantation, as is functionally significant chronic pulmonary insufficiency. Active nonskin malignancy is an absolute contraindication. Previously disseminated tuberculosis or coccidioidomycosis may be an absolute contraindication. Active hepatitis or advanced hepatic cirrhosis are probably absolute contraindications. Hepatitis B antigenemia does not adversely affect transplantation results. There is little experience with transplantation of patients known positive for HTLV III antibody (and presumably antigen) in the absence of signs or symptoms of disease. Active acquired immune deficiency syndrome (AIDS) must be regarded as

Table 19–3 Trends: United States Kidney Transplants Percent Change from Previous Calendar Year				
Year	**1981**	**1982**	**1983**	**1984**
Source				
Living donor	+14.4	+15.0	+ 7.0	− 5.1
Cadaver donor	+ 0.1	+ 7.4	+17.7	+21.5
Total	+ 5.1	+ 9.7	+14.4	+13.7

an absolute contraindication to renal transplantation.

Donor Selection

Having identified a suitable potential recipient, it is appropriate to consider a source of donation.

The recently demonstrated marked improvement in short-term patient survival with cadaver kidney transplantation, and the growing recent concern about the long-term consequences of living donor nephrectomy, cast doubt on both the medical need from the recipient's standpoint and the medical advisability from the donor's standpoint of performing any living donor transplantation. A few centers, mostly outside the United States, now refuse to perform any living donor transplants. Others restrict such transplantation to identical twins and HLA-identical siblings. At present, however, the lack of availability of sufficient cadaver organs would lead to fewer transplants and an even longer delay in transplantation of the ever-growing number of patients waiting for transplantation if living donor transplants were discontinued.

Sources of Living Donors

Nonhuman primate donors were used only in the very early experimental phase of renal transplantation. The experiment was abandoned because of dismal results and the progressive availability of other donor sources.

The use of unrelated prisoner volunteers and other unrelated living donors was also abandoned many years ago, since cadaver transplantation results were equally good and because of ethical concerns regarding imagined or real rewards for donation of an organ. The issue of use of unrelated living donor organs was recently revived when a Virginia doctor advertised a business to broker human kidneys for transplantation; this attracted considerable publicity and debate concerning the practical and moral aspects of buying and selling human organs. Virtually all kidney organizations publicly opposed this practice, as did the public, as indicated by passage of the Organ Procurement and Transplantation Act of 1984. This law specifically prohibits interstate commerce for this purpose.

The remaining source of living donors, then, is the patient's direct relatives. Distant relatives fail to offer any medical advantages compared with cadaver donors, so few uncle, aunt, or cousin transplants are or have been performed. Adult child-to-parent transplants are performed occasionally, but of all living transplants performed, over 98 percent are sibling to sibling or parent to child.[5]

The identification of potential donors for a suitable potential recipient, then, is a simple matter of inquiring concerning the existence, age, and apparent health of the potential recipient's parents and siblings, if any. The potential recipient is usually asked to contact family members initially to determine potential willingness to donate a kidney, with the nephrologist, transplant surgeon, and all other members of the team readily available to meet and speak with the potential donor and recipient, alone or together.

It must not be assumed that parents or siblings will necessarily wish to be considered as potential donors, even if of suitable age and without significant personal health problems. A request from one who is ill and dying of chronic renal failure is compelling, even coercive. The potential donor is torn between the feeling that he or she ought to help his or her close relative, and the responsibility to himself or herself and to others. In addition, there is a natural and not entirely inappropriate fear of major surgery. In the early days of renal transplantation family donors were more willing to donate. This apparent willingness probably represented the pragmatic assessment that there was no real alternative and that their son, daughter, brother, or sister would die if they refused to donate a kidney. More recently, with easily available dialysis and increasingly successful cadaver transplantation, suitable alternatives are available to preserve life, and the need for related donor transplantation is less coercive.

Evaluation of the Living Donor

It is best to meet with and answer questions of all potential donors for a potential recipient. At this point a rough screening can be achieved. Legal minors cannot donate, and probably should not except in very special circumstances. Donors should probably be age 50 or less because of the greater risk of operative morbidity in older patients; the natural progressive occurrence of glomerular sclerosis[10] and decline in renal function starting at age 40,[11] the lesser degree of functional compensatory hypertrophy in older people subject to nephrectomy,[12] and the decreased chance of func-

tional transplantation success seen with kidneys from those over age 50.[9] Donors with treated hypertension, prior nonskin malignancy, diabetes, or known renal disease can be excluded with a few simple questions.

Those who indicate a willingness and preliminary consent to donate can be medically evaluated as outlined in Figure 19-3. This scheme is designed to be medically ef-

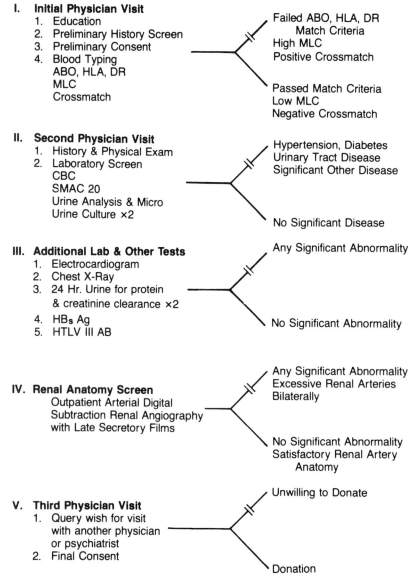

Figure 19-3. A decision tree helps in selection and evaluation of a living donor. The potential donor must pass each step before initiating the next step. Different criteria applied by different transplant centers, or changing criteria with changing technology and knowledge, can be accommodated readily by adding them to or eliminating them from the branches of the tree at the appropriate place.

ficient, to control costs, and to inconvenience and risk the potential donor as little as possible. It eliminates unsuitable donors at each step and provides all necessary information to identify a healthy donor with suitable donor-recipient tissue compatibility, anatomically, and functionally normal kidneys, and defined renal vascular anatomy. Most unsuitable donors will be identified with the initial meeting and preliminary medical screening, and most others will be eliminated by the early blood compatibility testing. Depending on how the initial pool of potential donors is defined, perhaps only one in three or four will emerge as both willing and medically suitable as donors. Most transplant programs offer potential donors a visit with a disinterested internist, psychologist, or psychiatrist to explore their feelings concerning donation and their willingness to donate. If they have substantial reservations, the recipient is informed that the potential donor has been found medically unsuitable for donation.

LONG-TERM FOLLOW-UP

Short-Term Consequences of Kidney Donation

The first successful unilateral nephrectomy was performed in 1861. Nearly 80 years later, Dr. C. L. Deming sought to answer two important questions now made most poignant by living donor nephrectomy: (1) "Can I live with one kidney?" (2) "What does the future hold in store for me?"[13] He immediately concluded that the answer to the first question was yes, since such had been observed many times by then. In his introduction he expressed that the answer to the second question was " . . . not so readily given" . . . and requires . . . "much thought and careful study." Nonetheless, he concluded from observations of 180 cases of unilateral nephrectomy, but only 8 following trauma, that "The young person whose kidney has been removed for . . . trauma . . . has a normal expectancy of life." Despite this conclusion, the answer to the second question remains in doubt today.

Deliberate unilateral nephrectomy of healthy adults between the ages of 21 and 55 with previously demonstrated normal renal function and anatomically normal kidneys was initiated in the late 1950s and especially the early 1960s for living organ donation. This practice afforded a unique opportunity to study the effects of unilateral nephrectomy in humans. Psychologic,[14] physiologic, and anatomic effects were studied. The remaining kidney was determined to be capable of maintaining fluid and electrolyte homeostasis,[15] and as expected from rat and dog studies,[16,17] underwent immediate functional hypertrophy and increase in mass.[18] Renal function in humans assessed by clearance of creatinine, inulin, and para-aminohippurate increases to about 70 percent of prenephrectomy values within a few days after nephrectomy.[19]

Perioperative risks and complications were also documented; these included short-term problems such as ileus, urinary tract infection, atelectasis, pleural effusion, and pneumothorax as well as problems with the potential for long-term disability such as brachial plexus injury, thrombophlebitis, incisional hernia, pulmonary embolism, and acute myocardial infarction.[18,20–22] Overall, the complication rate at the time of donation varied from 15 percent to 40 percent, depending in part on inclusion criteria for a complication. Interestingly, there are few reports of follow-up of perioperative complications or late complications in donors. There is sporadic mention of acute glomerulonephritis from several to many years after donation[20,23] and at least one report of urolithiasis after donation.[20] A systematic review of long-term satisfaction with organ donation demonstrated a continuing positive impact of donation on the donors' lives, particularly among those with surviving recipients.[24]

The critical role of the kidney in calcium and phosphorous homeostasis and vitamin D metabolism has received little study in donors, even though unilateral nephrectomy might be expected to alter significantly these aspects of kidney function. Friedlander[25] studied vitamin D metabolites, parathyroid hormone levels, serum calcium and phosphate, and urine calcium excretion in donors before and up to 6 months after nephrectomy and noted a significant increase in serum ionized calcium, a decrease in urine calcium, a marked increase in 1,25 $(OH)_2D_3$, an increase in 25

OHD_3, and an increase in C-terminal parathyroid hormone 6 months after nephrectomy. The results were most consistent with the effects of increased parathyroid activity and its associated stimulation of renal 1-hydroxylase 6 months but not 1 month after nephrectomy.

Intermediate Consequences of Kidney Donation

There are few studies of donor renal function in the few years following unilateral nephrectomy. Donadio and colleagues[26] found in four donors an average glomerular filtration rate (GFR) of 81 percent and renal plasma (RPF) of 71 percent of prenephrectomy values an average of 16 months after nephrectomy. These values were unchanged from those measured shortly after nephrectomy. In 1967 Ogden[12] studied 28 donors an average of 34 months and as long as 48 months after nephrectomy and found an average inulin clearance of 75.3 and PAH clearance of 348 ml per min per $1.73M^2$. In 17 of these donors GFR was 71.3 percent and ERPF was 66.3 percent of prenephrectomy values an average of 35.2 months after donation. In 1976 Slack and Wilson[27] reported renal function in 121 donors to be approximately 70 percent of initial function 2 weeks to 6 years after nephrectomy. Ogden[12] also first demonstrated a significant inverse relationship between age and postnephrectomy percent of prenephrectomy renal function.

Long-Term Consequences of Kidney Donation

Recently a great deal of attention has been focused on the physiologic and structural consequences of loss of renal mass on the remaining nephrons in experimental animals and humans.

In 1968, Rosen and colleagues[28] first postulated that a growth stimulus might potentiate spontaneous glomerular sclerosis in rats. In 1969, Striker and his associates[29] demonstrated a marked accentuation of pre-existing glomerulosclerosis in rats following uninephrectomy. In 1975, Shimamura and Morrison[30] suggested that the glomerular hyperfiltration of remaining nephrons that follows nephron loss might be responsible for the subsequent progressive glomerulosclerosis seen in rats and might also contribute to the glomerular lesions in late stages of various chronic renal diseases in humans. These investigators subjected rats to five-sixths nephrectomy and demonstrated progressive glomerulosclerosis in the ensuing 50 weeks, but without progressive renal insufficiency.

Age Changes in Structure and Function

These effects in experimental animals must be interpreted with caution, since for nearly 60 years substantial age changes in renal structure and function have been recognized in normal rats with intact kidneys.[31] These changes vary among different rat strains; tend to be most severe in male animals; are accelerated by a variety of toxins, radiation, and high-protein feedings; and are restricted in severity by food restriction. The changes are primarily glomerular, begin as early as 1 month of age, and are not associated with changes in blood vessels containing smooth muscle. The reader is referred to a recent review article for more detailed discussion and references.[32]

Age changes in renal structure and function also occur in humans. In a study of 122 victims of sudden death and acute illness and patients without known or recognized renal disease or hypertension, sclerotic glomeruli represented 1.1 percent of total glomeruli in those under 30 years of age; 2.1 percent in those aged 30 to 39 years; and 3.5 percent in those aged 40 to 49 years. By age 70 to 89, 11 percent of glomeruli were found to be sclerotic.[33] Cortical interstitium has been found to increase as a percentage of cortical mass in normotensive humans with normal renal function, and 30 percent of glomeruli were found to be sclerotic by age 70.[10] Concomitantly, significant disease of large and small blood vessels occurs in humans, although I am unaware of any study correlating these changes. Normal humans do not develop proteinuria or changes in glomerular membrane permeability with advancing age, as do rats,[34] despite the presence of "normal" glomerulosclerosis in humans. There is an associated age decline in renal function after the age of

40 in humans, such that by age 80 inulin, creatinine, and diodrast clearance and diodrast Tm are reduced about 40 percent.[11]

Hyperfiltration and Renal Function

In animal models of renal disease and following surgical ablation experiments in laboratory animals, once a critical mass of renal tissue is lost, progressive loss of function of the remaining diseased or normal kidney follows. An obvious parallel has been drawn with respect to human renal diseases, since in most patients with chronic renal insufficiency of any cause, renal function deteriorates predictably with time.[35]

Two mechanisms have been evoked to explain this phenomenon. Ibels and co-workers[36] postulated that alterations in calcium and phosphorus metabolism in renal insufficiency leads to renal calcification, inflammation, and fibrosis with accelerated decline in renal function. They then demonstrated increased renal calcium and phosphate both histologically and by tissue analysis in the rat remnant kidney model and the rat nephrotoxic serum model. This hypothesis remains unproven in human disease.

Brenner and coworkers[37] demonstrated marked increase in single-nephron GFR and filtration pressure within 1 week of eleven-twelfths surgical ablation of the renal mass in rats. They demonstrated temporally related changes in endothelial and epithelial cells and mesangial thickening. Of more importance, they found that protein restriction prevented the increases in single-nephron hyperfiltration and supernormal filtration pressures and flows, and largely prevented the glomerular structural changes. In another study[34] of the same rat model, they demonstrated the loss of both size and charge selectivity by the basement membrane of remnant glomeruli and suggested a causative role of increased transglomerular flux of plasma proteins with mesangial accumulation of protein, associated mesangial proliferation, and ultimate glomerulosclerosis.

It has been found that in rats with streptozocin-induced diabetes, unilateral nephrectomy accelerates the rate of diabetic glomerulosclerosis in the remaining kidney,[38] and in one patient with diabetes and unilateral renal artery stenosis, the kidney with the patent renal artery demonstrated typical Kimmelsteil-Wilson lesions, while the kidney with the stenotic artery did not.[39] Since glomerular hyperfiltration has been demonstrated in both experimental and human diabetes, these findings support a role of hyperfiltration in the genesis of glomerulosclerosis in diabetes. Based on these studies and others, Brenner and his colleagues[40] have suggested that in the presence of reduced renal mass of any cause, hyperfiltration and its associated changes in glomerular perfusion pressures and flows may lead to the progressive destruction of the remaining healthy nephrons in both experimental animals and humans. They further suggest[41] that high protein intake may contribute to this process, and specifically indicate that this ". . . progressive glomerulopathy may be initiated by the loss of only one kidney." This statement cast doubt on the wisdom of living donor transplantation and provoked additional studies of human renal donors.

Long-Term Renal Function

Since in the rat model an important correlate of glomerular hyperfiltration injury is increased urinary albumin excretion, and since microalbuminuria is predictive of subsequent development of overt diabetic nephropathy in humans,[42] Bertolatus and colleagues[43] studied renal function and microalbuminuria in renal donors serially for up to 3 years post nephrectomy. Both absolute and fractional albumin excretion rates, transiently elevated one week post nephrectomy, were not different from prenephrectomy values 1 month through 36 months after nephrectomy. They did document a significant increase in both systolic and diastolic blood pressures 24 and 36 months post nephrectomy.

In 1983 Ogden[32] reported a 19-year follow-up of a single donor. Creatinine clearance was 75.5 percent of the prenephrectomy value, and the donor remained normotensive. However, 24-hour protein excretion was 181 mg, over three times the normal value of 50 mg per 24 hours. Later the same year, Hakim and associates[44] reported results in 52 donors 10 to 28 years after unilateral nephrectomy. They found no deterioration in renal function assessed by serum creatinine or creatinine clearance but did find an increase in 24-hour total urinary protein; they also found hypertension in their male but not female donors compared with their prenephrectomy values and to age- and sex-matched inpatient and outpatient controls. The same year, Vincenti and his colleagues[45] reported results in 20 donors 14.5 to 18.5 years post nephrectomy. They found an insignificant trend of increasing creatinine clearance with time after nephrectomy and an increase in nonalbumin 24-hour urinary protein but no increase in 24-hour urine albumin compared with controls and no increase in blood pressure compared with prenephrectomy systolic or diastolic levels. Miller and colleagues[23] evaluated 46 donors an average of 6 years post nephrectomy by questionnaire and general laboratory follow up and found an increase in total 24-hour urine protein and an incidence of hypertension not significantly different from that of a control group. In a similar questionnaire-laboratory survey of 105 donors 10 to 20 years after donation, Anderson and associates[46] found no deterioration of renal function, a questionably normal 24-hour urinary total protein excretion, and hypertension similar to that of the area population. Smith and associates[47] studied a group of patients undergoing unilateral nephrectomy for a variety of causes. Evaluation in 40 patients with normal prenephrectomy serum creatinine and blood pressure demonstrated neither progression of renal insufficiency nor an incidence of hypertension greater than expected from the general population 5 to 30 years after nephrectomy. Weiland and colleagues[48] also failed to demonstrate a significant increase in blood pressure in 472 donors at various times up to 19 years after donation.

In a recent study[49] of 39 pregnancies in 23 donors who conceived 2 weeks to 9 years after unilateral nephrectomy, no hypertension was observed during pregnancy, and proteinuria did not occur with unexpected frequency. Evaluation of 13 of these donors 2 to 14 years after nephrectomy revealed a mean serum creatinine of 1.10 mg per dl; a GFR by creatinine clearance of 82.5 ml per min per $1.73M^2$; a 24-hour urinary protein of 50 mg per 24 hours; and mean blood pressure of 117 systolic and 72 diastolic. Thus, it would appear that no ad-

verse effects occurred either during or following the period of enhanced stimulus to glomerular hyperfiltration of pregnancy.

In many of these studies individual donors have developed significant proteinuria, albuminuria, hypertension, and even biopsy-documented glomerulonephritis with significant renal insufficiency. It is apparent, however, that from 10 to 20 years, and occasionally up to 30 years post nephrectomy, based on more than 750 donors evaluated, 24-hour total protein excretion but not 24-hour albumin excretion is increased; neither systolic nor diastolic hypertension occurs with greater than expected frequency; and progressive renal insufficiency does not occur in the absence of a specific cause other than uninephrectomy.

It cannot be assumed from these studies that glomerular hyperfiltration is of no consequence in humans. Human renal donors are subject to removal of only 50 percent of renal mass, and after perhaps 50 percent of their normal life span. Careful further studies of donors 20 to 40 years after unilateral nephrectomy may reveal deleterious effects of many years of hyperfiltration. It may also be that the effects of a diffusely damaging disease in both kidneys of humans are more prone to provoke progressive renal damage than the loss of the same number of nephrons by unilateral nephrectomy. Although changes of the glomerular basement membrane and mesangial changes have been observed in rats after unilateral nephrectomy, five-sixths nephrectomy, genetically determined disease processes, and experimentally provoked diffuse disease processes, rats cannot be assumed to behave like humans.

CONCLUSION

The practice of living related donor renal transplantation continues to be justified in view of the better long-term results to be anticipated than with cadaver renal transplantation and of the limited supply of cadaver organs for transplantation. The potential donor, however, must be medically suitable and must be carefully counseled concerning the perioperative risks and the current knowledge concerning potential long-term consequences. The question posed by Dr. Deming nearly 50 years ago concerning unilateral nephrectomy, "What does the future hold in store for me?" still demands further study.

REFERENCES

1. Shapiro, FL and Umen, A: Risk factors in hemodialysis patient survival. ASAIO J 6:176, 1983.
2. Blagg, CR, Wahl, PW, and Lamers, JY: Treatment of chronic renal failure at the Northwest Kidney Center, Seattle, from 1960 to 1982. ASAIO J 6:170, 1983.
3. Standards Committee of the American Society of Transplant Surgeons: Current results and expectations of renal transplantation. JAMA 246:1330, 1981.
4. Salvatierra, O Jr, et al: A seven-year experience with donor specific blood transfusions. Transplantation 40:654, 1985.
5. Terasaki, PI, et al: Patient, graft, and functional survival rates: An overview. In Terasaki, PI (ed): Clinical Kidney Transplants 1985. UCLA Tissue Typing Laboratory, Los Angeles, 1985.
6. Kahan, BD, et al: Clinical and experimental studies with cyclosporine in renal transplantation. Surgery 97:125, 1985.
7. Gutman, RA, Stead, WW, and Robinson, RR: Physical activity and employment status of patients on maintenance dialysis. N Eng J Med 304:309, 1981.
8. Starzl, TE, et al: Renal heterotransplantation from baboon to man: Experience with 6 cases. Transplantation 2:752, 1964.
9. Crosnier, J and Kreis, H: Donor and recipient selection in renal transplantation. In Suki, WN and Massry, SG (eds): Therapy of Renal Diseases and Related Disorders. Martinus Nijhoff, Netherlands, 1984.
10. Kappel, B and Olsen, S: Cortical interstitial tissue and sclerosed glomeruli in the normal human kidney, related to age and sex: A quantitative study. Virchows Arch [A] 387:271, 1980.
11. Davies, DF and Shock, NW: Age changes in glomerular filtration rate, effective renal plasma flow, and tubular excretory capacity in adult males. J Clin Invest 29:496, 1950.
12. Ogden, DA: Donor and recipient function 2 to 4 years after renal homotransplantation: A paired study of 28 cases. Ann Intern Med 67:998, 1967.
13. Deming, CL: The future of the unilaterally nephrectomized patient. J Urol 40:74, 1938.
14. Fellner, CH and Marshall, JR: Twelve kidney donors. JAMA 206:2703, 1968.
15. Bricker, NS, et al. Studies on the functional capacity of a denervated homotransplanted kidney in an identical twin with parallel observations in the donor. J Clin Invest 35:1364, 1956.
16. Potter, DE, et al: Early responses of glomerular filtration rate to unilateral nephrectomy. Kidney Int 5:131, 1974.
17. Rous, SN and Wakin, KG: Kidney function before, during and after compensatory hypertrophy. J Urol 98:30, 1967.
18. Ringden, O, et al: Living related kidney donors: Complications and long-term renal function. Transplantation 25:221–223, 1978.
19. Krohn, AG, Ogden, DA, and Holmes, JH: Renal function in 29 healthy adults before and after nephrectomy. JAMA 196:322, 1966.
20. Penn, I, et al: Use of living donors in kidney transplantation in man. Arch Surg 101:226, 1970.
21. Uehling, DT, Malek, GH, and Wear, JB: Complications of donor nephrectomy. J Urol 111:745, 1974.
22. Jacobs, SC, et al: Live donor nephrectomy. Urology 5:175, 1975.
23. Miller, IJ, et al: Impact of renal donation: Long-term clinical and biochemical follow-up of living donors in a single center. Am J Med 79:201, 1985.
24. Marshall, JR and Fellner, CH: Kidney donors revisited. Am J Psych 134:575, 1977.
25. Friedlander, MA, et al: The effect of uninephrectomy on circulating levels of immunoreactive parathyroid hormone and vitamin D metabolites in normal human kidney donors. In Vitamin D, Chemical, Biochemical and Clinical Endocrinology of Calcium Metabolism. Walter de Gruter, Berlin, New York, 1982, p 969.
26. Donadio, JV, et al: Renal function in donors and recipients of renal allotransplantation: Radioisotopic measurements. Ann Intern Med 66:105, 1967.
27. Slack, TK and Wilson, DM: Normal renal function: C_{IN} and C_{PAH} in healthy donors before and after nephrectomy. Mayo Clin Proc 51:296, 1976.
28. Rosen, VJ, et al: Ultrastructural studies of X-ray induced glomerular disease in rats subjected to uninephrectomy and food restriction. Lab Invest 18:260, 1968.
29. Striker, GE, et al: Response to unilateral nephrectomy in old rats. Arch Pathol Lab Med 87:439, 1969.
30. Shimamura, T and Morrison, AB: A progressive glomerulosclerosis occurring in partial five-sixths nephrectomized rats. Am J Pathol 79:95, 1975.
31. Newburgh, LH and Curtis, AC: Production of renal injury in the white rat by the pro-

tein of the diet. Arch Intern Med 42:801, 1928.

32. Ogden, DA: Consequences of renal donation in man. Am J Kidney Dis 2:501, 1983.
33. Kaplan, C, et al: Age-related incidence of sclerotic glomeruli in human kidneys. Am J Pathol 80:227, 1975.
34. Olson, JL, et al: Altered charge and size selective properties of the glomerular wall: A response to reduced renal mass. Kidney Int (abstr) 16:857, 1979.
35. Mitch, WE, et al: A simple method of estimating progression of chronic renal failure. Lancet 2:1326, 1976.
36. Ibels, LS, et al: Preservation of function in experimental renal disease by dietary restriction of phosphate. N Eng J Med 298:122, 1978.
37. Hostetter, TH, et al: Hyperfiltration in remnant nephrons: A potentially adverse response to renal ablation. Am J Physiol 241:F85, 1981.
38. Mauer, SM, Steffes, MW, and Brown, DM: The kidney in diabetes. Am J Med 70:603, 1981.
39. Berkman, J and Rifkin, H: Unilateral nodular diabetic glomerulosclerosis (Kimmelsteil-Wilson): Report of a case. Metabolism 22:715, 1973.
40. Hostetter, TH, Rennke, HG, and Brenner, BM: The case for intrarenal hypertension in the initiation and progression of diabetic and other glomerulopathies. Am J Med 72:375, 1982.
41. Brenner, BM, Meyer, TW, and Hostetter, TH: Dietary protein intake and the progressive nature of kidney disease: The role of hemodynamically mediated glomerular injury in the pathogenesis of progressive glomerular sclerosis in aging, renal ablation, and intrinsic renal disease. N Eng J Med 307:652, 1982.
42. Morgenson, CE: Microalbuminuria predicts clinical proteinuria and early mortality in clinical-onset diabetes. N Eng J Med 310:356, 1984.
43. Bertolatus, JA, et al: Urinary albumin excretion after donor nephrectomy. Am J Kidney Dis 5:165, 1985.
44. Hakim, RM, Goldszer, RC, and Brenner, BM: Hypertension and proteinuria: Long-term sequelae of uninephrectomy in humans. Kidney Int 25:930, 1984.
45. Vincenti, F, et al: Long-term renal function in kidney donors. Transplantation 36:626, 1983.
46. Anderson, CF, et al: The risks of unilateral nephrectomy: Status of kidney donors 10 to 20 years postoperatively. Mayo Clin Proc 60:367, 1985.
47. Smith, S, Laprad, P, and Grantham, J: Long-term effect of uninephrectomy on serum creatinine concentration and arterial blood pressure. Am J Kidney Dis 6:143, 1985.
48. Weiland, D, et al: Information on 628 living-related kidney donors at a single institution, with long-term follow-up in 472 cases. Transplant Proc 26:5, 1984.
49. Buszta, C, et al: Pregnancy after donor nephrectomy. Transplantation 40:651, 1985.

Chapter 20

Living Related Transplantation Results

OSCAR SALVATIERRA

The superior results in both patient and graft survival after living related donor transplantation as currently practiced suggests that this method be considered initially for patients with end-stage renal disease (ESRD) requiring transplantation.[1,2,3] Probably the strongest support for this strategy comes from the continuing shortage of cadaver kidneys. The advantages of a strategy supporting the continued use of living related transplantation is also strengthened by the very low morbidity and rare mortality amongst living related donors.[1,4,5]

It has been well recognized that an HLA-identical sibling match is the optimal immunologic situation. Only a few prospective transplant recipients have an ideally compatible related donor with good graft survival expectations, so that until recently a potential organ recipient had to rely primarily on cadaver transplantation. However with donor-specific blood transfusions (DST),[2,6,7] the advent of cyclosporine,[8] and even planned third-party blood transfusions[9,10] excellent results are being obtained with incompatible 1-haplotype matched donor-recipient pairs and even in 0-haplotype matched donor-recipient pairs with DSTs.[2,7]

DONOR-SPECIFIC BLOOD TRANSFUSIONS (DST)

In order to select MLC-incompatible 1-haplotype related donor-recipient pairs that might achieve better graft survival, and in an attempt to alter the recipient immune response, the DST protocol was introduced at the University of California at San Francisco (UCSF) in 1978.[11,12] Since donor blood given to recipients before renal allografting might result in sensitization to the donor and subsequent hyperacute rejection, physicians previously hesitated to employ this technique in renal transplantation. With the early good results, the indications for the DST protocol have been further expanded, and in addition, considerations for its use and for its maximum efficacy have been better defined.

In 1982 it was decided to pretreat all non-HLA-identical donor-recipient pairs with DST, regardless of the MLC, since the results in the DST-treated MLC-incompatible group were better than in the non-DST low-reactive MLC group.[13] In addition, DST pretreatment was extended to include a recent group of 0-haplotype-matched donor-recipient pairs; low-dose azathioprine coverage during DST administration was evaluated; and the effect of flow cytometry (fluorescence-activated cell sorter [FACS]) was studied.[2]

The DST procedure is essentially the same since its inception and involves administration of 200 ml of fresh whole blood or packed-cell equivalent on three separate occasions at 2-week intervals.[11,12] Small children receive blood volumes in proportion to their weight. Immunosuppression was not given during the transfusion process except when a recent group received DST under azathioprine coverage, with a maximum of 1 mg per kg azathioprine being administered beginning 1 week prior

to the first transfusion and continuing until the time of transplantation. The azathioprine dosage is titrated by the white cell count and is scaled down with evidence of leukopenia. Until the time of transplantation, potential recipient sensitization against blood donor lymphocytes is closely monitored by cross-match testing of weekly recipient sera obtained before, during, and after the blood transfusion period. The time of transplantation has generally been about 4 weeks after the last transfusion, and the criteria for proceeding with transplantation are a negative T-warm and a B-warm donor-specific cross-match, although recently it has been possible to select cases with a positive B-warm donor-specific cross-match where transplantation was possible with the use of flow cytometry.

Patient and graft survival are calculated without any exclusions, but when separate subset analyses, for example nondiabetic, are carried out, they are clearly indicated. Immunosuppression has primarily consisted of azathioprine, prednisone, and ATGAM or MALG for steroid-resistant rejection. The primary consideration in the use of immunosuppression at this center has been the placing of a ceiling on the amount of medication administered and a limitation on the number of rejection episodes treated.[14]

Graft and Patient Survival

Graft and patient survival in recipients pretreated with DST has been essentially the same as those achieved in the concur-

Table 20–1 Living Related Graft and Patient Survival (1978–1984)

	Graft Survival, %				
	6 Months	*1 Year*	*2 Years*	*3 Years*	*4 Years*
DST-1 and 0 haplotype (n = 221)	97±1	94±2	90±2	85±3	82±4
HLA-identical (n = 186)	92±2	90±2	87±3	85±3	84±3

	Patient Survival, %				
	6 Months	*1 Year*	*2 Years*	*3 Years*	*4 Years*
DST-1 and 0 haplotype (n = 221)	98±1	97±1	95±2	95±2	95±1
HLA-identical (n = 186)	99±1	97±1	95±2	94±2	93±2

Table 20–2 Nondiabetic Related Graft Survival, % (1978–1984)					
	6 Months	1 Year	2 Years	3 Years	4 Years
DST-1 and 0 haplotype (n = 174)	98 ± 1	96 ± 1	91 ± 1	88 ± 3	88 ± 3
HLA-identical (n = 143)	91 ± 2	89 ± 3	87 ± 3	85 ± 1	83 ± 4

rent HLA-identical group since the introduction of the DST protocol in 1978. Graft and patient survival rates in consecutive patients transplanted from 1978 through 1984 and with a minimum of 5 months of follow-up are shown in Table 20–1.[2]

Initially it was feared that the DST effect might dissipate with time, but a separate analysis of graft survival in 174 consecutive *nondiabetic* DST recipients with a minimum of 5 months of follow-up shows that the transfusion effect persists for at least 4 years[2] (Table 20–2). The corresponding graft function in this same group as determined by mean serum creatinine of functioning grafts through 4 years is excellent and remains stable[2] (Table 20–3).

These results have now been confirmed by a number of reports from other centers.[6,7,10,15–20]

DST with Living 0-Haplotype-Matched Pairs

Since only about one third of the 200 or more transplants performed yearly at UCSF have living related donors with either an HLA-identical match or with a 1-haplotype match with DST pretreatment, and because cadaver donor organs cannot meet an increasing waiting list of over 600 patients, an effort has been undertaken to use the DST protocol in well-informed 0-haplotype-matched donor-recipient pairs.

Graft survival in 24 such patients pretreated with DST has been 100 percent at 18 months. The Wisconsin group[7] also shows similar graft survival in a 0-haplotype-matched group.

Sensitization After DST

The incidence of donor-specific sensitization and changes in panel cytotoxins following DST were evaluated in the initial 172 patients who received blood from their potential kidney donors.[13,21] There were 157 potential recipients of first kidney grafts and 15 potential recipients of second or third grafts. Seventy percent of the initial patients who received DST prior to primary transplantation were accepted as potential recipients of a kidney from their blood donor on the basis of an appropriate negative T-warm and B-warm donor-specific cross-match. The sensitization rate was greater in patients who had already rejected a transplant. In essence, when sensitization occurred, the planned transplant was aborted and a suitable cadaver organ was used in most cases with similar results to those of patients who had not undergone DST.

Three patterns of donor-specific sensitization have emerged.

1. Approximately half of the patients sensitized to their blood donor had a positive T-warm cross-match pattern.

Table 20–3 Nondiabetic Related Graft Function (1978–1984): Serum Creatinine Levels					
	6 Months	1 Year	2 Years	3 Years	4 Years
DST-1 and 0 haplotype (n = 174)	1.4 ± 0.1	1.4 ± 0.1	1.5 ± 0.1	1.5 ± 0.1	1.4 ± 0.2
HLA-identical (n = 143)	1.4 ± 0.1	1.4 ± 0.1	1.3 ± 0.1	1.3 ± 0.1	1.2 ± 0.1

2. One-fourth had an initially positive B-warm cross-match that later converted to a positive T-warm cross-match.

3. Another fourth had a persistently positive B-warm cross-match.

There was approximately equal distribution of patients who developed a positive cross-match after the first, second, and third DST.

Serum samples were cross-matched against freshly isolated donor T cells first by a modification of the Amos technique and second by an anti-human-globulin technique using goat antihuman kappa light chain (Atlantic Antibodies, Scarborough, ME) antibody as the second antibody. B-lymphocyte cross-matches were performed on cells isolated by nylon-wool-packed plastic straws and further purified by rosetting with AET-treated sheep red blood cells. The isolated B cells were incubated at 37°C with patients' sera at dilutions of 1 to 1, 1 to 4, and 1 to 8 for 60 minutes followed by complement and incubation at room temperature for 120 minutes. Cross-match tests were considered positive when 20 percent or more cells were killed by the test serum.

Donor-Specific Versus PRA Panel Sensitization

It is important to define and separate the favorable effects of DST from the capacity to impart specific immunization to potential kidney recipients against the potential kidney donor and in addition to evaluate its effect on the PRA of the potential recipient. The same weekly sera evaluated for specific humoral response to the blood donor by cross-match testing were also prospectively screened against a panel of 30 potential unrelated donors (for PRA effect) in the first 131 patients undergoing DST prior to primary transplantation.[13,21] Only 4 percent of patients who received DST alone developed more than 10 percent increase in PRA T-warm panel cytotoxins from baseline compared with 23 percent of patients who received both DST and third-party transfusions (p = 0.01). Third-party transfusions were erratic, and in those who received them, neither the number nor the timing appeared to influence the rate of increased panel sensitization. Only the absence of any third-party transfusion history was significant. This suggests that when sensitization to DST alone occurs, it is usually specific and narrow, as might be expected from exposure to a limited number of transplantation antigens. However, exposure to a larger variety of foreign histocompatibility antigens, in the form of additional random third-party transfusions, has resulted in a greater degree of PRA panel sensitization in some patients. In final analysis, however, the DST process alone does not appear to produce an unfavorable degree of panel sensitization that would preclude transplantation from another donor source if necessary.

The interesting consideration that individuals exposed to other transfusions in addition to DST have a higher risk of developing increased levels of PRA T-warm panel cytotoxins is further corroborated by the study of Scornik and associates,[22] who demonstrated amplification of previous antigenic exposure by the development of broadly reactive cytotoxic antibodies following blood transfusions. It should also be noted that the DST protocol is not the only mechanism for the development of a positive cross-match between a potential kidney recipient and a potential donor. A group of 19 potential recipients developed a positive cross-match with their potential donor prior to the start of the DST protocol at USCF. All patients had demonstrated a negative cross-match at the initial evaluation, but administration of third-party transfusions in the interval between the negative and the positive cross-match most likely influenced the development of a positive cross-match to their potential kidney donor.

Influence of Azathioprine Coverage on DST Sensitization

Even though the donor-specific sensitization rate with DST should not by itself make patients nontransplantable, efforts to reduce this sensitization possibility are under way. Anderson and colleagues[15] and Glass and coworkers[6] have lowered their donor-sepcific sensitization rate to approximately 10 percent by using azathioprine during DST administration. The UCSF experience with azathioprine coverage has not produced the overall 10 percent sensitization rate; however, this is probably the result of the lower azathioprine dose, initially 1 mg per kg with an immediate decrease on manifestation of even mild leukopenia. Our dosage is approximately half the initial dose employed by the other two groups, but it has not been accompanied by any infections during the dialysis period when renal failure patients are at high risk.

Using our azathioprine dosage we evaluated the influence of azathioprine decreasing donor-specific sensitization in two concurrent groups receiving and not receiving azathioprine.[2] Of these patients, 91 received low-dose azathioprine and 93 received none during DST administration. Eighty-three patients in each group were considered for primary transplantation, while 8 were considered for secondary transplantation in the azathioprine group and 10 for secondary transplantation in the no-azathioprine group. Table 20–4 evaluates patients for primary transplantation and indicates a trend toward a beneficial effect in individuals with a PRA less than 10 percent prior to DST under azathioprine coverage.[2] Azathioprine conferred no beneficial effect in the smaller group of patients in whom the PRA was greater than 10 percent. Of the 7 patients in the sensitized azathioprine group with a positive cross-match, five had PRA levels of 50 percent or greater.

Following a high sensitization rate in a previous report of 15 patients receiving DST prior to second or third grafts,[13] a subsequent experience with 18 patients awaiting second or third transplants resulted in 50 percent becoming sensitized to their blood donor. Azathioprine conferred no beneficial effect in reducing the sensitization rate in this group. In the patients being considered for second or third transplants, PRA levels had no influence whatsoever on the subsequent development of a positive cross-match. What appeared to be most important was the fact that the patient had a failed first transplant.

From our results it appears that azathioprine has its maximum effect on patients undergoing their first transplantation with a pre-DST PRA less than 10 percent. Fortunately, this is the status of most patients at the time of initial consideration for transplantation and the largest group of patients to undergo DST. These results certainly encourage early DST and transplantation in this particular group of patients before third-party transfusions are administered and the PRA is increased. The azathioprine protocol does appear to have an attractive theoretic basis, since this agent interferes with DNA synthesis and may therefore inhibit the development of primary antibody responses in individuals without previous allogeneic exposure by preventing the proliferation of antigen-activated lymphocyte clones during the transient, repetitive exposure of blood from the potential kidney donor. Azathioprine coverage, however, does not appear to confer any beneficial effect on primary transplants with high pretransplantation PRAs or in individuals undergoing second or third transplants. In these cases blood transfusions (DST or third-party transfusions) seem only to amplify previous responses to exposed foreign histocompatibility antigens.

Positive B-Warm Cross-matches

The nature of B-warm antibodies per se, without further analysis, has until recently been uncertain. In the past most B-warm antibodies have been considered harmless in the non-DST situation, but it was difficult to proceed with transplantation after a positive B-warm cross-match following DST pretreatment without sorting out the nature of these antibodies. One fourth of

Table 20–4 Primary Living Donor Transplantation—DST Pretreatment		
PRA	Positive Cross-Match	
PRA <10% (n = 144)		
Azathioprine	9/74	12%
No azathioprine	15/70	21%
PRA >10% (n = 22)		
Azathioprine	7/9	78%
No azathioprine	4/13	31%
PRA: Percentage of reactive antibody against a panel of 40 selected cells.		

patients with a positive cross-match following DST pretreatment had B-warm antibodies alone.[13,21] In 1982, in an attempt to decrease the number of patients who might be excluded from subsequent transplantation because of a positive B-warm cross-match alone, we instituted flow cytometry in order to exclude with accuracy antidonor Class I antigen activity.[23]

From 1982 through 1985, 62 patients have demonstrated positive B-warm cross-matches alone, and these have been subsequently evaluated with cross-match testing by flow cytometry using the FACS. This procedure has provided a means of detecting previously unrecognized anti-T-lymphocyte (Class I antigen) activity in patients with a positive B-warm cross-match without requiring prior platelet absorption of sera or physical separation of T and B lymphocytes.[23] The latter feature was made possible by the presence of two peaks on FACS histograms. The first was a large low-intensity peak consisting of T lymphocytes, and the second was a smaller high-intensity peak of immunoglobulin-positive B cells. Binding of expressed B-warm antibody to T lymphocytes was considered indicative of anti-HLA-A, -B, or -C antibodies and was demonstrated by a rightward shift of the T cell peak proportional to the increased number of bound antibody molecules. Of the 62 patients with a positive B-warm cross-match alone, 45 (73 percent) had a subsequent negative FACS cross-match.[2] Of the FACS-negative cross-match patients, 44 of 45 had a B-warm antibody titer of 1 to 4 or less, while the other patient had a titer of 1 to 8. In those with a B-warm titer of 1 to 4 or less and a negative FACS cross-match, only one graft has been lost, whereas the single patient with a 1 to 8 titer lost his graft.

DST Advantages

For the potential kidney donors in the DST protocol, the process of preliminary blood donation has been harmless and has spared many donors the donation of a kidney that would probably later be rejected. The potential donor with a positive donor-specific cross-match has enjoyed increased self-esteem in actively participating as a family member in identifying a compatible kidney. For the blood transfusion donor who eventually undergoes an operation, the process of renal donation is being accomplished with excellent prospects of success, and the donor is able to approach the surgical procedure with more confidence and less anxiety. An additional advantage of the DST protocol is that the medical and family history of the blood donor are known with essentially no risk of hepatitis, AIDS, or other disease to the recipient.

In conclusion:

1. DST provides excellent long-term graft survival in 1-haplotype-matched pairs.

2. Excellent short-term graft survival has also been obtained in a limited 0-haplotype-matched experience.

3. Azathioprine coverage does appear to decrease DST sensitization to the blood donor in nonsensitized patients undergoing a first transplant, encouraging early DST and transplantation in this group.

4. Flow cytometry had been extremely helpful in excluding subliminal anti-class I antigen activity in patients with positive B-warm cross-matches.

5. DST in itself does not appear to preclude subsequent cadaveric transplantation in patients sensitized to their blood donor.

CYCLOSPORINE

The experience with cyclosporine in living related transplantation is limited and is primarily related to use in 1-haplotype-matched donor-recipient pairs. The largest reported single-center (Houston) experience in 62 1-haplotype-matched living related recipients shows a 3-year actuarial patient survival of 98 percent and a graft survival of 91 percent.[8] A recently reported collected experience of HCFA data in 407 patients shows a 1-year graft survival rate of 88 percent and patient survival rate of 95 percent.[24] At UCSF a 1-haplotype-matched group treated with cyclosporine shows an 85 ±8 percent survival at 1 year. In the only prospective randomized study, no difference in graft survival is shown in 1-haplotype-matched recipients treated with cyclosporine versus those pretreated with DST and with conventional immunosuppression posttransplantation.[25] Even though there are fewer than 20 patients in each of these two groups, there was a significant difference in creatinine levels with a higher mean creatinine level in the cyclosporine-treated group.[25]

Cyclosporine Versus DST

The question of whether DST or cyclosporine is the better therapy for incompatible donor-recipient pairs is probably settled with regards to 0-haplotype-matched donor-recipient pairs but remains to be established in 1-haplotype-matched living-related donor-recipient pairs, where only a prospective study of DST- and cyclosporine-treated patients with long-term follow-up will establish the optimum regimen. Of concern is the possible deleterious effect of cyclosporine on long-term kidney function because of its potential for nephrotoxicity.

What appears promising is the use of DST in 0-haplotype-matched donor-recipient pairs, which includes not only siblings but also distant relatives and spousal transplants. Our results of DSTs in this group and the Wisconsin series[7] shows graft survival similar to the DST-treated 1-haplotype-matched living-related donor-recipient pairs and HLA-identical siblings. The only experience with cyclosporine in a somewhat similarly matched group relates only to cadaver transplants, in which graft survival is lower. If long-term follow-up establishes that there is no significant attrition in graft survival in DST-pretreated 0-haplotype-matched pairs, this may be clearly the treatment of choice in this group. Quite promising is a recent report that shows excellent graft survival in diabetic recipients with DST regardless of matched grade: HLA-identical, 1-haplotype-match, or 0-haplotype-match.[26]

THIRD-PARTY BLOOD TRANSFUSIONS IN LIVING RELATED TRANSPLANTATION

The influence of random third-party blood transfusions before cadaveric renal transplantation with conventional immunosuppression is well established. Random third-party blood transfusions also appear to have a beneficial effect prior to trans-

plantation from living related donors with conventional immunosuppression. Opelz and associates[27] analyzed 314 HLA-identical siblings and 585 1-haplotype-matched transplant recipients and showed that pretransplantation third-party blood transfusions allowed a significant 10 percent improvement in 1-year graft survival in each of these living related categories when compared with nontransfused recipients. Brynger and colleagues[28] have also shown graft survival in 1-haplotype living related pairs to be significantly improved after random pretransplantation third-party blood transfusions. More current and similar studies evaluating single-haplotype living related recipients also show enhanced graft survival in this group.[9,10] In the large collected series of Opelz[10] graft survival in the transfused non-DST group was approximately 10 percent less than in the DST-treated group. None of the studies enumerated segregated 1-haplotype recipients by mixed lymphocyte culture (MLC). Most 1-haplotype donor-recipient pairs exhibit a high reactive MLC. In our own experience evaluation of the high reactive MLC group only showed a 56 percent 1-year graft survival, but when this group was analyzed according to pretransplantation third-party transfusions, there was a 73 percent one-year graft survival in the group that received third-party transfusions compared with an impaired graft survival in the nontransfused group ($p < 0.002$).

In regards to optimum number of random third-party transfusions to achieve a beneficial effect in 1-haplotype-matched donor-recipient pairs, Opelz[10] indicated that the maximum effect was seen when four or more were done.

Of great interest is the demonstration of a beneficial effect on HLA-identical siblings,[27] which was reconfirmed by a recent small series[29] in which 3-year graft survivals in the transfused and the nontransfused group were 92 percent and 78 percent, respectively.

All these studies relate to a transfusion effect with third-party blood transfusions in living-related transplantation without cyclosporine. There are now essentially no data in regard to a possible transfusion effect in living related transplantation treated with cyclosporine immunosuppression.

Complications of Blood Transfusions

The principal problem with third-party blood transfusions is the risk of sensitization and transfusion-induced disease such as hepatitis and AIDS. Most agree that multiple transfusions produce the greatest sensitization rate. According to Terasaki and associates[30] it was found that among cadaver graft recipients who were given more than 20 pretransplantation blood transfusions, 54 percent demonstrated lymphocytotoxic antibodies and about 26 percent had an antibody level of more than 80 percent. This study did not include those patients with more than 20 blood transfusions who may not have received transplants. Other studies have also shown that antibody levels increase progressively with additional third-party transfusions.[31,32]

Post-transfusion hepatitis remains a most serious complication of blood transfusions. Although fewer than 5 percent of transfused patients are expected to contract this disease, some of these patients may eventually develop severe chronic liver disease. This is particularly evident later, when the major cause of morbidity and mortality following transplantation appears to be hepatic dysfunction. Pirson and colleagues[33] have underscored the long-term consequences of chronic HBs antigenemia in renal transplant recipients. In their series HBs antigenemia was associated with a high incidence of severe liver disease and impaired patient and graft survival, primarily after the third year post-transplantation. However, the major cause of liver disease in patients with renal transplantation may be non-A, non-B hepatitis. It has been suggested that chronic liver disease, presumably caused by non-A, non-B hepatitis virus, is associated with modest morbidity and mortality.[34] These findings emphasize that screening of blood donors for hepatitis B antigen alone does not preclude the subsequent development of hepatic dysfunction and that some caution must be exercised in advocating a large number of pretransplantation third-party blood transfusions prior to transplantation.

The risk of AIDS is another consideration with random third-party blood transfusions. In the United States 15,948 cases of AIDS had been reported as of December 31, 1985, and at least 286 (1.8 percent) were related to transfusions. Theoretically recipients of kidney transplants are at increased risk for AIDS because of frequent blood transfusions and immunosuppression. Kidney transplants can undoubtedly serve as a vehicle of transmission as well. The risk of AIDS and other adverse conditions in recipients of kidney transplants is probably very small in spite of direct and indirect exposure to numerous blood transfusions, immunosuppression, and the possibility that some transplantation donors have the AIDS virus (although present methods of screening should exclude this occurrence). However, in view of the apparently long incubation period for AIDS, it will undoubtedly be years before the validity of this statement can be proved. When AIDS does occur in the kidney transplantation recipient, the patient's course is likely to be adversely affected by immunosuppression.

CONCLUSION AND TRANSPLANTATION STRATEGY

In contrast to past experiences with living related transplantation, when the HLA-identical sibling was the only match grade that assured excellent graft and patient survival, in the mid-1980s there are several good alternative therapies that will produce similar excellent results regardless of the degree of incompatibility between a living donor and the kidney recipient. DST, cyclosporine, and third-party blood transfusions all have demonstrated efficacy, but each also has some risk, in some cases small and in others of a greater degree.

As a strategy for preparing a patient with ESRD for a living related transplant, choosing an HLA-identical sibling match is ideal. Pretransplantation blood transfusions appear to be beneficial in this group, and DST pretreatment may provide the transfusion benefit without the risks posed by third-party blood transfusions, but this will have to be determined. If third-party blood transfusions are to be used, it is preferable to use designated blood donors whose medical and family history is well known.

In the 1-haplotype-matched group, DST

with azathioprine coverage is probably preferable in nonsensitized or low-sensitized patients being considered for a first transplantation. In highly sensitized patients DST may be used, but probably without azathioprine, or the use of cyclosporine may be considered. In patients being evaluated for second or third transplants, cyclosporine may be the therapy of choice. If a living-related or unrelated transplant is to be considered with a 0-haplotype match, DST with azathioprine appears to be the only logical consideration.

REFERENCES

1. Salvatierra, O: Advantages of continued use of kidney transplant from living donors. Transplant Proc 17(2):18, 1985.
2. Salvatierra, O, et al: A seven-year experience with donor-specific blood transfusions: Results and considerations for maximum efficacy. Transplantation 40:654, 1985.
3. Krakauer, H, et al: The recent U.S. experience in the treatment of end-stage renal disease by dialysis and transplantation. N Engl J Med 308:1558, 1983.
4. Vincenti, F, et al: Long-term renal function in kidney donors. Transplantation 36:626, 1983.
5. Sutherland, DER: Living-related donors should be used whenever possible. Transplant Proc 17:1503, 1985.
6. Glass, NR, et al: Comparative analysis of the DST and Imuran-plus-DST protocol for live donor renal transplantation. Transplantation 36:636, 1983.
7. Sollinger, HW, et al: Donor-specific transfusions in unrelated and related HLA-mismatched donor-recipient combinations. Transplantation 38:612, 1984.
8. Flechner, SM, et al: The use of cyclosporine in living-related renal transplantation. Transplantation 38:685, 1984.
9. Pfaff, WW, et al: Planned random donor blood transfusions in preparation for transplantation. Transplantation 38:701, 1984.
10. Opelz, G: Comparison of random transfusions with donor-specific transfusions for pretreatment of HLA 1-haplotype-matched related donor kidney transplant recipients. Transplant Proc 17(6):2357, 1985.
11. Salvatierra, O, et al: Deliberate donor-specific blood transfusions prior to living related transplantation: A new approach. Ann Surg 192:543, 1980.
12. Salvatierra, O, et al: Pretreatment with donor-specific blood transfusions in related recipients with high MLC. Transplant Proc 13:142, 1981.
13. Salvatierra, O, et al: Four-year experience with donor-specific blood transfusions. Transplant Proc 15:924, 1983.
14. Salvatierra, O, et al: Improved patient survival in renal transplantation. Surgery 79:166, 1976.
15. Anderson, CB, et al: Pretreatment of renal allograft recipients with immunosuppression and donor-specific blood. Transplantation 38:664, 1984.
16. Leivestad, T, et al: Effect of pretransplant donor-specific transfusions in renal transplantation. Transplant Proc 14:370, 1982.
17. Mendez, R, et al: Antibody response and allograft outcome with deliberate donor-specific blood transfusions. Transplant Proc 14:378, 1982.
18. Takahashi, I, et al: Prolonged graft survival by donor-specific blood transfusion (DSBT). Transplant Proc 14:367, 1982.
19. Whelchel, JD, et al: The effect of pretransplant stored donor-specific blood transfusion on renal allograft survival in one-haplotype living-related transplant recipients. Transplantation 38:654, 1984.
20. Balakrishnan, K, et al: Donor-specific transfusions: Sensitization patterns. Transplant Proc 17(6):2354, 1985.
21. Salvatierra, O, et al: Incidence, characteristics and outcome of recipients sensitized after donor-specific blood transfusions. Transplantation 32:528, 1981.
22. Scornik, JC, et al: Assessment of the risk for broad sensitization by blood transfusions. Transplantation 37:249, 1984.
23. Garovoy, M, et al: Flow cytometry cross-matching for donor-specific transfusion recipients and cadaveric transplantation. Transplantation Proc 17:693, 1985.
24. Spees, EK, et al: The current experience with cyclosporine in the United States: Living related kidney transplant recipients. Transplantation Proc 17(6):2657, 1985.
25. Sommer, BG and Ferguson, RM: Mismatched living related donor renal transplantation: A prospective randomized study. Surgery 98:267, 1985.
26. Belzer, FO, et al: Two haplotype mismatched live donor renal transplantation in diabetics. Transplant Proc 18:1730, 1986.
27. Opelz, G, Mickey, MR, and Terasaki, PI: Blood transfusions and kidney transplants: Remaining controversies. Transplant Proc 13:136, 1981.
28. Brynger, H, et al: Graft survival and blood transfusions. In Robinson, BHB (ed): Proceedings of the XIVth Congress of the European Dialysis and Transplant Associa-

tion. Pitman Medical Publishing, Kent, England, 1977, p 290.

29. Norman, DJ, et al: Blood transfusions are beneficial in HLA-identical sibling kidney transplants. Transplant Proc 17(6):2347, 1985.

30. Terasaki, PI, et al: Reduction of accelerated failures by transfusion. Transplant Proc 14:251, 1982.

31. Fehrman, I, et al: Improved renal graft survival in transfused uremics. Transplantation 30:324, 1980.

32. Werner-Favre, C, et al: Blood transfusions, cytotoxic antibodies, and kidney graft survival. Transplantation 28:343, 1979.

33. Pirson, Y, Alexandre, GP and van Ypersele de Strihou, C: Long-term effect of HBs antigenemia on patient survival after renal transplantation. N Engl J Med 296:194, 1977.

34. LaQuaglia, MP, et al: Impact of hepatitis on renal transplantation. Transplantation 32:504, 1981.

Epilogue

Future Prospects in Kidney Transplantation

Optimizing the Availability and Use of Organs for Transplantation
  Increasing Awareness
  Donor Cards
  Required Request Legislation
  Standardizing Criteria for Brain Death
  National Computerized Registry
  International Organ Sharing and Common Laws
  Living Nonrelated Donors
Improving Transplantation Results
  Future of Organ Preservation
  Improving Immunosuppression
Ethical Issues
  Sale of Organs
  Transplantation for Foreign National Recipients
Financial Considerations

In the past decade kidney transplantation has become viewed as a nearly routine procedure at many medical centers. With improved immunosuppressive protocols using drugs such as cyclosporine, the transplant patient can expect to keep his or her graft functioning far longer and with fewer complications than with the previously used steroid therapy. Considerations for those involved in renal transplantation include increasing public awareness of the importance of transplantation; increasing the number of organs available for transplantation; improving preservation techniques and organ viability assessment; tailoring immunosuppressive protocols for the needs of individual patients; improvement of immunologic monitoring techniques; and ethical, moral, and financial issues.

OPTIMIZING THE AVAILABILITY AND USE OF ORGANS FOR TRANSPLANTATION

Increasing Awareness

Transplantable organs are often lost because potential donors are not identified by medical or paramedical personnel, because consent is not obtained, and/or because the kidneys are not retrieved. It has been estimated that there are between 12,000 and 27,000 potential donors each year, depending on the age criteria used. However, fewer than 40 percent become kidney donors.[1] In addition, most individuals are not aware of the great need for kidneys for transplantation. Each year 10,000 Americans with end-stage renal disease (ESRD) are in need of renal transplants, but only half of these patients actually receive one. Therefore, a continued effort to educate both the general public and the medical community as to the need for organs is important.

Donor Cards

Another means of potentially increasing organ donation is through the use of signed donor cards. The Uniform Anatomical Gift Act, which was enacted by all 50 states, provides for a wallet-sized organ donor card.[2] This card may be signed by any adult individual and two witnesses to indicate his or her intention to donate organs or tissues upon death. Although these cards are legal documents, family wishes regarding the disposition of the organs and body of the deceased individual take precedence despite the existence of a signed card. Studies show that unless signing of donor cards is mandatory, less than 5 percent of the public actually sign the cards on the back of their driver's license. Therefore, donor cards have not had very much impact on the number of organs retrieved. They may, however, encourage some conversation regarding organ donation and transplantation.

Required Request Legislation

Several states have recently enacted or are considering required request laws.[3] These laws require that when death occurs in a hospital to a person who meets the criteria for organ donation and who has not made an anatomic gift, the hospital administrator or designated representative is required to request consent from the decedent's family for organ donation. The intent of these laws is to increase the supply of available organs by requiring medical personnel to ask for organ donation. The actual impact of these laws, however, may not be apparent for some time.

Standardizing Criteria for Brain Death

One of the ethical issues that remains to be standardized in transplantation is the determination of donor death. As discussed in Chapter 2, the criteria for brain death have been changed over the years and have not been the same at all transplantation centers nor in all states. The adoption by each state of well-defined uniform criteria for brain death would allow physicians to make the determination more readily. This would lead to improved quality of transplantable organs and increase the number of organs available for transplantation. In the future it will be important for legislators and physicians to be aware of the new medical advances that may alter these criteria.

National Computerized Registry

The Task Force on Organ Transplantation[4] suggested that distribution of organs in the future would be facilitated by a national computerized registry of all waiting recipients and transplantation centers. This would help to eliminate the differences in waiting times that now exist between centers. Theoretically, each kidney could be transplanted into the most suitable transplantation candidate. The recent National Organ Transplant Act[5] has mandated the establishment of an organ procurement and transplantation network to provide these services under the direction of the Department of Health and Human Services. Private interests in the United States have also begun to pursue this type of endeavor. The United Network for Organ Sharing (UNOS) has begun to computerize all recipients on a national basis.

International Organ Sharing and Common Laws

Although there has been some international organ sharing, this process has not been well organized in the past. The Task Force on Organ Transplantation has suggested that exportation and importation of donor organs be prohibited except when the distribution is arranged or coordinated by the Organ Procurement and Transplantation Network.[2] Then documentation will be required that demonstrates that all appropriate efforts have been made to locate a recipient in the United States and/or Canada. Ideally, international organ sharing would also be facilitated if all countries adopted similar reciprocal laws.

Living Nonrelated Donors

Some renal transplantation centers have considered transplantation from living nonrelated donors such as spouses and friends of the potential recipient as a means of reducing the depletion of the cadaver kidney pool. This has not been followed by most centers, however, because the histocompatibility disparity is the same as for cadaver transplantation. If cadaver results are to equal those of live related transplants, the doubts might disappear and live nonrelated transplantation might be a more definite possibility. If enough cadaver donors were able to maintain the supply of needed recipients, the potential of nonrelated transplantation would be remote. However, we believe that live nonrelated transplantation will eventually become well accepted as more evidence for better results is seen and as evidence for safe unilateral nephrectomy of living nonrelated donors is apparent.

IMPROVING TRANSPLANTATION RESULTS

Future of Organ Preservation

Improvement in organ preservation techniques and a lengthening of preservation times should be seen in the near future, as research continues to explore the physiologic and biochemical changes involved in hypothermia, tissue and organ ischemia, and reperfusion injury. New methods for viability assessment will assist in the evaluation of kidneys prior to transplantation, especially those that have been hypothermically stored. New preservation solutions will be tailored the better to protect organs, especially those that are exposed to prolonged warm ischemia and/or preserved for extended periods.

Improving Immunosuppression

Although cyclosporine, in general and in combination with azathioprine, prednisolone, and ALG/ATG, has greatly improved cadaver kidney allograft survival, the same immunosuppressive protocol cannot be used for all transplant recipients. Development of even better immunosuppressive protocols and new immunologic monitoring techniques that will prognosticate rejection will help to tailor immunosuppression for both high and low responders and for high-risk patients.

ETHICAL ISSUES

Sale of Organs

There has been considerable discussion in the past few years regarding organ donation or solicitation for economic gain. This concept is in direct contrast to the intention of the Uniform Anatomic Gift Act of 1968.[2] It has also been opposed by the Committee on Morals and Ethics of the Transplantation Society[6,7] and the American Society of Transplant Surgeons.[6] This issue has recently been put to rest in the United States by passage of the National Organ Transplantation Act of 1984.[5] This law provides for a maximum penalty of $50,000 or 5 years in prison or both for the purchase of human organs for use in transplantation.

Transplantation for Foreign National Recipients

The Task Force on Organ Transplantation has recommended that nonimmigrant aliens not comprise more than 10 percent of the total number of kidney transplant recipients at each transplantation center until the Organ Procurement and Transplantation Network has had an opportunity to review the issue.[2] Some individuals feel that kidneys should only be transplanted into individuals from other countries after all possible candidates in this country have been eliminated. It has been the practice of some programs, however, to solicit and advertise for nonimmigrant aliens as kidney recipients without regard to the waiting list. The Task Force on Organ Transplantation has called for this practice to cease.

FINANCIAL CONSIDERATIONS

The future of renal transplantation will undoubtedly be affected by decisions of governmental agencies and private health insurers in the areas of cost and effectiveness of the procedure. The transplantation community should consider the present and future role that government and private insurers might play in determining patient selection criteria, procedures for organ donation and procurement, distribution of organs, and the course of postoperative care. Recent legislation proposed by Senator Hatch seeks to provide government support for the purchase of immunosuppressive drugs to be distributed to transplantation centers that meet minimum standards to assure quality of care.[8]

SUMMARY

It appears that the next decade or so will be both an exciting and challenging time for individuals involved in renal transplantation. The status of renal transplantation as we approach the twenty-first century will be determined by the factors mentioned in this chapter, some of which we can affect and others of which we cannot.

REFERENCES

1. Bart, KJ, et al: Cadaveric kidneys for transplantation: A paradox of shortage in the face of plenty. Transplantation 31:379, 1981.
2. Uniform Anatomical Gift Act, 8A ULA 16 (1983).
3. Organ Donation and the Impact of Required Request Legislation, American Hospital Association, September 18, 1986.
4. Report of the Task Force on Organ Transplantation: Organ Transplantation—Issues and Recommendations. Government Printing Office, Washington, D.C., April 1986.
5. United States National Organ Transplantation Act: Public Law 98-507. 1984 Oct. 19. 98:2339.
6. Joint Announcement from the Transplantation Society, American Society of Transplant Surgeons, and the American Society of Transplant Physicians. Transplant Proceedings, Vol 16, Front Matter.
7. Transplantation Society. Council on Commercialization in Transplantation: The problems and some guidelines for practice. Lancet 2:715, 1985.
8. Immunosuppressive Drug Therapy Act. S. 2536 and S. 2540.

Index